D0116245

THE JOHNS HOPKINS
MEDICAL HANDBOOK

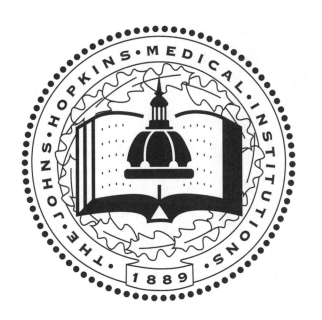

The Johns Hopkins Medical Handbook

New Updated Edition

The 100 Major Medical Disorders of People Over the Age of 50

PLUS A DIRECTORY
OF THE LEADING TEACHING HOSPITALS,
RESEARCH ORGANIZATIONS, TREATMENT
CENTERS, AND SUPPORT GROUPS

Medical Editor
Simeon Margolis, M.D., Ph.D.

Prepared by the Editors of
The Johns Hopkins Medical Letter
HEALTH AFTER 50

PUBLISHED BY
REBUS, INC. NEW YORK

DISTRIBUTED BY RANDOM HOUSE, INC.

THE JOHNS HOPKINS MEDICAL LETTER
HEALTH AFTER 50

THE JOHNS HOPKINS MEDICAL HANDBOOK *is the definitive home medical reference for adults, from America's top research hospital.*

THE JOHNS HOPKINS MEDICAL LETTER HEALTH AFTER 50, *our monthly eight-page newsletter, provides the same kind of timely information for everyone concerned with taking control of his or her own health and medical care. From the century-old tradition of Johns Hopkins excellence,* HEALTH AFTER 50 *uses clear, nontechnical language that is easy to understand. For information on how to order this unique newsletter, write to Medletter Associates, Inc., Department 1102, 632 Broadway, New York, New York 10012.*

This book is not intended as a substitute for the advice of a physician. Readers who suspect they may have specific medical problems should consult a physician about any suggestions made in this book.

New Updated Edition
Copyright © 1999 Medletter Associates, Inc.
Illustrations © The Johns Hopkins University

All rights reserved.
No part of this book may be reproduced or transmitted in any form or by any means, electronic, mechanical, photocopying, recording, or otherwise, without the prior written permission of the publisher.

For information about permission to reproduce selections from this book, write to Permissions, Medletter Associates, Inc., 632 Broadway, New York, New York 10012.

Library of Congress Cataloging-in-Publication Data
The Johns Hopkins medical handbook : the 100 major medical disorders of people over the age of 50 : plus a directory to the leading teaching hospitals, research organizations, treatment centers, and support groups / medical editor, Simeon Margolis ; prepared by the editors of the Johns Hopkins medical letter health after 50.
p.   cm.
New updated ed. originally published in 1995.
Includes index.
ISBN 0-929661-51-6 (hardcover). — ISBN 0-929661-54-0
1. Geriatrics Handbooks, manuals, etc. 2. Aged—Diseases Handbooks, manuals, etc. 3. Aged—Medical care Handbooks, manuals, etc. I. Margolis, Simeon, 1931- . II. Johns Hopkins medical letter health after 50.
[RC952.55.J64 1999]
616'.0084'4—dc21
                          99-14516
                          CIP
Printed in the United States of America
10 9 8 7 6 5 4 3 2 1
Distributed by Random House, Inc.

Johns Hopkins Medical Books
are published under the auspices of
The Johns Hopkins Medical Letter
HEALTH AFTER 50.

RODNEY FRIEDMAN
Editor and Publisher

EVAN HANSEN
Executive Editor

NATASHA RAYMOND
Managing Editor

PATRICE BENNEWARD
Senior Writer

TINA PAVANE, R.N.
Medical Researcher

TOM R. DAMRAUER, M.L.S.
Chief of Information Resources

ELLEN TULCHINSKY, M.L.S.
Librarian

LESLIE MALTESE-McGILL
Copy Editor

HELEN MULLEN
Circulation Director

BARBARA MAXWELL O'NEILL
Associate Publisher

DAVID ALEXANDER
Circulation Manager

JERRY LOO
Product Manager

DEBORAH BOYER
Promotions Manager

LISA NATOLI
Special Sales

The Johns Hopkins Medical Handbook

EVAN HANSEN
Editorial Director

EDWARD PETONIAK
Executive Editor

JEREMY D. BIRCH
Managing Editor

TIMOTHY JEFFS
Art Director

YOHEVED GERTZ
Designer

JOHN P. LYNCH
Assistant Editor

HELEN C. DUNN
Copy Editor

ROBERT DUCKWALL
Medical Illustrator

CARNEY W. MIMMS III
Directory Database Programmer

JOHN VASILIADIS
Trafficking Database Programmer

MARK MINEART
Computer Support Technician

The Johns Hopkins Medical Institutions
Baltimore, Maryland 21205

MEDICAL EDITOR

SIMEON MARGOLIS, M.D., PH.D.
Professor, Medicine &
Biological Chemistry

EDITORIAL BOARD OF ADVISORS

MARTIN D. ABELOFF, M.D.
Professor, Oncology
Director, Oncology Center

BARBARA DE LATEUR, M.D.
Professor & Director
Physical Medicine & Rehabilitation

JOHN A. FLYNN, M.D.
Assistant Professor, Medicine
Clinical Director, Division of General
Internal Medicine

LINDA P. FRIED, M.D., M.P.H.
Professor, Medicine & Epidemiology
Director, Center on Aging & Health

H. FRANKLIN HERLONG, M.D.
Associate Dean, School of Medicine
Associate Professor, Medicine

KEITH D. LILLEMOE, M.D.
Professor & Vice-Chairman, Surgery

PETER RABINS, M.D.
Professor, Psychiatry
Director, Division of Geriatric & Neuropsychiatry

ANDREW P. SCHACHAT, M.D.
Professor, Ophthalmology
Director, Retinal Vascular Center

EDWARD E. WALLACH, M.D.
Professor, Gynecology & Obstetrics

PATRICK C. WALSH, M.D.
Professor & Chairman, Urology

JAMES WEISS, M.D.
Professor, Medicine
Cardiology Division

OFFICE OF COMMUNICATIONS
& PUBLIC AFFAIRS

ELAINE FREEMAN
Executive Director

JOANN RODGERS
Deputy Director

KRISTIN BRUNNWORTH
Editorial Assistant

The following organizations have cooperated with Johns Hopkins in providing material for this Handbook:

AMERICAN ACADEMY OF DERMATOLOGY

AMERICAN ACADEMY OF OPHTHALMOLOGY

AMERICAN ACADEMY OF OTOLARYNGOLOGY

AMERICAN COLLEGE OF OBSTETRICIANS AND GYNECOLOGISTS

AMERICAN DIABETES ASSOCIATION

AMERICAN HEART ASSOCIATION

AMERICAN LIVER FOUNDATION

AMERICAN LUNG ASSOCIATION

AMERICAN PSYCHIATRIC ASSOCIATION

AMERICAN SLEEP DISORDERS ASSOCIATION

NATIONAL CANCER INSTITUTE

NATIONAL INSTITUTE OF DENTAL RESEARCH

NATIONAL INSTITUTE OF DIABETES AND DIGESTIVE AND KIDNEY DISEASES

NATIONAL INSTITUTE OF NEUROLOGICAL DISORDERS AND STROKE

NATIONAL INSTITUTE ON AGING

NATIONAL KIDNEY FOUNDATION

THYROID FOUNDATION OF AMERICA

U.S. DEPARTMENT OF HEALTH AND HUMAN SERVICES

WARREN GRANT MAGNUSON CLINICAL CENTER

CONTENTS

INTRODUCTION

The *Johns Hopkins Medical Handbook* is intended to provide a compendium of the 100 major medical disorders of people over the age of 50—along with a directory of the American medical care system. It has been prepared with the cooperation of some of the leading medical societies and health information organizations in the United States, and we are honored to have them associated with us in this endeavor.

While many medical encyclopedias are available to the general public, none specifically address the major health concerns of people over 50, and none have a directory like this one.

The entries are taken from the most recent publications prepared for the public by the organizations listed on page 7. Each of these organizations has already subjected its material to an extensive review process by doctors who are recognized authorities in their fields. We then took that material and asked our specialists at Johns Hopkins to give it an additional review. Our doctors have added further comments and explanations about the text; these are identified in the Handbook by either the "Hopkins dome" symbol (⌂) or the signature "The Editors."

The purpose of this Handbook is to provide a ready reference source of available knowledge rather than to report the most recent advances in each field. Of course, the information presented is not meant to substitute for the advice of your own physician.

We believe, however, that the entries in this Handbook will help you gain a familiarity with the vocabulary of the disorder that concerns you, provide you with helpful and detailed explanations of the basics, and serve as a good starting point for further conversations with your physicians or with health-care organizations—such as those listed in the Directory—that can provide additional information and assistance. We expect that, in this way, the Handbook will prove to be a valuable asset to you in taking control of your own health and medical care.

The Editors

Cancer

OVERVIEW

Cancer is a group of more than 100 different diseases. Cancer occurs when cells become abnormal and keep dividing and forming more cells without control or order.

All organs of the body are made up of cells. Normally, cells divide to produce more cells only when the body needs them. This orderly process helps keep us healthy. If cells keep dividing when new cells are not needed, a mass of tissue forms. This mass of extra tissue, called a growth or tumor, can be benign or malignant.

- Benign tumors are not cancer. They can usually be removed and, in most cases, they do not come back. Most important, cells from benign tumors do not spread to other parts of the body. Benign tumors are rarely a threat to life.
- Malignant tumors are cancer. Cancer cells can invade and damage nearby tissues and organs. Also, cancer cells can break away from a malignant tumor and enter the bloodstream or the lymphatic system. This is how cancer spreads from the original (primary) tumor to form new tumors in other parts of the body. The spread of cancer is called metastasis.

Most cancers are named for the type of cell or the organ in which they begin. When cancer spreads, the new tumor has the same kind of abnormal cells and the same name as the primary tumor. For example, if lung cancer spreads to the liver, the cancer cells in the liver are lung cancer cells. The disease is called metastatic lung cancer (it is not liver cancer).

EARLY DETECTION

In many cases, the sooner cancer is diagnosed and treated, the better a person's chance for a full recovery. If you develop cancer, you can improve the chance that it will be detected early if you have regular medical checkups and do certain self-exams. Often a doctor can find early cancer during a physical exam or with routine tests—even if a person has no symptoms. Some important medical exams, tests, and self-exams are discussed below and on the next page. The doctor may suggest other exams for people at increased risk for cancer.

Ask your doctor about your cancer risk, about problems to watch for, and about a schedule of regular checkups. The doctor's advice will be based on your age, medical history, and other risk factors. The doctor also can help you learn about self-exams.

Many local health departments have information about cancer screening or early detection programs. The Cancer Information Service (1-800-4-CANCER) also can tell you about such programs.

Exams for Both Men and Women

Skin. The doctor should examine your skin during regular checkups for signs of skin cancer. You should also check regularly for new growths, sores that do not heal, changes in the size, shape, or color of any moles, or any other changes on the skin. Warning signs like these should be reported to the doctor right away.

Colon and Rectum. Beginning at age 50, you should have a yearly fecal occult blood test. This test is a check for hidden (occult) blood in the stool. A small amount of stool is placed on a plastic slide or on special paper. It may be tested in the doctor's office or sent to a lab. This test is done because cancer of the colon and rectum may cause bleeding. However, noncancerous conditions may also cause bleeding, so having blood in the stool does not necessarily mean a person has cancer. If blood is found, the doctor orders more tests to help make a diagnosis.

To check for cancer of the rectum, the doctor inserts a gloved finger into the rectum and feels for any bumps or abnormal areas. A digital rectal exam should be done during regular checkups. Every three to five years after age 50, you should have sigmoidoscopy. In this exam, the doctor uses a thin, flexible tube with a light to look inside the rectum and colon for abnormal areas.

Mouth. Your doctor and dentist should examine your mouth at regular visits. Also, by looking in a mirror, you can check inside your mouth for changes in the color of the lips, gums, tongue, or inner cheeks, and for scabs, cracks, sores, white patches, swelling, or bleeding. It is often possible to see or feel changes in the mouth that might be cancer or a condition that might lead to cancer. Any symptoms in your mouth should be checked by a doctor or dentist. Oral exams are especially important for people who use alcohol or tobacco products and for anyone over age 50.

Exams for Men

Prostate. Men over age 40 should have a yearly digital rectal exam to check the prostate gland for hard or lumpy areas. The doctor feels the prostate through the wall of the rectum.

Testicles. Testicular cancer occurs most often between ages 15 and 34. Most of these cancers are found by men themselves, often by doing a testicular self-exam. If you find a lump or notice another change, such as heaviness, swelling, unusual tenderness, or pain, you should see your doctor. Also, the doctor should examine the testicles as part of regular medical checkups.

Exams for Women

Breast. When breast cancer is found early, a woman has more treatment choices and a good chance of complete recovery. So it is important that breast cancer be detected as early as possible. The National Cancer Institute encourages women to take an active part in early detection. They should talk to their doctor about this disease, the symptoms to watch for, and an appropriate schedule of checkups. Women should ask their doctor about:

- Mammograms (x-rays of the breast)
- Breast exams by a doctor or nurse
- Breast self-examination (BSE)

A mammogram can often show tumors or changes in the breast before they can be felt or cause symptoms. However, mammograms cannot find every abnormal area in the breast. This is especially true in the breasts of young women. Another important step in early detection is for women to have their breasts examined regularly by a doctor or a nurse.

Between visits to the doctor, women should examine their breasts every month. By doing BSE, women learn what looks and feels normal for their breasts, and they are more likely to find a change. Any changes should be reported to the doctor. Most breast lumps are not cancer, but only a doctor can make a diagnosis.

Cervix. Regular pelvic exams and Pap tests are important to detect early cancer of the cervix. In a pelvic exam, the doctor feels the uterus, vagina, ovaries, fallopian tubes, bladder, and rectum for any change in size or shape.

For the Pap test, a sample of cells is collected from the upper vagina and cervix with a small brush or a flat wooden stick. The sample is placed on a glass slide and checked under a microscope for cancer or other abnormal cells. Women should start having a Pap test every year after they turn 18 or become sexually active. If the results are normal for three or more years in a row, a woman may have this test less often, based on her doctor's advice.

SYMPTOMS OF CANCER

You should see your doctor for regular checkups and not wait for problems to occur. But you should also know that the following symptoms may be associated with cancer: changes in bowel or bladder habits, a sore that does not heal, unusual bleeding or discharge, thickening or lump in the breast or any other part of the body, indigestion or difficulty swallowing, obvious change in a wart or mole, or nagging cough or hoarseness. These symptoms are not always a sign of cancer. They can also be caused by less serious conditions. Only a doctor can make a diagnosis. It is important to see a doctor if you have any of these symptoms. Don't wait to feel pain: Early cancer usually does not cause pain.

DIAGNOSIS

If you have a sign or symptom that might mean cancer, the doctor will do a physical exam and ask about your medical history. In addition, the doctor usually orders various tests and exams. These may include imaging procedures, which produce pictures of areas inside the body; endoscopy, which allows the doctor to look directly inside certain organs; and laboratory tests. In most cases, the doctor also orders a biopsy, a procedure in which a sample of tissue is removed. A pathologist examines the tissue under a microscope to check for cancer cells.

Imaging

Images of areas inside the body help the doctor tell whether a tumor is present. These images can be made in several ways. In many cases, the doctor uses a special dye so that certain organs show up better on film. The dye may be swallowed or put into the body through a needle or a tube.

X-rays are the most common way doctors make pictures of the inside of the body. A special kind of x-ray imaging called a CT scan uses a computer linked to an x-ray machine to make a series of detailed pictures.

In radionuclide scanning, the patient swallows or is given an injection of a mildly radioactive substance. A machine (scanner) measures radioactivity levels in certain organs and prints a picture on paper or film. By looking at the amount of radioactivity in the organs, the doctor can find abnormal areas.

Ultrasonography is another procedure for viewing the inside of the body. High-frequency sound waves that cannot be heard by humans enter the body and bounce back. Their echoes produce a picture called a sonogram. These pictures are shown on a monitor like a TV screen and can be printed on paper.

In MRI, a powerful magnet linked to a computer is used to make detailed pictures of areas in the body. These pictures are viewed on a monitor and can also be printed.

Endoscopy

Endoscopy allows the doctor to look into the body through a thin, lighted tube called an endoscope. The exam is named for the organ involved (for example, colonoscopy to look inside the colon). During the exam, the doctor may collect tissue or cells for closer examination.

Laboratory Tests

Although no single test can be used to diagnose cancer, laboratory tests such as blood and urine tests give the doctor important information. If cancer is present, lab work may show the effects of the disease on the body. In some cases, special tests are used to measure the amount of certain substances in the blood, urine, other body fluids, or tumor tissue. The levels of these substances may become abnormal when certain kinds of cancer are present.

Biopsy

The physical exam, imaging, endoscopy, and lab tests can show that something abnormal is present, but a biopsy is the only sure way to know whether the problem is cancer. In a biopsy, the doctor removes a sample of tissue from the abnormal area or may remove the whole tumor. A pathologist examines the tissue under a microscope. If cancer is present, the pathologist can usually tell what kind of cancer it is and may be able to judge whether the cells are likely to grow slowly or quickly.

Staging

When cancer is found, the patient's doctor needs to know the stage, or extent, of the disease to plan the best treatment. The doctor may order various tests and exams to find out whether the cancer has spread and, if so, what parts of the body are affected. In some cases, lymph nodes near the tumor are removed and checked for cancer cells. If cancer cells are found in the lymph nodes, it may mean that the cancer has spread to other organs.

TREATMENT

Cancer is treated with surgery, radiation therapy, chemotherapy, hormonal therapy, or biological therapy. Patients with cancer are often treated by a team of specialists, which may include a medical oncologist (specialist in cancer treatment), a surgeon, a radiation oncologist (specialist in radiation therapy), and others. The doctors may decide to use one treatment method or a combination of methods. The choice of treatment depends on the type and location of the cancer, the stage of the disease, the patient's age and general health, and other factors.

Some cancer patients take part in a clinical trial (research study) using new treatment methods. Such studies are designed to improve cancer treatment. (Additional information about clinical trials is on page 20.)

Getting a Second Opinion

Before starting treatment, the patient may want another doctor to review the diagnosis and treatment plan. Some insurance companies require a second opinion; others may pay for a second opinion if the patient requests it.

There are a number of ways to find specialists to consult for a second opinion:

- The patient's doctor may suggest a specialist for a second opinion.
- The Cancer Information Service, at 1-800-4-CANCER, can tell callers about treatment facilities, including cancer centers and other programs in their area supported by the National Cancer Institute.
- Patients can get the names of doctors from their local medical society, a nearby hospital, or a medical school.

Preparing for Treatment

Many people with cancer want to learn all they can about their disease and their treatment choices so they can take an active part in decisions about their medical care. Often it helps to make a list of questions to ask the doctor. Patients may take notes or, with the doctor's consent, tape record the discussion. Some patients also find it helps to have a family member or friend with them when they talk with the doctor—to take part in the discussion, to take notes, or just to listen.

When a person is diagnosed with cancer, shock and stress are natural reactions. These feelings may make it difficult to think of every question to ask the doctor. Patients may find it hard to remember everything the doctor says. They should not feel they need to ask all their questions or remember all the answers at one time. They will have other chances for the doctor to explain things that are not clear and to ask for more information.

Methods of Treatment

Surgery. Surgery is local treatment to remove the tumor. Tissue around the tumor and nearby lymph nodes may also be removed during the operation.

Radiation therapy. In radiation therapy (also called radiotherapy), high-energy rays are used to damage cancer cells and stop them from growing and dividing. Like surgery, radiation therapy is a local treatment; it can affect cancer cells only in the treated area. Radiation may come from a machine (external radiation). It also may come from an implant (a small container of radioactive material) placed directly into or near the tumor (internal radiation). Some patients get both kinds of radiation therapy.

External radiation therapy is usually given on an outpatient basis in a hospital or clinic five days a week for several weeks. Patients are not radioactive during or after the treatment.

For internal radiation therapy, the patient stays in the hospital for a few days. The implant may be temporary or permanent. Because the level of radiation is highest during the hospital stay, patients may not be able to have visitors or may have visitors only for a short time. Once an implant is removed, there is no radioactivity in the body. The amount of radiation in a permanent implant goes down to a safe level before the patient leaves the hospital.

Chemotherapy. Treatment with drugs to kill cancer cells is called chemotherapy. Most anti-cancer drugs are injected into a vein (IV) or a muscle; some are given by mouth. Chemotherapy is systemic treatment, meaning that the drugs flow through the bloodstream to nearly every part of the body.

Often patients who need many doses of IV chemotherapy receive the drugs through a catheter (a thin flexible tube). One end of the catheter is placed in a large vein in the chest. The other end is outside the body or attached to a small device just under the skin. Anti-cancer drugs are given through the catheter. This can make chemotherapy more comfortable for the patient. Patients and their families are shown how to care for the catheter and keep it clean. For some types of cancer, doctors are studying whether it helps to put anti-cancer drugs directly into the affected area.

Chemotherapy is generally given in cycles: A treatment period is followed by a recovery period, then another treatment period, and so on. Usually a patient has chemotherapy as an outpatient—at the hospital, at the doctor's office, or at home. However, depending on which drugs are given and the patient's general health, the patient may need to stay in the hospital for a short time.

Hormonal therapy. Some types of cancer, including most breast and prostate cancers, depend on hormones to grow. For this reason, doctors may recommend therapy that prevents cancer cells from getting or using the hormones they need. Sometimes the patient has surgery to remove organs (such as the ovaries or testicles) that make the hormones; in other cases, the doctor uses drugs to stop hormone production or change the way hormones work. Like chemotherapy, hormonal therapy is a systemic treatment; it affects cells throughout the body.

Biological therapy. Biological therapy (also called immunotherapy) is a form of treatment that uses the body's natural ability (immune system) to fight infection and disease or to protect the body from some of the side effects of treatment. Monoclonal antibodies, interferon, interleukin-2 (IL-2), and several types of colony-stimulating factors (CSF, GM-CSF, G-CSF) are forms of biological therapy.

Side Effects of Cancer Treatment

It is hard to limit the effects of treatment so that only cancer cells are removed or destroyed. Because treatment also damages healthy cells and tissues, it often causes unpleasant side effects. The side effects of cancer treatment vary. They depend mainly on the type and extent of the treatment. Also, each person reacts differently. Doctors try to plan the patient's therapy to keep side effects to a minimum and they can help with any problems that occur.

Surgery. The side effects of surgery depend on the location of the tumor, the type of operation, the patient's general health, and other factors. Although patients are often uncomfortable during the first few days after surgery, this pain can be controlled with medicine. Patients should feel free to discuss pain relief with the doctor or nurse. It is also common for patients to feel tired or weak for a while.

The length of time it takes to recover from an operation varies for each patient.

Radiation therapy. With radiation therapy, the side effects depend on the treatment dose and the part of the body that is treated. The most common side effects are tiredness, skin reactions (such as a rash or redness) in the treated area, and loss of appetite. Radiation therapy also may cause a decrease in the number of white blood cells, cells that help protect the body against infection. Although the side effects of radiation therapy can be unpleasant, the doctor can usually treat or control them. It also helps to know that, in most cases, they are not permanent.

Chemotherapy. The side effects of chemotherapy depend mainly on the drugs and the doses the patient receives. Generally, anticancer drugs affect cells that divide rapidly. These include blood cells, which fight infection, help the blood to clot, or carry oxygen to all parts of the body. When blood cells are affected by anticancer drugs, patients are more likely to get infections, may bruise or bleed easily, and may have less energy.

Cells that line the digestive tract also divide rapidly. As a result of chemotherapy, patients may have side effects such as loss of appetite, nausea and vomiting, hair loss, or mouth sores. For some patients, the doctor may prescribe medicine to help with side effects, especially with nausea and vomiting. Usually, these side effects gradually go away during the recovery period or after treatment stops.

Hair loss, another side effect of chemotherapy, is a major concern for many patients. Some chemotherapy drugs only cause the hair to thin out, but others may result in the loss of all body hair. Patients may feel better if they decide how to handle hair loss before starting treatment.

In some men and women, chemotherapy drugs cause changes that may result in a loss of fertility (the ability to have children). Loss of fertility may be temporary or permanent depending on the drugs used and the patient's age. For men, sperm banking before treatment may be a choice. Women's menstrual periods may stop, and they may have hot flashes and vaginal dryness. Periods are more likely to return in young women.

In some cases, bone marrow transplantation and peripheral stem cell support are used to replace the tissue that forms blood cells when that tissue has been destroyed by the effects of chemotherapy or radiation therapy.

Hormonal therapy. Hormonal therapy can cause a number of side effects. Patients may have nausea and vomiting, swelling or weight gain, and, in some cases, hot flashes. In women, hormonal therapy also may cause interrupted menstrual periods, vaginal dryness, and sometimes, loss of fertility. Hormonal therapy in men may cause impotence, loss of sexual desire, or loss of fertility. These changes may be temporary, long lasting, or permanent.

Biological therapy. The side effects of biological therapy depend on the type of treatment. Often these treatments cause flu-like symptoms such as chills, fever, muscle aches, weakness, loss of appetite, nausea, vomiting, and diarrhea. Some patients get a rash, and some bleed or bruise easily. In addition, interleukin therapy can cause swelling.

Depending on how severe these problems are, patients may need to stay in the hospital during treatment. These side effects are usually short-term; they gradually go away after treatment stops. Doctors and nurses can explain the side effects of cancer treatment and help with any problems that occur.

NUTRITION FOR CANCER PATIENTS

Some patients lose their appetite and find it hard to eat well. In addition, the common side effects of treatment, such as nausea, vomiting, or mouth sores, can make it difficult to eat. For some patients, foods taste different. Also, people may not feel like eating when they are uncomfortable or tired.

Eating well means getting enough calories and protein to help prevent weight loss and regain strength. Patients who eat well during treatment often feel better and have more energy. In addition, they may be better able to handle the side effects of treatment. Doctors, nurses, and dietitians can offer advice for healthy eating during cancer treatment.

CLINICAL TRIALS

When laboratory research shows that a new treatment method has promise, cancer patients can receive the treatment in carefully controlled trials. These trials are designed to find out whether the new approach is both safe and effective and to answer scientific questions. Often clinical trials compare a new treatment with a standard approach so that doctors can learn which is more effective.

Researchers also look for ways to reduce the side effects of treatment and improve the quality of patients' lives. Patients who take part in clinical trials make an important contribution to medical science. These patients take certain risks, but they also may have the first chance to benefit from improved treatment methods.

Clinical trials offer important options for many patients. Cancer patients who are interested in taking part in a clinical trial should talk with their doctor.

One way to learn about clinical trials is through PDQ, a computerized resource developed by the National Cancer Institute. PDQ contains information about cancer treatment and about clinical trials in progress all over the country. The Cancer Information Service (1-800-4-CANCER) can provide PDQ information to doctors, patients, and the public.

SUPPORT FOR CANCER PATIENTS

Living with a serious disease is difficult. Cancer patients and those who care about them face many problems and challenges. Coping with these problems is often easier when people have helpful information and support services.

Cancer patients may worry about holding their job, caring for their family, or keeping up daily activities. Worries about tests, treatments, hospital stays, and medical bills are also common. Doctors, nurses, and other members of the health-care team can answer questions about treatment, working, or daily activities. Meeting with a social worker, counselor, or member of the clergy also can be helpful to patients who want to talk about their feelings or discuss their concerns about the future or about personal relationships.

Friends and relatives, especially those who have had personal experience with cancer, can be very supportive. Also, it helps many patients to meet with others who are facing problems like theirs. Cancer patients often get together in support groups, where they can share what they have learned about cancer and its treatment and about coping with the disease. It is important to keep in mind, however, that each patient is different. Treatments and ways of dealing with cancer that work for one person may not be right for another even if both have the same kind of cancer. It is always a good idea to discuss the advice of friends and family members with the doctor.

Often a social worker at the hospital or clinic can suggest groups that help with rehabilitation, emotional support, financial aid, transportation, or home care. The American Cancer Society has many services for patients and families. Local offices of the American Cancer Society are listed in the white pages of the telephone directory. In addition, the public library has many books and articles on living with cancer. The Cancer Information Service also has information on local resources.

CAUSES AND PREVENTION OF CANCER

The number of new cases of cancer in the United States is going up each year. People of all ages get cancer, but nearly all types are more common in middle-aged and elderly people than in young people. Skin cancer is the most common type of cancer for both men and women. The next most common type among men is prostate cancer; among women, it is breast cancer. Lung cancer, however, is the leading cause of death from cancer for both men and women in the United States. Brain cancer and leukemia are the most common cancers in children and young adults.

The more we can learn about what causes cancer, the more likely we are to find ways to prevent it. Scientists study patterns of cancer in the population to look for factors that affect the risk of developing this disease. In the laboratory, they explore possible causes of cancer and try to determine what actually happens when normal cells become cancerous.

Our current understanding of the causes of cancer is incomplete, but it is clear that cancer is not caused by an injury, such as a bump or bruise. And although being infected with certain viruses may increase the risk of some types of cancer, cancer is not contagious. No one can "catch" cancer from another person.

Cancer develops gradually as a result of a complex mix of factors related to environment, lifestyle, and heredity. Scientists have identified many risk factors that increase the chance of getting cancer. They estimate that about 80 percent of all cancers are related to the use of tobacco products, to what we eat and drink, or, to a lesser extent, to exposure to radiation or cancer-causing agents (carcinogens) in the environment and the workplace. Some people are more sensitive than others to factors that can cause cancer.

Many risk factors can be avoided. Others, such as inherited risk factors, are unavoidable. It is helpful to be aware of them, but it is also important to keep in mind that not everyone with a particular risk factor for cancer actually gets the disease; in fact, most do not. People at risk can help protect themselves by avoiding risk factors where possible and by getting regular checkups so that, if cancer develops, it is likely to be found early.

These are some of the factors that are known to increase the risk of cancer:

Tobacco. Tobacco causes cancer. In fact, smoking tobacco, using "smokeless" tobacco, and being regularly exposed to environmental tobacco smoke without actually smoking are responsible for one-third of all cancer deaths in the United States each year. Tobacco use is the most preventable cause of death in this country.

Smoking accounts for more than 85 percent of all lung cancer deaths. If you smoke, your risk of getting lung cancer is affected by the number and type of cigarettes you smoke and how long you have been smoking. Overall, for those who smoke one pack a day, the chance of getting lung cancer is about 10 times greater than for nonsmokers. Smokers are also more likely than nonsmokers to develop several other types of cancer (such as oral cancer and cancers of the larynx, esophagus, pancreas, bladder, kidney, and cervix). The risk of cancer begins to decrease when a smoker quits, and the risk continues to decline gradually each year after quitting.

The use of smokeless tobacco (chewing tobacco and snuff) causes cancer of the mouth and throat. Precancerous conditions, or tissue changes that may lead to cancer, begin to go away after a person stops using smokeless tobacco.

Exposure to environmental tobacco smoke, also called involuntary smoking, increases the risk of lung cancer for nonsmokers. The risk goes up 30 percent or more for a nonsmoking spouse of a person who smokes. Involuntary smoking causes about 3,000 lung cancer deaths in this country each year.

If you use tobacco in any form and you

need help quitting, talk with your doctor or dentist, or join a smoking cessation group sponsored by a local hospital or voluntary organization. For information on such groups or other programs, call the Cancer Information Service or the American Cancer Society.

Diet. Your choice of foods may affect your chance of developing cancer. Evidence points to a link between a high-fat diet and certain cancers, such as cancer of the breast, colon, uterus, or prostate. Being seriously overweight appears to be linked to increased rates of cancer of the prostate, pancreas, uterus, colon, or ovary, and to breast cancer in older women. On the other hand, studies suggest that foods containing fiber and certain nutrients help protect us against some types of cancer.

You may be able to reduce your cancer risk by making some simple food choices. Try to have a varied, well-balanced diet that includes generous amounts of foods that are high in fiber, vitamins, and minerals.

At the same time, try to cut down on fatty foods. You should eat five servings of fruits and vegetables each day, choose more whole-grain breads and cereals, and cut down on eggs, high-fat meat, high-fat dairy products (such as whole milk, butter, and most cheeses), salad dressings, margarine, and cooking oils.

Sunlight. Ultraviolet radiation from the sun and from other sources (such as sunlamps and tanning booths) damages the skin and can cause skin cancer. Repeated exposure to ultraviolet radiation increases the risk of skin cancer, especially if you have fair skin or you freckle easily. The sun's ultraviolet (UV) rays are strongest in summer between roughly 11 a.m. and 3 p.m. (daylight saving time). The risk is greatest at this time, when the sun is high overhead. As a rule, it is best to avoid the sun when your shadow is shorter than you are.

Protective clothing, such as a hat and long sleeves, can help block the sun's harmful rays. You can also use sunscreens to help protect yourself. Sunscreens are rated in strength according to their SPF (sun protection factor), which ranges from 2 to 30 and higher. Those rated 15 to 30 block most of the sun's harmful rays.

Alcohol. Drinking large amounts of alcohol increases the risk of cancers of the mouth, throat, esophagus, and larynx. (People who smoke cigarettes and drink alcohol have an especially high risk of getting these cancers.) Alcohol can damage the liver and increase the risk of liver cancer. Some studies suggest that drinking alcohol also increases the risk of breast cancer. So if you drink at all, do so in moderation—not more than one or two drinks a day.

Radiation. Exposure to large doses of radiation from medical x-rays can increase the risk of cancer. X-rays used for diagnosis expose you to very little radiation and the benefits nearly always outweigh the risks. However, repeated exposure can be harmful, so it is a good idea to talk with your doctor or dentist about the need for each x-ray and ask about the use of shields to protect other parts of your body.

Before 1950, x-rays were used to treat noncancerous conditions (such as an enlarged thymus, enlarged tonsils and adenoids, ringworm of the scalp, and acne) in children and young adults. People who have received radiation to the head and neck have a higher-than-average risk of developing thyroid cancer years later. People with a history of such treatments should report it to their doctor and should have a careful exam of the neck every one or two years.

Chemicals and other substances in the workplace. Being exposed to substances such as metals, dust, chemicals, or pesticides at work can increase the risk of cancer. Asbestos, nickel, cadmium, uranium, radon, vinyl chloride, benzidine, and benzene are well-known examples of carcinogens in the workplace. These may act alone or along with another carcinogen, such as cigarette smoke. For example, inhaling asbestos fibers increases the risk of lung diseases, including cancer, and the cancer risk is especially high for asbestos workers who smoke. It is important to follow work and safety rules to avoid contact with dangerous materials.

Hormone replacement therapy. Many women use estrogen therapy to control the hot flashes, vaginal dryness, and osteoporosis (thinning of the bones) that may occur during menopause. However, studies show that estrogen use increases the risk of cancer of the uterus. Other studies suggest an increased risk of breast cancer among women who have used high doses of estrogen or have used estrogen for a long time. At the same time, taking estrogen may reduce the risk of heart disease and osteoporosis.

The risk of uterine cancer appears to be less when progesterone is used with estrogen than when estrogen is used alone. But some scientists are concerned that the addition of progesterone may also increase the risk of breast cancer.

Researchers are still studying and finding new information about the risks and benefits of taking replacement hormones. A woman considering hormone replacement therapy should discuss these issues with her doctor.

Diethylstilbestrol (DES). DES is a form of estrogen that doctors prescribed from the early 1940s until 1971 to try to prevent miscarriage. In some daughters of women who were given DES during pregnancy, the uterus, vagina, and cervix do not develop normally. DES-exposed daughters also have an increased chance of developing abnormal cells (dysplasia) in the cervix and vagina. In addition, a rare type of

QUESTIONS A PATIENT MAY WANT TO ASK THE DOCTOR
- What is my diagnosis?
- What is the stage of the disease?
- What are my treatment choices? Which do you recommend for me? Why?
- What are the chances that the treatment will be successful?
- Would a clinical trial be appropriate for me?
- What are the risks and possible side effects of each treatment?
- How long will treatment last?
- Will I have to change my normal activities?
- What is the treatment likely to cost?

vaginal and cervical cancer has been found in a small number of DES-exposed daughters. Women who took DES during pregnancy may have a slightly increased risk of developing breast cancer. DES-exposed mothers and daughters should tell their doctor about this exposure. DES-exposed daughters should have regular special pelvic exams by a doctor familiar with conditions related to DES.

Exposure to DES before birth does not appear to increase the risk of cancer in DES-exposed sons; however, reproductive and urinary system problems may occur. These men should tell the doctor and should have regular medical checkups.

Close relatives with certain types of cancer. A small number of cancers (including melanoma and cancers of the breast, ovary, and colon) tend to occur more often in some families than in the rest of the population. It is not always clear whether a pattern of cancer in a family is due to heredity, factors in the family's environment, or chance. Still, if close relatives have been affected by cancer, it is important to let your doctor know this and then to follow his or her advice about cancer prevention and checkups to detect problems early.

The National Cancer Institute

23

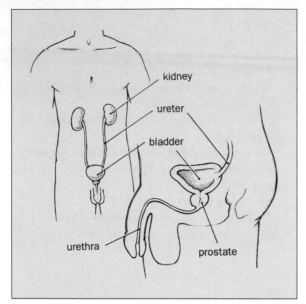 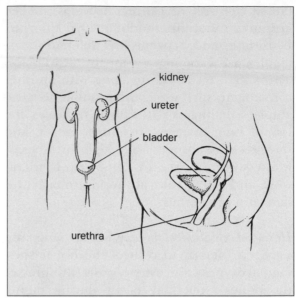

The bladder (essentially the same in both men and women) holds urine, which descends from the kidneys, until it is ready to be excreted. Most cases of bladder cancer originate in the cells that line the organ.

BLADDER CANCER

The bladder is a hollow organ in the lower abdomen. It stores urine, the waste that is produced when the kidneys filter the blood. The bladder has a muscular wall that allows it to get larger and smaller as urine is stored or emptied. The wall of the bladder is lined with several layers of transitional cells.

Urine passes from the two kidneys into the bladder through two tubes called ureters. Urine leaves the bladder through another tube, the urethra.

Most cancers are named for the part of the body or type of cells in which they begin. About 90 percent of bladder cancers are transitional cell carcinomas, cancers that begin in the cells lining the bladder. Cancer that is confined to the lining of the bladder is called superficial bladder cancer. After treatment, superficial bladder cancer can recur; if this happens, most often it recurs as another superficial cancer.

In some cases, cancer that begins in the transitional cells spreads through the lining of the bladder and invades the muscular wall of the bladder. This is known as invasive bladder cancer. Invasive cancer may grow through the bladder wall and spread to nearby organs.

Bladder cancer cells may also be found in the lymph nodes surrounding the bladder. If the cancer has reached these nodes, it may mean that cancer cells have spread to other lymph nodes and to distant organs, such as the lungs. The cancer cells in the new tumor are still bladder cancer cells. The new tumor is called metastatic bladder cancer rather than lung cancer because it has the same kind of abnormal cells found in the bladder.

SYMPTOMS

Some common symptoms of bladder cancer include: blood in the urine (slightly rusty to deep red in color), pain during urination, and frequent urination, or feeling the need to urinate without results.

When symptoms occur, they are not sure signs of bladder cancer. They may also be caused by infections, benign tumors, bladder stones, or other problems. Only a doctor can make a diagnosis. (People with symptoms like these generally see their family doctor or a urologist, a doctor who specializes in diseases of the urinary system.) It is important to see a doctor so that any illness can be diagnosed and treated as early as possible.

DIAGNOSIS AND STAGING

To find the cause of symptoms, the doctor asks about the patient's medical history and does a physical exam. The physical will include a rectal or vaginal exam that allows the doctor to check for tumors that can be felt. In addition, urine samples are sent to the laboratory for testing to check for blood and cancer cells.

The doctor may use an instrument to look directly into the bladder, a procedure called cystoscopy. This procedure may be done with local or general anesthesia. The doctor inserts a thin, lighted tube (called a cystoscope) into the bladder through the urethra to examine the lining of the bladder. The doctor can remove samples of tissues through this tube. The sample is then examined under a microscope by a pathologist. The removal of tissue to look for cancer cells is called a biopsy. In many cases, performing a biopsy is the only sure way to tell whether cancer is present. If the entire cancer is removed during the biopsy, bladder cancer can be diagnosed and treated in a single procedure.

Once bladder cancer is diagnosed, the doctor will want to learn the grade of the cancer and the stage, or extent, of the disease. Grade is important because it tells how closely the cancer resembles normal tissue and suggests how fast the cancer is likely to grow. Low-grade cancers more closely resemble normal tissue and are likely to grow and spread more slowly than high-grade cancers.

Staging is a careful attempt to find out whether the cancer has spread and, if so, what parts of the body are affected. The stage of bladder cancer may be determined at the time of diagnosis, or it may be necessary to perform other tests, including imaging tests such as a CT scan, MRI, sonogram, intravenous pyelography (IVP), bone scan, or chest x-ray.

TREATMENT

Treatment for bladder cancer depends on the stage of the disease (particularly if, or how deeply, the cancer has invaded the bladder wall), the grade of the cancer, the patient's general health, and other factors. People with bladder cancer are often treated by a team of specialists, which may include a urologist, oncologist, and radiation oncologist. The doctors develop a treatment plan to fit each patient's needs.

Depending on its stage and grade, bladder cancer may be treated with surgery, radiation therapy, chemotherapy, or biological therapy. Doctors may recommend one treatment method or a combination of methods. It is important for patients to discuss the treatment plan with their doctors. (See page 20 for more on Support for Cancer Patients.)

Methods of Treatment

Transurethral resection (TUR). Surgery is a common form of treatment for bladder cancer. Early (superficial) bladder cancer may be treated at the time of diagnosis through a procedure called transurethral resection (TUR). During TUR, the doctor inserts a cystoscope into the bladder through the urethra. The doctor then uses a tool with a small wire loop on the end to remove the cancer or to burn away cancer cells with an electric current (fulguration). TUR requires anesthesia and may be done in the hospital.

Cystectomy. Surgery to remove part or all of the bladder is called cystectomy. The most common form of surgery for invasive bladder cancer is radical cystectomy. This surgery may be done when the bladder cancer invades the muscle wall, or when superficial cancer involves a large part of the bladder.

Radical cystectomy removes the entire bladder, nearby lymph nodes, and any surrounding organs that contain cancerous cells. In men, the nearby organs that are removed include the prostate and the seminal vesicles. In women, the uterus, the ovaries, and part of the vagina are removed. Sometimes when the cancer has spread outside the bladder and cannot be completely removed, surgery to remove only the bladder may be done to relieve urinary symptoms caused by the cancer. When the bladder must be removed, the doctor creates another way for urine to leave the body.

In some cases, patients may have part of the bladder removed in an operation called segmental cystectomy. This type of surgery may be done when a patient has a low-grade cancer that has invaded the wall of the bladder but is limited to one area of the organ. Because most of the bladder remains intact, a patient urinates normally after recovering.

Radiation therapy. In radiation therapy, high-energy rays are used to kill cancer cells. Like surgery, radiation therapy is local therapy; it affects cancer cells only in the treated area. Sometimes radiation is given before or after surgery or along with anticancer drugs. When bladder cancer has spread to other organs, radiation therapy may be used to relieve symptoms caused by the cancer.

Radiation may come from a machine outside the body (external radiation) or from a small container of radioactive material, called a radiation implant, placed directly into the bladder (internal radiation). Some patients have both kinds of radiation therapy.

Chemotherapy. Chemotherapy is the use of drugs to kill cancer cells. The doctor may use one drug or a combination of drugs. Chemotherapy may be used alone or after TUR with fulguration to treat superficial bladder cancer. In a treatment called intravesical chemotherapy, anticancer drugs are placed in the bladder through a tube called a catheter, which is inserted through the urethra. When given in this way, the anticancer drugs, which remain in the bladder for several hours, affect mainly the cells of the bladder. The treatment is usually done once a week for several weeks. Sometimes the treatments continue once or several times a month for up to a year.

To help control the disease when cancer cells have deeply invaded the bladder or spread to lymph nodes or other organs, the anticancer drugs are usually given by injection into a vein (IV); some may be given by mouth. This form of chemotherapy is systemic therapy, meaning that the drugs flow through the bloodstream to nearly every part of the body. The drugs are usually given in cycles: a treatment period followed by a recovery period, then another treatment period, and so on.

Biological therapy. A form of treatment that uses the body's natural ability (immune system) to fight cancer, biological therapy for bladder cancer is most often used when the disease is superficial. Like chemotherapy, biological therapy may be used alone to treat bladder cancer or after TUR with fulguration to help prevent the cancer from recurring. This form of treatment involves placing a solution of BCG, a substance that stimulates the immune system, into the bladder. The medicine stays in the bladder for about two hours before the patient is allowed to empty the bladder by urinating. This treatment is usually done once a week for six weeks and may need to be prolonged or repeated. Doctors are also studying the use of other forms of biological therapy for other stages of bladder cancer.

Side Effects of Treatment

It is hard to limit the effects of cancer therapy so that only cancer cells, not healthy cells, are removed or destroyed. Because treatment can damage healthy cells and tissues, it frequently causes side effects.

These side effects depend mainly on the type and extent of the cancer treatment. Also, the effects may not be the same for each person, and they may even change from one treatment to the next. Doctors and nurses can explain the possible side effects of treatment, and they can help relieve symptoms that may occur during and after treatment.

TUR causes few problems. Patients may have some blood in their urine and difficulty or pain when urinating for a few days afterward.

After any bladder surgery, particularly radical cystectomy, patients are often uncomfortable during the first few days. However, this pain can be controlled with medicine. Patients should feel free to discuss pain relief with the doctor or nurse. It is also common for patients to feel tired or weak for a while. The length of time it takes to recover from an operation varies for each patient.

After segmental cystectomy, patients may not be able to hold as much urine in their bladder. In most cases, this problem is temporary, but some patients may have long-lasting changes in bladder capacity.

When the bladder is removed, the patient needs a new way to store and pass urine. Various methods are used. In one common method, the surgeon uses a piece of the person's small intestine to form a new tube through which urine can pass. The ureters are attached to one end, and the other end is brought out through an opening in the wall of the abdomen. This new opening is called a stoma. A flat bag fits over the stoma to collect urine, and special adhesive holds it in place. The patient will be taught how to care for the stoma. The surgical procedure to create a stoma is called a urostomy or an ostomy. One method uses part of the small intestine to make a new storage pouch (called a continent reservoir) inside the body. Urine collects there instead of emptying into a bag. The pouch is connected either to a stoma or to the urethra. The patient learns to use a catheter to drain the urine through the stoma or urethra.

Women who have had a radical cystectomy are not able to have children because their uterus has been removed. In addition, the vagina may be narrower or shallower, which may make sexual intercourse difficult.

In the past, nearly all men were impotent after radical cystectomy, but improvements in surgery have made it possible to prevent this side effect is some cases. However, men who have had their prostate gland and seminal vesicles removed no longer produce semen, so they do not ejaculate when they have an orgasm and are not able to father children.

With radiation therapy, the side effects depend mainly on the treatment dose and the part of the body that is treated. Patients are likely to become very tired during radiation therapy, especially in the later weeks of treatment. Resting is important, but doctors usually advise patients to try to stay as active as they can.

With external radiation, there may be permanent darkening or "bronzing" of the skin in the treated area. In addition, it is common to lose hair in the treated area and for the skin to become red, dry, tender, and itchy. These problems are temporary, and the doctor may be able to suggest ways to relieve them.

Radiation therapy to the abdomen may cause nausea, vomiting, diarrhea, or urinary discomfort. Radiation therapy also may cause a decrease in the number of white blood cells, cells that help protect the body against infection. Usually, the doctor can suggest certain diet changes or medicine to ease these problems. For both men and women, radiation treatment for bladder cancer can affect sexuality. Women may experience vaginal dryness, and men may have difficulty with erections.

Although side effects of radiation therapy can be distressing, the doctor can usually treat or control them. It also helps to know that, in most cases, side effects are not permanent.

The side effects of chemotherapy depend mainly on the drugs and the doses the patient receives, as well as how the drugs are given. In addition, as with other types of treatment, side effects vary from person to person.

Anticancer drugs that are placed in the bladder may irritate the bladder for a few days after treatment, causing some discomfort or bleeding. Some drugs, if they come into contact with the skin or genitals, may cause a rash.

Systemic chemotherapy affects rapidly dividing cells throughout the body. These cells include blood cells, which fight infection, help the blood to clot, or carry oxygen to all parts of the body. When blood cells are affected by anticancer drugs, patients are more likely to get infections, may bruise or bleed easily, and may have less energy.

Cells in hair roots and cells that line the digestive tract also divide rapidly. As a result, patients may lose their hair and may have other side effects such as poor appetite, nausea and vomiting, or mouth sores. Usually, these side effects go away gradually during the recovery periods between treatments or after treatment is over.

Certain drugs used in the treatment of bladder cancer also may cause kidney damage. Patients are given large amounts of fluid while taking these drugs. Anticancer drugs can also cause tingling in the fingers, ringing in the ears, or hearing loss. These problems may not clear up after treatment stops.

Treatment with BCG can irritate the bladder for a few days after treatment. This may cause pain, especially while urinating, and the feeling of an urgent need to urinate. Patients also may have some blood in their urine, have a low fever, or feel tired or nauseated.

Other types of biological therapy may cause flu-like symptoms such as chills, fever, muscle aches, weakness, loss of appetite, nausea, vomiting, and diarrhea. Patients also may bleed or bruise easily, get a rash, or have swelling. These problems can be severe, but they go away after the treatment stops.

To help withstand the side effects of treatment in general, it is important that patients maintain good nutrition (see Nutrition for Cancer Patients, page 19).

FOLLOW-UP CARE

It is important for people who have had cancer to have regular follow-up examinations after their treatment is over. For people with bladder cancer who have not had their bladder removed, the doctor will check the bladder with a cystoscope and remove any superficial tumors that may have recurred. Patients also may have urine tests to check for cancer cells. Care may also include blood tests, a CT scan, a chest x-ray, or other tests.

LIVING WITH CANCER

The diagnosis of bladder cancer can change the lives of cancer patients and the people who care about them. These changes in daily life can be difficult to handle. (See Support for Cancer Patients, page 20.)

WHAT THE FUTURE HOLDS

Each year, more than 47,000 Americans will find out they have bladder cancer. The outlook for patients diagnosed with early bladder cancer is very good. The chances of recovery from more advanced bladder cancer are improving as researchers continue to look for better ways to treat this disease.

The National Cancer Institute

BREAST CANCER

Each breast has six to nine overlapping sections called lobes. Within each lobe are many smaller lobules, which end in dozens of tiny bulbs that can produce milk. The lobes, lobules, and bulbs are all linked by thin tubes called ducts, which lead to the nipple in the center of a dark area of skin called the areola. Fat fills the spaces between lobules and ducts.

There are no muscles in the breast, but muscles lie under each breast and cover the ribs.

Each breast also contains blood vessels and vessels that carry colorless fluid called lymph. The lymph vessels lead to small bean-shaped organs called lymph nodes, clusters of which are found under the arm, above the collarbone, and in the chest. Lymph nodes are also found in many other parts of the body.

TYPES OF BREAST CANCER

There are several types of breast cancer. The most common one begins in the lining of the ducts and is called ductal carcinoma. Another type, called lobular carcinoma, arises in the lobules. Cancers that begin in other tissues in the breast are rare and are not discussed here.

When breast cancer spreads outside the breast, cancer cells are often found in the lymph nodes under the arm. If the cancer has reached these nodes, it may mean that cancer cells have spread to other parts of the body—other lymph nodes and other organs, such as the bones, liver, or lungs.

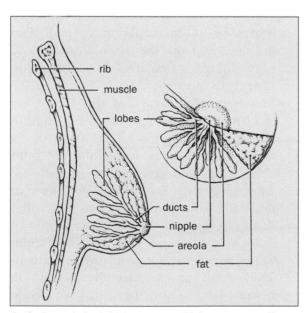

In the breast's fatty tissue are several lobes, many smaller lobules, and dozens of milk-producing bulbs and connecting ducts. Most breast cancers begin in the ducts or lobules.

Cancer that spreads is the same disease and has the same name as the original (primary) cancer. When breast cancer spreads, it is called metastatic breast cancer, even though the secondary tumor is in another organ. Doctors sometimes call this "distant" disease.

EARLY DETECTION

Women can take an active part in the early detection of breast cancer. They should talk with their doctor about the symptoms to watch for and an appropriate schedule of checkups. The doctor's advice will be based on the woman's age, medical history, and other factors. Women should ask the doctor about:

- Mammograms (x-rays of the breast)
- Breast exams by a doctor or nurse
- Breast self-examination (BSE)

A mammogram is a special kind of x-ray. It is different from a chest x-ray or x-rays of other parts of the body. Mammography uses very low levels of radiation and usually involves two x-rays of each breast, one taken from the side and one from the top. The breast must be squeezed between two plates for the pictures to be clear. While this squeezing may be a bit uncomfortable, it lasts only a few seconds.

In many cases, mammograms can show breast tumors before they cause symptoms or can be felt. A mammogram can also show small deposits of calcium in the breast. A cluster of very tiny specks of calcium (called microcalcifications) may be an early sign of cancer.

Mammography should be done only by specially trained medical staff using machines designed just for taking x-rays of the breast. A qualified doctor, called a radiologist, should read the mammogram. Women should talk with their doctor or call the Cancer Information Service (1-800-4-CANCER) for help in finding a certified mammography facility.

For women of all ages, a breast exam by a

IMPORTANT QUESTIONS

These are some questions a woman may want to ask her doctor before having surgery:

• What kind of operation will it be?

• How will I feel after the operation? If I have pain, how will you help me?

• Where will the scars be? What will they look like?

• If I decide to have plastic surgery to rebuild my breast, when can that be done?

• Will I have to do any special exercises?

• When can I get back to my normal activities?

doctor or nurse (called a clinical breast exam) is usually part of the regular medical checkup. Also, many women choose to examine their own breasts once a month. For more information on breast self-examination, see page 439.

Ideal breast cancer screening for women age 40 and over includes a monthly self-exam and an annual clinical exam and mammogram.

It's important to remember that every woman's breasts are different and that they change because of age, the menstrual cycle, pregnancy, menopause, or taking birth control pills or other hormones. It is normal for the breasts to feel lumpy and uneven. Also, it is common for a woman's breasts to be swollen and tender right before or during her menstrual period. A woman should contact her doctor about any unusual changes in her breasts, whether she notices them during breast self-exam or at another time.

SYMPTOMS

Early breast cancer usually does not cause pain. In fact, when it first develops, breast cancer may cause no symptoms at all. But as the cancer grows, it can cause changes that women should watch for:

• A lump or thickening in or near the breast or in the underarm area

• A change in the size or shape of the breast

• A discharge from the nipple

• A change in the color or feel of the skin of the breast, areola, or nipple (dimpled, puckered, or scaly)

A woman should talk with her doctor if she notices any of these changes. Usually they are not cancer, but only a doctor can tell for sure.

DIAGNOSIS

An abnormal area on a mammogram, a lump, or other changes in the breast can be caused by cancer or by other, less serious problems. To find out the cause of any of these signs or symptoms, a woman's doctor does a careful physical exam and asks about her personal and family medical history. In addition to checking general signs of health, the doctor may do one or more of the breast exams described below to help make a diagnosis.

• *Palpation.* The doctor can tell a lot about a lump—its size, its texture, and whether it moves easily—by palpation, carefully feeling the lump and the tissue around it. Benign lumps often feel different from cancerous ones.

• *Mammography.* X-rays of the breast can give the doctor important information about a breast lump. If an area on the mammogram looks suspicious or is not clear, additional views may be needed.

• *Ultrasonography.* Sometimes the doctor orders ultrasonography, which can often show whether a lump is solid or filled with fluid. This exam uses high-frequency sound waves, which cannot be heard by humans. The sound waves enter the breast and bounce back. The pattern of their echoes produces a picture called a sonogram, which is displayed on a screen. This exam is often used along with mammography.

Based on these exams, the doctor may decide that no further tests are needed and no treatment is necessary. In such cases, the doctor may want to check the woman regularly to watch for any changes. Often, however, the doctor must remove fluid or tissue from the breast to make a diagnosis.

- *Aspiration or needle biopsy.* The doctor uses a needle to remove fluid or a small amount of tissue from a breast lump. This procedure may show whether the lump is a fluid-filled cyst (not cancer) or a solid mass (which may or may not be cancer). Tissues can be removed with a needle from an area that is suspicious on a mammogram but cannot be felt; it goes to a lab to be checked for cancer cells.
- *Surgical biopsy.* The doctor cuts out part or all of a lump or suspicious area. A pathologist examines the tissue under a microscope to check for cancer cells.

When Cancer Is Found

When cancer is present, the pathologist can tell what kind of cancer it is (whether it began in a duct or a lobule) and whether it is invasive (has invaded nearby tissues in the breast).

Special laboratory tests of the tissue help the doctor learn more about the cancer. For example, hormone receptor tests (estrogen and progesterone receptor tests) can show whether the cancer is sensitive to hormones. Positive test results mean hormones help the cancer grow and the cancer is likely to respond to hormonal treatment (see page 32). Other lab tests are sometimes done to help the doctor predict whether the cancer is likely to grow slowly or quickly.

The patient's doctor may refer her to doctors who specialize in treating cancer. Treatment generally begins within a few weeks after the diagnosis. There will be time for the woman to talk with the doctor about her treatment choices, to get a second opinion, and to prepare herself and her loved ones. (See page 17 for more information about getting a second opinion and planning treatment.)

TREATMENT

Methods of treatment for breast cancer are local or systemic. Local treatments are used to remove, destroy, or control the cancer cells in a specific area. Surgery and radiation therapy are local treatments. Systemic treatments are used to destroy or control cancer cells anywhere in the body. Chemotherapy and hormonal therapy are systemic treatments. A patient may have just one form of treatment or a combination. Different forms of treatment may be given at the same time or one after another.

Surgery is the most common treatment for breast cancer. Several types of surgery may be used. The doctor can explain them in detail, can discuss the benefits and risks of each type, and can describe how each will affect the woman's appearance.

An operation to remove the breast is a mastectomy; an operation to remove the cancer but not the breast is called breast-sparing surgery. Lumpectomy and segmental mastectomy are types of breast-sparing surgery and usually are followed by radiation therapy to destroy any cancer cells that may remain in the area. In most cases, the surgeon also removes lymph nodes under the arm to help determine whether cancer cells have entered the lymph system.

- *In lumpectomy,* the surgeon removes just the breast tumor and some normal tissue around it.
- *In partial (segmental) mastectomy,* the surgeon removes the tumor, some of the normal breast tissue around it, and the lining over the chest muscles below the tumor.
- *In total (simple) mastectomy,* the surgeon removes the whole breast.

31

- **In modified radical mastectomy,** the surgeon removes the breast, some of the lymph nodes under the arm, and the lining over the chest muscles. Sometimes the smaller of the two chest muscles is removed.
- **In radical mastectomy** (also called Halsted radical mastectomy), the surgeon removes the breast, the chest muscles, all of the lymph nodes under the arm, and some additional fat and skin. For many years, this operation was the standard one, but it is very rarely necessary and seldom used now.

Radiation therapy (also called radiotherapy) is the use of high-energy x-rays to damage cancer cells and stop them from growing. The rays may come from radioactive material outside the body (external radiation) directed at the breast by a machine or from radioactive material placed directly in the breast in thin plastic tubes (implant radiation). Sometimes the patient receives both kinds of radiation.

Patients go to the hospital or clinic each day for external radiation treatments. When this therapy follows breast-sparing surgery, the treatments are given five days a week for five to six weeks. At the end of that time, an extra "boost" of radiation is often given to the tumor site. The boost may be either external or internal (using an implant). Patients stay in the hospital for a short time for implant radiation.

Chemotherapy is the use of drugs to kill cancer cells. Chemotherapy for breast cancer is usually a combination of drugs. The drugs may be given by mouth or by injection. Either way, chemotherapy is a systemic therapy, because the drugs enter the bloodstream and travel through the body.

Chemotherapy is given in cycles: a treatment period followed by a recovery period, then another treatment, and so on. Most patients have chemotherapy in an outpatient part of the hospital, at the doctor's office, or at home. Depending on which drugs are given

and the woman's general health, however, she may need to stay in the hospital during her treatment.

Hormonal therapy is used to keep cancer cells from getting the hormones they need to grow. This treatment may include the use of drugs that change the way hormones work or surgery to remove the ovaries, which make female hormones. Like chemotherapy, hormonal therapy is a systemic treatment; it can affect cancer cells throughout the body.

Treatment Choices
Treatment decisions are complex. These decisions are affected by the judgment of the doctor and by the desires of the patient. A patient's treatment options depend on a number of factors. These factors include her age and menopausal status, her general health, the location of the tumor, and the size of her breasts. Certain features of the cancer cells (such as whether they depend on hormones to grow) are also considered. The most important factor is the stage of the disease. The stage is based on the size of the tumor and whether it has spread. Below are brief descriptions of the treatments most often used for each stage of breast cancer. (Other treatments may sometimes be appropriate.)

- **Lobular carcinoma in situ** (LCIS) refers to abnormal cells in the lining of a lobule. Although these abnormal cells seldom become invasive cancer, their presence is a sign that a woman has a higher-than-average risk of developing breast cancer in either breast. Some patients with LCIS may have no treatment, but return to the doctor regularly for checkups. Others may have surgery to remove both breasts to prevent cancer from developing. Underarm lymph nodes are not usually removed.
- **Ductal carcinoma in situ,** or intraductal carcinoma (DCIS), refers to abnormal cells in the lining of a duct. The cells have not bro-

ken through the duct or invaded nearby tissue. Occasionally, however, DCIS becomes invasive cancer, and the cells can spread. Patients with DCIS may have a mastectomy or they may have breast-sparing surgery followed by radiation therapy. Underarm lymph nodes are not usually removed.

- **Stage I and stage II** are early stages of breast cancer, but the cancer has invaded nearby tissue. Stage I means that cancer cells have not spread beyond the breast and the tumor is no more than about an inch across. Stage II means that cancer has spread to underarm lymph nodes and/or that the size of the tumor is one to two inches across.

Women with early stage breast cancer may have breast-sparing surgery followed by radiation therapy as their primary local treatment, or they may have a mastectomy. These treatments are equally effective.

With either approach, lymph nodes under the arm generally are removed. Some women with stage I and most with stage II breast cancer have chemotherapy or hormonal therapy or both. This added treatment is called adjuvant therapy. Adjuvant therapy is given to prevent the cancer from recurring.

- **Stage III** is also called locally advanced cancer. The tumor in the breast is large (more than two inches across), the cancer is extensive in the underarm lymph nodes, or it has spread to other lymph node areas or to other tissues near the breast. Inflammatory breast cancer is a stage III cancer.

Patients with stage III breast cancer usually have both local treatment to remove or destroy the cancer in the breast and systemic treatment to stop the disease from spreading. The local treatment may be surgery and/or radiation therapy to the breast and underarm. The systemic treatment may be chemotherapy, hormonal therapy, or both; it may be given before local treatment.

- **Stage IV** is metastatic cancer. The cancer has spread from the breast to other organs of the body. Women who have stage IV breast cancer receive chemotherapy and/or hormonal therapy to shrink the tumor or destroy cancer cells. They may have surgery or radiation therapy to control the cancer in the breast. Radiation may also be useful to control tumors in other parts of the body.

- **Recurrent cancer** means the disease has come back in spite of the initial treatment. Even when a tumor in the breast seems to have been completely removed or destroyed, the disease sometimes returns because undetected cancer cells remain in the area after treatment or because the disease had already spread before treatment. Most recurrences appear within the first two or three years after treatment, but can appear many years later.

Cancer that returns only in the area of the surgery is called a local recurrence. If the disease returns in another part of the body, it is called metastatic breast cancer (or distant disease). The patient may have one type of treatment or a combination of therapies.

Side Effects of Treatment

It is hard to limit the effects of cancer treatment so that only cancer cells are removed or destroyed. Because healthy cells and tissues may also be damaged, treatment often causes unpleasant side effects.

After surgery, the skin in the breast area may be tight, and the muscles of the arm and shoulder may feel stiff. For most women, reduced strength and limited movement are temporary.

The doctor, nurse, or physical therapist can recommend exercises to help a woman regain movement and strength in her arm and shoulder. A woman may have numbness and tingling in the chest, underarm, shoulder, and arm. In most of these patients, some numbness may be permanent.

Mastectomy is usually easier to recover from physically than psychologically. Fortunately, many women today can be treated with breast-sparing surgery, such as lumpectomy or partial mastectomy.

Removing the lymph nodes under the arm slows the flow of lymph. In some women, lymph builds up in the arm and hand and causes swelling (lymphedema). Women need to protect the arm and hand on the treated side from injury. They should ask the doctor how to handle any cuts, scratches, insect bites, or other injuries that may occur. Also, they should contact the doctor if an infection develops in the arm or hand.

The radiation oncologist will explain the possible side effects of radiation therapy for breast cancer—including uncommon side effects that may involve the heart, lungs, or ribs. One of the common side effects is fatigue, especially in the later weeks of treatment. Resting is important, but doctors usually advise their patients to try to stay reasonably active. Women should match their activities to their energy level.

Another common side effect is for the skin in the treated areas to become red, dry, tender, and itchy. Toward the end of treatment, the skin may become moist and "weepy." This area should be exposed to the air as much as possible. Patients should avoid wearing a bra or clothes that may rub; loose-fitting cotton clothes are usually best. Good skin care is important at this time, but patients should not use any lotions or creams without the doctor's advice and should not use any deodorant on the treated side. The effects of radiation therapy on the skin are temporary. The area will heal when the treatment is over.

For most women, the breast will look and feel about the same after radiation therapy.

Occasionally, the treated breast may be firmer. Also, it may be larger (due to fluid buildup) or smaller (because of tissue changes) than before. For some women, the breast skin is more sensitive after radiation treatment; for others, it is less sensitive.

The side effects of chemotherapy depend mainly on the drugs the patient receives. As with other types of treatment, side effects vary from person to person. In general, anticancer drugs affect rapidly dividing cells. These include blood cells, which fight infection, cause the blood to clot, and carry oxygen to all parts of the body.

When blood cells are affected by anticancer drugs, patients are more likely to get infections, bruise or bleed easily, and have less energy. Cells in hair follicles and cells that line the digestive tract also divide rapidly. As a result of chemotherapy, patients may lose their hair and may have other side effects, such as loss of appetite, nausea, vomiting, diarrhea, or mouth sores.

Many of chemotherapy's side effects can be controlled with medicine, and they generally are short-term problems. They gradually go away during the recovery part of the chemotherapy cycle or after the treatment is over. With modern chemotherapy, long-term side effects are fortunately quite rare, but there have been cases in which the heart is weakened, and second cancers such as leukemia have occurred.

Some anticancer drugs can damage the ovaries. If the ovaries fail to produce hormones, the woman may experience symptoms of menopause, such as vaginal dryness and hot flashes. Her periods may become irregular or may stop, and she may not be able to become pregnant. In women over the age of 35 or 40, some of these effects, such as infertility, are likely to be permanent.

Hormonal therapy can cause a number of side effects. They depend largely on the specific drug or type of treatment, and they vary from patient to patient.

Tamoxifen is the most commonly used form of hormonal treatment. This drug blocks the body's use of estrogen but does not stop estrogen production. Tamoxifen may cause hot flashes, vaginal discharge or irritation, and irregular periods. Any unusual bleeding should be reported to the doctor. Serious side effects of tamoxifen are rare, but the drug can cause blood clots in the veins, especially the legs. In a very small number of women, tamoxifen has caused cancer of the lining of the uterus. The doctor may do biopsies or other tests of the uterus lining to monitor for this condition.

Young women whose ovaries are removed to deprive the cancer cells of estrogen experience menopause immediately. The side effects they have—including hot flashes and vaginal dryness—are likely to be more severe than those of natural menopause.

To help withstand the side effects of treatment, it is important that patients maintain good nutrition (see Nutrition for Cancer Patients, page 19).

After Treatment

Rehabilitation is a very important part of breast cancer treatment. The health-care team makes every effort to help women return to their normal activities as soon as possible. Recovery will be different for each woman, depending on the extent of the disease, the treatment she had, and other factors.

Exercising after surgery can help a woman regain motion and strength in her arm and shoulder. It can also reduce pain and stiffness in her neck and back. Carefully planned exercises should be started as soon as the doctor says the woman is ready, often within a day or so after surgery. Exercising begins slowly and gently and can even be done in bed.

Gradually, exercising can be more active, and regular exercise should become part of a woman's normal routine. Women who have a mastectomy and immediate breast reconstruction (plastic surgery to rebuild a breast)

need special exercises, which the doctor or nurse can explain and demonstrate.

Often lymphedema after surgery can be reduced or prevented with certain exercises and by resting with the arm propped up on a pillow. If lymphedema occurs later on, the doctor may suggest exercises and other ways to deal with this problem, such as wearing an elastic sleeve or using an elastic cuff to improve lymph circulation.

After a mastectomy, some women decide to wear a breast form (prosthesis). Others prefer to have breast reconstruction either at the same time as the mastectomy or later on. Each has its pros and cons, and what is right for one woman may not be right for another.

What is important is that nearly every woman treated for breast cancer has choices. It may be helpful to talk with a plastic surgeon before the mastectomy, but reconstruction is still possible later on.

Various procedures are used to reconstruct the breast. Some use implants; others use tissue moved from another part of the woman's body. The woman should ask the plastic surgeon to explain the risks and benefits of each type of reconstruction. The Cancer Information Service (1-800-4-CANCER) can suggest sources of printed information about breast reconstruction and can tell callers about breast cancer support groups. Members of such groups are often willing to share their personal experiences about breast reconstruction.

FOLLOW-UP CARE

Regular follow-up exams are very important after breast cancer treatment. The doctor will continue to check closely to be sure that the cancer has not returned. Regular checkups usually include exams of the chest, underarm, and neck. Occasionally, the woman has a complete physical exam and a mammogram.

A woman who has had cancer in one breast has a slightly higher-than-average risk of developing cancer in her other breast. She should report any changes to her doctor right away.

Also, a woman who has had breast cancer should tell her doctor about other physical problems if they come up, such as pain, loss of appetite or weight, changes in menstrual periods, unusual vaginal bleeding, or blurred vision. She should also report dizziness, headaches, backaches, coughing or hoarseness, or digestive problems that seem unusual or that don't go away. These symptoms may be a sign that the cancer has returned, but they can also be signs of many other problems. Only the doctor can tell for sure.

LIVING WITH CANCER

The diagnosis of breast cancer can change a woman's life and the lives of those close to her. These changes can be hard to handle. It's common for the woman and her family and friends to have many different and sometimes confusing emotions.

At times, patients and their loved ones may be frightened, angry, or depressed. These are normal reactions when people face a serious health problem. Many people find it helps to share their thoughts and feelings with loved ones. Sharing can help everyone feel more at ease and can open the way for others to show their concern and offer their support.

Sometimes women who have had breast cancer may be concerned that breast cancer and its treatment will affect their sexual relationships. Many couples find that talking about these concerns helps them find ways to express their love during and after treatment. Some seek counseling or a couples' support group.

Finding the strength to deal with the changes brought about by breast cancer can be easier for patients and those who love them when they have appropriate support services.

Information about programs and services for breast cancer patients and their families is available through the Cancer Information Service. (See page 20 for more on Support for Cancer Patients.)

WHAT THE FUTURE HOLDS

Researchers are always looking for better ways to detect and treat breast cancer, and the chances of recovery keep improving. Still, it is natural for patients to be concerned about their future.

Sometimes patients use statistics they have heard to try to figure out their own chances of being cured. It is important to remember, however, that statistics are averages based on large numbers of patients. They can't be used to predict what will happen to a particular woman because no two cancer patients are alike. The doctor who takes care of the patient and knows her medical history is in the best position to talk with her about the chance of recovery (prognosis).

Women should feel free to ask the doctor about their prognosis, but they should keep in mind that not even the doctor knows exactly what will happen. Doctors often talk about surviving cancer, or they may use the term "remission." Doctors use these terms because, although many breast cancer patients will be cured, the disease can recur.

THE PROMISE OF CANCER RESEARCH

Doctors and researchers at hospitals and medical centers all across the country are studying breast cancer. They are trying to learn more about what causes this disease and how to prevent it. They are also looking for better ways to diagnose and treat it.

Causes and Prevention

Doctors can seldom explain why one person gets this disease and another doesn't. It is clear, however, that breast cancer is not caused by bumping, bruising, or touching the breast. And this disease is not contagious; no one can "catch" breast cancer from another person.

By studying large numbers of women all over the world, researchers have found certain risk factors that increase a woman's chance of developing breast cancer. There may be other risk factors we do not know about. Having these risk factors means having a higher-than-average chance of getting this disease. However, studies also show that most women with known risk factors do not get breast cancer. And many women who get breast cancer have none of the risk factors we know about, other than the risk that comes with growing older. The following are some of the known risk factors for this disease:

- *Age*. The risk of breast cancer increases as a woman gets older. Most breast cancers occur in women over the age of 50; the risk is especially high for women over 60. This disease is uncommon in women under the age of 35.
- *Family history*. The risk of getting breast cancer increases for a woman whose mother, sister, or daughter has had the disease. The woman's risk increases more if her relative's cancer developed before menopause or if it affected both breasts.
- *Personal history*. Women who have had breast cancer face an increased risk of getting breast cancer again. As many as 10 to 15 percent of women treated for breast cancer or DCIS get a second breast cancer later on. The risk is also greater for women who have had LCIS.

Other risk factors for breast cancer include starting to menstruate at an early age (before 12) or having a late menopause (after 55). The risk is also greater in women who had their first child after the age of 30 and those who never had children. These factors are all related to a woman's natural hormones. At this time, no one knows whether the risk of breast cancer is affected by taking medicines that contain hormones (for birth control, to treat infertility, or as estrogen replacement therapy to control symptoms of menopause), especially if women take them for many years. At this time, no one knows for sure whether taking hormones affects the risk of breast cancer. Scientists hope to find the answer to this important question by studying a large number of women taking part in hormone-related research.

Some studies suggest a slightly higher risk of breast cancer among women who drink alcohol. The risk appears to go up with the amount of alcohol consumed, so women who drink should do so only in moderation.

Many women are concerned about benign breast conditions. For most women, the ordinary "lumpiness" they feel in their breasts does not increase their risk of breast cancer. However, women who have had breast biopsies that show certain benign changes in breast tissues, such as atypical hyperplasia, do have an increased risk of breast cancer.

Some scientists believe that choosing a low-fat diet, eating plenty of fruits and vegetables, and maintaining an ideal body weight may lower a woman's risk. Recent studies suggest that regular exercise may decrease risk in younger women.

Detection

At present, regular mammography is the most effective tool to detect breast cancer. However, mammography is not always accurate. (A woman who feels something is wrong with her breasts should not assume a normal mammogram rules out a problem. She should discuss her concerns with her doctor.) Mammography cannot reveal every breast cancer at an early stage, and it sometimes arouses suspicion when no cancer is present. Researchers are looking for ways to make mammography more accurate. They are also exploring other techniques to produce detailed pictures of the tissues in the breast.

In addition, researchers are studying tumor markers, substances that may be present in abnormal amounts in the blood or urine of a woman with breast cancer. Some markers are used to follow women who have already been diagnosed with breast cancer. At this time, however, no blood or urine test is reliable enough to reveal early breast cancer.

Treatment

Researchers also are looking for more effective ways to treat breast cancer. In addition, they are exploring ways to reduce the side effects of treatment and improve the quality of patients' lives. When laboratory research shows that a new treatment method has promise, cancer patients receive the treatment in clinical trials. These trials are designed to answer scientific questions and to find out whether the new approach is both safe and effective. Often clinical trials compare a new treatment with a standard approach. Patients who take part in clinical trials make an important contribution to medical science and may have the first chance to benefit from improved treatment methods. (See page 20 for more information on participating in clinical trials.)

Trials to study new treatments for patients with all stages of breast cancer are under way. Researchers are testing new treatment methods, new chemotherapy doses and treatment schedules, and new ways of combining treatments. They are working with various anticancer drugs and drug combinations as well as types of hormonal therapy. They are also exploring new ways to combine chemotherapy with hormonal therapy and radiation therapy. Some trials include biological therapy, treatment with substances that boost the immune system's response to cancer or help the body recover from treatment side effects.

In a number of trials, doctors are trying to learn whether very high doses of anticancer drugs are more effective than the usual doses in destroying breast cancer cells. Because these higher doses seriously damage the patient's bone marrow, where blood cells are formed, researchers are developing and testing ways to replace the bone marrow or to help it recover.

The National Cancer Institute

CERVICAL CANCER

The cervix is the lower, narrow part of the uterus (womb). The uterus, a hollow, pear-shaped organ, is located in a woman's lower abdomen, between the bladder and the rectum. The cervix forms a canal that opens into the vagina, which leads to the outside of the body.

Cancer of the cervix also may be called cervical cancer. Like most cancers, it is named for the part of the body in which it begins. Cancers of the cervix also are named for the type of cell in which they begin. Most cervical cancers are squamous cell carcinomas. Squamous cells are thin, flat cells that form the surface of the cervix.

PRECANCEROUS CONDITIONS AND CANCER OF THE CERVIX

Cells on the surface of the cervix sometimes appear abnormal but not cancerous. Scientists believe that some abnormal changes in cells on the cervix are the first step in a series of slow changes that can lead to cancer years later. That is, some abnormal changes are precancerous; they may become cancerous with time.

Over the years, doctors have used different terms to refer to abnormal changes in the cells on the surface of the cervix. One term now used is squamous intraepithelial lesion (SIL). (The word "lesion" refers to an area of abnormal tissue; "intraepithelial" means that the abnormal cells are present only in the sur-

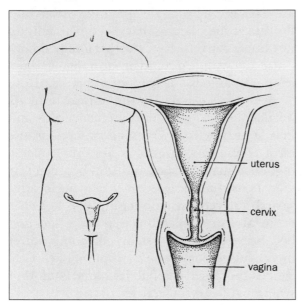

The cervix, at the end of the vaginal canal, marks the opening to the uterus. Cervical cancer is the most common cancer of the female reproductive system.

face layer of cells.) Changes in these cells can be divided into two categories:

- *Low-grade SIL* refers to early changes in the size, shape, and number of cells that form the surface of the cervix. Some low-grade lesions go away on their own. However, with time, others may grow larger or become more abnormal, forming a high-grade lesion. Precancerous low-grade lesions also may be called mild dysplasia or cervical intraepithelial neoplasia 1 (CIN 1). Such early changes in the cervix most often occur in women between ages 25 and 35 but can appear in women of other ages as well.
- *High-grade SIL* means there are a large number of precancerous cells; they look very different from normal cells. Like low-grade SIL, these precancerous changes involve only cells on the surface of the cervix. The cells will not become cancerous and invade deeper layers of the cervix for many months, perhaps years. High-grade lesions also may be called moderate or severe dysplasia, CIN 2 or 3, or carcinoma in situ.

They develop most often in women between the ages of 30 and 40 but can occur at other ages as well.

If abnormal cells spread deeper into the cervix or to other tissues or organs, the disease is then called cervical cancer, or invasive cervical cancer. It occurs most often in women over the age of 40.

EARLY DETECTION

If all women had regular pelvic exams and Pap tests (also called Pap smears), most precancerous conditions would be detected and treated before cancer develops. That way, most invasive cancers could be prevented. Any invasive cancer that does occur would likely be found at an early, curable stage.

In a pelvic exam, the doctor checks the uterus, vagina, ovaries, fallopian tubes, bladder, and rectum. The doctor feels these organs for any abnormality in their shape or size. A speculum is used to widen the vagina so that the doctor can see the upper part of the vagina and the cervix.

The Pap test is a simple, painless test to detect abnormal cells in and around the cervix. A woman should have this test when she is not

ATYPICAL PAP SMEARS

Occasionally, abnormal cells known as atypical squamous cells of undetermined significance (ASCUS) are found on a Pap test (or Pap smear). The proper management of such findings should include:
- Biopsy of any suspicious lesion
- Treatment of specific infections
- A repeat test in at least three to six months
- Colposcopy and biopsy if either: a) two or more such reports are positive for ASCUS; or b) any high risk factors are present, including HPV (human papilloma virus) infection, HIV (human immunodeficiency virus) infection, smoking, or multiple sexual partners

The Editors

menstruating; the best time is between 10 and 20 days after the first day of her menstrual period. For about two days before a Pap test, she should avoid douching or using spermicidal foams, creams, or jellies or vaginal medicines (except as directed by a physician), which may wash away or hide any abnormal cells.

A Pap test can be done in a doctor's office or a health clinic. A wooden scraper (spatula) and/or a small brush is used to collect a sample of cells from the cervix and upper vagina. The cells are placed on a glass slide and sent to a medical laboratory to be checked for abnormal changes.

The current method of describing Pap test results is called the Bethesda System. Changes are described as low-grade or high-grade SIL. Many doctors believe that the Bethesda System provides more useful information than an older system, which uses numbers ranging from class 1 to class 5. (In class 1, the cells in the sample are considered normal; class 5 refers to invasive cancer.) Women should ask their doctor to explain the system used for their Pap test.

Women should have regular checkups, including a pelvic exam and a Pap test, if they are or have been sexually active or if they are age 18 or older. Those who are at increased risk of developing cancer of the cervix should be especially careful to follow their doctor's advice about checkups.

A pelvic exam and Pap test should be performed annually for women at increased risk of developing cervical cancer. Older women, particularly those who haven't had a pelvic exam in several years, should continue to be screened because 25 percent of cervical cancer cases occur in women over age 65.

Women who have had a hysterectomy (surgery to remove the uterus, including the cervix) should ask their doctor's advice about having pelvic exams and Pap tests.

SYMPTOMS

Precancerous changes of the cervix usually do not cause pain. In fact, they generally do not cause any symptoms and are not detected unless a woman has a pelvic exam and a Pap test.

Symptoms usually do not appear until abnormal cervical cells become cancerous and invade nearby tissue. When this happens, the most common symptom is abnormal bleeding. Bleeding may start and stop between regular menstrual periods, or it may occur after sexual intercourse, douching, or a pelvic exam. Menstrual bleeding may last longer and be heavier than usual. Bleeding after menopause also may be a symptom of cervical cancer. Increased vaginal discharge is another symptom of cervical cancer.

These symptoms may be caused by cancer or by other health problems. Only a doctor can tell for sure. It is important for a woman to see her doctor if she has any symptoms.

DIAGNOSIS

The pelvic exam and Pap test allow the doctor to detect abnormal changes in the cervix. If these exams show an infection is present, the doctor treats the infection and then repeats the Pap test at a later time. If the exam or Pap test suggests something other than an infection, the doctor may repeat the Pap test and do other tests to find out what the problem is.

Colposcopy is a widely used method to check the cervix for abnormal areas. The doctor applies a vinegar-like solution to the cervix and then uses an instrument much like a microscope (called a colposcope) to look closely at the cervix.

The doctor may remove a small amount of cervical tissue for examination by a pathologist. This procedure is called a biopsy. In one type of biopsy, the doctor uses an instrument to pinch off small pieces of cervical tissue. Another method used to do a biopsy is called loop electrosurgical excision procedure (LEEP). In this procedure, the doctor uses an electric wire loop to slice off a thin, round piece of tissue. These types of biopsies may be done in the doctor's office using local anesthesia.

The doctor also may want to check inside the opening of the cervix, an area that cannot be seen during colposcopy. In a procedure called endocervical curettage (ECC), the doctor uses a curette (a small, spoon-shaped instrument) to scrape tissue from inside the cervical opening.

These procedures for removing tissue may cause some bleeding or other discharge. However, healing usually occurs quickly. Women also often experience some pain similar to menstrual cramping, which can be relieved with medicine.

These tests may not show for sure whether the abnormal cells are present only on the surface of the cervix. In that case, the doctor will then remove a larger, cone-shaped sample of tissue. This procedure, called conization or cone biopsy, allows the pathologist to see whether the abnormal cells have invaded tissue beneath the surface of the cervix. Conization also may be used as treatment for a precancerous lesion if the entire abnormal area can be removed. The procedure requires either local or general anesthesia and may be done in the doctor's office or in the hospital.

In a few cases, it may not be clear whether an abnormal Pap test or a woman's symptoms are caused by problems in the cervix or in the endometrium (the lining of the uterus). In this situation, the doctor may do dilatation and curettage (D&C). The doctor stretches the cervical opening and uses a curette to scrape tissue from the lining of the uterus as well as from the cervical canal. Like conization, this procedure requires local or general anesthesia and may be done in the doctor's office or in the hospital.

TREATING PRECANCEROUS CONDITIONS
Treatment for a precancerous lesion of the cervix depends on a number of factors. These factors include whether the lesion is low or high grade, whether the woman wants to have children in the future, the woman's age and general health, and the preference of the woman and her doctor. A woman with a low-grade lesion may not need further treatment, especially if the abnormal area was completely removed during biopsy, but she should have a Pap test and pelvic exam regularly. When a precancerous lesion requires treatment, the doctor may use cryosurgery (freezing), cauterization (burning, also called diathermy), or laser surgery to destroy the abnormal area without harming nearby healthy tissue. The doctor also can remove the abnormal tissue by LEEP or conization. Treatment for precancerous lesions may cause cramping or other pain, bleeding, or a watery discharge.

In some cases, a woman may have a hysterectomy, particularly if abnormal cells are found inside the cervix opening. This surgery is more likely to be done when the woman does not want to have children in the future.

TREATING CANCER OF THE CERVIX
The choice of treatment for cervical cancer depends on the location and size of the tumor, the state (extent) of the disease, the woman's age and general health, and other factors.

Staging
Staging is a careful attempt to find out whether the cancer has spread and, if so, what parts of the body are affected. Blood and urine tests usually are done. The doctor also may do a thorough pelvic exam in the operating room with the patient under anesthesia. During this exam, the doctor may do procedures called cystoscopy and proctosigmoidoscopy. In cystoscopy, the doctor looks inside the bladder with a thin, lighted instrument. Proctosigmoidoscopy is a procedure in which a lighted instrument is used to check the rectum and the lower part of the large intestine.

Because cervical cancer may spread to the bladder, rectum, lymph nodes, or lungs, the doctor also may order x-rays or tests to check those areas. For example, the woman may have a series of x-rays of the kidneys and bladder, called an intravenous pyelogram. The doctor also may check the intestines and rectum using a barium enema.

To look for lymph nodes that may be enlarged because they contain cancer cells, the doctor may order a CT scan, a series of x-rays put together by a computer to make detailed pictures of areas inside the body. Other procedures that may be used to check organs inside the body are ultrasonography and MRI.

Methods of Treatment

Most often, treatment for cervical cancer involves surgery and radiation therapy. Sometimes chemotherapy or biological therapy is used. Patients are often treated by a team of specialists. (See page 17 for more information about getting a second opinion and planning treatment.) The team may include gynecologic oncologists and radiation oncologists. The doctors may decide to use one treatment method or a combination of methods. Some patients take part in a clinical trial (research study) using new treatment methods. More information about clinical trials appears on page 20.

Surgery is local therapy to remove abnormal tissue in or near the cervix. If the disease has invaded deeper layers of the cervix but has not spread beyond the cervix, the doctor may perform an operation to remove the tumor but leave the uterus and the ovaries. In other cases, however, a woman may need to have a hysterectomy or may choose to have this surgery, especially if she is not planning to have children in the future. In this procedure, the doctor removes the entire uterus, including the cervix; sometimes the ovaries and fallopian tubes also are removed. In addition,

the doctor may remove lymph nodes near the uterus to learn whether the cancer has spread to these organs.

Radiation therapy (also called radiotherapy) uses high-energy rays to damage cancer cells and stop them from growing. Like surgery, radiation therapy is local therapy; the radiation can affect cancer cells only in the treated area. The radiation may come from a large machine (external radiation) or from radioactive materials placed directly into the cervix (implant radiation). Some patients receive both types of radiation therapy.

A woman receiving external radiation therapy goes to the hospital or clinic each day for treatment. Usually treatments are given five days a week for five to six weeks. At the end of that time, the tumor site very often gets an extra "boost" of radiation.

For internal or implant radiation, a capsule containing radioactive material is placed directly in the cervix. The implant puts cancer-killing rays close to the tumor while sparing most of the healthy tissue around it. It is usually left in place for one to three days, and the treatment may be repeated several times over the course of one to two weeks. The patient stays in the hospital while the implants are in place.

In certain cases, chemotherapy may be given along with radiation therapy to increase the effectiveness of radiotherapy.

Chemotherapy is the use of drugs to kill cancer cells. It is most often used when cervical cancer has spread to other parts of the body. The doctor may use just one drug or a combination of drugs.

Anticancer drugs used to treat cervical cancer may be given by injection into a vein or by mouth. Either way,

chemotherapy is systemic treatment, meaning that the drugs flow through the body in the bloodstream.

Chemotherapy is given in cycles: a treatment period followed by a recovery period, then another treatment period, and so on. Most patients have chemotherapy as an outpatient (at the hospital, at the doctor's office, or at home). Depending on which drugs are given and the woman's general health, however, she may need to stay in the hospital during her treatment.

Biological therapy is treatment using substances to improve the way the body's immune system fights disease. It may be used to treat cancer that has spread from the cervix to other parts of the body. Interferon is the most common form of biological therapy for this disease; it may be used in combination with chemotherapy. Most patients who receive interferon are treated as outpatients.

SIDE EFFECTS OF TREATMENT
It is hard to limit the effects of therapy so that only cancer cells are removed or destroyed. Because treatment also damages healthy cells and tissues, it often causes unpleasant side effects.

The side effects of cancer treatment depend mainly on the type and extent of the treatment. Also, each patient reacts differently. Doctors and nurses can explain the possible side effects of treatment, and they can help relieve symptoms that may occur during and after treatment. It is important to let the doctor know if any side effects occur.

Surgery
Methods for removing small cancers on the cervix are similar to those used to treat precancerous lesions. Treatment may cause cramping or other pain, bleeding, or a watery discharge.

Hysterectomy is major surgery. For a few days after the operation, the woman may have pain in her lower abdomen. The doctor can order medicine to control the pain. A woman may have difficulty emptying her bladder and may need to have a catheter inserted into the bladder to drain the urine for a few days after surgery. She also may have trouble having normal bowel movements. For a period of time after the surgery, the woman's activities should be limited to allow healing to take place. Normal activities, including sexual intercourse, usually can be resumed in four to eight weeks.

Women who have had their uterus removed no longer have menstrual periods. However, sexual desire and the ability to have intercourse usually are not affected by hysterectomy. On the other hand, many women have an emotionally difficult time after this surgery. A woman's view of her own sexuality may change, and she may feel an emotional loss because she is no longer able to have children. An understanding partner is important at this time. Women may want to discuss these issues with their doctor, nurse, medical social worker, or member of the clergy.

Radiation Therapy
Patients are likely to become very tired during radiation therapy, especially in the later weeks of treatment. Resting is important, but doctors usually advise patients to try to stay as active as they can. With external radiation, it is common to lose hair in the treated area and for the skin to become red, dry, tender, and itchy. There may be permanent darkening or "bronzing" of the skin in the treated area. This area should be exposed to the air when possible but protected from the sun, and patients should avoid wearing clothes that rub the treated area. Patients will be shown how to keep the area clean. They should not use any lotion or cream on their skin without the doctor's advice.

Usually, women are told not to have intercourse during radiation therapy or while an implant is in place. However, most women can have sexual relations within a few weeks after treatment ends. Sometimes after radiation treatment, the vagina becomes narrower and less flexible, and intercourse may be painful. Patients may be taught how to use a dilator as well as a water-based lubricant to help minimize these problems.

Patients who receive external or internal radiation therapy also may have diarrhea and frequent, uncomfortable urination. The doctor can make suggestions or order medicines to control these problems.

Chemotherapy

The side effects of chemotherapy depend mainly on the drugs and the doses the patient receives. In addition, as with other types of treatment, side effects vary from person to person. Generally, anticancer drugs affect cells that divide rapidly. These include blood cells, which fight infection, help the blood to clot, or carry oxygen to all parts of the body. When blood cells are affected by anticancer drugs, patients are more likely to get infections, may bruise or bleed easily, and may have less energy. Cells in hair roots and cells that line the digestive tract also divide rapidly. When chemotherapy affects these cells, patients may lose their hair and may have other side effects, such as poor appetite, nausea, vomiting, or mouth sores. The doctor may be able to give medicine to help with side effects. Side effects gradually go away during the recovery periods between treatments or after treatment is over.

Biological Therapy

The side effects caused by biological therapies vary with the type of treatment the patient receives. These treatments may cause flu-like symptoms such as chills, fever, muscle aches, weakness, loss of appetite, nausea, vomiting, and diarrhea. Sometimes patients get a rash, and they may bleed or bruise easily. These problems can be severe, but they gradually go away after the treatment stops.

To help withstand the side effects of treatment, it is important that patients maintain good nutrition (see Nutrition for Cancer Patients, page 19).

FOLLOW-UP CARE

Regular follow-up exams—including a pelvic exam, a Pap test, and other laboratory tests—are very important for any woman who has been treated for precancerous changes or for cancer of the cervix. The doctor will do these tests and exams frequently for several years to check for any sign that the condition has returned.

Cancer treatment may cause side effects many years later. For this reason, patients should continue to have regular checkups and should report any health problems that appear.

WHAT THE FUTURE HOLDS

The outlook for women with precancerous changes of the cervix or very early cancer of the cervix is excellent; nearly all patients with these conditions can be cured. Researchers continue to look for new and better ways to treat invasive cervical cancer.

Patients and their families are naturally concerned about what the future holds. Sometimes patients use statistics to try to figure out their chances of being cured. It is important to remember, however, that statistics are averages based on large numbers of patients. They cannot be used to predict what will happen to a particular woman because no two patients are alike; treatments and responses vary greatly. The doctor who takes care of the patient and knows her medical history is in the best position to talk with her about her chance of recovery (prognosis).

Doctors often talk about surviving cancer, or they may use the term "remission" rather than "cure." Although many women with cervical cancer recover completely, doctors use these terms because the disease can recur. (The return of cancer is called a recurrence.)

CAUSE AND PREVENTION

By studying large numbers of women all over the world, researchers have identified certain risk factors that increase the chance that cells in the cervix will become abnormal or cancerous. They believe that, in many cases, cervical cancer develops when two or more risk factors act together.

Research has shown that women who began having sexual intercourse before age 18 and women who have had many sexual partners have an increased risk of developing cervical cancer. Women also are at increased risk if their partners began having sexual intercourse at a young age, have had many sexual partners, or were previously married to women who had cervical cancer.

Scientists do not know exactly why the sexual practices of women and their partners affect the risk of developing cervical cancer. However, research suggests that some sexually transmitted viruses can cause cells in the cervix to begin the series of changes that can lead to cancer. Women who have had many sexual partners or whose partners have had many sexual partners may have an increased risk for cervical cancer at least in part because they are more likely to get a sexually transmitted virus.

Scientists are studying the effects of sexually transmitted human papilloma viruses (HPVs). Some sexually transmitted HPVs cause genital warts (condylomata acuminata). In addition, scientists believe that some of these viruses may cause the growth of abnormal cells in the cervix and may play a role in cancer development. They have found that women who have HPV or whose partners have HPV have a higher-than-average risk of developing cervical cancer. However, most women who are infected with HPV do not develop cervical cancer, and the virus is not present in all women who

have this disease. For these reasons, scientists believe that other factors act together with HPVs. Further research is needed to learn the exact role of these viruses and how they act together with other factors in the development of cervical cancer.

There are many varieties of the human papilloma virus (HPV). Certain strains, such as HPV-16 and HPV-18, are more highly associated with the eventual development of cervical cancer than others. Testing for the specific type of HPV involved may ultimately help in determining which women are at greater risk.

Smoking also increases the risk of cancer of the cervix, although it is not clear exactly how or why. The risk appears to increase with the number of cigarettes a woman smokes each day and with the number of years she has smoked.

Women whose mothers were given the drug diethylstilbestrol (DES) during pregnancy to prevent miscarriage also are at increased risk. (This drug was used for this purpose from about 1940 to 1970.) A rare type of vaginal and cervical cancer has been found in a small number of women whose mothers used DES.

Several reports suggest that women whose immune system is weakened are more likely than others to develop cervical cancer. For example, women who have the human immunodeficiency virus (HIV), which causes AIDS, are at increased risk. Also, organ transplant patients, who receive drugs that suppress the immune system to prevent rejection of the new organ, are more likely than others to develop precancerous lesions.

Some researchers believe that there is an increased risk of cervical cancer in women who use oral contraceptives (the pill). However, scientists have not found that the pill directly causes cancer of the cervix. This relationship is hard to prove because the two main risk factors for cervical cancer—intercourse at an early age and multiple sex partners—may be more common among women who use the pill than among those who do not. Still, oral contraceptive labels warn of this possible risk and advise women who use them to have yearly Pap tests.

Some research has shown that vitamin A may play a role in stopping or preventing cancerous changes in cells like those on the surface of the cervix. Further research with forms of vitamin A may help scientists learn more about preventing cancer of the cervix.

At present, early detection and treatment of precancerous tissue remain the most effective ways of preventing cervical cancer. Women should talk with their doctor about an appropriate schedule of checkups. The doctor's advice will be based on such factors as the women's age, medical history, and risk factors.

The National Cancer Institute

COLORECTAL CANCER

The colon and rectum are part of the digestive system. Together, they form a long, muscular tube called the large intestine (also called the large bowel). The colon is the upper five to six feet of the large intestine, and the rectum is the last six to eight inches.

After food is digested in the stomach and small intestine, it moves into the colon, where any remaining water is absorbed into the body, leaving solid waste (called stool). Stool moves through the colon and rectum and leaves the body through the anus.

EARLY DETECTION

Most health problems respond best to treatment when they are diagnosed and treated as early as possible. This is especially true for colorectal cancer. Treatment is most effective before the disease spreads. People can take an active role in the early detection of col-

orectal cancer by adhering to the following guidelines:

- During regular checkups, have a digital rectal exam. For this exam, the doctor inserts a lubricated, gloved finger into the rectum and feels for abnormal areas.
- Beginning at age 50, have an annual fecal occult blood test. This test is a check for hidden (occult) blood in the stool. A small amount of stool is placed on a plastic slide or on special paper. The stool may be tested in the doctor's office or sent to a lab. The test is done because colorectal cancer may cause bleeding that cannot be seen. However, other conditions also may cause bleeding, so having blood in the stool does not necessarily mean a person has cancer.
- Beginning at age 50, have sigmoidoscopy every three to five years. The doctor looks through a thin, lighted tube to check for polyps, tumors, or other abnormalities in the rectum and lower colon.

People who may be at a greater than average risk for colon cancer (see Cause and Prevention, page 51) should discuss a schedule for these or other tests with their doctor.

SYMPTOMS

Colorectal cancer can cause many symptoms. Warning signs to watch for include:

- A change in bowel habits
- Diarrhea or constipation
- Blood in or on the stool (either bright red or very dark in color)
- Stools that are narrower than usual
- General stomach discomfort (bloating, fullness, and/or cramps)
- Frequent gas pains
- A feeling that the bowel does not empty completely
- Weight loss with no known reason
- Constant tiredness

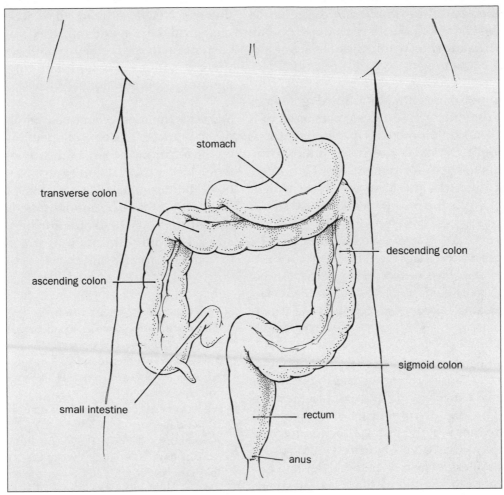

About 75 percent of all colorectal cancers and polyps occur in the rectum or in the sigmoid portion of the colon—the segments easiest to examine and treat.

These symptoms also can be caused by other problems—such as ulcers, an inflamed colon, or hemorrhoids. Only a doctor can determine the cause. People who have any of these symptoms should see their doctor. The doctor may refer them to a doctor who specializes in diagnosing and treating digestive problems (a gastroenterologist).

DIAGNOSIS

To find the cause of symptoms, the doctor asks about the patient's personal and family medical history, does a physical exam, and may order laboratory tests. In addition to the exams described previously, the doctor may also order the following tests:

• *Lower GI series.* In this procedure, x-rays of the colon and rectum (the lower gastrointestinal tract) are taken after the patient is given an enema with a white, chalky solution containing barium. (This test is sometimes called a barium enema.) The barium outlines the colon and rectum on the x-rays, helping the doctor find tumors or other abnormal areas. To make small tumors easier to see, the doctor may expand the colon by carefully pumping in air during the test.

47

• *Colonoscopy*. An examination of the inside of the entire colon using a colonoscope, an instrument similar to a flexible sigmoidoscope, but longer.

If a polyp or other abnormal growth is found, the doctor can remove part or all of it through a sigmoidoscope or colonoscope. A pathologist examines the tissue under a microscope to check for cancer cells. This procedure is called a biopsy. Most polyps are benign, but a biopsy is the only way to know for sure.

If the pathologist finds cancer, the patient's doctor needs to learn the stage, or extent, of the disease. Staging exams and tests help the doctor find out whether the cancer has spread and, if so, what parts of the body are affected. Treatment decisions depend on these findings.

Staging may include x-rays, ultrasonography, or CT scans of the lungs and liver because colorectal cancer tends to spread to these organs. The doctor may order blood tests to measure how well the liver is functioning. The doctor also may do a blood test called a CEA assay. This test measures the blood level of carcinoembryonic antigen (CEA), a substance that is sometimes found in higher than normal amounts in people who have colorectal cancer, especially when the disease has spread.

TREATMENT

The doctor develops a treatment plan to fit each patient's needs. Treatment for colorectal cancer depends on the size and location of the tumor, the stage of the disease, the patient's general health, and other factors. (See page 17 for more information about getting a second opinion and planning treatment.)

Methods of Treatment

Colorectal cancer is generally treated with surgery, chemotherapy, and/or radiation therapy. New treatment approaches such as biological therapy and improved ways of using current methods are being studied in clinical trials. A patient may have one form of treatment or a combination.

Surgery is the most common treatment for colorectal cancer. The type of operation depends on the location and size of the tumor. Most patients have a partial colectomy. In this operation, the surgeon takes out the part of the colon or rectum that contains the cancer and a small amount of surrounding healthy tissue. Surgery is often the only treatment needed for early colorectal cancer.

IMPORTANT QUESTIONS

These are some questions a patient may want to ask the doctor before surgery:
• What kind of operation will it be?
• How will I feel afterward? If I have pain, how will you help me?
• Will I need a colostomy? Will it be temporary or permanent?
• How long will I be in the hospital?
• Will I have to be on a special diet? Who will teach me about my diet?
• When can I return to my normal activities?
• Will I need additional treatment?

Usually, lymph nodes near the tumor are removed during surgery to help the doctor be more accurate about the stage of the cancer. A pathologist examines the lymph nodes under a microscope to see whether they contain cancer cells. If the cancer has reached these nodes, the disease may also have spread to other parts of the body, and the patient may need further treatment.

In most cases, the surgeon reconnects the healthy sections of the colon or rectum. This part of the surgery is called anastomosis. If the healthy sections of the colon or rectum cannot be reconnected, the doctor performs a colostomy, creating an opening (stoma) in the abdomen through which solid waste leaves the body. The patient uses a special bag to cover the stoma and collect waste. A colostomy may be temporary or permanent.

- A temporary colostomy is sometimes needed to allow the lower colon or the rectum to heal after surgery. Later, in a second operation, the surgeon reconnects the healthy sections of the colon or rectum and closes the colostomy. The patient's bowel functions soon return to normal.
- A permanent colostomy may be necessary when the tumor is in the rectum. A few patients who have cancer in the lower colon may also require a permanent colostomy. Overall, however, only about 15 percent of patients with colorectal cancer need a permanent colostomy.

Although it may take some time to adjust to a colostomy, most patients return to their normal lifestyle. A nurse or an enterostomal therapist teaches the patient how to care for a colostomy and suggests ways to continue with normal activities. Support groups, such as those offered through the United Ostomy Association, may also be helpful.

Chemotherapy is the use of drugs to kill cancer cells. Chemotherapy is sometimes given after surgery for colorectal cancer to try to prevent the disease from spreading. This additional treatment is called adjuvant therapy. Chemotherapy also may be given to relieve symptoms of the disease in patients whose primary tumor cannot be completely removed or to control the growth of new tumors. The doctor may use one drug or a combination of drugs.

Chemotherapy is usually given in cycles: a treatment period followed by a recovery period, then another treatment period, and so on. Anticancer drugs may be taken by mouth or given by injection into a blood vessel or body cavity. Chemotherapy is a systemic therapy,

meaning that the drugs enter the bloodstream and travel through the body.

In clinical trials, researchers are studying ways of putting chemotherapy drugs directly into the area to be treated. (For more information on clinical trials and how to participate in one, see page 20.) For colorectal cancer that has spread to the liver, drugs can be injected into a blood vessel that leads directly to the liver. This treatment is called intrahepatic chemotherapy. Researchers are also investigating a method called intraperitoneal chemotherapy in which the doctor puts anticancer drugs directly into the abdomen through a thin tube.

Usually a person has chemotherapy as an outpatient at the hospital, at the doctor's office, or at home. However, depending on which drugs are given, how they are given, and the patient's general health, a short hospital stay may be necessary.

Radiation therapy (also called radiotherapy) is the use of high-energy rays to damage cancer cells and stop them from growing. Like surgery, radiation therapy is local therapy; it can affect cancer only in the treated area. Radiation therapy is sometimes used before surgery to shrink a tumor so that it is easier to remove. More often, radiation therapy is given after surgery to destroy any cancer cells that may remain in the area. It may also be given to relieve pain or other problems in patients whose tumors cannot be surgically removed. Radiation therapy is usually given on an outpatient basis in a hospital or clinic five days a week for several weeks.

Researchers are conducting clinical trials to look for more effective ways of using radiation therapy. For example, some are studying the benefits of using radiation both before and after surgery ("sandwich" technique), and others are giving radiation during surgery (intraoperative radiation). Doctors are also exploring the use of radiation therapy alone (instead of surgery) for rectal cancer that has not spread.

Biological therapy is a cancer treatment that helps the body's immune (defense) system attack and destroy cancer cells. For some patients, biological therapy may be combined with chemotherapy as adjuvant treatment after surgery. New types of biological therapy are being used to treat patients in clinical trials. Patients may need to stay in the hospital while receiving some types of biological therapy.

SIDE EFFECTS OF TREATMENT

It is often hard to limit the effects of therapy so that only cancer cells are removed or destroyed. Because healthy tissue also may be damaged, treatment can cause unpleasant side effects.

The side effects of cancer treatment are different for each person, and they may even be different from one treatment to the next. Doctors try to plan treatment in ways that keep side effects to a minimum, and they can help with any problems that occur. For this reason, it is very important to let the doctor know about any health problems during or after treatment.

Surgery

Surgery for colorectal cancer (including colostomy) may cause temporary constipation or diarrhea. The doctor can prescribe medicine or suggest a diet to help relieve these problems.

Patients who have pain after surgery should tell their doctor so that medicine can be given to relieve their discomfort. For a period of time after the surgery, the person's activity will be limited to allow for healing.

Colostomy patients may have irritation on the skin around the stoma. The doctor, nurse, or enterostomal therapist can teach the patient how to clean the area to prevent irritation and infection.

Chemotherapy

The side effects of chemotherapy depend mainly on the drugs the patient is given. As with any other type of treatment, side effects vary from person to person. In general, anticancer drugs affect rapidly dividing cells. These include blood cells, which fight infection, cause the blood to clot, or carry oxygen throughout the body. When blood cells are affected by anticancer drugs, patients are more likely to get infections, may bruise or bleed easily, and may have less energy. Cells in hair roots and cells that line the digestive tract also divide rapidly. For these reasons, chemotherapy can cause hair loss and problems such as poor appetite, mouth sores, nausea, vomiting, and diarrhea. The doctor can prescribe medicines or suggest other ways to prevent or reduce many of these effects. The side effects of chemotherapy gradually go away during the recovery period or after treatment stops.

Radiation Therapy

Patients who receive radiation therapy to the abdomen may have nausea, vomiting, and diarrhea. The doctor can prescribe medicine or suggest dietary changes to relieve these problems. Radiation therapy for colorectal cancer may cause hair loss in the pelvic area; the loss may be temporary or permanent. The skin in the treated area also may become red, dry, tender, and itchy. Patients should avoid wearing clothes that rub; loose-fitting cotton clothes are usually best. It is important for patients to take good care of their skin during treatment, but they should not use lotions or creams without the doctor's advice.

During radiation therapy, patients may become very tired, especially in the later weeks of treatment. Although resting is important, doctors usually suggest that patients continue as many of their normal activities as possible.

Biological Therapy

The side effects of biological therapy vary with the type of treatment. Often these treatments cause flu-like symptoms, such as chills, fever, weakness, nausea, vomiting, and diarrhea. Sometimes patients also get a rash.

To help withstand the side effects of treatment in general, it is important that patients maintain good nutrition (see Nutrition for Cancer Patients, page 19).

Other Side Effects

Sometimes treatment for colorectal cancer interferes with patients' ability to have sexual intercourse. Depending on the location of the tumor, surgery may damage the nerves that control a man's erection or the arteries that carry blood to the penis, causing temporary or permanent impotence. Also, radiation therapy to the abdomen sometimes causes problems with erection. Women who have had surgery to remove a colorectal tumor may have discomfort during sexual intercourse. Radiation therapy also may cause temporary vaginal dryness or tightness. The doctor or nurse can offer suggestions for dealing with these problems.

Patients who have a colostomy may have special concerns about sexuality. It may take time to adjust to the colostomy before they are ready for sexual intimacy. Many patients find that sharing their thoughts and feelings with a partner, close friend, or therapist helps them deal with these concerns. An enterostomal therapist can help patients adjust to the colostomy and can suggest ways to prevent it from interfering with sexuality.

FOLLOW-UP CARE

Regular follow-up exams are very important after treatment for colorectal cancer. The cancer can recur at or near the site of the original tumor or can spread to another area of the body. The doctor will continue to check closely so that, if the cancer comes back, it can be treated again as soon as possible.

Checkups often include a physical exam, a fecal occult blood test, sigmoidoscopy, colonoscopy, chest x-ray, and blood tests, including the CEA assay. Often the CEA level in a patient's blood is high before surgery and returns to normal within several weeks after the tumor has been removed. If the level of CEA begins to rise again, it may mean the cancer has come back. Other tests must also be done, because conditions other than cancer can cause the level to rise.

In addition to follow-up exams to check for a recurrence of colorectal cancer, patients may want to ask their doctor about checking for other types of cancer. Women who have had colorectal cancer have an increased risk of developing cancer of the breast, ovary, or cervix. Men who have had colorectal cancer appear to be at increased risk for developing prostate cancer.

In a small number of patients, cancer treatment may cause side effects many years later. Patients may wish to discuss these possible effects with their doctor. Patients should continue to have checkups and should report any problem as soon as it appears.

CAUSE AND PREVENTION

Colorectal cancer is one of the most common types of cancer in the United States. Scientists are trying to learn more about what causes the disease and how it can be prevented.

Although doctors do not yet know why one person gets colorectal cancer and another does not, they do know that no one can catch colorectal cancer from another person. Cancer is not contagious.

Some people are more likely to develop colorectal cancer than others. Studies have found that certain factors increase a person's risk. The following are risk factors for this disease:

- *Polyps*. Most—perhaps all—colorectal cancers develop in polyps. Polyps are benign, but they may become cancerous over time. Removing polyps is an important way to prevent colorectal cancer.
- *Age*. Colorectal cancers occur most often

in people who are over the age of 50, and the risk increases as people get older.

- *Family history*. Close relatives of a person who has had colorectal cancer have a higher-than-average risk of developing the disease. The risk for colon cancer is even higher among members of a family in which many relatives have had it. (In such cases, the disease is called familial colon cancer.)
- *Familial polyposis*. This is an inherited condition in which hundreds of polyps develop in the colon and rectum. Over time, these polyps can become cancerous. Unless the condition is treated, a person who has familial polyposis is almost sure to develop colorectal cancer.
- *Diet*. The risk of developing colon cancer seems to be higher in people whose diet is high in fat, low in fruits and vegetables, and low in high-fiber foods such as whole-grain breads and cereals.
- *Ulcerative colitis*. This disease causes inflammation of the lining of the colon. The risk of colon cancer is much greater than average for people who have this disease, and the risk increases with the length of time they have had it.

Researchers have found some trends in the incidence of colorectal cancer. For example, colorectal cancer occurs most often among people who live in cities. Colon cancer occurs slightly more often among blacks, and rectal cancer is more common among whites.

People can lower their risk of getting colorectal cancer. For example, those who have colorectal polyps should talk with the doctor about having them removed. People also can change their eating habits to cut down on fat in their diet. Major sources of fat are meat, eggs, dairy products, and oils used in cooking and salad dressings. People should increase the amount of fiber (roughage) in their diet. Fiber comes from vegetables, fruits, and whole-grain breads and cereals. The National

Cancer Institute recommends a low-fat, high-fiber diet that includes at least five servings of fruits and vegetables each day. Additional information about a healthy diet is available from the Cancer Information Service (1-800-4-CANCER).

People who think they are at risk for developing colorectal cancer should discuss this concern with their doctor. The doctor may suggest ways to decrease the risk and can plan an appropriate schedule for checkups.

The National Cancer Institute

HODGKIN'S DISEASE

Hodgkin's disease is a type of lymphoma. Lymphomas are cancers that develop in the lymphatic system, part of the body's immune system. The job of the lymphatic system is to help fight diseases and infection.

The lymphatic system is made up of a network of thin tubes that branch, like blood vessels, into all the tissues of the body. Lymphatic vessels carry lymph, a colorless, watery fluid that contains infection-fighting cells called lymphocytes. Along this network of vessels are groups of small, bean-shaped organs called lymph nodes that filter the lymph fluid as it passes through the nodes. Clusters of lymph nodes are found in the underarm, groin, neck, and abdomen. Other parts of the lymphatic system are the spleen, thymus gland, tonsils, and bone marrow.

Like all types of cancer, Hodgkin's disease affects the body's cells. Healthy cells grow, divide, and replace themselves in an orderly manner. This process keeps the body in good repair. In Hodgkin's disease, cells in the lymphatic system grow abnormally and can spread to other organs. As the disease progresses, the body is less able to fight infection.

Hodgkin's disease is rare. It accounts for less than 1 percent of all cases of cancer in the

United States. It is most often seen in young people aged 15 to 34 and in people over the age of 55.

SYMPTOMS

The most common symptom of Hodgkin's disease is a painless swelling in the lymph nodes in the neck, underarm, or groin. Other symptoms may include fevers, night sweats, tiredness, weight loss, or itching skin. However, these symptoms are not sure signs of cancer. They may also be caused by many common illnesses, such as the flu or other infections. But it is important to see a doctor if any of these symptoms lasts longer than two weeks. Any illness should be diagnosed and treated as early as possible, and this is especially true of Hodgkin's disease.

DIAGNOSIS

If Hodgkin's disease is suspected, the doctor will ask about the patient's medical history and will conduct a thorough physical exam. Blood tests and x-rays of the chest, bones, liver, and spleen will also be done.

Tissue from an enlarged lymph node will be removed. This is known as a biopsy. It is the only sure way to tell if cancer is present.

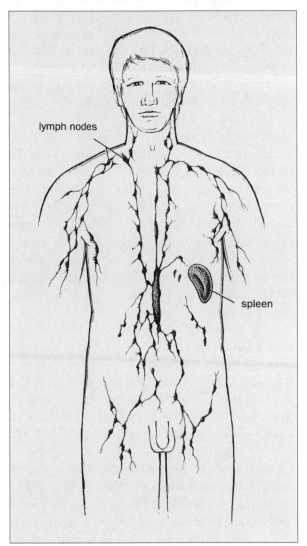

Hodgkin's disease causes swelling in the glands or nodes of the lymphatic system, located throughout the body. The spleen is actually a large lymph gland.

A pathologist will look at the tissue under the microscope for Reed-Sternberg cells, abnormal cells usually found with Hodgkin's disease. When Hodgkin's disease is diagnosed, the doctor needs to know the stage, or extent, of the disease. Knowing the stage is very important for planning treatment. The stage indicates where the disease has spread and how much tissue is affected. In staging, the doctor checks:

- The number and location of affected lymph nodes
- Whether the affected lymph nodes are above, below, or on both sides of the diaphragm (the thin muscle under the lungs and heart that separates the chest from the abdomen)
- Whether the disease has spread to the bone marrow, spleen, or to places outside the lymphatic system, such as the liver

In staging, the doctor usually orders several tests, including biopsies of the lymph nodes, liver, and bone marrow. Another test is computed tomography (also called CT scan), a series of x-rays of cross sections of the body.

TREATMENT

Treatment decisions for Hodgkin's disease are complex. Before starting treatment, the patient might want another doctor to review the diagnosis and treatment plan. (See also Preparing for Treatment, page 17.)

Methods of Treatment

Treatment for Hodgkin's disease usually includes radiation therapy or chemotherapy. Sometimes both are given. Treatment decisions are made depending on the stage of disease, its location in the body, which symptoms are present, and the general health and age of the patient. Often patients are referred to doctors or medical centers that specialize in the different treatments of Hodgkin's disease.

Radiation therapy uses high-energy rays to damage cancer cells and stop their growth. Radiation therapy is generally given in a hospital or clinic. Most often, patients receive radiation therapy five days a week for several weeks as outpatients.

Chemotherapy is the use of drugs to kill cancer cells. To treat Hodgkin's disease, the doctor prescribes a combination of drugs that work together. The drugs may be given in different ways: some by mouth; others injected into an artery, vein, or muscle. The drugs travel through the bloodstream to almost every part of the body. Chemotherapy is usually given in cycles: a treatment period followed by a rest period, then another treatment period, and so on.

Side Effects of Treatment

The methods used to treat Hodgkin's disease are very powerful. That's why the treatment often causes side effects—both short-term and permanent. Side effects depend on the type of treatment and on the part of the body being treated. Also, each patient may respond differently.

During radiation therapy, patients may become unusually tired as therapy continues. Getting enough rest is important. Skin reactions (redness or dryness) in the area being treated are also common. Patients should be gentle with the treated area of skin. Lotions and creams should not be used without the doctor's advice.

When the chest is treated, patients may have a dry, sore throat and may have trouble swallowing. Sometimes they have shortness of breath or a dry cough. Radiation treatment to the lower abdomen may cause nausea, vomiting, or diarrhea. Some patients have tingling or numbness in their arms, legs, and lower back. These side effects gradually disappear when treatment is over.

The side effects of chemotherapy depend mainly on the drugs given. In general, anticancer drugs affect rapidly growing cells, such as blood cells that fight infection, cells that line the digestive tract, and cells in hair follicles. As a result, patients may have side effects such as hair loss, lowered resistance to infection, loss of appetite, nausea and vomiting, and mouth sores. These side effects usually end after chemotherapy is finished.

Treatment for Hodgkin's disease can cause fertility problems. Women's menstrual periods may stop. Periods are more likely to return in younger women. In men, both Hodgkin's disease and its treatment can affect fertility. Younger men are more likely to regain their fertility. Sperm banking before treatment may be an option for some men.

Effects on fertility vary greatly with the particular chemotherapy drugs used.

To help withstand the side effects of treatment, it is important that patients maintain good nutrition (see Nutrition for Cancer Patients, page 19).

FOLLOW-UP CARE

Regular follow-up exams are very important for anyone who has been treated for Hodgkin's disease. The doctor will continue to watch the patient closely for several years. Generally, checkups include a careful physical exam, x-rays, blood tests, and other laboratory tests.

Patients treated for Hodgkin's disease have an increased risk of developing other types of cancer later in life, especially leukemia. Patients should follow their doctor's recommendations on health care and checkups. Having regular checkups allows problems to be detected and treated promptly if they should arise.

LIVING WITH CANCER

When people have cancer, life can change for them and for the people who care about them. These changes in daily life can be difficult to handle. (See Support for Cancer Patients, page 20.)

WHAT THE FUTURE HOLDS

More than 8 million Americans living today have had some type of cancer. Thirty years ago, few patients with Hodgkin's disease recovered from their illness. Now, because of modern radiation therapy and combination chemotherapy, more than 75 percent of all newly diagnosed Hodgkin's disease patients are curable. The chances for recovery continue to improve as scientists find new treatments.

The National Cancer Institute

KIDNEY CANCER

The kidneys are two reddish brown, bean-shaped organs located just above the waist, one on each side of the spine. They are part of the urinary system.

Their main function is to filter blood and produce urine to rid the body of waste. As blood flows through the kidneys, they remove waste products and unneeded water. The resulting liquid, urine, collects in the middle of each kidney in an area called the renal pelvis. Urine drains from each kidney through a long tube, the ureter, into the bladder, where it is stored. Urine leaves the body through another tube, called the urethra.

The kidneys also produce substances that help control blood pressure and regulate the formation of red blood cells.

TYPES OF KIDNEY CANCER

Several types of cancer can develop in the kidney. Renal cell cancer, the most common form of kidney cancer in adults, is discussed here. Transitional cell cancer (carcinoma), which affects the renal pelvis, is a less common form of kidney cancer. It is similar to cancer that occurs in the bladder and is often treated like bladder cancer.

SYMPTOMS

In its early stages, kidney cancer usually causes no obvious signs or troublesome symptoms. However, as a kidney tumor grows, symptoms may occur. These may include:

- Blood in the urine. Blood may be present one day and not the next. In some cases, a person can actually see the blood, or traces of it may be found in urinalysis, a lab test often performed as part of a regular medical checkup.
- A lump or mass in the kidney area.

Other less common symptoms may include fatigue, loss of appetite, weight loss, recurrent fevers, a pain in the side that doesn't go away, and a general feeling of poor health. High blood pressure or a lower than normal number of red cells in the blood (anemia) may also signal a kidney tumor; however, these symptoms occur less often.

55

These symptoms may be caused by cancer or by other, less serious problems such as an infection or a cyst. Only a doctor can make a diagnosis. People with any of these symptoms may see their family doctor or a urologist, a doctor who specializes in diseases of the urinary system. Usually, early cancer does not cause pain; it is important not to wait to feel pain before seeing a doctor. In most cases, the earlier cancer is diagnosed and treated, the better a person's chance for a full recovery.

DIAGNOSIS

To find the cause of symptoms, the doctor asks about the patient's medical history and does a physical exam. The doctor may perform blood and urine tests and carefully feel the abdomen for lumps or irregular masses.

The doctor usually orders tests that produce pictures of the kidneys and nearby organs. These pictures can often show changes in the kidney and surrounding tissue.

- *An IVP (intravenous pyelogram)* is a series of x-rays of the kidneys, ureters, and bladder after the injection of a dye to show changes in the shape of these organs.
- *Arteriography* is a series of x-rays of the blood vessels around the kidney after the injection of a dye.
- *A CT scan* is another x-ray procedure that gives detailed, computer-created pictures of cross sections of the body.
- *Ultrasound* is a test that sends high-frequency sound waves, which cannot be heard by humans, into the kidney to create a picture called a sonogram.
- *MRI (magnetic resonance imaging)* uses a very strong magnet linked to a computer to create pictures of the kidney.

If test results suggest kidney cancer may be present, a biopsy may be performed; it is the only sure way to diagnose cancer. During a biopsy for kidney cancer, a thin needle is inserted into the tumor and a sample of tissue is withdrawn. A pathologist then examines the tissue under a microscope to check for cancer cells.

Once kidney cancer is diagnosed, the doctor will want to learn the stage, or extent, of the disease. Staging is a careful attempt, through additional tests, to find out whether the cancer has spread and, if so, what parts of the body are affected. This information is needed to plan a patient's treatment.

TREATMENT

Treatment for kidney cancer depends on the disease stage, the patient's general health and age, and other factors. The doctor develops a treatment plan to fit each patient's needs. (See Preparing for Treatment, page 17.)

Methods of Treatment

Surgery is the most common treatment for kidney cancer. An operation to remove the kidney is called a nephrectomy. Most often, the surgeon removes the whole kidney along with the adrenal gland and the tissue around the kidney. Some lymph nodes in the area may also be removed. This procedure is called a radical nephrectomy.

In some cases, the surgeon removes only the kidney (simple nephrectomy). The remaining kidney generally is able to perform the work of both kidneys. In another procedure called partial nephrectomy the surgeon removes just the part of the kidney that contains the tumor.

In arterial embolization small pieces of a special gelatin sponge or other material are injected through a catheter to clog the main renal blood vessel. This procedure shrinks the tumor by depriving it of the oxygen-carrying blood and other substances it needs to grow. It is sometimes used before an operation to make surgery easier. It also may be used to provide relief from pain or bleeding when removal of the tumor is not possible.

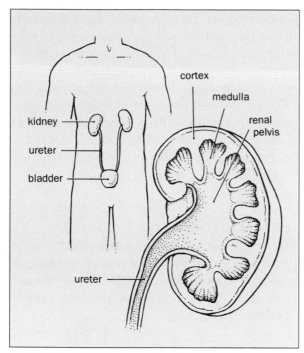

The kidneys eliminate wastes, chemicals, and excess water from the blood and produce urine. Tumors of the kidney tend to form on the organ's top outer edge.

Radiation therapy (also called radiotherapy) uses high-energy rays to kill cancer cells. Doctors sometimes use radiation therapy to relieve pain (palliative therapy) when kidney cancer has spread to the bone.

Radiation therapy for kidney cancer involves external radiation, which comes from radioactive material outside the body. A machine aims the rays at a specific area of the body. Most often, treatment is given on an outpatient basis in a hospital or clinic five days a week for several weeks. This schedule helps protect normal tissue by spreading out the total dose of radiation. The patient does not need to stay in the hospital for radiation therapy, and patients are not radioactive during or after treatment.

Biological therapy (also called immunotherapy) is a form of treatment that uses the body's natural ability (immune system) to fight cancer. Interleukin-2 and interferon are types of bio-

logical therapy used to treat advanced kidney cancer. Clinical trials continue to examine better ways to use biological therapy while reducing the side effects patients may experience. Many people having biological therapy stay in the hospital during treatment so that these side effects can be monitored.

Chemotherapy is the use of drugs to kill cancer cells. Although useful in the treatment of many other cancers, chemotherapy has shown limited effectiveness against kidney cancer.

Hormonal therapy is used in a small number of patients with advanced kidney cancer. Some kidney cancers may be treated with hormones to try to control the growth of cancer cells. More often it is used to relieve pain.

Side Effects of Treatment

The side effects of cancer therapy depend mainly on the type and extent of the treatment. Also, side effects may not be the same for each person, and they may even change from one treatment to the next. Doctors and nurses can explain the possible side effects of therapy, and they can help relieve problems that may occur during and after treatment. Patients should notify a doctor of the side effects they are having, as some may require immediate medical attention.

The side effects of kidney surgery depend on the type of operation, the patient's general health, and other factors. Nephrectomy is major surgery, and after the operation most people have pain and discomfort. Patients may find it difficult to breathe deeply due to discomfort from surgery; they may have to do special coughing and breathing exercises to help keep their lungs clear. It is also common for patients who have had surgery to feel tired or weak for a while.

In addition, patients may need intravenous (IV) feeding and fluids for several days before and after the operation. When a kidney is removed, the one remaining kidney takes over the work of both. Nurses will monitor the amount of fluid a person takes in and the amount of urine produced. The length of time it takes to recover from an operation varies from person to person.

Arterial embolization can cause pain, fever, nausea, or vomiting. Often people need IV fluids as the body recovers from this procedure.

With radiation therapy, the side effects depend on the treatment dose and the part of the body that is treated. Patients are likely to become very tired, especially in the later weeks of treatment. Resting is important, but doctors usually advise patients to try to stay as active as they can.

It is common for the skin in the treated area to become red, dry, tender, and itchy. There may be permanent darkening or "bronzing" of the skin in the treated area. Radiation to the kidney and nearby areas may cause nausea, vomiting, diarrhea, or urinary discomfort. It may also cause a decrease in the number of white blood cells, cells that help protect the body against infection.

The side effects caused by biological therapy vary with the type of treatment. These treatments may cause flu-like symptoms such as chills, fever, muscle aches, weakness, loss of appetite, nausea, vomiting, and diarrhea.

The side effects of chemotherapy depend on the drugs that are given. In general, patients may have side effects such as lower resistance to infection, loss of appetite, nausea, vomiting, or mouth sores. They may also have less energy and may lose their hair.

The side effects of hormonal therapy are usually mild. Progesterone is the hormone most often used to treat kidney cancer. Drugs containing progesterone may cause changes in appetite and weight. They may also cause swelling or fluid retention. These side effects generally go away after treatment.

To help withstand the side effects of treatment, it is important that patients maintain good nutrition (see Nutrition for Cancer Patients, page 19).

FOLLOW-UP CARE

Regular follow-up is very important after treatment for kidney cancer. Checkups may include exams, chest x-rays, and lab tests. The doctor sometimes also orders scans (special x-rays) and other tests.

LIVING WITH CANCER

The diagnosis of kidney cancer can change the lives of cancer patients and the people who care about them. These changes can be difficult to handle. (See Support for Cancer Patients, page 20.)

The National Cancer Institute

LEUKEMIA

Leukemia is cancer of the blood cells. To understand leukemia, it is helpful to know about normal blood cells and what happens to them when leukemia develops.

Normal Blood Cells

The blood is made up of fluid called plasma and three types of cells. Each type has special functions.

- *White blood cells* (also called WBCs or leukocytes) help the body fight infections and other diseases.
- *Red blood cells* (also called RBCs or erythrocytes) carry oxygen from the lungs to the body's tissues and take carbon dioxide from the tissues back to the lungs. The red blood cells give blood its color.
- *Platelets* (also called thrombocytes) help form blood clots that control bleeding.

Blood cells are formed in the bone marrow, the soft, spongy center of bones. New (immature) blood cells are called blasts. Some blasts stay in the marrow to mature. Some travel to other parts of the body to mature. Normally, blood cells are produced in an orderly, controlled way, as the body needs them. This process helps keep us healthy.

Leukemia Cells

When leukemia develops, the body produces large numbers of abnormal blood cells. In most types of leukemia, the abnormal cells are white blood cells. The leukemia cells usually look different from normal blood cells, and they do not function properly.

TYPES OF LEUKEMIA

There are several types of leukemia. They are grouped in two ways. One way is by how quickly the disease develops and gets worse. The other is by the type of blood cell that is affected.

Leukemia is either acute or chronic. In acute leukemia, the abnormal blood cells are blasts that remain very immature and cannot carry out their normal functions. The number of blasts increases rapidly, and the disease gets worse quickly. In chronic leukemia, some blast cells are present, but in general, these cells are more mature and can carry out some of their normal functions. Also, the number of blasts increases less rapidly than in acute leukemia. As a result, chronic leukemia gets worse gradually.

Leukemia can arise in either of the two main types of white blood cells: lymphoid cells or myeloid cells. When leukemia affects lymphoid cells, it is called lymphocytic leukemia. When myeloid cells are affected, the disease is called myeloid or myelogenous leukemia. These are the most common types of leukemia:

- *Acute lymphocytic leukemia* (ALL) is the most common type of leukemia in young children. This disease also affects adults, especially those age 65 and older.
- *Acute myeloid leukemia* (AML) occurs in both adults and children. This type of leukemia is sometimes called acute nonlymphocytic leukemia (ANLL).
- *Chronic lymphocytic leukemia* (CLL) most often affects adults over the age of 55. It sometimes occurs in younger adults, but it almost never affects children.
- *Chronic myeloid leukemia* (CML) occurs mainly in adults. A very small number of children also develop this disease.

Hairy cell leukemia is an uncommon type of chronic leukemia. This and other uncommon types of leukemia are not discussed here. The Cancer Information Service (1-800-4-CANCER) can supply information about them.

SYMPTOMS

Leukemia cells are abnormal cells that cannot do what normal blood cells do. They cannot help the body fight infections. For this reason, people with leukemia often get infections and have fevers.

Also, people with leukemia often have less than the normal amount of healthy red blood cells and platelets. As a result, there are not enough red blood cells to carry oxygen through the body. With this condition, called anemia, patients may look pale and feel weak and tired. When there are not enough platelets, patients bleed and bruise easily.

Like all blood cells, leukemia cells travel through the body. Depending on the number of abnormal cells and where these cells collect, patients with leukemia may have a number of symptoms.

In acute leukemia, symptoms appear and get worse quickly. People with this disease go to their doctor because they feel sick. In chronic leukemia, symptoms may not appear for a long time; when symptoms do appear, they generally are mild at first and get worse gradually. Doctors often find chronic leukemia during a routine checkup—before there are any symptoms. These are some of the common symptoms of leukemia:

- Fever, chills, and other flu-like symptoms
- Weakness and fatigue
- Frequent infections
- Loss of appetite and/or weight
- Swollen or tender lymph nodes, liver, or spleen
- Easy bleeding or bruising
- Tiny red spots (called petechiae) under the skin
- Swollen or bleeding gums
- Sweating, especially at night
- Bone or joint pain

In acute leukemia, the abnormal cells may collect in the brain or spinal cord (also called the central nervous system or CNS). The result may be headaches, vomiting, confusion, loss of muscle control, and seizures. Leukemia cells also can collect in the testicles and cause swelling. In addition, some patients develop sores in the eyes or on the skin. Leukemia also can affect the digestive tract, kidneys, lungs, or other parts of the body.

In chronic leukemia, the abnormal blood cells may gradually collect in various parts of the body. Chronic leukemia may affect the skin, central nervous system, digestive tract, kidneys, and testicles.

DIAGNOSIS

To find the cause of a person's symptoms, the doctor asks about the patient's medical history and does a physical exam. In addition to checking general signs of health, the doctor feels for swelling in the liver, the spleen, and in the lymph nodes under the arms, in the groin, and in the neck.

Blood tests also help in the diagnosis. A sample of blood is examined under a microscope to see what the cells look like and to de-termine the number of mature cells and blasts. Although blood tests may reveal that a patient has leukemia, they may not show what type of leukemia it is.

To check further for leukemia cells or to tell what type of leukemia a patient has, a hematologist, oncologist, or pathologist examines a sample of bone marrow under a microscope. The doctor withdraws the sample by inserting a needle into a large bone (usually the hip) and removing a small amount of liquid bone marrow. This procedure is called bone marrow aspiration. A bone marrow biopsy is performed with a larger needle and removes a small piece of bone and bone marrow.

If leukemia cells are found in the bone marrow sample, the patient's doctor orders other tests to find out the extent of the disease. A spinal tap (lumbar puncture) checks for leukemia cells in the fluid that fills the spaces in and around the brain and spinal cord (cerebrospinal fluid). Chest x-rays can reveal signs of disease in the chest.

TREATMENT

Treatment for leukemia is complex. It varies with the type of leukemia and is not the same for all patients. The doctor plans the treatment to fit each patient's needs. The treatment depends not only on the type of leukemia, but also on certain features of the leukemia cells, the extent of the disease, and whether the leukemia has been treated before. It also depends on the patient's age, symptoms, and general health. (See page 17 for more information about getting a second opinion and planning treatment.)

Whenever possible, patients should be treated at a medical center that has doctors who have experience in treating leukemia. If this is not possible, the patient's doctor should discuss the treatment plan with a specialist at such a center. Also, patients and their doctors can call the Cancer Information Service at 1-800-4-CANCER to request up-to-date treat-

IMPORTANT QUESTIONS

Here are some questions patients and their families may want to ask the doctor before treatment begins:

• What type of leukemia is it?

• What are the treatment choices? Which do you recommend? Why?

• Would a clinical trial be appropriate?

• What are the expected benefits of each kind of treatment?

• What are the risks and possible side effects of each treatment?

• If I have pain, how will you help me?

• Will I have to change my normal activities?

• How long will treatment last?

• What is the treatment likely to cost? How can I find out what my insurance will cover?

ment information from the National Cancer Institute's PDQ database.

Acute leukemia needs to be treated right away. The goal of treatment is to bring about a remission. Then, when there is no evidence of the disease, more therapy may be given to prevent a relapse. Many people with acute leukemia can be cured.

Chronic leukemia patients who do not have symptoms may not require immediate treatment. However, they should have frequent checkups so the doctor can see whether the disease is progressing. When treatment is needed, it can often control the disease and its symptoms.

Many patients and their families want to learn all they can about leukemia and the treatment choices so they can take an active part in decisions about medical care. The doctor is the best person to answer these questions. When discussing treatment, the patient (or, in the case of a child, the patient's family) may want to talk with the doctor about research studies of new treatment methods. Such studies, called clinical trials, are designed to improve cancer treatment. (For more information about clinical trials, see page 20.)

When a person is diagnosed with leukemia, shock and stress are natural reactions. These feelings may make it difficult to think of every question to ask the doctor. Also, patients may find it hard to remember everything the doctor says.

Often it helps to make a list of questions to ask the doctor. Taking notes or, if the doctor agrees, using a tape recorder can make it easier to remember the answers. Some people find that it also helps to have a family member or friend with them—to take part in the discussion, to take notes, or just to listen. Patients do not need to ask all their questions or remember all the answers at one time. They will have other chances for the doctor to explain things that are not clear and to ask for more information.

Methods of Treatment

Most patients with leukemia are treated with chemotherapy. Some also may have radiation therapy and/or bone marrow transplantation (BMT) or biological therapy. In some cases, surgery to remove the spleen (an operation called a splenectomy) may be part of the treatment plan.

Chemotherapy is the use of drugs to kill cancer cells. Depending on the type of leukemia, patients may receive a single drug or a combination of two or more drugs.

Some anticancer drugs can be taken by mouth. Most are given by IV injection (injected into a vein). Often patients who need to have many IV treatments receive the drugs through a catheter. One end of this thin, flexible tube is placed in a large vein, often in the upper chest. Drugs are injected into the catheter, rather than directly into a vein, to avoid the discomfort of repeated injections and injury to the skin.

Anticancer drugs given by IV injection or taken by mouth enter the bloodstream and affect leukemia cells in most parts of the body. However, the drugs often do not reach cells in the central nervous system because they are stopped by the blood-brain barrier. This protective barrier is formed by a network of blood vessels that filter blood going to the brain and spinal cord. To reach leukemia cells in the central nervous system, doctors use intrathecal chemotherapy. In this type of treatment, anticancer drugs are injected directly into the cerebrospinal fluid.

Intrathecal chemotherapy can be given in two ways. Some patients receive the drugs by injection into the lower part of the spinal column. Others, especially children, receive intrathecal chemotherapy through a special type of catheter. This device is placed under the scalp, where it provides a pathway to the cerebrospinal fluid. Injecting anticancer drugs into the reservoir instead of into the spinal column can make intrathecal chemotherapy easier and more comfortable for the patient.

Chemotherapy is given in cycles: a treatment period followed by a recovery period, then another treatment period, and so on. In some cases, the patient has chemotherapy as an outpatient at the hospital, at the doctor's office, or at home. However, depending on which drugs are given and the patient's general health, a hospital stay may be necessary.

Radiation therapy is used along with chemotherapy for some kinds of leukemia. Radiation therapy (also called radiotherapy) uses high-energy rays to damage cancer cells and stop them from growing. The radiation comes from a large machine.

Radiation therapy for leukemia may be given in two ways. For some patients, the doctor may direct the radiation to one specific area of the body where there is a collection of leukemia cells, such as the spleen or testicles. Other patients may receive radiation that is directed to the whole body. This type of radiation therapy, called total-body irradiation, usually is given before a bone marrow transplant.

Bone marrow transplantation also may be used for some patients. The patient's leukemia-producing bone marrow is destroyed by high doses of drugs and radiation and is then replaced by healthy bone marrow. The healthy bone marrow may come from a donor, or it may be marrow that has been removed from the patient and stored before the high-dose treatment. If the patient's own bone marrow is used, it may first be treated outside the body to remove leukemia cells.

Chronic leukemias can seldom be cured without bone marrow transplantation.

Patients who have a bone marrow transplant usually stay in the hospital for several weeks. Until the transplanted bone marrow begins to produce enough white blood cells, patients have to be carefully protected from infection.

Biological therapy involves treatment with substances that affect the immune system's response to cancer. Interferon is a form of biological therapy that is used against some types of leukemia.

Supportive Care
Leukemia and its treatment can cause a number of complications and side effects. Patients receive supportive care to prevent or control these problems and to improve their comfort and quality of life during treatment.

Because leukemia patients get infections very easily, they may receive antibiotics and other drugs to help protect them from infections. They are often advised to stay out of crowds and away from people with colds and other infectious diseases. If an infection develops, it can be serious and should be treated promptly. Patients may need to stay in the hospital to treat the infection.

Anemia and bleeding are other problems

that often require supportive care. Transfusions of red blood cells may be given to help reduce the shortness of breath and fatigue that anemia can cause. Platelet transfusions can help reduce the risk of serious bleeding.

Dental care also is very important. Leukemia and chemotherapy can make the mouth sensitive, easily infected, and likely to bleed. Doctors often advise patients to have a complete dental exam before treatment begins. Dentists can show patients how to keep their mouth clean and healthy during treatment.

SIDE EFFECTS OF TREATMENT

It is hard to limit the effects of therapy so that only leukemia cells are destroyed. Because treatment also damages healthy cells and tissues, it causes side effects.

The side effects of cancer treatment vary. They depend mainly on the type and extent of the treatment. Also, each person reacts differently. Side effects may even be different from one treatment to the next. Doctors try to plan the patient's therapy to keep side effects to a minimum. Doctors and nurses can explain the side effects of treatment and can suggest medicine, diet changes, or other ways to deal with them.

Chemotherapy

The side effects of chemotherapy depend mainly on the drugs the patient receives. In addition, as with other types of treatment, side effects may vary from person to person. Generally, anticancer drugs affect dividing cells. Cancer cells divide more often than healthy cells and are more likely to be affected by chemotherapy. Still, some healthy cells also may be damaged. Healthy cells that divide often, including blood cells, cells in hair roots, and cells in the digestive tract, are likely to be damaged.

When chemotherapy affects healthy cells, it may lower patients' resistance to infection, and patients may have less energy and may bruise or bleed easily. They may lose their hair. They also may have nausea, vomiting, and mouth sores. Most side effects go away gradually during the recovery periods between treatments or after treatment stops.

Some anticancer drugs can affect a patient's fertility. Women's periods may become irregular or stop, and women may have symptoms of menopause, such as hot flashes and vaginal dryness. Men may stop producing sperm. Because these changes may be permanent, some men choose to have their sperm frozen and stored. Most children treated for leukemia appear to have normal fertility when they grow up. However, depending on the drugs and doses used and on the age of the patient, some boys and girls may not be able to have children when they mature.

Radiation Therapy

Patients receiving radiation therapy may become very tired. Resting is important, but doctors usually suggest that patients remain as active as they can.

When radiation is directed to the head, patients often lose their hair. Radiation can cause the scalp or the skin in the treated area to become red, dry, tender, and itchy. Patients will be shown how to keep the skin clean. They should not use any lotion or cream on the treated area without the doctor's advice. Radiation therapy also may cause nausea, vomiting, and loss of appetite. These side effects are temporary, and doctors and nurses can often suggest ways to control them until the treatment is over.

However, some side effects may be lasting. Children (especially young ones) who receive radiation to the brain may develop problems with learning and coordination. For this reason, doctors use the lowest possible doses of radiation, and they give this treatment only to children who cannot be treated successfully with chemotherapy alone.

Also, radiation to the testicles is likely to affect both fertility and hormone production. Most boys who have this form of treatment are not able to have children later on. Some may need to take hormones.

Bone Marrow Transplantation

Patients who have a bone marrow transplant face an increased risk of infection, bleeding, and other side effects from the large doses of chemotherapy and radiation they receive. In addition, graft-versus-host disease (GVHD) may occur in patients who receive bone marrow from a donor. In GVHD, the donated marrow reacts against the patient's tissues (most often the liver, the skin, and the digestive tract). GVHD can be mild or very severe. It can occur any time after the transplant (even years later). Drugs may be given to reduce the risk of GVHD and to treat the problem if it occurs.

To help withstand the side effects of treatment in general, it is important that patients maintain good nutrition (see Nutrition for Cancer Patients, page 19).

FOLLOW-UP CARE

Regular follow-up exams are very important after treatment for leukemia. The doctor will continue to check the patient closely to be sure that the cancer has not returned. Checkups usually include exams of the blood, bone marrow, and cerebrospinal fluid. From time to time, the doctor does a complete physical exam.

Cancer treatment may cause side effects many years later. Patients should continue to have regular checkups and promptly report any health changes or problems to their doctor.

WHAT THE FUTURE HOLDS

Researchers are finding better ways to treat leukemia, and the chances of recovery keep improving. Still, it is natural for patients and their families to be concerned about the future.

Sometimes people use rates of survival and other statistics to try to figure out whether a patient will be cured or how long the patient will live. It is important to remember, howev-

er, that statistics are averages based on large numbers of patients. They cannot be used to predict what will happen to a certain patient because no two patients are alike; treatments and responses vary greatly. The doctor who takes care of the patient is in the best position to discuss the chance of recovery (prognosis). Patients and their families should feel free to ask the doctor about the prognosis, but they should keep in mind that not even the doctor knows exactly what will happen. Doctors often talk about surviving cancer, or they may use the term "remission," rather than "cure." Even though many leukemia patients are cured, doctors use these terms because the disease can recur.

POSSIBLE CAUSES

At this time, we do not know what causes leukemia. Researchers are trying to solve this problem. Scientists know that leukemia occurs in males more often than in females and in white people more often than in black people. However, they cannot explain why one person gets leukemia and another does not.

By studying large numbers of people all over the world, researchers have found certain risk factors that increase a person's risk of getting leukemia. For example, exposure to large amounts of high-energy radiation increases the risk of getting leukemia. Such radiation was produced by the atomic bomb explosions in Japan during World War II. In nuclear power plants, strict safety rules protect workers and the public from exposure to harmful amounts of radiation.

Some research suggests that exposure to electromagnetic fields is a possible risk factor for leukemia. (Electromagnetic fields are a type of low-energy radiation that comes from power lines and electric appliances.) However, more studies are needed to prove this link.

Certain genetic conditions can increase the risk for leukemia. One such condition is Down syndrome; chil-

dren born with this syndrome are more likely to get leukemia than other children.

Workers exposed to certain chemicals over a long period of time are at higher risk for leukemia. Benzene is one of these chemicals. Also, some of the drugs used to treat other types of cancer may increase a person's risk of getting leukemia. However, this risk is very small when compared with the benefits of chemotherapy.

Scientists have identified a virus that seems to increase the risk for one very uncommon type of leukemia. However, this virus has no known association with common forms of leukemia. Scientists throughout the world continue to study viruses and other possible risk factors for leukemia. By learning what causes this disease, researchers hope to better understand how to prevent and treat it.

The National Cancer Institute

LUNG CANCER

The lungs, a pair of cone-shaped organs made up of spongy pinkish gray tissue, are part of the respiratory system. They take up most of the space in the chest and are separated from each other by the mediastinum, an area that contains the heart, trachea (windpipe), esophagus, and many lymph nodes. The right lung has three sections, called lobes; it is a little larger than the left lung, which has two lobes.

When we breathe, air enters the body through the nose or the mouth. The air travels down the throat, through the larynx (voice box) and trachea, and into the lungs through tubes called main-stem bronchi. One main-stem bronchus leads to the right lung and one to the left lung. In the lungs, the main-stem bronchi divide into smaller bronchi and then into even smaller tubes called bronchioles.

The bronchioles end in tiny air sacs called alveoli. The lungs take in oxygen, which cells need to live and carry out their normal functions. The lungs also get rid of carbon dioxide, a waste product of the body's cells.

Lung cancer often spreads to lymph nodes or other tissues in the chest (including the other lung). In many cases, lung cancer also spreads to other organs of the body, such as the bones, brain, or liver. Cancer that spreads is the same disease and has the same name as the original (primary) cancer. In other words, lung cancer that spreads to the brain (or another organ) is called metastatic lung cancer, even though the new tumor is in the brain (or another organ).

WHAT CAUSES LUNG CANCER?

Most lung cancer is caused by cigarette smoking. Tobacco smoke contains many carcinogens—harmful substances that damage cells. Over time, these cells can become cancerous. The more a person smokes, the higher the risk of getting cancer—not just lung cancer, but also cancers of the mouth, throat, esophagus, larynx, bladder, kidney, cervix, and pancreas.

The risk of lung cancer begins decreasing slowly as soon as a person quits smoking. Although quitting early is best, smokers should know that it is never too late to benefit from quitting—even if they have lung cancer. Lung cancer patients who stop smoking are less likely to get a second lung cancer than are patients who continue to smoke.

Many programs are available to help people stop smoking. The Cancer Information Service, the American Cancer Society, and the American Lung Association can offer advice about quitting and can give you information about programs in your area.

Although smoking is by far the major cause of lung cancer, it is not the only cause. Exposure to other people's tobacco smoke (environmental tobacco smoke) increases the risk of lung cancer among nonsmokers. Scientists have found that nonsmokers who live or work with smokers have a higher lung cancer risk than nonsmokers who do not face this type of exposure to environmental tobacco smoke.

Exposure to certain carcinogens in the workplace, such as asbestos, also increases the risk of lung cancer. (The risk is especially high for workers who smoke.) People should carefully follow work and safety rules to reduce their exposure to workplace carcinogens.

Workers (especially smokers) who are exposed to high levels of radon, a radioactive gas, have an increased risk of developing lung cancer. High levels of radon are found in some types of underground mines (for example, underground uranium mines).

Radon also can build up in some homes, but the levels in homes are generally much lower than in mines. Researchers are studying whether exposure to radon in the home can increase lung cancer risk. The United States Environmental Protection Agency can provide information about radon exposure and testing for radon in the home.

TYPES OF LUNG CANCER

Nearly all lung cancers are carcinomas. A carcinoma is a cancer that begins in the lining or covering tissues of an organ. Lung cancers are generally divided into two types: nonsmall cell lung cancer and small cell lung cancer. The tumor cells of each type of lung cancer grow and spread differently, and each type needs different treatment.

Nonsmall cell lung cancer is more common than small cell lung cancer. The three main kinds of nonsmall cell lung cancer are named for the type of cells in the tumor:

- *Squamous cell carcinoma,* also called epidermoid carcinoma, is the most common type of lung cancer in men. It often begins in the bronchi and usually does not spread as quickly as other types of lung cancer.

- *Adenocarcinoma* usually begins along the outer edges of the lungs and under the lining of the bronchi. This is the most common type of lung cancer in women and in people who have never smoked.
- *Large cell carcinomas* are a group of cancers with large, abnormal-looking cells. These tumors usually begin along the outer edges of the lungs.

Small cell lung cancer is sometimes called oat cell cancer because the cancer cells may look like oats when viewed under a microscope. This type of lung cancer grows rapidly and quickly spreads to other organs.

SYMPTOMS

Lung cancer usually does not cause symptoms when it first develops. Doctors sometimes discover lung cancer in a person with no symptoms after the individual has a chest x-ray for another medical reason. Usually, however, lung cancer is found after the growing tumor causes symptoms to appear.

A cough is the most common symptom of lung cancer. It is likely to occur when a tumor irritates the lining of the airways or blocks the passage of air. The person may have a "smoker's cough" that becomes worse. Another symptom is constant chest pain. Other symptoms may include shortness of breath, wheezing, repeated bouts of pneumonia or bronchitis, coughing up blood, or hoarseness. A tumor that presses on large blood vessels near the lung can cause swelling of the neck and face. If the tumor presses on certain nerves near the lung, it can cause pain and weakness in the shoulder, arm, or hand.

In addition, there may be symptoms that do not seem to be at all related to the lungs. Like all cancers, lung cancer can cause fatigue, loss of appetite, and loss of weight. If the cancer spreads to other parts of the body, it may cause headache, pain, or bone fractures.

Other symptoms can be caused by sub-

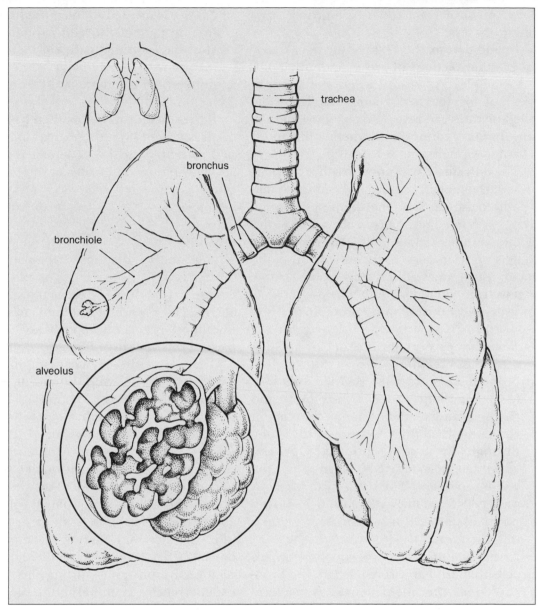

The trachea divides into two bronchi, one in each lung. These branch out into bronchioles and culminate in tiny air sacs, or alveoli. The most common type of lung cancer begins in the bronchi.

stances made by lung cancer cells. Doctors often refer to these symptoms as a paraneoplastic syndrome. For example, certain lung cancer cells produce a substance that causes a sharp drop in the level of salt (sodium) in the blood. A decrease in the sodium level can cause many symptoms, including confusion and sometimes even coma. None of these symptoms is a sure sign of lung cancer. Only a

doctor can tell whether a patient's symptoms are caused by cancer or by another problem.

DIAGNOSIS

To find the cause of any of these symptoms, the doctor asks about the patient's personal and family medical background, as well as smoking and work history. The doctor also

67

does a physical exam and usually orders x-rays and other tests.

In addition to chest x-rays, the doctor may order other pictures of areas inside the body. For example, a CT scan is a series of x-ray images put together by a computer. These detailed pictures can reveal that a tumor is in the lung, but they cannot show whether the tumor is benign or malignant.

The only sure way to know whether cancer is present is to obtain cells from the lungs so that a pathologist can examine them under a microscope. Sometimes cancer cells can be found in the sputum, a thick fluid that the patient coughs up from deep in the airways. Also, the doctor usually does a biopsy to remove a sample of cells from the lung. To do a biopsy, the doctor uses one of the following procedures:

- *Bronchoscopy* permits the doctor to look into the breathing passages through a bronchoscope (a thin, lighted tube). A local anesthetic reduces discomfort and gagging, and medicine helps the patient relax as the doctor inserts the tube through the nose or mouth. (A general anesthetic may be used instead to put the patient to sleep.) The doctor can brush or wash cells from the walls of bronchi or snip off small pieces of tissue for study under a microscope.
- *Needle aspiration* is a procedure to remove cells that are hard to reach with the bronchoscope. After the patient is given a local anesthetic, the doctor inserts a needle through the chest into the tumor to withdraw a small sample of tissue. Most often, the doctor uses fluoroscopy or CT scans to locate the tumor.
- *Examination of fluid from the pleura* (the fluid-filled sac that surrounds the lungs) sometimes reveals lung cancer. Using a needle, the doctor removes a sample of the fluid in the pleura and checks it for cancer cells. For this procedure, called thoracentesis, the patient receives a local anesthetic.

- *Surgery* is needed to diagnose lung cancer in some patients. Surgery to open the chest (for diagnosis or treatment) is called thoracotomy. This is major surgery and is done under a general anesthetic.

If the doctor can feel swollen lymph nodes or an enlarged liver, these areas may be biopsied to help with the diagnosis. The doctor also may biopsy other sites of the body where cancer is suspected.

STAGING

If lung cancer is diagnosed, the patient's doctor needs to learn the stage, or extent, of the disease so that proper treatment can be given. Staging is a careful attempt to find out whether the cancer has spread and, if so, what parts of the body are affected.

To find out whether a patient's lung cancer has spread to the lymph nodes in the chest, the doctor removes a sample of tissue. In some patients, this can be done with a needle; in others, the doctor will need to perform surgery. Surgery to biopsy lymph nodes in the chest can often be done through a small incision near the breastbone. This procedure is called mediastinoscopy when the incision is above the breastbone and mediastinotomy when the incision is on one side of the breastbone. If a thoracotomy is planned, the doctor removes lymph nodes during the operation. Patients receive a general anesthetic for any of these operations.

Doctors may order CT scans to detect the spread of lung cancer to the lymph nodes and other parts of the body. Radionuclide scans of the bones, brain, or liver also may help doctors find out whether the cancer has spread. In these tests, a small amount of radioactive material is injected into a vein. A machine then scans the body to measure the radiation and reveal abnormal areas.

In another technique, called MRI (magnetic resonance imaging), a strong magnet linked to a computer is used to produce images. Doctors may order MRI to see whether lung cancer has spread to the brain or spinal cord.

TREATMENT

The doctor develops a treatment plan to fit each patient's needs. This plan depends on many factors, including the type of lung cancer, the size and location of the tumor, and the stage of the disease. The doctor also considers the patient's age, medical history, and general health. (See page 17 for more information about getting a second opinion and planning treatment.)

Most people with cancer want to learn all they can about their disease and their treatment choices so they can take an active part in decisions about their medical care. The doctor is the best person to answer questions about the extent of the cancer, how it can be treated, how successful the treatment is likely to be, and how much it is likely to cost.

The patient also may want to talk with the doctor about taking part in a research study of new treatment methods. Such studies, called clinical trials, are designed to find ways to improve cancer treatment. (For more information about clinical trials, see page 20.)

Many patients find it helps to make a list of questions before seeing the doctor. Taking notes during visits can make it easier to remember what the doctor says. Some patients also find that it helps to have a family member or friend with them—to take part in the discussion, to take notes, or just to listen.

There is a lot to learn about cancer and its treatment. Patients should not feel that they need to understand everything at once. They will have many chances to ask the doctor to explain things that are not clear and to ask for more information. (See page 20 for more on Support for Cancer Patients.)

Methods of Treatment

Surgery, radiation therapy, and chemotherapy are the usual treatments for lung cancer. Surgery is done when it is likely that all of the tumor can be removed. Radiation therapy (also called radiotherapy) is the use of high-energy rays to damage cancer cells and stop them from growing and dividing. Chemotherapy is the use of drugs to kill cancer cells. A patient may have just one form of treatment or a combination, depending on his or her needs. Several specialists may work together as a team to provide treatment.

Three main types of surgery are used in lung cancer treatment. The choice depends on the size and location of the tumor, the extent of the cancer, the general health of the patient, and other factors.

An operation to remove only a small part of the lung is called a segmental or wedge resection. When the surgeon removes an entire lobe of the lung, the procedure is a lobectomy. Pneumonectomy is the removal of an entire lung.

Like surgery, radiation therapy is local treatment; it can affect cancer only in the treated area. The radiation, which comes from a large machine, is usually given five days a week for several weeks. The patient goes to the hospital or clinic each day to receive the treatments.

Chemotherapy is systemic treatment, meaning that the drugs flow through the bloodstream to nearly every part of the body. Most anticancer drugs are injected into a blood vessel or a muscle; some are given by mouth. Chemotherapy is most often given in cycles: a treatment period followed by a recovery period, then another treatment period, and so on.

Usually a patient has chemotherapy as an outpatient at the hospital, at the doctor's office, or at home. However, depending on which drugs the doctor orders and on the patient's health, the patient may need to stay in the hospital for a few days so that the drugs' side effects can be watched.

Treating Nonsmall Cell Lung Cancer

Patients with nonsmall cell lung cancer may be treated in several ways. The choice of treatment depends mainly on the extent of the disease.

Surgery is the usual treatment for patients whose cancer is in only one lung or in one lung and the closest lymph nodes. Patients who cannot have surgery because of other medical problems and patients with large tumors often receive radiation therapy. Radiation therapy also is the usual treatment for patients whose cancer has spread within the chest—to more distant lymph nodes or other tissues. Some patients have both surgery and radiation therapy.

Doctors may use radiation therapy and chemotherapy to treat patients whose cancer has spread from the lung to other parts of the body. Although it is very hard to control lung cancer that has spread, treatment can often shrink the tumors. This can help relieve pain and other symptoms.

Treating Small Cell Lung Cancer

Small cell lung cancer spreads quickly. In most cases, cancer cells have already spread to distant parts of the body when the disease is diagnosed. To be sure that treatment affects all cancer cells, doctors generally use chemotherapy, even when the disease appears to be limited to the lung and nearby lymph nodes. Usually, chemotherapy for small cell lung cancer includes a combination of two or more anticancer drugs.

In many cases, treatment also includes radiation therapy—to shrink or destroy the primary tumor in the lung or tumors elsewhere in the body (such as in the brain). Some patients have radiation therapy to the brain even though no cancer is found there. This treatment, called prophylactic cranial irradiation or PCI, is given to prevent tumors from forming in the brain. Usually, PCI is reserved for patients whose lung tumor has responded well to treatment.

Surgery also can be part of the treatment plan for small cell lung cancer. This treatment is appropriate only for a small number of patients.

SIDE EFFECTS OF TREATMENT

It is hard to limit the effects of cancer therapy so that only cancer cells are removed or destroyed. Because treatment also damages healthy cells and tissues, it often causes unpleasant side effects.

The side effects of cancer treatment vary. They depend mainly on the type and extent of the treatment. Also, each person reacts differently to treatment. Doctors try to plan the patient's therapy to keep side effects to a minimum. Doctors and nurses can explain the side effects of cancer treatment and can suggest ways to deal with them.

Surgery

Surgery for lung cancer is a major operation. It may take several weeks or months for patients to regain their energy and strength. This recovery time differs from patient to patient. The doctor and nurse will explain what will happen and what they and the patient can do to make recovery easier.

Doctors can prescribe medicine to control pain after surgery. The doctor or nurse also may suggest other ways to reduce discomfort. Patients should feel free to ask what can be done to relieve their pain or discomfort.

After lung surgery, air and fluid tend to collect in the chest. The air and fluid are drained out through flexible tubes put in place during surgery. Patients also are helped to turn, cough, and breathe deeply. All of these procedures are important for recovery because they help expand the remaining lung tissue and get rid of excess air and fluid.

Generally, patients who have had lung surgery receive respiratory therapy—treatments and exercises to keep the lungs expanded and prevent fluid buildup. Patients may feel short of breath because they have less

lung tissue to supply the body with oxygen. For this reason, they may have to limit their activities for some time. In most cases, the remaining lung tissue gradually expands somewhat, making it easier to breathe.

After surgery, the muscles of the chest and the arm on the affected side may become weak. Special exercises can help the patient regain strength in these muscles.

Radiation Therapy

Patients often become very tired during radiation therapy, especially in the later weeks of treatment. Resting is important, but doctors usually advise their patients to try to stay as active as they can.

It also is common for the skin in the treated area to become red, dry, tender, and itchy. There may be permanent darkening or "bronzing" in the treated area. The skin should be exposed to the air but protected from the sun, and patients should avoid wearing clothes that rub or irritate the treated area. Good skin care is important at this time, and patients will be shown how to keep the area clean. They should not use any lotion or cream on the skin without the doctor's advice.

During radiation therapy for lung cancer and for a short time afterward, patients may have a dry, sore throat, and it may be difficult to swallow. Many find it helpful to eat soft foods and drink extra liquids until these problems go away.

Radiation therapy to the lungs can cause certain permanent changes in lung tissues. These changes, called radiation fibrosis, tend to occur several months after the treatment is over. Fibrosis, which is similar to scarring, can interfere with the ability of the lung to supply the body with oxygen. Patients who have this problem may have to limit their activities.

Chemotherapy

The side effects of chemotherapy depend mainly on the drugs the patient is given. In addition, as with other types of treatment, side effects vary from person to person. Generally, anticancer drugs affect cells that divide rapidly. These include blood cells, which fight infection, help the blood to clot, or carry oxygen to all parts of the body. When blood cells are affected by anticancer drugs, patients are more likely to get infections, may bruise or bleed easily, and may have less energy. Cells in hair roots and cells that line the digestive tract also divide rapidly. When chemotherapy affects these cells, it can cause hair loss and other problems such as nausea and vomiting. Usually these side effects go away gradually during the recovery period or after treatment stops.

To help withstand the side effects of treatment in general, it is important that patients maintain good nutrition (see Nutrition for Cancer Patients, page 19).

THE PROMISE OF CANCER RESEARCH

Researchers at hospitals and medical centers all across the country are studying lung cancer. They are learning more about what causes this disease and how to prevent it. They also are looking for better ways to detect and treat it.

Cause and Prevention

Scientists are continuing to identify factors that may increase the risk for lung cancer. For example, certain genetic traits make some people very sensitive to carcinogens. Smokers with these traits may be more likely than other smokers to develop lung cancer.

Researchers also are studying ways to help people lower their risk of lung cancer. An important area of study is chemoprevention—the use of natural and synthetic substances to prevent or delay cancer. Vitamin A and substances like it may offer some protection against lung cancer. Other substances also are being studied. However, more research is needed, and some vitamins can be dangerous if taken in large doses. It is best to get a doctor's advice before taking vitamins or other nutrients.

Currently, the best way to prevent lung cancer is not to smoke. The National Cancer Institute, the American Cancer Society, and other organizations have programs designed to reduce the number of smokers. If these efforts are successful, far fewer people will develop and die of lung cancer each year.

Detection

The earlier cancer is detected, the more successful treatment is likely to be. However, lung cancer is difficult to diagnose at an early stage. For this reason, scientists are studying ways of checking for lung cancer in people who have no symptoms of the disease. This is called screening. The goal of screening is to detect lung cancer before symptoms appear so that it can be treated as early as possible. Whether successful screening methods for this disease can be developed is not yet known.

Treatment

Because lung cancer is so hard to control, researchers are looking for more effective treatments. They also are exploring ways to reduce the side effects of treatment and improve the quality of patients' lives. When laboratory research shows that a new method has promise, cancer patients can receive the treatment in clinical trials. These trials are designed to find out whether the new approach is both safe and effective and to answer scientific questions. Some clinical trials compare a new treatment with a standard approach. Patients who take part in clinical trials make an important contribution to medical science and may have the first chance to benefit from improved treatment methods.

Trials are under way to study new treatments for patients with all stages of lung cancer. Some trials involve treatments to shrink or destroy the primary tumor. In others, scientists are testing ways to prevent lung cancer from coming back in the chest or spreading to other parts of the body after the primary tumor has been treated. Still others involve treatments to slow or stop the spread of lung cancer.

Researchers are studying the timing of treatments and new ways to combine various types of treatment. They also are trying new anticancer drugs and drug combinations, new forms of radiation therapy, and drugs that make cancer cells more sensitive to radiation. Another method under study is photodynamic therapy. In this treatment, cancer cells are destroyed with a combination of laser light and light-sensitive drugs. Other types of laser therapy are being studied as a way to open the airways in patients whose tumors block the bronchi. Some researchers also are working with biological therapy. This type of treatment includes efforts to help the body's immune system fight cancer more effectively or to protect the body from some of the side effects of treatment.

The National Cancer Institute

MULTIPLE MYELOMA

Multiple myeloma is a type of cancer that affects certain white blood cells called plasma cells. To understand multiple myeloma, it is helpful to know about normal cells, especially plasma cells, and what happens when they become cancerous.

Normal Cells

The body is made up of many kinds of cells. Each type of cell has special functions. Normal cells are produced in an orderly, controlled way as the body needs them. This process keeps us healthy.

Plasma cells and other white blood cells are part of the immune system, which helps protect the body from infection and disease. All white blood cells begin their development in the bone marrow, the soft, spongy tis-

sue that fills the center of most bones. Certain white blood cells leave the bone marrow and mature in other parts of the body. Some of these develop into plasma cells when the immune system needs them to fight substances that cause infection and disease.

Plasma cells produce antibodies, proteins that move through the bloodstream to help the body get rid of harmful substances. Each type of plasma cell responds to only one specific substance by making a large amount of one kind of antibody. These antibodies find and act against that one substance. Because the body has many types of plasma cells, it can respond to many substances.

Cancerous Cells

Cancer is a group of diseases with one thing in common: Cells become abnormal and are produced in large amounts. Cancerous cells interfere with the growth and functions of normal cells. In addition, they can spread from one part of the body to another.

Myeloma Cells

When cancer involves plasma cells, the body keeps producing more and more of these cells. The unneeded plasma cells—all abnormal and all exactly alike—are called myeloma cells.

Myeloma cells tend to collect in the bone marrow and in the hard, outer part of bones. Sometimes they collect in only one bone and form a single mass, or tumor, called a plasmacytoma. In most cases, however, the myeloma cells collect in many bones, often forming many tumors and causing other problems. When this happens, the disease is called multiple myeloma.

It is important to keep in mind that cancer is classified by the type of cell or the part of the body in which the disease begins. Although plasmacytoma and multiple myeloma affect the bones, they begin in cells of the immune system. These cancers are different from bone cancer, which actually begins in cells that form the hard, outer part of bone.

This fact is important because the diagnosis and treatment of plasmacytoma and multiple myeloma are different from the diagnosis and treatment of bone cancer.

Because multiple myeloma patients have an abnormally large number of identical plasma cells, they also have too much of one type of antibody. These myeloma cells and antibodies can cause serious medical problems.

- As myeloma cells increase in number, they damage and weaken bones, causing pain and sometimes fractures. Bone pain can make it difficult for patients to move.
- When bones are damaged, calcium is released into the blood. This may lead to hypercalcemia (too much calcium in the blood). Hypercalcemia can cause loss of appetite, nausea, thirst, fatigue, muscle weakness, restlessness, and confusion.
- Myeloma cells prevent the bone marrow from forming normal plasma cells and other white blood cells that are important to the immune system. Patients may not be able to fight infection and disease.
- The cancer cells also may prevent the growth of new red blood cells, causing anemia. Patients with anemia may feel unusually tired or weak.
- Multiple myeloma patients may have serious problems with their kidneys. Excess antibody proteins and calcium can prevent the kidneys from filtering and cleaning the blood properly.

In certain cases, excess antibody proteins can increase the blood's viscosity, causing problems with oxygen delivery to the tissues.

SYMPTOMS

Symptoms of multiple myeloma depend on how advanced the disease is. In the earliest stage of the disease, there may be no symptoms. When symptoms do occur, patients commonly have bone pain, often in the back or ribs. Patients also may have broken bones, weakness, fatigue, weight loss, or repeated infections. When the disease is advanced, symptoms may include nausea, vomiting, problems with urination, constipation, and weakness or numbness in the legs. These are not sure signs of multiple myeloma; they can be symptoms of other types of medical problems. A person should see a doctor if these symptoms occur. Only a doctor can determine what is causing a patient's symptoms.

DIAGNOSIS

Multiple myeloma may be found as part of a routine physical exam before patients have symptoms of the disease. When patients do have symptoms, the doctor asks about their personal and family medical history and does a complete physical exam. In addition to checking general signs of health, the doctor may order a number of tests to determine the cause of the symptoms. If a patient has bone pain, x-rays can show whether any bones are damaged or broken. Samples of the patient's blood and urine are checked to see whether they contain high levels of antibody proteins that doctors call M proteins. The doctor also may do a bone marrow aspiration and/or a bone marrow biopsy to check for myeloma cells.

In an aspiration, the doctor inserts a needle into the hip bone or breast bone to withdraw a sample of fluid and cells from the bone marrow. To do a biopsy, the doctor uses a larger needle to remove a sample of solid tissue from the marrow. A pathologist examines the samples under a microscope to see whether myeloma cells are present.

To plan a patient's treatment, the doctor needs to know the stage, or extent, of the disease. Staging is a careful attempt to find out what parts of the body are affected by the cancer. Treatment decisions depend on these

findings. Results of the patient's exam, blood tests, and bone marrow tests can help doctors determine the stage of the disease. In addition, staging usually involves a series of x-rays to determine the number and size of tumors in the bones. In some cases, a patient will have an imaging test (MRI) if close-up views of the bones are needed.

TREATMENT

Treatment depends on the extent of the cancer and the patient's symptoms. The doctor also considers the person's age and general health. The doctor may want to discuss the patient's case with other doctors who treat multiple myeloma. (See page 17 for more information about getting a second opinion and planning treatment.) Also, the patient may want to talk with the doctor about taking part in a research study of new treatment methods. Such studies, called clinical trials, are designed to improve the treatment of this type of cancer. (For more information about clinical trials, see page 20.)

Methods of Treatment

Plasmacytomas and multiple myeloma are very hard to cure. Although patients who have a plasmacytoma may be free of symptoms for a long time after treatment, many eventually develop multiple myeloma. For those who have multiple myeloma, treatment can improve the quality of a patient's life by controlling the symptoms and complications of the disease.

People who have multiple myeloma but do not have symptoms of the disease usually do not receive treatment. For these patients, the risks and side effects of treatment are likely to outweigh the possible benefits. However, these patients are watched closely, and they begin treatment when symptoms appear. Patients who need treatment for multiple myeloma usually receive chemotherapy and sometimes radiation therapy.

Chemotherapy is the use of drugs to treat cancer. It is the main treatment for multiple myeloma. Doctors may prescribe two or more drugs that work together to kill myeloma cells. Many of these drugs are taken by mouth; others are injected into a blood vessel. Either way, the drugs travel through the bloodstream, reaching myeloma cells in many parts of the body. For this reason, chemotherapy is called systemic therapy.

Anticancer drugs often are given in cycles: a treatment period followed by a rest period, then another treatment and rest period, and so on. Most patients take their chemotherapy at home, as outpatients at the hospital, or at the doctor's office. However, depending on their health and the drugs being given, patients may need to stay in the hospital during treatment.

Radiation therapy (also called radiotherapy) uses high-energy rays to damage cancer cells and stop them from growing. In this form of treatment, a large machine aims the high-energy rays at a tumor and the area close to it. Treatment with radiation is local therapy; it affects only the cells in the treated area.

Radiation therapy is the main treatment for people who have a single plasmacytoma. They usually receive radiation therapy on weekdays for four to five weeks in the outpatient department of a hospital or clinic.

People who have multiple myeloma sometimes receive radiation therapy in addition to chemotherapy. The purpose of the radiation therapy is to help control the growth of tumors in the bones and relieve the pain that these tumors cause. Treatment usually lasts for one to two weeks.

Treatment Studies

Because multiple myeloma is so hard to control, many researchers are looking for more effective treatments. They also are looking for treatments that have fewer side effects and for better ways to care for patients who have complications caused by this disease. When laboratory research shows that a new method has promise, doctors use it to treat cancer patients in clinical trials. These trials are designed to answer scientific questions and to find out whether the new approach is both safe and effective. Patients who take part in clinical trials make an important contribution to medical science and may have the first chance to benefit from improved treatment methods.

Many clinical trials of new treatments for multiple myeloma are under way. In some studies, doctors are testing new drugs and new drug combinations. In others, they are using chemotherapy along with biological therapy, treatment with substances that boost the immune system's response to cancer.

Researchers also are testing new approaches to cancer treatment that allow the use of very high doses of anticancer drugs, sometimes along with radiation. Doctors believe that higher doses of anticancer drugs and radiation might be more effective than the usual doses in destroying myeloma cells.

However, higher doses also cause greater damage to healthy bone marrow. New approaches to treatment may help the healthy marrow recover or may allow doctors to replace marrow that is destroyed. Patients interested in taking part in a clinical trial should discuss this option with their doctor.

Side Effects of Treatment

The methods used to treat multiple myeloma are very powerful. Treatment can help patients feel better by relieving symptoms such as bone pain. However, it is hard to limit the effects of therapy so that only cancer cells are destroyed. Because healthy cells also may be damaged, treatment can cause unpleasant side effects.

The side effects that patients have during cancer treatment vary for each person. They may even be different from one treatment to the next. Doctors try to plan treatment to keep side effects to a minimum. They also monitor patients very carefully so they can help with any problems that occur.

The side effects of chemotherapy depend on the drugs that are given. In general, anti-cancer drugs affect rapidly growing cells, such as blood cells that fight infection, cells that line the digestive tract, and cells in hair follicles. As a result, patients may have lower resistance to infection, loss of appetite, nausea, vomiting, or mouth sores. Patients also may have less energy and may lose their hair. One drug used to treat multiple myeloma, called prednisone, may cause swelling of the face and feet, burning indigestion, mood swings, restlessness, and acne. The side effects of chemotherapy usually go away over time after treatment stops.

During radiation therapy, the patient may be more tired than usual. Resting as much as possible is important. Also, the skin in the treated area may become red or dry. The skin should be exposed to the air but protected from the sun, and patients should avoid wearing clothes that rub the treated area. They should not use any lotion or cream on the skin without the doctor's advice.

Patients may have other side effects, depending upon the areas treated. For example, radiation to the lower back may cause nausea, vomiting, or diarrhea because the lower digestive tract is exposed to radiation. The doctor often can prescribe medicine or suggest changes in diet to ease these problems. Side effects usually disappear gradually after radiation therapy is over.

To help withstand the side effects of treatment in general, it is important that patients maintain good nutrition (see Nutrition for Cancer Patients, page 19).

SUPPORTIVE CARE

The complications of multiple myeloma can affect many parts of the body. Chemotherapy and radiation therapy often can help control complications such as pain, bone damage, and kidney problems. However, from time to time, most patients need additional treatment to manage these and other problems caused by the disease. This type of treatment, called supportive care, is given to improve patients' comfort and quality of life.

Multiple myeloma patients frequently have pain caused by bone damage or by tumors pressing on nerves. Doctors often suggest that patients take pain medicine and/or wear a back or neck brace to help relieve their pain. Some patients find that techniques such as relaxation and imagery can reduce their pain.

Preventing or treating bone fractures is another important part of supportive care. Because exercise can reduce the loss of calcium from the bones, doctors and nurses encourage patients to be active, if possible. They may suggest appropriate forms of exercise.

If a patient has a fracture or a breakdown of certain bones, especially those in the spine, a surgeon may need to operate to remove as much of the cancer as possible and to strengthen the bone.

Patients who have hypercalcemia may be given medicine to reduce the level of calcium in the blood. They also are encouraged to drink large amounts of fluids every day; some may need intravenous (IV) fluids. Getting plenty of fluids helps the kidneys get rid of excess calcium in the blood. It also helps prevent problems that occur when calcium collects in the kidneys.

If the kidneys aren't working well, dialysis or plasmapheresis may be necessary. In dialysis, the patient's blood passes through a machine that removes wastes, and the blood is then returned to the patient. Plasmapheresis is used to remove excess antibodies produced by the myeloma cells. This thins the blood, making it easier for the kidneys and the heart to function.

Multiple myeloma weakens the immune system. Patients must be very careful to protect themselves from infection. It is important that they stay out of crowds and away from people with colds or other infectious diseases. Any sign of infection (fever, sore throat, cough) should be reported to the doctor right away. Patients who develop infections are treated with antibiotics or other drugs.

Patients who have anemia may have transfusions of red blood cells. Transfusions can help reduce the shortness of breath and fatigue that can be caused by anemia. (See page 20 for more on Support for Cancer Patients.)

FOLLOW-UP CARE

Regular follow-up is very important for anyone who has multiple myeloma. Checkups generally include a physical exam, x-rays, and blood and urine tests. Regular follow-up exams help doctors detect and treat problems promptly if they should arise. It is also important for the patient to tell the doctor about any new symptoms or problems that develop between checkups.

POSSIBLE CAUSES

Scientists at hospitals, medical schools, and research laboratories across the country are studying multiple myeloma. At this time, we do not know what causes this disease or how to prevent it. However, we do know that no one can "catch" multiple myeloma from another person; cancer is not contagious.

Although scientists cannot explain why one person gets multiple myeloma and another doesn't, we do know that most multiple myeloma patients are between the ages of 50 and 70. This disease affects blacks more often than whites and men more often than women.

Some research suggests that certain risk factors increase a person's chance of getting multiple myeloma. For example, a person's family background appears to affect the risk of developing multiple myeloma; children or brothers and sisters of patients who have this disease have a slightly increased risk. Farmers and petroleum workers exposed to certain chemicals also seem to have a higher-than-average chance of getting multiple myeloma.

In addition, people exposed to large amounts of radiation (such as survivors of the atomic bomb explosions in Japan) have an increased risk for this disease. Scientists have some concern that smaller amounts of radiation (such as those radiologists and workers in nuclear plants are exposed to) also may increase the risk. At this time, however, scientists do not have clear evidence that large numbers of medical x-rays increase the risk for multiple myeloma. In fact, most people receive a fairly small number of x-rays, and scientists believe that the benefits of medical x-rays far outweigh the possible risk for multiple myeloma.

In most cases, people who develop multiple myeloma have no clear risk factors. The disease may be the result of several factors (known and/or unknown) acting together.

The National Cancer Institute

NON-HODGKIN'S LYMPHOMAS

"Lymphoma" is a general term for cancers that develop in the lymphatic system. They account for about 4 percent of all cases of cancer in this country.

The most common type of lymphoma is called Hodgkin's disease. All other lymphomas are grouped together and are called non-Hodgkin's lymphomas.

The lymphatic system is part of the body's immune defense system. Its job is to help fight diseases and infection. The lymphatic system is made up of a network of thin tubes that branch, like blood vessels, into tissues throughout the body.

Lymphatic vessels carry lymph, a colorless, watery fluid that contains infection fighting cells called lymphocytes. Along this network of vessels are groups of small, bean-shaped organs called lymph nodes. Clusters of lymph nodes are found in the underarm, groin, neck, chest, and abdomen.

Other parts of the lymphatic system are the spleen, thymus gland, tonsils, and bone marrow. Lymphatic tissue is also found in other parts of the body, including the stomach, intestines, and skin.

Like all types of cancer, lymphomas are diseases of the body's cells. Healthy cells grow, divide, and replace themselves in an orderly manner. This process keeps the body in good repair.

In the non-Hodgkin's lymphomas, cells in the lymphatic system begin growing abnormally. They divide too rapidly and grow without any order or control. Too much tissue is formed, and tumors begin to grow. The cancer cells can also spread to other organs.

SYMPTOMS

The most common symptom of non-Hodgkin's lymphomas is a painless swelling in the lymph nodes in the neck, underarm, or groin. Other symptoms may include fevers, night sweats, tiredness, weight loss, itching, and reddened patches on the skin. Sometimes there is nausea, vomiting, or abdominal pain. As lymphomas progress, the body is less able to fight infection.

These symptoms are not sure signs of cancer, however. They may also be caused by many common illnesses, such as the flu or other infections. But it is important to see a doctor if any of these symptoms lasts longer than two weeks. Any illness should be diagnosed and treated as early as possible.

DIAGNOSIS

The doctor asks about the patient's medical history and does a thorough physical exam. The only sure way to tell whether cancer is present is with a biopsy. Tissue from an enlarged lymph node will be removed. By examining these tissues under the microscope, a pathologist can identify the cancer cells and tell whether the lymphoma is the kind that usually grows slowly or rapidly.

There are at least 10 types of non-Hodgkin's lymphomas. Often they are grouped into three categories by how fast they grow: low grade (slow growing), intermediate grade, and high grade (rapidly growing).

When lymphoma is diagnosed, the doctor needs to know what kind it is and the stage, or extent, of the disease. This information is very important for planning treatment. The stage indicates where the disease has spread and how much tissue is affected. The doctor checks:

• The number and location of affected lymph nodes
• Whether the affected lymph nodes are above, below, or on both sides of the diaphragm (the thin muscle under the lungs and heart that separates the chest from the abdomen)
• Whether the disease has spread to the bone marrow or organs outside the lymphatic system, such as the liver

In staging, the doctor usually orders blood tests and x-rays of the chest, bones, liver, and spleen. Other special tests include additional biopsies of the lymph nodes, bone marrow, and other sites. Most patients have lymphangiograms, x-rays of the lymphatic system using a special dye to outline the lymph nodes and vessels. The doctor may also order a CT scan, a series of x-rays put together by a computer. Ultrasonography may also be used. This test creates pictures of internal organs using echoes of high-frequency sound waves.

TREATMENT

Treatment decisions for non-Hodgkin's lymphomas are complex. Before starting treatment, the patient might want a specialist who treats lymphomas to review the diagnosis and treatment plan. (See also Preparing for Treatment, page 17.)

Methods of Treatment

Treatment planning takes into account the type of lymphoma, the stage of disease, whether it is likely to grow slowly or rapidly, and the general health and age of the patient. Often patients are referred to medical centers that specialize in treating lymphomas.

For low-grade lymphomas that usually grow very slowly and cause few symptoms, the doctor may decide to wait until the disease shows signs of spreading before starting treatment.

Treatment for intermediate or high-grade lymphomas usually involves chemotherapy, with or without radiation therapy. In addition, surgery may be needed to remove a large tumor.

Chemotherapy is the use of drugs to kill cancer cells. Chemotherapy for non-Hodgkin's lymphomas usually consists of a combination of several drugs. Some drugs are given by mouth; others are injected into a blood vessel or muscle. The drugs travel through the bloodstream to almost every part of the body. Chemotherapy is usually given in cycles: a treatment period followed by a rest period, then another treatment period, and so on.

Radiation therapy uses high-energy rays to damage cancer cells and stop their growth. Radiation therapy is generally given in the outpatient department of a hospital or clinic. Most often, patients receive radiation therapy five days a week for five to six weeks.

Side Effects of Treatment

The methods used to treat lymphomas are very powerful. That's why treatment often causes side effects. Fortunately, most side effects are temporary.

The side effects of chemotherapy depend on the drugs given and the individual response of the patient. Chemotherapy commonly affects rapidly growing cells, such as blood-forming cells and cells that line the digestive tract. As a result, patients may have side effects, such as lowered resistance to infection, loss of appetite, nausea and vomiting, and mouth sores. They may also lose their hair. These side effects usually end after chemotherapy is finished.

During radiation therapy, patients may notice a number of side effects. They may become unusually tired as the treatment continues. Getting enough rest is important. Skin reactions (redness or dryness) in the area being treated are also common. Patients should be gentle with the treated area of skin. Lotions and creams should not be used without the doctor's advice. When the chest and neck area is treated, patients may have a dry, sore throat, and may have some trouble swallowing. Sometimes they have shortness of breath or a dry cough. Radiation therapy to the abdomen may cause nausea, vomiting, or diarrhea. Some patients may have tingling or numbness in their arms, legs, and lower back. These side effects gradually disappear when treatment is over.

To help withstand the side effects of treatment, it is important that patients maintain good nutrition (see Nutrition for Cancer Patients, page 19).

FOLLOW-UP CARE

Regular follow-up exams are very important for anyone who has been treated for non-Hodgkin's lymphoma. Most relapses occur in the first two years after therapy.

Generally, checkups include a careful physical exam, x-rays, blood tests, and other laboratory tests. Patients should follow their doctor's recommendations on health care and checkups. Having regular checkups allows problems to be detected and treated promptly if they should arise.

LIVING WITH CANCER

When people have cancer, life can change for them and for the people who care about them. These changes in daily life can be difficult to handle. (See Support for Cancer Patients, page 20.)

WHAT THE FUTURE HOLDS

More than 8 million Americans living today have had some type of cancer. Thirty years ago, few patients recovered from non-Hodgkin's lymphoma. Because of advances in combination chemotherapy and radiation therapy, about half of all non-Hodgkin's lymphoma patients now survive. As scientists find new and more effective treatments, the chances for recovery continue to improve.

The National Cancer Institute

ORAL CANCER

Cancer may originate in the oral cavity (mouth) and the oropharynx (the part of the throat at the back of the mouth). The oral cavity includes many parts: the lips; the lining inside the lips and cheeks, called the buccal mucosa; the teeth; the bottom (floor) of the mouth under the tongue; the front two-thirds of the tongue; the bony top of the mouth (hard palate); the gums; and the small area behind the wisdom teeth. The oropharynx includes the back one-third of the tongue, the soft palate, the tonsils, and the back of the throat. Salivary glands throughout the oral cavity make saliva, which keeps the mouth moist and helps digest food.

When oral cancer spreads, it usually travels through the lymphatic system. Cancer cells that enter the lymphatic system are carried along by lymph, an almost colorless, watery fluid containing cells that help the body fight infection and disease. Along the lymphatic channels are groups of small, bean-shaped organs called lymph nodes (sometimes called lymph glands). Oral cancer that spreads usually travels to the lymph nodes in the neck. It can also spread to other parts of the body. Cancer that spreads is the same disease and has the same name as the original (primary) cancer.

EARLY DETECTION

Regular checkups that include an examination of the entire mouth can detect precancerous conditions or the early stages of oral cancer. Your doctor and dentist should check the tissues in your mouth as part of your routine exams.

SYMPTOMS

Oral cancer usually occurs in people over the age of 45 but can develop at any age. These are some warning signs to watch for:

- A sore in the mouth that does not heal
- A lump on the lip or in the mouth or throat
- Unusual bleeding, pain, or numbness in the mouth
- A white or red patch on the gums, tongue, or lining of the mouth
- Sore throat that does not go away, or a feeling that something is caught in the throat
- Difficulty or pain chewing or swallowing
- A change in the voice or pain in the ear
- Swelling of the jaw that causes dentures to fit poorly or become uncomfortable

Any of these symptoms may be caused by cancer or by other, less serious problems. It is important to see a dentist or doctor about any symptoms like these, so that the problem can be diagnosed and treated as early as possible.

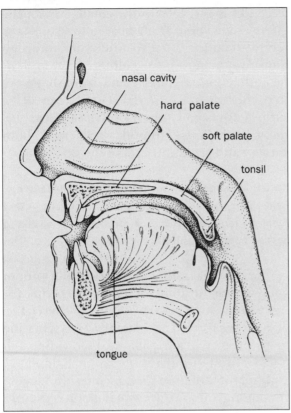

nasal cavity

hard palate

soft palate

tonsil

tongue

Cancer may develop anywhere within the oral cavity. Oral cancers are rare among people under 40; they are most likely to develop in those over 60.

DIAGNOSIS

If an abnormal area has been found in the oral cavity, a biopsy is the only way to know whether it is cancer. Usually, the patient is referred to an oral surgeon or an ear, nose, and throat surgeon, who removes part or all of the lump or abnormal-looking area. A pathologist examines the tissue under a microscope to check for cancer cells.

Almost all oral cancers are squamous cell carcinomas. Squamous cells line the oral cavity. If the pathologist finds oral cancer, the patient's doctor needs to know the stage, or extent, of the disease in order to plan the best treatment. Staging tests and exams help the doctor find out whether the cancer has spread and what parts of the body are affected.

Staging generally includes dental x-rays and x-rays of the head and chest. The doctor may also want the patient to have a CT scan. A CT scan is a series of x-rays put together by a computer to form detailed pictures of areas inside the body. Ultrasonography is another way to produce pictures of areas in the body. High-frequency sound waves (ultrasound), which cannot be heard by humans, are bounced off organs and tissue. The pattern of echoes produced by these waves creates a picture called a sonogram.

Sometimes the doctor asks for MRI (magnetic resonance imaging), a procedure in which pictures are created using a magnet linked to a computer. The doctor also feels the lymph nodes in the neck to check for swelling or other changes. In most cases, the patient will have a complete physical examination before treatment begins. (See page 17 for more information about getting a second opinion and planning treatment.)

TREATMENT

After diagnosis and staging, the doctor develops a treatment plan to fit each patient's needs. Treatment for oral cancer depends on a number of factors. Among these are the location, size, type, and extent of the tumor and the stage of the disease. The doctor also considers the patient's age and general health. Treatment involves surgery, radiation therapy, or, in many cases, a combination of the two. Some patients receive chemotherapy, treatment with anticancer drugs.

For most patients, it is important to have a complete dental exam before cancer treatment begins. Because cancer treatment may make the mouth sensitive and more easily infected, doctors often advise patients to have any needed dental work done before treatment begins.

Most people with cancer want to learn all they can about their disease and their treatment choices so they can take an active part in decisions about their medical and dental care. The doctor is the best person to answer their questions. Also, the patient may want to talk with the doctor about taking part in a research study (clinical trial) of new treatment methods.

Methods of Treatment

Patients with oral cancer may be treated by a team of specialists. The medical team may include an oral surgeon; an ear, nose, and throat surgeon; a medical oncologist; a radiation oncologist; a prosthodontist; a general dentist; a plastic surgeon; a dietitian; a social worker; a nurse; and a speech therapist.

Surgery to remove the tumor in the mouth is the usual treatment for patients with oral cancer. If there is evidence that the cancer has spread, the surgeon may also remove lymph nodes in the neck. If the disease has spread to muscles and other tissues in the neck, the operation may be more extensive.

Radiation therapy (also called radiotherapy) is the use of high-energy rays to damage cancer cells and stop them from growing. Like surgery, radiation therapy is local therapy; it affects only the cells in the treated area. The energy may come from a large machine (external radiation). It can also come from radioactive materials placed directly into or near the tumor (internal radiation). Radiation therapy is sometimes used instead of surgery for small tumors in the mouth. Patients with large tumors may need both surgery and radiation therapy.

Radiation therapy may be given before or after surgery. Before surgery, radiation can shrink the tumor so that it can be removed. Radiation after surgery is used to destroy cancer cells that may remain.

For external radiation therapy, the patient goes to the hospital or clinic each day for treatments. Usually, treatment is given five days a week for five to six weeks. This schedule helps protect healthy tissues by dividing the total amount of radiation into small doses.

Implant radiation therapy puts tiny "seeds" containing radioactive material directly into the tumor or in tissue near it. Generally, an implant is left in place for several days, and the patient will stay in the hospital in a private room. The length of time nurses and other caregivers, as well as visitors, can spend with the patient will be limited. The implant is removed before the patient goes home.

Chemotherapy is the use of drugs to kill cancer cells. Researchers are looking for effective drugs or drug combinations to treat oral cancer. They are also exploring ways to combine chemotherapy with other forms of cancer treatment to help destroy the tumor and prevent the disease from spreading.

Clinical Trials

Researchers are conducting clinical trials to study the timing of treatments and new ways to combine various types of treatment. For example, they are trying to increase the effectiveness of radiation therapy by giving treatments twice a day instead of once a day.

IMPORTANT QUESTIONS

Before surgery, the patient may want to ask the doctor these questions:

- **What kind of operation will it be?**
- **How will I feel after the operation? If I have pain, how will you help me?**
- **Will I have trouble eating?**
- **Where will the scars be? What will they look like?**
- **Do you expect that there will be long-term effects from the surgery?**
- **Will there be permanent changes in my appearance?**
- **Will I lose any teeth? Can they be replaced? How soon?**
- **If I need to have plastic surgery, when can that be done?**
- **Will I need to see a specialist for help with my speech?**
- **When can I get back to my normal activities?**

They are also working with hyperthermia (heat) and with drugs called radiosensitizers to try to make cancer cells more sensitive to radiation. Researchers are also using drugs to help protect normal cells from radiation damage. In addition, they are exploring various new anticancer drugs and drug combinations.

People who have had oral cancer have an increased risk of getting a new cancer of the mouth or another part of the head or neck. Doctors are trying to find ways to prevent these new cancers. Some research has shown that a substance related to vitamin A may prevent a new cancer from developing in someone who has already been successfully treated for oral cancer. Oral cancer patients who are interested in taking part in a trial should talk with their doctor. (For more information about clinical trials, see page 20.)

SIDE EFFECTS OF TREATMENT
It is hard to limit the effects of cancer treatment so that only cancer cells are removed or destroyed. Because healthy cells and tissues may also be damaged, treatment often causes unpleasant side effects.

The side effects of cancer treatment vary. They depend mainly on the type and extent of the treatment and the specific area being treated. Also, each person reacts differently. Some side effects are temporary; others are permanent. Doctors try to plan the patient's therapy to keep side effects to a minimum. They also watch patients very carefully so they can help with any problems that occur.

Surgery to remove a small tumor in the mouth usually does not cause any lasting problems. For a larger tumor, however, the surgeon may need to remove part of the palate, tongue, or jaw. Such surgery is likely to change the patient's ability to chew, swallow, or talk. The patient may also look different.

After surgery, the patient's face may be swollen. This swelling usually goes away within a few weeks. However, removing lymph nodes can slow the flow of lymph, which may collect in the tissues; this swelling may last for a long time.

Before starting radiation therapy, a patient should see a dentist who is familiar with the changes this therapy can cause in the mouth. Radiation therapy can make the mouth sore. It can also cause changes in the saliva and may reduce the amount of saliva, making it hard to chew and swallow. Because saliva normally protects the teeth, mouth dryness can promote tooth decay. Good mouth care can help keep the teeth and gums healthy and can make the patient feel more comfortable. The health-care team may suggest the use of a special kind of toothbrush or mouthwash. The dentist usually suggests a special fluoride program to keep the teeth healthy.

To help relieve mouth dryness, the health-care team may suggest the use of artificial saliva and other methods to keep the mouth moist. Mouth dryness from radiation therapy goes away in some patients, but it can be permanent.

An oral medication, pilocarpine (Salagen), can be prescribed during radiation therapy to stimulate the saliva glands and help reduce mouth dryness.

Weight loss can be a serious problem for patients being treated for oral cancer, because a sore mouth may make eating difficult. Your doctor may suggest ways to maintain a healthy diet. In many cases, it helps to have food and beverages in very small amounts. Many patients find that eating several small meals and snacks during the day works better than trying to have three large meals. Often it is easier to eat soft, bland foods that have been moistened with sauces or gravies; thick soups, puddings, and high-protein milkshakes are nourishing and easy to swallow. It may be helpful to prepare other foods in a blender. The doctor may also suggest special liquid dietary supplements for patients who have trouble chewing. Drinking lots of fluids helps keep the mouth moist and makes it easier to eat.

Some patients are able to wear their dentures during radiation therapy. Many, however, will not be able to wear dentures for up to a year after treatment. Because the tissues in the mouth that support the denture may change during or after treatment, dentures may no longer fit properly. After treatment is over, a patient may need to have dentures refitted or replaced.

Radiation therapy can also cause sores in the mouth and cracked and peeling lips. These usually heal in the weeks after treatment is completed. Often good mouth care can help prevent these sores. Dentures should not be worn until the sores have healed.

During radiation therapy, patients may become very tired, especially in the later weeks of treatment. Resting is important, but doctors usually advise their patients to try to stay reasonably active. Patients should match their activities to their energy level. It's common for radiation to cause the skin in the treated area to become red, dry, tender, and itchy. Toward the end of treatment, the skin may become moist and "weepy." There may be permanent darkening or "bronzing" of the skin in the treated area. This area should be exposed to the air as much as possible but should also be protected from the sun. Good skin care is important at this time, but patients should not use any lotions or creams without the doctor's advice.

Men may lose all or part of their beard, but facial hair generally grows back after treatment is done. Usually, men shave with an electric razor during treatment to prevent cuts that may lead to infection.

Most effects of radiation therapy on the skin are temporary. The area will heal when the treatment is over.

The side effects of chemotherapy depend on the drugs that are given. In general, anticancer drugs affect rapidly growing cells, such as blood cells that fight infection, cells that line the mouth and the digestive tract, and cells in hair follicles. As a result, patients may have side effects such as lower resistance to infection, loss of appetite, nausea, vomiting, or mouth sores. They also may have less energy and may lose their hair.

The side effects of cancer treatment are different for each person, and they may even be different from one treatment to the next. Doctors, nurses, and dietitians can explain the side effects of cancer treatment and can suggest ways to deal with them. (See page 20 for more on Support for Cancer Patients.)

REHABILITATION

Rehabilitation is a very important part of treatment for patients with oral cancer. The goals of rehabilitation depend on the extent of the disease and the treatment a patient has received. The health-care team makes every effort to help the patient return to normal activities as soon as possible. Rehabilitation may include dietary counseling, surgery, a dental prosthesis, speech therapy, and other services.

Sometimes a patient needs reconstructive and plastic surgery to rebuild the bones or tissues of the mouth. If this is not possible, a prosthodontist may be able to make an artificial dental or facial part (prosthesis). Patients may need special training to use the device.

Speech therapy generally begins as soon as possible for a patient who has trouble speaking after treatment. Often a speech therapist visits the patient in the hospital to plan therapy and teach speech exercises. Speech therapy usually continues after the patient returns home.

FOLLOW-UP CARE

Regular follow-up exams are very important for anyone who has been treated for oral cancer. The physician and the dentist watch the patient closely to check the healing process and to look for signs that the cancer may have returned. Patients with mouth dryness from radiation therapy should have dental exams three times a year.

The patient may need to see a dietitian if weight loss or eating problems continue. Most doctors urge their patients to stop using tobacco and alcohol to reduce the risk of developing a new cancer.

WHAT THE FUTURE HOLDS

Patients and their families are naturally concerned about what the future holds. Sometimes they use statistics to try to figure out whether the patient will be cured or how long he or she will live. It is important to remember, however, that statistics are averages based on large numbers of patients. They cannot be used to predict what will happen to a certain patient because no two cancer patients are alike. The doctor who takes care of the patient knows his or her medical history and is in the best position to discuss the person's outlook (prognosis).

People should feel free to ask the doctor about their chance of recovery, but not even the doctor knows for sure what will happen. When doctors talk about surviving cancer, they may use the term "remission," rather than "cure." Even though many patients with oral cancer recover completely, doctors use this term because oral cancer can recur.

CAUSES AND PREVENTION

Scientists at hospitals and medical centers all across the country are studying this disease to learn more about what causes it and how to prevent it. Doctors do know that no one can "catch" cancer from another person: it is not contagious. Two known causes of oral cancer are tobacco and alcohol use.

Tobacco use—smoking cigarettes, cigars, or pipes; chewing tobacco; or dipping snuff—accounts for 80 to 90 percent of oral cancers. A number of studies have shown that cigar and pipe smokers have the same risk as cigarette smokers.

Studies indicate that smokeless tobacco users are at particular risk of developing oral cancer. For long-time users, the risk is much greater, making the use of snuff or chewing tobacco among young people a special concern.

People who stop using tobacco—even after many years of use—can greatly reduce their risk of oral cancer. Special counseling or self-help groups may be useful for those who are trying to give up tobacco. Some hospitals have groups for people who want to quit. Also, the Cancer Information Service and the American Cancer Society may have information about groups in local areas to help people quit using tobacco.

Chronic and/or heavy use of alcohol also increases the risk of oral cancer, even for people who do not use tobacco. However, people who use both alcohol and tobacco have an especially high risk of oral cancer. Scientists believe that these substances increase each other's harmful effects.

Cancer of the lip can be caused by exposure to the sun. The risk can be avoided with the use of a lotion or lip balm containing a sunscreen. Wearing a hat with a brim can also block the sun's harmful rays. Pipe smokers are especially prone to cancer of the lip.

Some studies have shown that many people who develop oral cancer have a history of leukoplakia, a whitish patch inside the mouth. The causes of leukoplakia are not well understood, but it is commonly associated with heavy use of tobacco and alcohol. The condition often occurs in irritated areas, such as the gums and mouth lining of smokeless tobacco users and the lower lip of pipe smokers.

Another condition, erythroplakia, appears as a red patch in the mouth. Erythroplakia occurs most often in people 60 to 70 years of age. Early diagnosis and treatment of leukoplakia and erythroplakia are important because cancer may develop in these patches.

People who think they might be at risk for developing oral cancer should discuss this concern with their doctor or dentist, who may be able to suggest ways to reduce the risk and plan an appropriate schedule for checkups.

The National Cancer Institute

OVARIAN CANCER

The ovaries are a pair of female reproductive organs. They are located in the pelvis one on each side of the uterus. Each ovary is about the size and shape of an almond. The ovaries have two functions: They produce eggs and female hormones.

Each month, during the menstrual cycle, an egg is released from one ovary. The egg travels from the ovary through a fallopian tube to the uterus. The ovaries are the main source of female hormones (estrogen and progesterone). These hormones control the development of female body characteristics, such as the breasts, body shape, and body hair. They also regulate the menstrual cycle and pregnancy.

Like all other organs of the body, the ovaries are made up of many types of cells. Normally, cells divide to produce more cells only when the body needs them. This orderly process helps keep us healthy. If cells keep dividing when new cells are not needed, a mass of tissue forms. This mass of extra tissue, called a growth, or tumor, can be benign or malignant.

SYMPTOMS

Ovarian cancer is hard to find early. Often there are no symptoms in the early stages and in many cases the cancer has spread by the time it is found. The cancer may grow for some time before it causes pressure, pain, or other problems. Even when symptoms appear, they may be so vague that they are ignored.

As the tumor grows, the woman may feel swollen or bloated, or may have general discomfort in the lower abdomen. The disease may cause a loss of appetite or a feeling of fullness, even after a light meal. Other symptoms may include gas, indigestion, nausea, and weight loss. A large tumor may press on nearby organs, such as the bowel or bladder, causing diarrhea or constipation, or frequent urination. Less often, bleeding from the vagina is a symptom of ovarian cancer.

Ovarian cancer may cause swelling due to a buildup of fluid in the abdomen (ascites). Fluid also may collect around the lungs causing shortness of breath. These symptoms may be caused by cancer or by other, less serious conditions. Only a doctor can tell for sure.

DIAGNOSIS AND STAGING

To find the cause of any symptoms the doctor asks about the woman's medical history and does a careful physical exam including a pelvic exam. The doctor feels the vagina, rectum, and lower abdomen for masses or growths. A Pap smear (a common test for cancer of the cervix) is often part of the pelvic exam, but it is not a reliable way to find or diagnose ovarian cancer. The doctor may also order other tests:

- *Ultrasonography* is the use of highfrequency sound waves. These waves, which cannot be heard by humans, are aimed at the ovaries. The pattern of the echoes they produce creates a picture called a sonogram. Healthy tissues, fluid-filled cysts, and tumors produce different echoes.
- *A CT scan* is a series of x-rays put together by a computer.
- *A lower GI series,* or barium enema, is a series

of x-rays of the colon and rectum. The pictures are taken after the patient is given an enema with a white chalky solution containing barium. The barium outlines the colon and rectum on the x-ray, which helps the doctor see tumors or other abnormal areas.

• *An intravenous pyelogram (IVP)* is an x-ray of the kidneys and ureters taken after the injection of a dye.

Often the doctor orders a blood test to measure a substance in the blood called CA-125. This substance, called a tumor marker, can be produced by ovarian cancer cells. However, CA-125 is not always present in women with ovarian cancer, and it may be present in women who have benign ovarian conditions. Thus, this blood test cannot be used alone to diagnose cancer.

Indeed, a National Institutes of Health consensus conference concluded that neither sonography nor the CA-125 blood test are reliable screening tests for ovarian cancer.

The only sure way to know if cancer is present is for a pathologist to examine a sample of tissue under the microscope. Removing tissue from the body for this examination is called a biopsy. To obtain the tissue, the surgeon does an operation called a laparotomy. If cancer is suspected, the surgeon removes the entire ovary (oophorectomy). This is important because, if the problem is cancer, cutting through the outer layer of the ovary could allow cancer cells to escape and cause the disease to spread. If cancer is found at this time, the surgeon proceeds with surgery, as described on page 88.

During surgery, the surgeon removes nearby lymph nodes, and takes samples of tissue from the diaphragm and other organs in the abdomen. The surgeon also collects fluid from the abdomen. All of these samples are

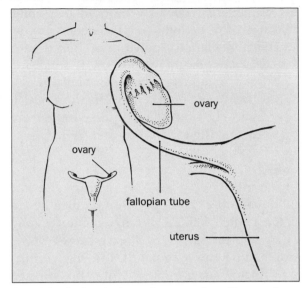

The abdominal cavity is spacious enough to allow ovarian tumors to grow for quite some time before they produce any symptoms.

examined by a pathologist to check for cancer cells. This process, called surgical staging, is needed to find out whether the cancer has spread. Staging is important in the planning of follow-up treatment.

TREATMENT
Treatment for ovarian cancer depends on a number of individual factors, including the stage of the disease and the woman's age and general health. Treatment for ovarian cancer is best planned by doctors who specialize in the diagnosis and treatment of this disease. (See page 17 for more information about getting a second opinion and planning treatment. Also see page 20 for information on Support for Cancer Patients.)

Methods of Treatment
Ovarian cancer may be treated with surgery, radiation therapy, or chemotherapy. The doctor may use just one method or combine them.

• *Surgery* is the initial treatment for almost every woman with ovarian cancer.

- *Radiation therapy* may be used in a small number of patients to kill cancer cells that may remain in the pelvic area after surgery.
- *Chemotherapy* may be used following surgery as adjuvant therapy, to kill any cancer cells that may remain in the body. It may also be used at a later time if there are signs that the cancer has recurred.

Surgery for ovarian cancer usually involves removal of the ovaries, the uterus, and the fallopian tubes. This operation is called hysterectomy with bilateral salpingo-oophorectomy. (If a woman has a very early slow-growing tumor and wants to remain able to have a child, the doctor may remove only the affected ovary.) If the cancer has spread, the surgeon removes as much of the cancer as possible in a procedure called tumor debulking. Tumor debulking reduces the amount of cancer to be treated with chemotherapy or radiation therapy.

Radiation therapy (also called radiotherapy) is the use of high-energy rays to damage cancer cells and stop them from growing. Radiation may come from a machine (external radiation) or from radioactive material placed into or near the tumor (internal radiation). Like surgery, radiation therapy is local therapy; it affects cancer cells only in the treated area.

For external radiation therapy, the patient goes to the hospital or clinic each day. Usually, the treatments are given five days a week for about five weeks.

Some women receive a type of internal radiation called intraperitoneal irradiation. Radioactive liquid is put into the abdomen through a catheter. A short hospital stay may be necessary for this treatment.

Chemotherapy for ovarian cancer often involves a combination of drugs. Anticancer drugs are usually given by injection into a vein or by mouth. Either way, chemotherapy is considered systemic therapy because the drugs travel throughout the body in the bloodstream. Chemotherapy is usually given in cycles: a treatment period followed by a recovery period, then another treatment period, and so on. A woman may receive chemotherapy as an outpatient at the hospital, at the doctor's office, or at home. Depending on which drugs are used, how they are given, and her general health, a woman may need to stay in the hospital while receiving chemotherapy.

Doctors are studying another way of giving anticancer drugs called intraperitoneal chemotherapy. In this approach, the drugs are put directly into the abdomen through a catheter. In this way, drugs reach the cancer directly. This treatment is given in the hospital.

Clinical Trials

Various trials for ovarian cancer patients are under way. Doctors are studying new drugs, new drug combinations, and different treatment schedules. They also are exploring drugs designed to make radiation therapy more effective, and other ways of combining different types of treatment. Biological therapy, the use of substances that boost the immune system's response to cancer or protect the body from some of the side effects of treatment, is under study in patients with recurrent or advanced ovarian cancer. A woman with ovarian cancer who is interested in participating in a trial should talk with her doctor. (For more information about clinical trials, see page 20.)

SIDE EFFECTS OF TREATMENT

It is hard to limit the effects of therapy so that only cancer cells are destroyed. Because treatment often damages healthy cells and tissues, it can cause unpleasant side effects.

The side effects of cancer treatment vary, depending on the type of treatment. Also, each woman reacts differently. Doctors try to keep side effects to a minimum, but problems may occur.

Surgery

Surgery for ovarian cancer is a major operation. For several days after surgery, the patient may have difficulty emptying her bladder and having normal bowel movements. Drugs may be given to relieve pain and to prevent or treat infection. A woman should ask the doctor or nurse for medicine to relieve pain. For a period of time after the surgery, some of the woman's normal activities are limited to let healing take place.

In younger women, when the ovaries are removed, the body's natural source of estrogen is lost and menopause starts. Symptoms of menopause are likely to appear soon after the surgery. Hormone replacement therapy is commonly used to ease such symptoms as hot flashes and vaginal dryness in menopausal women. However, the use of hormone replacement therapy has not been studied in women who have had ovarian cancer. Deciding whether to use it is an individual matter; ovarian cancer patients should discuss the possible risks and benefits of hormone replacement therapy with their doctor.

Chemotherapy

The side effects of chemotherapy depend mainly on which drugs the patient receives. In addition, side effects vary from patient to patient. In general, anticancer drugs affect rapidly dividing cells. These include blood cells, which fight infection, cause the blood to clot, and carry oxygen to all parts of the body. When blood cells are affected by anticancer drugs, women are more likely to get infections, bruise or bleed easily, and have less energy. Cells in hair roots and cells that line the digestive tract also divide rapidly. As a result, women may lose their hair and may have other side effects, such as nausea, vomiting, or mouth sores. Usually the doctor can suggest diet changes or medications to ease these problems. Most side effects of chemotherapy gradually go away during the recovery period or after treatment stops.

Certain drugs used in the treatment of ovarian cancer can cause kidney damage. To help protect the kidneys while taking these drugs, patients are given large amounts of fluid. These drugs also may cause tingling in the fingers or toes, ringing in the ears, or difficulty hearing. These problems may continue after treatment stops.

Radiation Therapy

Patients are likely to become very tired during radiation therapy, especially in the later weeks of treatment. Resting is important, but doctors usually advise patients to try to stay as active as they can.

It is also common for the skin in the treated area to become red, dry, tender, and itchy. There may be permanent darkening or "bronzing" of the skin in the treated area. This area should be exposed to the air as much as possible, but protected from sunlight. Patients should avoid wearing clothes that rub the treated area. The radiation therapist or nurse will give advice about keeping the skin clean. Patients should not use any lotion or cream on their skin without checking with the doctor or nurse.

Radiation treatment to the lower abdomen may cause nausea, vomiting, diarrhea, or urinary discomfort. Usually the doctor can suggest diet changes or medicines to ease these problems.

Radiation therapy for ovarian cancer also can cause vaginal dryness and interfere with intercourse. Women may be advised not to have intercourse during treatment. However, most women are able to resume sexual activity a few weeks after radiation treatment ends.

To help withstand the side effects of treatment in general, it is important that patients maintain good nutrition (see Nutrition for Cancer Patients, page 19).

FOLLOW-UP CARE

In some cases, doctors recommend "second-look" surgery after chemotherapy has been

89

completed. This allows the doctor to examine the abdomen directly and take fluid and tissue samples to see whether the treatment has been successful. If cancer is found, additional treatment is needed.

When treatment is over, regular checkups generally include a physical exam, as well as a pelvic exam and Pap smear.

Sometimes doctors also order chest x-rays, a CT scan of the abdomen, and laboratory tests such as urinalysis, a complete blood count, and the CA-125 assay. Often the CA-125 level in a patients blood is high before surgery and returns to normal within several weeks after the tumor has been removed. If the CA-125 level begins to rise again, it may mean the cancer has come back.

Depending on the drugs she has received, a woman treated for ovarian cancer with chemotherapy may have an increased risk of developing leukemia later in life. However, it is important to keep in mind that the benefits of receiving treatment for ovarian cancer far outweigh the risks of future disease.

Women should carefully follow their doctor's advice on health care and checkups, and should report any problem to the doctor as soon as it appears.

THE PROMISE OF CANCER RESEARCH

Scientists at hospitals and medical centers all across the country are studying ovarian cancer. They are trying to learn more about what causes this disease and how to prevent it. They are also looking for ways to detect it earlier and to treat it more effectively.

Cause and Prevention

About one in every 70 women in the United States will develop ovarian cancer during her lifetime. Most cases occur in women over the age of 50, but it can also affect younger women. The disease is more common in white women than in black women, but doctors do not know why.

Scientists do not know what causes ovarian cancer. It is clear, however, that this disease is not contagious; no one can "catch" ovarian cancer from another person.

By studying large numbers of women all over the world, researchers have found certain risk factors that increase a woman's chance of developing ovarian cancer. However, studies also show that most women with these risk factors do not get ovarian cancer, and many women who do get the disease have none of the risk factors we know about.

The following are some of the known risk factors for ovarian cancer:

Family medical history. The risk of getting ovarian cancer increases for a woman whose close relative (mother, sister, daughter) has had the disease. The risk is especially high if two or more close relatives have had the disease. The risk is not quite as high for women with other relatives (grandmother, aunt, or cousin) who have had ovarian cancer.

Women with more than one first-degree relative who has had ovarian cancer may wish to talk to their doctor about the option of prophylactic oophorectomy (preemptive removal of the ovaries before cancer has had a chance to develop).

Childbearing. Women who have never been pregnant are more likely to develop ovarian cancer than are women who have had children. In fact, the more times a woman has been pregnant, the less likely she is to develop ovarian cancer. Also, women who use oral contraceptives (birth control pills) are less likely to develop ovarian cancer than are women who do not. A possible reason is that the pill creates hormone levels in the body that are similar to those during pregnancy.

Age. The risk of developing ovarian cancer increases as a woman gets older. Most ovarian cancers occur in women over the age of 50; the risk is especially high for women over 60.

Personal medical history. Women who have had breast cancer are twice as likely to develop ovarian cancer as are women who have not had breast cancer.

Recent research raises the question of whether infertile women who take fertility drugs and do not become pregnant may be at an increased risk of developing ovarian cancer. But this possible link has not been proven. Further research is under way to determine whether ovarian cancer is related to infertility and/or to the use of fertility drugs.

Although certain drugs used to improve fertility by promoting ovulation (gonadotropins, clomiphene) have been reported to heighten one's risk of developing ovarian cancer, this association has never been confirmed. Currently, epidemiological studies (that is, those that evaluate significantly large representative samples of the population) are under way to investigate whether or not such an association exists.

Women who think they may be at risk for developing ovarian cancer should discuss this concern with their doctor, who can plan an appropriate schedule of checkups.

Early Detection
Most health problems respond best to treatment when they are found early. Women who have regular pelvic exams increase the chance that, if ovarian cancer occurs, it will be found before the disease causes symptoms.

However, pelvic exams often cannot find ovarian cancer at an early stage. Scientists are trying to find better ways to detect ovarian cancer earlier, when treatment may be more successful.

The National Cancer Institute

PANCREATIC CANCER

The pancreas is located in the abdomen. About six inches long, it is shaped like a long, flattened pear—wide at one end and narrow at the other. The wide part of the pancreas is called the head, the narrow end is the tail. The pancreas is a gland that has two main functions. It makes pancreatic juices, and it produces several hormones, including insulin.

Pancreatic juices contain proteins called enzymes that help digest food. The pancreas releases these juices, as they are needed, into a system of ducts. The main pancreatic duct joins the common bile duct from the liver and gallbladder. (The common bile duct carries bile, a fluid that helps digest fat.) Together these ducts form a short tube that empties into the duodenum, the first section of the small intestine.

Pancreatic hormones help the body use or store the energy that comes from food. For example, insulin helps control the amount of sugar (a source of energy) in the blood. The pancreas releases insulin and other hormones when they are needed.

SYMPTOMS
Pancreatic cancer has been called a "silent" disease because it usually does not cause symptoms early on. If the tumor blocks the common bile duct and bile cannot pass into the digestive system, the skin and whites of the eyes may become yellow, and the urine may become darker. This condition is called jaundice.

As the cancer grows and spreads, pain often develops in the upper abdomen and sometimes spreads to the back. The pain may become worse after the person eats or lies down. Cancer of the pancreas can also cause nausea, loss of appetite, weight loss, and weakness.

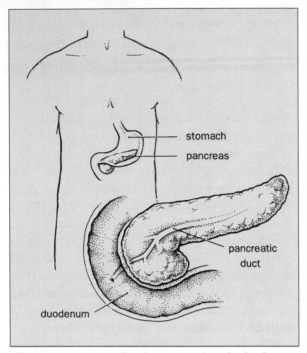

The pancreas secretes digestive enzymes into the duodenum and makes insulin and glucagon, hormones essential in maintaining blood sugar levels.

A rare type of pancreatic cancer, called islet cell cancer, can cause the pancreas to make too much insulin or hormones. When this happens, the patient may feel weak or dizzy and may have chills, muscle spasms, or diarrhea. These symptoms may be caused by cancer or by other less serious problems. Only a doctor can tell for sure.

DIAGNOSIS AND STAGING

To find the cause of a person's symptoms, the doctor performs a physical exam and asks about the patient's medical history. In addition to checking general health signs, the physician may also perform blood, urine, and stool tests.

The doctor usually orders procedures that produce pictures of the pancreas and the area around it. Pictures can help the doctor diagnose cancer of the pancreas. They also can help the doctor determine the stage, or extent, of the disease by showing whether the cancer affects nearby organs. Pictures that show the location and extent of the cancer help the doctor decide how to treat it. Procedures to produce pictures of the pancreas and nearby organs may include:

- *An upper GI series.* Sometimes called a barium swallow, the test consists of a series of x-rays of the upper digestive system taken after the patient drinks a barium solution. The barium shows an outline of the digestive organs on the x-rays.
- *CT scans.* An x-ray machine linked to a computer is used to produce various x-ray images. The computer puts the images together to produce detailed pictures.
- *MRI.* Using a powerful magnet linked to a computer, an MRI machine is very large, with space for the patient to lie in a tunnel inside the magnet. The machine measures the body's response to the magnetic field; the computer uses this information to make detailed pictures of the body.
- *Ultrasound.* An instrument sends sound waves into the patient's abdomen. The echoes that the sound waves produce as they bounce off internal organs create a picture called a sonogram. Healthy tissues and tumors produce different echoes.
- *Endoscopic retrograde cholangiography (ERCP).* The doctor passes a long, flexible tube (endoscope) down the throat, through the stomach, and into the small intestine. The doctor then injects dye into the ducts and takes x-rays of the common bile duct and pancreatic ducts.
- *Percutaneous transhepatic cholangiography (PTC).* A thin needle is put into the liver through the skin on the right side of the abdomen. Dye is injected into the bile ducts in the liver so that blockages in the ducts can be seen on x-rays.

A biopsy is the only sure way for the doctor to learn whether cancer is present. In a biopsy, the doctor removes a tissue sample. A pathologist looks at the tissue under a microscope to check for cancer cells.

One way to remove tissue is called a needle biopsy. The doctor inserts a long needle through the skin into the pancreas. Doctors use x-rays or ultrasound to guide the placement of the needle.

Another type of biopsy is a brush biopsy. This is done during the ERCP. The doctor inserts a very small brush through the endoscope into the opening from the bile duct and main pancreatic duct to rub off cells to examine under a microscope.

Sometimes the biopsy to diagnose pancreatic cancer is done during surgery. In one type, called laparoscopy, the doctor inserts a lighted instrument shaped like a thin tube into the abdomen through a small incision. In addition to removing tissue samples to be examined under the microscope, the doctor can see inside the abdomen to determine the location and extent of the disease. During the laparoscopy, the doctor can decide whether a larger operation called a laparotomy is needed to remove the tumor or relieve symptoms caused by the cancer.

TREATMENT

The choice of treatment depends on the type of cancer, the location and size of the tumor, the extent (stage) of the disease, the person's age and general health, and other factors. Cancer that begins in the pancreatic ducts may be treated with surgery, radiation therapy, or chemotherapy. Doctors sometimes use combinations of these treatments. Researchers are also studying biological therapy to see whether it can help when pancreatic cancer has spread to other parts of the body or has recurred. (See also Preparing for Treatment, page 17.)

Methods of Treatment

Cancer of the pancreas is very hard to control. This disease can be cured only when it is found at an early stage, before it has spread. However, treatment can improve the quality of a person's life by controlling the symptoms and complications of this disease.

Surgery may be done to remove all or part of the pancreas and other nearby tissue. The type of surgery depends on the type of pancreatic cancer, the location of the tumor in the pancreas, the person's symptoms, whether the cancer involves other organs, and whether the cancer can be completely removed. In the Whipple procedure, the surgeon removes the head of the pancreas, the duodenum, part of the stomach, and other nearby tissue. A total pancreatectomy is surgery to remove the entire pancreas as well as the duodenum, common bile duct, gallbladder, spleen, and nearby lymph nodes.

Sometimes the cancer cannot be completely removed. However, surgery can help to relieve symptoms that occur if the duodenum or bile duct is blocked. To relieve such symptoms, the surgeon creates a bypass around the blockage.

Radiation therapy (also called radiotherapy) is the use of high-energy rays to damage cancer cells and stop them from growing and dividing. Like surgery, radiation therapy is local treatment; the radiation can affect cancer cells only in the treated area. The radiation to treat pancreatic cancer comes from a machine that aims the rays from radioactive material at a specific area of the body.

Chemotherapy is the use of drugs to kill cancer cells. It may be given alone or along with radiation therapy to relieve symptoms of the disease if the cancer cannot be removed. When the cancer can be removed, doctors sometimes give chemotherapy after surgery to help control the growth of cancer cells that may remain in the body. The doctor may use one drug or a combination of drugs. Chemotherapy is usually given in cycles: a treatment period followed by a recovery period, then another treatment period, and so on.

Biological therapy (also called immunotherapy) is a form of treatment that uses the body's natural ability (immune system) to fight disease or to protect the body from treatment side effects. Researchers are testing several types of biological therapy, alone or in combination with chemotherapy. These treatments may be used when pancreatic cancer has spread to other organs or when it has recurred. People receiving biological therapy may need to stay in the hospital so that the side effects of their treatment can be watched.

Side Effects of Treatment

It is hard to limit the effects of therapy so that only cancer cells are removed or destroyed. Because treatment also damages healthy cells and tissues, it often causes unpleasant side effects. The side effects of cancer treatment depend mainly on the type and extent of the treatment. Also, they may not be the same for each person, and they may even change from one treatment to the next.

Surgery for cancer of the pancreas is a major operation. During recovery from surgery, a patient's diet and weight are checked carefully. At first, patients may be fed only liquids and may be given extra nourishment by IV. Foods are added gradually.

When the entire pancreas is removed, and even sometimes when only part of the pancreas is removed, people with pancreatic cancer may not have enough pancreatic juices or hormones. When a patient does not have enough pancreatic juices, problems with digestion may occur. The doctor can suggest an appropriate diet and prescribe medicine to help relieve diarrhea or other problems such as pain, feelings of fullness, or cramping.

Patients who do not have enough pancreatic hormones may develop other problems. For example, those who do not have enough insulin may develop diabetes. The doctor can treat this problem by giving patients hormones to replace those no longer produced by the pancreas.

During radiation therapy people are likely to become very tired, especially in the later weeks of treatment. Getting plenty of rest is important. It is common to lose hair in the treated area and for the skin to become red, tender, and itchy.

Radiation therapy to the pancreas and nearby tissues and organs may cause nausea, vomiting, diarrhea, or problems with digestion. Usually, the doctor can suggest certain diet changes or medicine to treat or control these problems. In most cases, side effects go away when treatment is over.

The side effects of chemotherapy depend on the drugs that are given. In addition, each person reacts differently. Chemotherapy affects rapidly growing cells, such as blood-forming cells, those that line the digestive tract, and those in the skin and hair. As a result, patients may have side effects such as lower resistance to infection, less energy, loss of appetite, nausea, vomiting, or mouth sores. Patients may also lose their hair.

The side effects caused by biological therapy vary with the type of treatment. These treatments may cause flu-like symptoms such as chills, fever, muscle aches, weakness, loss of appetite, nausea, vomiting, and diarrhea. Patients also may bleed or bruise easily, get a rash, or have swelling. These problems can be severe, but they usually go away after the treatment stops.

PAIN CONTROL

Pain is a common problem for people with pancreatic cancer, especially when the cancer grows outside the pancreas and presses against nerves and other organs. In most cases, the doctor prescribes medicine to control pain. Sometimes a combination of pain medicines is needed. Medicines that relieve pain may make people drowsy and constipated, but resting and taking laxatives can help.

In some cases, pain medicine is not enough. The doctor may use other treatments that affect nerves in the abdomen. For example, the doctor may inject alcohol into the area around certain nerves to block the feeling of pain. Sometimes the doctor cuts nerves in the abdomen during surgery to block the feeling of pain. In addition, radiation therapy can help relieve pain by shrinking the tumor.

WHAT THE FUTURE HOLDS

Patients should talk with the doctor about their chance of recovery (prognosis). When doctors talk about surviving cancer, they may use the term "remission," rather than "cure." Even though pancreatic cancer can be cured, doctors use these terms because of the chance that the disease can recur.

The National Cancer Institute

PROSTATE CANCER

The prostate is a male sex gland. It produces a thick fluid that forms part of semen. The prostate is about the size of a walnut. It is located below the bladder and in front of the rectum. The prostate surrounds the upper part of the urethra, the tube that empties urine from the bladder.

The prostate needs male hormones to function. The main male hormone is testosterone, which is made by the testicles. Other male hormones are produced in small amounts by the adrenal glands.

The prostate, like all other organs of the body, is made up of many types of cells. Normally, cells divide to produce more cells only when they are needed. This orderly process helps keep the body healthy. When cells divide without control, they form too much

tissue. This tissue can be benign (noncancerous) or malignant (cancerous). When cancer spreads outside the prostate, it often shows up in nearby lymph nodes (also called lymph glands). Prostate cancer can also spread to the bones, liver, bladder, rectum, and other organs.

SYMPTOMS

Early prostate cancer often does not cause symptoms. When symptoms of prostate cancer do occur, they may include any of the following problems:

- A need to urinate frequently, especially at night
- Difficulty starting urination or holding back urine
- Inability to urinate
- Weak or interrupted flow of urine
- Painful or burning urination
- Painful ejaculation
- Blood in urine or semen
- Frequent pain or stiffness in the lower back, hips, or upper thighs

Any symptoms may be caused by cancer or by other, less serious health problems, such as benign prostatic hyperplasia (BPH) or an infection. Only a doctor can tell the cause. A man who has symptoms like these should see his family doctor or a urologist (a doctor who specializes in treating diseases of the genitourinary system). Do not wait to feel pain; early prostate cancer does not cause pain.

DIAGNOSIS

If symptoms occur, the doctor asks about the patient's medical history, performs a physical exam, and may order laboratory tests. These exams and tests may include the following:

- *Digital rectal exam.* The doctor inserts a gloved, lubricated finger into the rectum

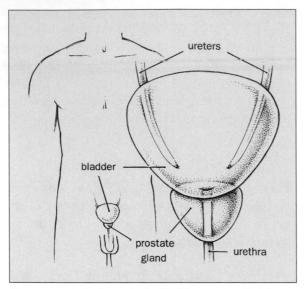

The prostate is just beneath the bladder, surrounding the urethra. Prostate enlargement, common in men over 50, is usually unrelated to prostate cancer.

and feels the prostate through the rectal wall to check for hard or lumpy areas.

• *Blood tests.* A lab measures the levels of prostate-specific antigen (PSA) and prostatic acid phosphatase (PAP) in the blood. The level of PSA in the blood may rise in men who have prostate cancer, BPH, or an infection in the prostate. The level of PAP rises above normal in many prostate cancer patients, especially if the cancer has spread beyond the prostate. The doctor cannot diagnose prostate cancer with these tests alone because elevated PSA or PAP levels may also indicate other, non-cancerous problems. However, the doctor will take the results of these tests into account in deciding whether to check the patient further for signs of cancer.

• *Urine test.* A lab checks the urine for blood or infection.

The doctor may order other tests to learn more about the cause of symptoms and to help determine whether conditions of the prostate are benign or malignant. In one procedure, transrectal ultrasonography,

sound waves that cannot be heard by humans (ultrasound) are sent out by a probe inserted into the rectum. The waves bounce off the prostate, and a computer uses the echoes to create a picture called a sonogram. The patient also may have an intravenous pyelogram, a series of x-rays of the organs of the urinary tract. In addition, the doctor may order a procedure called cystoscopy, in which he or she looks into the urethra and bladder through a thin, lighted tube.

If test results suggest that cancer may be present, the patient will need to have a biopsy. A biopsy is the only sure way to know whether a problem is cancer.

During the biopsy procedure, an ultrasound device is inserted into the rectum to help doctors view the parts of the prostate they wish to sample. Prostate tissue is obtained using a device that pushes six needles through the wall of the rectum and extracts samples of tissue from six portions of the prostate gland (sextant biopsy). Though brief, the procedure can be uncomfortable and can cause temporary rectal bleeding or blood in the seminal fluid.

Even if the physical exam and test results do not suggest cancer, the doctor may recommend medicine to reduce the symptoms caused by an enlarged prostate. Surgery is another way to relieve these symptoms. The surgery used in such cases is transurethral resection of the prostate (TURP or TUR). In TURP, an instrument is inserted through the penis to remove prostate tissue that is pressing against the upper part of the urethra.

STAGING

If cancer is found in the prostate, the doctor needs to know the stage, or extent, of the disease. Staging is a careful attempt to find out whether the cancer has spread and, if so, what parts of the body are affected. The doctor may use various blood and imaging tests to learn the stage of the disease. Treatment decisions depend on these findings.

The results of these tests help the doctor decide which of the following stages best describes a patient's disease:

- *Stage I (A).* Cancer cannot be detected by rectal exam and causes no symptoms. The cancer is usually found during surgery to relieve problems with urination. Stage I tumors may be in more than one area of the prostate, but there is no evidence of spread outside the prostate.
- *Stage II (B).* The tumor is felt during a rectal exam or detected by a blood test, with no evidence of spread beyond the prostate.
- *Stage III (C).* The cancer has spread outside the prostate to nearby tissues.
- *Stage IV (D).* Cancer cells have spread to lymph nodes or to other parts of the body.

TREATMENT OPTIONS

Treatment for prostate cancer depends on the stage of the disease and the grade of the tumor (how fast the cells are likely to grow or spread to other organs). Other factors in planning treatment are the man's age and general health and his feelings about the treatments and their possible side effects. (See page 17 for more information about getting a second opinion and planning treatment. Also see the section on Support for Cancer Patients, page 20.)

Methods of Treatment

Many men whose prostate cancer is slow growing and found at an early stage may not need treatment. Treatment may not be advised for older men or men with other serious medical problems. For these men, the possible side effects and the risks of treatment may outweigh the benefits of treatment. Instead, the doctor may suggest "watchful waiting:" following the patient closely and treating him later for

symptoms that may arise. Researchers are studying men with early stage prostate cancer to determine when and in whom treatment may be necessary and effective.

Treatment for prostate cancer may involve surgery, radiation therapy, or hormonal therapy. Sometimes patients receive a combination of these treatments.

Surgery is a common treatment for the early stages of prostate cancer. Surgery to remove the entire prostate is called radical prostatectomy. It is done in one of two ways. In retropubic prostatectomy, the prostate and nearby lymph nodes are removed through an incision in the abdomen. In perineal prostatectomy, an incision is made between the scrotum and the anus to remove the prostate. Nearby lymph nodes sometimes are removed through a separate incision in the abdomen. If the pathologist finds cancer cells in the lymph nodes, it may mean that the disease has spread to other parts of the body.

Radiation therapy is another way to treat prostate cancer. In radiation therapy (also called radiotherapy), high-energy rays are used to damage cancer cells and stop them from growing and dividing. Like surgery, radi-

---

IMPORTANT QUESTIONS

Here are some questions patients may want to ask the doctor:
- What are my treatment choices?
- Would a clinical trial be appropriate for me?
- What are the expected benefits of each kind of treatment?
- What are the risks and possible side effects of each treatment?
- How will treatment affect my sex life?
- If I have pain, how will you help me?
- Will I need to change my normal activities? If so, for how long?
- How often will I need to have checkups?

ation therapy is local therapy; it affects only the cells in the treated area. In early stage prostate cancer, radiation can be used instead of surgery, or it may be used after surgery to destroy any cancer cells that may remain in the area. In advanced stages, it may be given to relieve pain or other problems.

Radiation may be directed at the body by a machine (external radiation), or it may come from a small container of radioactive material placed directly into or near the tumor (internal radiation). Some patients receive both kinds of radiation therapy.

For external radiation therapy for prostate cancer, the patient goes to an outpatient department of a hospital or clinic. Treatment generally is given five days a week for five to seven weeks. This schedule helps protect healthy tissues by spreading out the total dose of radiation. The radiation is aimed at the pelvic area. At the end of treatment, an extra "boost" of radiation is often given to a smaller area of the pelvis, where most of the tumor was found.

For internal (or implant) radiation therapy, a brief stay in the hospital may be needed when the radioactive material is implanted. The implant may be temporary or permanent. When a temporary implant is removed, there is no radioactivity in the body. The amount of radiation in a permanent implant is not generally dangerous to other people, but patients may be advised to avoid prolonged close contact with others for a time.

Hormonal therapy prevents the prostate cancer cells from getting the male hormones they need to grow. When a man undergoes hormonal therapy, the level of male hormones is decreased. This drop in hormone level can affect all prostate cancer cells, even if they have spread to other parts of the body. For this reason, hormonal therapy is a systemic therapy.

There are several forms of hormonal therapy. One is surgery to remove the testicles. This operation, called orchiectomy, elimi-

BETTER PROSTATE CANCER PREDICTIONS

Elevated levels of PSA may be due to prostate cancer, benign prostatic hyperplasia (BPH), or prostatitis (inflammation of the prostate). Several approaches may help to distinguish when a PSA is elevated due to prostate cancer rather than to these other conditions:

- *PSA density* is determined by dividing the PSA value by the volume of the prostate (as determined by ultrasound). The higher the PSA density, the greater the chance of cancer because the elevated PSA is less likely due to a greatly enlarged prostate. Several studies indicate that a PSA density greater than 0.15 ng/ml suggests a high risk of cancer.

- *PSA velocity* involves annual or semiannual monitoring of changes in PSA values, which increase more rapidly in men with prostate cancer than in others. A study from Johns Hopkins and the National Institutes of Health found that an increase in PSA values greater than 0.75 ng/ml a year was an early predictor of prostate cancer.

- *The free PSA measurement* takes advantage of the fact that blood PSA is either bound to proteins or free (unbound). The two forms of PSA can be distinguished in the laboratory, and men with prostate cancer have a lower percentage of free PSA than men with BPH. Studies have shown that a PSA greater than 24 percent of the total is unlikely to be due to prostate cancer in men with a total PSA between 4 and 10 ng/ml.

The Editors

nates the main source of male hormones.

The use of luteinizing hormone-releasing hormone (LHRH) agonist is another type of hormonal therapy. LHRH agonists prevent the testicles from producing testosterone.

In another form of hormonal therapy, patients take the female hormone estrogen to stop the testicles from producing testosterone.

After orchiectomy or treatment with an LHRH agonist or estrogen, the body no longer gets testosterone from the testicles. However, the adrenal glands still produce small amounts of male hormones. Sometimes the patient is also given an antiandrogen, a drug that blocks the effect of any remaining male hormones. This combination of treatment is known as a total androgen blockade.

Prostate cancer that has spread to other parts of the body usually can be controlled with hormonal therapy for a period of time, often several years. Eventually, however, most prostate cancers are able to grow with very little or no male hormones. When this happens, hormonal therapy is no longer effective, and the doctor may suggest other forms of treatment that are under study.

Clinical Trials

Researchers are looking for treatment methods that are more effective and have fewer side effects. When laboratory research shows that a new treatment has promise, doctors test the new method by using it to treat cancer patients in clinical trials. (For more information about clinical trials, see page 20.)

SIDE EFFECTS OF TREATMENT

Although doctors plan treatment very carefully, it is hard to limit the effects of treatment so that only cancer cells are removed or destroyed. Because treatment also damages healthy cells and tissues, it often causes unwanted and sometimes serious side effects.

The side effects of cancer treatment depend mainly on the type and extent of the treatment. Also, each patient reacts differently. Doctors and nurses can explain the possible side effects of treatment, and they can often suggest ways to help relieve symptoms that may occur during and after treatment. It is important to let the doctor know if any side effects occur.

Surgery. Although patients are often uncomfortable during the first few days after surgery, their pain can be controlled with medicine. Patients should feel free to discuss pain relief with the doctor or nurse. It is also common for patients to feel tired or weak for a while. The length of time it takes to recover from an operation varies for each patient.

Surgery to remove the prostate may cause permanent impotence and sometimes causes urinary incontinence. These side effects are somewhat less common than in the past.

Some surgeons use new methods, especially when removing small tumors. These techniques, called nerve-sparing surgery, may prevent permanent injury to the nerves that control erection and damage to the opening of the bladder.

When this surgery is fully successful, impotence and urinary incontinence are only temporary. However, men who have a prostatectomy no longer produce semen, so they have dry orgasms.

Radiation therapy. Radiation therapy may cause patients to become very tired as treatment continues. Resting is important, but doctors usually advise patients to try to stay as active as they can. Patients may have diarrhea or frequent and uncomfortable urination. In addition, when patients receive external radiation therapy, it is common for the skin in the treated area to become red, dry, and tender. Radiation therapy can also cause hair loss in the pelvic area. The loss may be temporary or permanent, depending on the amount of radiation used.

Radiation therapy causes impotence in some men. This does not occur as often with internal radiation therapy as with external radiation therapy; internal radiation therapy is not as likely to damage the nerves that control erection.

Hormonal therapy. Orchiectomy, LHRH agonists, and estrogen often cause side effects such as loss of sexual desire, impotence, and hot flashes. When first taken, an LHRH ago-nist tends to increase tumor growth and make the patient's symptoms worse. This temporary problem is called "tumor flare." Gradually, however, the drug causes a man's testosterone level to fall. Without testos-terone, tumor growth slows down and the pa-tient's condition improves. Prostate cancer patients who receive estrogen or an antian-drogen may have nausea, vomiting, or ten-derness and swelling of the breasts. (Estrogen is used less now than in the past because it increases a man's risk of heart problems. This form of treatment is not ap-propriate for men who have a history of heart disease.)

Chemotherapy. The side effects of chemothera-py depend mainly on the specific drugs that are used. To help withstand the side effects of chemotherapy and treatment in general, it is important that patients maintain good nutri-tion (See Nutrition for Cancer Patients for more information, page 19).

FOLLOW-UP CARE

Regular follow-up exams are important for any man who has had prostate cancer. The doctor will suggest an appropriate follow-up schedule. The doctor will examine the patient regularly to be sure that the disease has not re-turned or progressed, and decide what other medical care may be needed. Follow-up exams may include x-rays, scans, and labora-tory tests, including the PSA blood test.

CAUSES AND PREVENTION

The causes of prostate cancer are not yet un-derstood. Researchers are looking at factors that may increase the risk of this disease. The more they can learn about these factors, the better the chance of finding ways to prevent and treat prostate cancer.

Studies in the United States show that prostate cancer is found mainly in men over age 55; the average age of patients at the time of diagnosis is 72. This disease is more com-mon in black men than in white men. In fact, black men in the United States have the high-est rate of prostate cancer in the world. Doc-tors cannot explain why one man gets prostate cancer and another does not, but they do know that no one can "catch" prostate cancer from another person. Prostate cancer is not contagious.

Some studies have shown that a man has a higher risk for prostate cancer if his father or brother has had the disease. However, re-searchers are uncertain why some families have a higher incidence of prostate cancer.

Scientists are studying the effects of diet. Some evidence suggests that a diet high in fat increases the risk of prostate cancer, and a diet high in fruits and vegetables decreases the risk, but these links have not been proven.

Researchers have studied whether having a vasectomy increases a man's risk for prostate cancer. Some studies suggest there may be such a link, but other studies have not sup-ported this claim.

Additional studies show that farmers and workers exposed to the metal cadmium dur-ing welding, electroplating, or making batter-ies may have an increased risk of getting this disease. Also, workers in the rubber industry appear to develop prostate cancer more often than members of the general public. Howev-er, more research is needed to confirm these results.

Scientists are also doing studies to deter-mine whether BPH or a sexually transmitted virus increases the risk for prostate cancer. At this time, they do not have clear evidence of increased risk in either case.

DETECTION

Men should talk with their doctor about prostate cancer, the symptoms to watch for, and an appropriate schedule of checkups.

The doctor's advice will be based on the risks and benefits of diagnosis and treatment, the man's age, medical history, and other factors.

The National Cancer Institute

SKIN CANCER

The skin is the body's outer covering. It protects us against heat, light, injury, and infection. It regulates body temperature and fluid balance, manufactures vitamin D, and overlies fat tissue. Weighing about six pounds, the skin is the body's largest organ. It is made up of two main layers: the outer epidermis and the inner dermis.

The epidermis (outer layer of skin) is mostly made up of flat, scalelike cells called squamous cells. Under the squamous cells are round cells called basal cells. The deepest part of the epidermis also contains melanocytes. These cells produce melanin, which gives the skin its color.

The dermis (inner layer of skin) contains blood and lymph vessels, hair follicles, and glands. These glands produce sweat, which helps regulate body temperature, and sebum, an oily substance that helps keep the skin from drying out. Sweat and sebum reach the skin's surface through tiny openings called pores.

TYPES OF SKIN CANCER

The two most common kinds of skin cancer are basal cell carcinoma and squamous cell carcinoma. (Carcinoma is cancer that begins in the cells that cover or line an organ.)

Basal cell carcinoma accounts for more than 90 percent of all skin cancers in the United States. It is a slow-growing cancer that seldom spreads to other parts of the body. Squamous cell carcinoma also rarely spreads.

Basal cell carcinoma and squamous cell car-

cinoma are sometimes called nonmelanoma skin cancer. Another type of cancer that occurs in the skin is melanoma, which begins in the melanocytes.

Although basal and squamous cell carcinomas grow slowly, it is best to detect them early, when they are smaller and require less surgery to remove.

CAUSE AND PREVENTION

Skin cancer is the most common type of cancer in the United States. According to present estimates, 40 to 50 percent of Americans who live to age 65 will have skin cancer at least once. Although anyone can get skin cancer, the risk is greatest for people who have fair skin that freckles easily—often those with red or blond hair and blue or light-colored eyes.

Ultraviolet (UV) radiation from the sun is the main cause of skin cancer. Artificial sources of UV radiation, such as sunlamps and tanning booths, can also cause skin cancer.

The risk of developing skin cancer is also affected by where a person lives. People who live in areas that get high levels of UV radiation from the sun are more likely to get skin cancer.

In the United States skin cancer is more common in Texas than it is in Minnesota, where the sun is not as strong. Worldwide, the highest rates of skin cancer are found in South Africa and Australia, areas that receive high amounts of UV radiation.

In addition, skin cancer is related to lifetime exposure to UV radiation. Most skin cancers appear after age 50, but the sun's damaging effects begin at an early age. Therefore, protection should start in childhood to prevent skin cancer later in life.

Whenever possible, people should avoid exposure to the midday sun (from 10 a.m. to

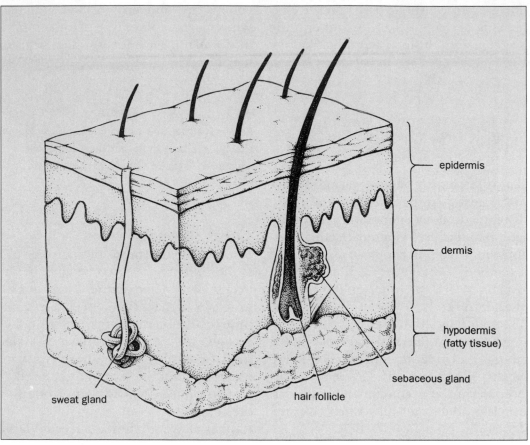

epidermis

dermis

hypodermis
(fatty tissue)

sebaceous gland

sweat gland

hair follicle

Skin cancers originate almost exclusively in the uppermost layer of skin, the epidermis. Within this layer are melanocytes and the basal and squamous cells.

2 p.m. standard time, or from 11 a.m. to 3 p.m. daylight saving time). Keep in mind that protective clothing, such as sun hats and long sleeves, can block out the sun's harmful rays. Also, lotions that contain sunscreens can protect the skin. Sunscreens are rated in strength according to a sun protection factor (SPF), which ranges from 2 to 30 or higher. Those rated 15 to 30 block most of the sun's harmful rays.

SYMPTOMS

The most common warning sign of skin cancer is a change on the skin, especially a new growth or a sore that doesn't heal. Skin cancers do not all look the same. For example, the cancer may start as a small, smooth, shiny, pale, or waxy lump. Or it can appear as a firm red lump. Sometimes the lump bleeds or develops a crust. Skin cancer can also start as a flat, red spot that is rough, dry, or scaly.

Both basal and squamous cell cancers are found mainly on areas of the skin that are exposed to the sun—the head, face, neck, hands, and arms. However, skin cancer can occur anywhere.

An actinic keratosis appears as a rough, red patch on the skin. It is called a precancerous condition because it sometimes develops into squamous cell cancer. Like skin cancer, it usually appears on sun-exposed areas.

Changes in the skin are not sure signs of cancer; however, it is important to see a doctor if any symptom lasts longer than two weeks. Don't wait for the area to hurt because skin cancers seldom cause pain.

HOW TO DO A SKIN SELF-EXAM

You can improve your chances of finding skin cancer promptly by performing a simple skin self-examination each month.

The best time to do a skin self-examination is after a shower or bath. A skin self-exam should be done in a well-lighted room with a full-length mirror and a hand-held mirror. It's best to begin by learning where your birthmarks, moles, and blemishes are located and how they usually look. Check for anything new: A change in the size, texture, or color of a mole, or a sore that does not heal should be noted.

Check all areas of the skin, including the back, scalp, buttocks, and genital area.

(1) Look at the front and back of your body in the mirror, then raise your arms and look at the left and right sides.

(2) Bend your elbows and look carefully at the palms, the forearms (including the undersides), and the upper arms.

(3) Examine the back and front of your legs. Also look between the buttocks and around the genital area.

(4) Sit and closely examine your feet, including the soles and spaces between the toes.

(5) Look at your face, neck, and scalp. You may want to use a comb or a blow dryer to move hair so that you can see better.

By checking your skin regularly, you will become familiar with what is normal. (See also Mole Inspection—Learning Your ABCDs, page 419.) If you find anything unusual, see your doctor right away. Remember, the earlier skin cancer is found, the better the chance for cure.

DETECTION AND DIAGNOSIS
Detection

The cure rate for skin cancer could be 100 percent if all skin cancers were brought to a doctor's attention before they had a chance to spread. Therefore, people should check themselves regularly for new growths or other changes in the skin. Any new, colored growths or any changes in growths that are already present should be reported to the doctor without delay. Doctors should also look at the skin during routine physical exams. Persons who have already had skin cancer should be sure to have regular exams so that the doctor can check the skin—both the treated areas and other places where cancer may develop.

It is important to note that half of all people with a new skin cancer will develop a second skin cancer within five years.

Diagnosis

Basal cell carcinoma and squamous cell carcinoma are generally diagnosed and treated in the same way. When an area of skin does not look normal, the doctor may remove all or part of the growth. This is called a biopsy. To check for cancer cells, the tissue is examined under a microscope by a pathologist or a dermatologist. A biopsy is the only sure way to tell if the problem is cancer.

Doctors generally divide skin cancer into two stages: local (affecting only the skin) or metastatic (spreading beyond the skin). Because skin cancer rarely spreads, a biopsy often is the only test needed to determine the stage. In cases where the growth is very large or has been present for a long time, the doctor will carefully check the lymph nodes in the area. In addition, the patient may need to have additional tests, such as special x-rays, to find out whether the cancer has spread to other parts of the body. Knowing the stage of a skin cancer helps the doctor plan the best treatment.

TREATMENT

In treating skin cancer, the doctor's main goal is to remove or destroy the cancer completely with as small a scar as possible. To plan the best treatment, the doctor considers the location and size of the cancer, the risk of scarring, and the person's age, general health, and medical history.

It is sometimes helpful to have the advice of more than one doctor before starting treatment. It may take several weeks to arrange for a second opinion. But this short delay will not reduce the chance that treatment will be successful. For a second opinion, your doctor may be able to suggest a dermatologist or a plastic surgeon, who has a special interest in skin cancer.

Surgery

Treatment for skin cancer usually involves some type of surgery. Many skin cancers can be cut from the skin quickly and easily. In some cases, doctors suggest radiation therapy or chemotherapy. Sometimes a combination of these methods is used.

Curettage and Electrodesiccation

Doctors commonly use a type of surgery called curettage. After a local anesthetic numbs the area, the cancer is scooped out with a curette, an instrument with a sharp, spoon-shaped end. The area is also treated by electrodesiccation. An electric current from a special machine is used to control bleeding and kill any cancer cells remaining around the edge of the wound. Most patients develop a flat, white scar.

Mohs' Surgery

Mohs' technique is a special type of surgery used for skin cancer. Its purpose is to remove all of the cancerous tissue and as little of the healthy tissue as possible.

This method is also used to remove large tumors, those in hard-to-treat places, and cancers that have recurred. The patient is given a local anesthetic, and the cancer is shaved off one thin layer at a time. Each layer is checked under a microscope until the entire tumor is removed. The degree of scarring depends on the location and size of the treated area. This method should be used only by doctors who are specially trained in this type of surgery.

Mohs' surgery is especially helpful when the skin cancer is on a curved surface, such as the ear, nose, eyelid, or lip.

Grafting

Sometimes, especially when a large cancer is removed, a skin graft is needed to close the wound and reduce the amount of scarring. For this procedure, the doctor takes a piece of healthy skin from another part of the body to replace the skin that was removed.

Cryosurgery

Extreme cold may be used to treat precancerous skin conditions, such as actinic keratosis, as well as certain small skin cancers. In cryosurgery, liquid nitrogen is applied to the growth to freeze and kill the abnormal cells. After the area thaws, the dead tissue falls off. More than one freezing may be needed to remove the growth completely. A white scar may form in the treated area.

Cryosurgery may produce a burning sensation during the first 10 to 30 seconds or more of freezing and for a few minutes thereafter. Over the next week, the area will feel like any other sore.

Topical Chemotherapy

Topical chemotherapy is the use of anticancer drugs in a cream or lotion applied to the skin. Actinic keratoses can be treated effectively with the anticancer drug fluorouracil (also called 5-FU). This treatment is also useful for cancers limited to the top layer of skin. The

5-FU is applied daily for several weeks. Intense inflammation is common during treatment, but scars usually do not occur.

Laser Therapy

Laser therapy uses a narrow beam of light to remove or destroy cancer cells. This approach is sometimes used for cancers that involve only the outer layer of skin.

Radiation

Skin cancer responds well to radiation therapy, which uses high-energy rays to damage cancer cells. Doctors often use this treatment for cancers that occur in areas that are hard to treat with surgery. For example, radiation therapy might be used for cancers of the eyelid, the tip of the nose, or the ear. Several treatments may be needed to destroy all of the cancer cells. Radiation therapy may cause a rash or make the skin in the area dry or red. Changes in skin color and/or texture may develop after the treatment is over and may become more noticeable many years later.

Clinical Trials

In clinical trials (research studies with patients), doctors are studying new treatments for skin cancer. For example, they are exploring photodynamic therapy, a treatment that destroys cancer cells with a combination of laser light and drugs that make the cells sensitive to light. Biological therapy (also called immunotherapy) is a form of treatment to improve the body's natural ability to fight cancer. Interferon and tumor necrosis factor are types of biological therapy under study for skin cancer.

FOLLOW-UP CARE

Even though most skin cancers are cured, the disease can recur in the same place. Also, people who have been treated for skin cancer have a higher-than-average risk of developing a new cancer of the skin. That's why it's so important for them to continue to examine themselves regularly, to visit their doctor for regular checkups, and to follow their doctor's instructions on how to reduce their risk of developing skin cancer again.

LIVING WITH CANCER

When people have cancer, life can change for them and for the people who care about them. These changes in daily life can be difficult to handle. (See Support for Cancer Patients, page 20.)

WHAT THE FUTURE HOLDS

Skin cancer has a better prognosis, or outcome, than most other types of cancer. Although skin cancer is the most common type of cancer in the United States, it accounts for much less than 1 percent of all cancer deaths. It is cured in 85 to 95 percent of all cases.

The National Cancer Institute

STOMACH CANCER

The stomach is part of the digestive system. It is located in the upper abdomen, under the ribs. The upper part of the stomach connects to the esophagus, and the lower part leads into the small intestine.

When food enters the stomach, muscles in the stomach wall create a rippling motion that mixes and mashes the food. This motion is called peristalsis. At the same time, juices made by glands in the lining of the stomach help digest the food. After about three hours, the food becomes a liquid and moves into the small intestine, where digestion continues.

Stomach cancer (also called gastric cancer) can develop in any part of the stomach and may spread throughout the stomach and to other organs. It may grow along the stomach wall into the esophagus or small intestine.

It also may extend through the stomach wall and spread to nearby lymph nodes, and to organs such as the liver, pancreas, and colon. Stomach cancer also may spread to distant organs, such as the lungs, lymph nodes above the collar bone, and the ovaries.

When cancer spreads to another part of the body, the new tumor has the same kind of abnormal cells and the same name as the primary tumor. For example, if stomach cancer spreads to the liver, the cancer cells in the liver are stomach cancer cells. The disease is metastatic stomach cancer; it is not liver cancer. However, when stomach cancer spreads to an ovary, the tumor in the ovary is called a Krukenberg tumor. (This tumor, named for a doctor, is not a different disease; it is metastatic stomach cancer. The cancer cells in a Krukenberg tumor are stomach cancer cells, the same as the cancer cells in the primary tumor.)

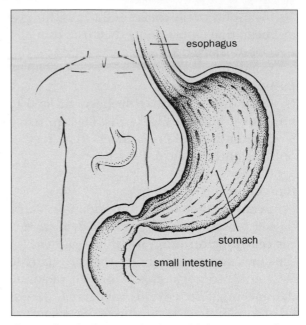

Contractions in the stomach, along with its enzymes and acid, promote digestion. Stomach cancer usually starts as an ulcer in the lining of the stomach.

SYMPTOMS

Stomach cancer can be hard to find early. Often there are no symptoms in the early stages and, in many cases, the cancer has spread before it is found. When symptoms do occur, they are often so vague that the person ignores them. Stomach cancer can cause:

- Indigestion or a burning sensation (heartburn)
- Discomfort or pain in the abdomen
- Nausea and vomiting
- Diarrhea or constipation
- Bloating of the stomach after meals
- Loss of appetite
- Weakness and fatigue
- Bleeding (vomiting blood or having blood in the stool)

Any of these symptoms may be caused by cancer or by other, less serious health problems, such as a stomach virus or an ulcer. Only a doctor can tell the cause. People who have any of these symptoms should see their doctor. They may be referred to a gastroenterologist, a doctor who specializes in diagnosing and treating digestive problems. These doctors are sometimes called gastrointestinal (GI) specialists.

DIAGNOSIS

To find the cause of symptoms, the doctor asks about the patient's medical history, does a physical exam, and may order laboratory studies. The patient may also have one or all of the following exams:

- *Fecal occult blood test,* a check for hidden (occult) blood in the stool. This test is done by placing a small amount of stool on a plastic slide or on special paper. It may be tested in the doctor's office or sent to a laboratory. This test is done because stomach cancer sometimes causes bleeding that cannot be seen. However, noncancerous conditions also may cause bleeding, so having blood in the stool does not necessarily mean that a person has cancer.

- **Upper GI series,** x-rays of the esophagus and stomach (the upper gastrointestinal, or GI, tract). The x-rays are taken after the patient drinks a barium solution, a thick chalky liquid. (This test is sometimes called a barium swallow.) The barium outlines the stomach on the x-rays, helping the doctor find tumors or other abnormal areas. During the test, the doctor may pump air into the stomach to make small tumors easier to see.

- **Endoscopy,** an exam of the esophagus and stomach using a thin, lighted tube called a gastroscope, which is passed through the mouth and esophagus to the stomach. The patient's throat is sprayed with a local anesthetic to reduce discomfort and gagging. Patients also may receive medicine to relax them. Through the gastroscope, the doctor can look directly at the inside of the stomach. If an abnormal area is found, the doctor can remove some tissue through the gastroscope. Another doctor, a pathologist, examines the tissue under a microscope to check for cancer cells. This procedure—removing tissue and examining it under a microscope—is called a biopsy. A biopsy is the only sure way to know whether cancer cells are present.

STAGING

If the pathologist finds cancer cells in the tissue sample, the patient's doctor needs to know the stage, or extent, of the disease. Staging exams and tests help the doctor find out whether the cancer has spread and, if so, what parts of the body are affected. Because stomach cancer can spread to the liver, the pancreas, and other organs near the stomach as well as to the lungs, the doctor may order a CT scan, an ultrasound exam, or other tests to check these areas.

Staging may not be complete until after surgery. The surgeon removes nearby lymph nodes and may take samples of tissue from other areas in the abdomen. All of these samples are examined by a pathologist to check for cancer cells. Decisions about treatment after surgery depend on these findings.

TREATMENT

The doctor develops a treatment plan to fit each patient's needs. Treatment for stomach cancer depends on the size, location, and extent of the tumor, the stage of the disease, the patient's general health, and other factors.

Many people who have cancer want to learn all they can about the disease and their treatment choices so they can take an active part in decisions about their medical care. (For information about Getting a Second Opinion and Preparing for Treatment, see page 17.)

When talking about treatment choices, the patient may want to ask about taking part in a research study. Such studies, called clinical trials, are designed to improve cancer treatment. (For more information about clinical trials, see page 20.)

Methods of Treatment

Cancer of the stomach is difficult to cure unless it is found in an early stage (before it has begun to spread). Unfortunately, because early stomach cancer causes few symptoms, the disease is usually advanced when the diagnosis is made. However, advanced stomach cancer can be treated, and the symptoms can be relieved. Treatment for stomach cancer may include surgery, chemotherapy, and/or radiation therapy. New treatment approaches such as biological therapy and improved ways of using current methods are being studied in clinical trials. A patient may have one form of treatment or a combination of treatments.

Surgery is the most common treatment for stomach cancer. The operation is called gastrectomy. The surgeon removes part (subtotal or partial gastrectomy) or all (total gastrectomy) of the stomach, as well as some of the tissue around the stomach. After a subtotal gastrectomy, the doctor connects the remaining part of the stomach to the esophagus or the small intestine. After a total gastrectomy, the doctor connects the esophagus directly to the small intestine. Because cancer can spread through the lymphatic system, lymph nodes near the tumor are often removed during surgery so that the pathologist can check them for cancer cells. If cancer cells are in the lymph nodes, the disease may have spread to other parts of the body.

Chemotherapy is the use of drugs to kill cancer cells. This type of treatment is called systemic therapy because the drugs enter the bloodstream and travel through the body.

Clinical trials are in progress to find the best ways to use chemotherapy to treat stomach cancer. Scientists are exploring the benefits of giving chemotherapy before surgery to shrink the tumor, or as adjuvant therapy after surgery to destroy remaining cancer cells. Combination treatment with chemotherapy and radiation therapy is also under study. Doctors are testing a treatment in which anticancer drugs are put directly into the abdomen (intraperitoneal chemotherapy). Chemotherapy also is being studied as a treatment for cancer that has spread, and as a way to relieve symptoms of the disease.

Most anticancer drugs are given by injection; some are taken by mouth. The doctor may use one drug or a combination of drugs. Chemotherapy is given in cycles: a treatment period followed by a recovery period, then another treatment, and so on. Usually a person receives chemotherapy as an outpatient (at the hospital, at the doctor's office, or at home). However, depending on which drugs are given and the patient's general health, a short hospital stay may be needed.

Radiation therapy (also called radiotherapy) is the use of high-energy rays to damage cancer cells and stop them from growing. Like surgery, it is local therapy; the radiation can affect cancer cells only in the treated area. Radiation therapy is sometimes given after surgery to destroy cancer cells that may remain in the area. Researchers are conducting clinical trials to find out whether it is helpful to give radiation therapy during surgery (intraoperative radiation therapy). Radiation therapy may also be used to relieve pain or blockage.

The patient goes to the hospital or clinic each day for radiation therapy. Usually treatments are given five days a week for five to six weeks.

Biological therapy (also called immunotherapy) is a form of treatment that helps the body's immune system attack and destroy cancer cells; it may also help the body recover from some of the side effects of treatment. In clinical trials, doctors are studying biological therapy in combination with other treatments to try to prevent a recurrence of stomach cancer. In another use of biological therapy, patients who have low blood cell counts during or after chemotherapy may receive colony-stimulating factors to help restore the blood cell levels. Patients may need to stay in the hospital while receiving some types of biological therapy.

SIDE EFFECTS OF TREATMENT

It is hard to limit the effects of therapy so that only cancer cells are removed or destroyed. Because healthy cells and tissues also may be damaged, treatment can cause unpleasant side effects.

The side effects of cancer treatment are different for each person, and they may even be different from one treatment to the next. Doctors try to plan treatment in ways that keep side effects to a minimum; they can help with any problems that occur. For this reason, it is very important to let the doctor know about any problems during or after treatment.

Surgery

Gastrectomy is major surgery. For a period of time after the surgery, the person's activities are limited to allow healing to take place. For the first few days after surgery, the patient is fed intravenously (through a vein). Within several days, most patients are ready for liquids, followed by soft, then solid, foods. Those who have had their entire stomach removed cannot absorb vitamin B_{12}, which is necessary for healthy blood and nerves, so they need regular injections of this vitamin. Patients may have temporary or permanent difficulty digesting certain foods, and they may need to change their diet. Some gastrectomy patients will need to follow a special diet for a few weeks or months, while others will need to do so permanently. The doctor or a dietitian (a nutrition specialist) will explain any necessary dietary changes.

Some gastrectomy patients have cramps, nausea, diarrhea, and dizziness shortly after eating because food and liquid enter the small intestine too quickly. This group of symptoms is called the dumping syndrome. Foods containing high amounts of sugar often make the symptoms worse. The dumping syndrome can be treated by changing the patient's diet.

Doctors often advise patients to eat several small meals throughout the day, to avoid foods that contain sugar, and to eat foods high in protein. To reduce the amount of fluid that enters the small intestine, patients are usually encouraged not to drink at mealtimes. Medicine also can help control the dumping syndrome. The symptoms usually disappear in three to 12 months, but they may be permanent.

Following gastrectomy, bile in the small intestine may back up into the remaining part of the stomach or into the esophagus, causing the symptoms of an upset stomach. The patient's doctor may prescribe medicine or suggest over-the-counter products to control such symptoms.

Chemotherapy

The side effects of chemotherapy depend mainly on the drugs the patient receives. As with any other type of treatment, side effects also vary from person to person. In general, anticancer drugs affect cells that divide rapidly. These include blood cells, which fight infection, help the blood to clot, or carry oxygen to all parts of the body. When blood cells are affected by anticancer drugs, patients are more likely to get infections, may bruise or bleed easily, and may have less energy. Cells in hair roots and cells that line the digestive tract also divide rapidly. As a result of chemotherapy, patients may have side effects such as loss of appetite, nausea, vomiting, hair loss, or mouth sores. For some patients, the doctor may prescribe medicine to help with side effects, especially with nausea and vomiting. These effects usually go away gradually during the recovery period between treatments or after the treatments stop.

Radiation Therapy

Patients who receive radiation to the abdomen may have nausea, vomiting, and diarrhea. The doctor can prescribe medicine or suggest dietary changes to relieve these problems. The skin in the treated area may become red, dry, tender, and itchy. Patients should avoid wearing clothes that rub; loose-fitting cotton clothes are usually best. It is important for patients to take good care of their skin during treatment, but they should not use lotions or creams without the doctor's advice.

Patients are likely to become very tired during radiation therapy, especially in the later weeks of treatment. Resting is important, but doctors usually advise patients to try to stay as active as they can.

Biological Therapy

The side effects of biological therapy vary with the type of treatment. Some cause flu-like symptoms, such as chills, fever, weakness, nausea, vomiting, and diarrhea. Patients sometimes get a rash, and they may bruise or bleed easily. These problems may be severe, and patients may need to stay in the hospital during treatment.

To help withstand the side effects of treatment in general, it is important that patients maintain good nutrition (see Nutrition for Cancer Patients, page 19).

CAUSES OF STOMACH CANCER

The stomach cancer rate in the United States and the number of deaths from this disease have gone down dramatically over the past 60 years. Still, stomach cancer is a serious disease, and scientists all over the world are trying to learn more about what causes this disease and how to prevent it. At this time, doctors cannot explain why one person gets stomach cancer and another does not. They do know, however, that stomach cancer is not contagious; no one can "catch" cancer from another person.

Researchers have learned that some people are more likely than others to develop stomach cancer. The disease is found most often in people over age 55. It affects men twice as often as women, and is more common in black people than in white people. Also, stomach cancer is more common in some parts of the world—such as Japan, Korea, parts of Eastern Europe, and Latin America—than in the United States. People in these areas eat many foods that are preserved by drying, smoking, salting, or pickling. Scientists believe that eating foods preserved in these ways may play a role in the development of stomach cancer. On the other hand, fresh foods (especially fresh fruits and vegetables and properly frozen or refrigerated fresh foods) may protect against this disease.

Stomach ulcers do not appear to increase a person's risk of getting stomach cancer. However, some studies suggest that a type of bacteria, *Helicobacter pylori*, which may cause stomach inflammation and ulcers, may be an important risk factor for this disease. Also, research shows that people who have had stomach surgery or have pernicious anemia, achlorhydria, or gastric atrophy (which generally result in lower than normal amounts of digestive juices) have an increased risk of stomach cancer.

Exposure to certain dusts and fumes in the workplace has been linked to a higher-than-average risk of stomach cancer. Also, some scientists believe smoking may increase stomach cancer risk.

People who think they might be at risk for stomach cancer should discuss this concern with their doctor. The doctor can suggest an appropriate schedule of checkups so that, if cancer appears, it can be detected as early as possible.

The National Cancer Institute

UTERINE CANCER

The uterus is a hollow, pear-shaped organ. It is located in a woman's lower abdomen between the bladder and the rectum. Attached to either side of the top of the uterus are the fallopian tubes, which extend from the uterus to the ovaries.

The narrow, lower portion of the uterus is the cervix; the broad, middle part is the corpus; and the dome-shaped upper portion is the fundus. The walls of the uterus are made of two layers of tissue: the inner layer or lining (endometrium) and the outer layer or muscle (myometrium).

Normally, cells grow and divide to produce more cells only when the body needs them.

This orderly process helps keep the body healthy. Sometimes cells keep dividing when new cells are not needed. A mass of extra tissue forms, and this mass is called a growth or tumor. Tumors can be benign or malignant.

Benign tumors are not cancer. They can usually be removed and, in most cases, they do not come back. Cells from benign tumors do not spread to other parts of the body. Most important, benign tumors are rarely a threat to life.

Fibroids are common benign tumors of the uterine muscle. These tumors do not develop into cancer. Fibroids are found mainly in women in their forties. Women may have many fibroid tumors at the same time. In most cases, fibroids cause no symptoms and require no treatment, although they should be checked by a doctor. Symptoms sometimes occur and may include irregular bleeding, vaginal discharge, and frequent urination. When fibroids cause heavy bleeding or press against nearby organs and cause pain, surgery or other treatment may be recommended. When a woman reaches menopause, fibroids may become smaller and sometimes disappear.

Endometriosis is another benign condition that affects the uterus. It does not develop into cancer. Endometriosis is seen mostly in women in their thirties and forties, particularly in women who have never been pregnant. It occurs when endometrial tissue begins to grow on the outside of the uterus and on nearby organs. This condition may cause painful menstrual periods, abnormal vaginal bleeding, and sometimes loss of fertility (ability to produce children). Treatment options generally include hormonal therapy and surgery.

Endometrial hyperplasia, also a benign condition, is an increase in the number of cells lining the uterus. Although it is not cancer, endometrial hyperplasia is considered a precancerous condition; in some cases, it may develop into cancer. Heavy menstrual periods, bleeding between periods, and bleeding after menopause are common symptoms of hyperplasia. The treatment is usually hysterectomy or hormonal therapy with progesterone, depending on the extent of the condition and whether a woman wants to have children.

Malignant tumors are cancer. Cancer cells can invade and damage tissues and organs near the tumor. Also, cancer cells can break away from a malignant tumor and enter the bloodstream or lymphatic system. This is how cancer spreads from the original (primary) tumor to form new tumors in other parts of the body. The spread of cancer is called metastasis.

Most cancers are named for the part of the body in which they begin. The most common type of cancer of the uterus begins in the endometrium. This type of cancer is called endometrial or uterine cancer. A different type of cancer, uterine sarcoma, develops in the uterine muscle. Cancer that begins in the cervix is also a different type of cancer.

SYMPTOMS

Abnormal vaginal bleeding, especially after menopause, is the most common symptom of uterine cancer of the uterus. Bleeding may start as a watery, blood-streaked flow that gradually contains more blood. Although uterine cancer usually occurs after menopause, it sometimes occurs around the time menopause begins. Abnormal bleeding should not be considered simply part of menopause and should be checked by a doctor.

A woman should see a doctor if she has any of the following symptoms: unusual vaginal bleeding or discharge; difficult or painful urination; pain during intercourse; or pain in the pelvic area.

DIAGNOSIS

If a woman has symptoms, her doctor asks about her medical history and conducts a physical exam. In addition to checking gener-

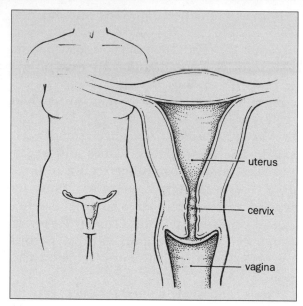

After menopause, the lining of the uterus thins and menstruation ceases. At this time of life, the risk of uterine cancer increases significantly.

al signs of health, the doctor usually performs blood and urine tests and one or more of the following procedures:.

- **Pelvic exam.** The doctor thoroughly examines the uterus, vagina, ovaries, bladder, and rectum. The doctor feels these organs for any abnormality in their shape or size. A speculum is used to widen the opening of the vagina so that the doctor can look at the upper portion of the vagina and the cervix.
- **Pap test.** The doctor uses a wooden scraper (spatula) or small brush to collect a sample of cells from the cervix and upper vagina. The cells are then sent to a medical laboratory to be checked for abnormal changes. Because uterine cancer begins inside the uterus, it may not show up on a Pap test; a biopsy is necessary to help the doctor make a diagnosis
- **Biopsy.** A biopsy can usually be done in the doctor's office. The doctor removes a sample of tissue from the uterine lining.
- **D&C.** This procedure is usually same-day

surgery done in a hospital with anesthesia. The opening of the cervix is widened and the doctor scrapes tissue from the lining of the uterus. A pathologist examines the tissue for cancer cells, hyperplasia, or other conditions. Women may have cramps and vaginal bleeding during healing.

STAGING

Once uterine cancer is diagnosed, the doctor needs to know the stage, or extent, of the disease in order to plan the best treatment. Staging procedures help the doctor find out whether the cancer has spread and, if so, what parts of the body are affected. For most women, staging procedures include blood and urine tests and chest x-rays. Doctors may also order a CT scan, MRI, sigmoidoscopy, colonoscopy, ultrasonography, or other x-rays.

TREATMENT

The choice of treatment depends on the size of the tumor, the stage of the disease, whether female hormones affect tumor growth, and tumor grade, which tells how closely the cancer resembles normal cells and suggests how fast the cancer is likely to grow. Other factors, including the woman's age and general health, are also considered when planning treatment. (See also Preparing for Treatment, page 17.)

Methods of Treatment

Most women with uterine cancer are treated with surgery. Some have radiation therapy. A smaller number of women may be treated with hormonal therapy or chemotherapy. Another treatment option for women with uterine cancer is to take part in treatment studies called clinical trials (see page 20).

Surgery to remove the uterus (hysterectomy) and the fallopian tubes and ovaries (bilateral salpingo-oophorectomy) is the treatment recommended for most women with uterine cancer. Lymph nodes near the tumor may also be removed during surgery to see if they contain cancer. If cancer cells have reached the lymph nodes, it may mean that the disease has spread to other parts of the body. If cancer cells have not spread beyond the endometrium, the disease can usually be cured with surgery alone.

In radiation therapy (also called radiotherapy), high-energy rays are used to kill cancer cells. Radiation therapy may be used in addition to surgery to treat women with certain stages of uterine cancer. Radiation may be used before surgery to shrink the tumor or after surgery to destroy any cancer cells that remain in the area. Also, for a small number of women who cannot have surgery, radiation treatment is sometimes used instead.

Hormonal therapy is the use of drugs, such as progesterone, that prevent cancer cells from getting or using the hormones they may need to grow. Women who are unable to have surgery or who have metastatic or recurrent endometrial cancer are sometimes treated with hormonal therapy.

Chemotherapy is the use of drugs to kill cancer cells. Anticancer drugs may be taken by mouth or given by injection into a blood vessel or a muscle. Like hormonal therapy, chemotherapy is a systemic therapy; it can kill cancer cells throughout the body.

Side Effects of Treatment

In treating cancer, it is hard to limit the effects of treatment so that only cancer cells are removed or destroyed. Because treatment also damages healthy cells and tissues, it often causes side effects.

After a hysterectomy, women usually have some pain and general fatigue. In some cases, patients may have nausea and vomiting following surgery, and some women may have problems returning to normal bladder and bowel function.

Women who have had a hysterectomy no longer have menstrual periods. When the ovaries are removed, menopause occurs immediately. Hot flashes and other symptoms of menopause caused by surgery may be more severe than those caused by natural menopause. In the general population, estrogen replacement therapy (ERT) is often prescribed to relieve these problems. However, ERT is not commonly used for women who have had endometrial cancer. Because estrogen has been linked to the development of uterine cancer, many doctors are concerned that ERT may cause uterine cancer to recur. Other doctors point out that there is no scientific evidence that ERT increases the risk of recurrence. A large research study is being conducted to determine whether women who have had early stage endometrial cancer can safely take estrogen.

With radiation therapy, the side effects depend largely on the treatment dose and the part of the body that is treated. During radiation therapy, people are likely to become very tired, especially in the later weeks of treatment. Resting is important, but doctors usually advise patients to stay as active as they can.

Radiation therapy for uterine cancer commonly causes dry, reddened skin and hair loss in the treated area, loss of appetite, fatigue, diarrhea or frequent and uncomfortable urination. It also may cause a decrease in the number of white blood cells that help protect the body against infection. Some women have dryness, itching, tightening, and burning in the vagina. Women may be advised not to have intercourse during treatment, but most can resume sexual activity within a few weeks after treatment ends. Women may be taught how to use a dilator, as well as a water-soluble lubricant, to help minimize these problems.

Hormonal therapy can cause a number of side effects. Women taking progesterone may experience fatigue and changes in appetite and weight, and they may retain fluid. Premenopausal women may have changes in their menstrual periods. Women may wish to discuss the side effects of hormonal therapy with their doctor.

The side effects of chemotherapy depend mainly on the drugs and the doses received. In addition, as with other types of treatment, side effects vary for each individual. When blood cells are affected by anticancer drugs, patients are more likely to get infections, may bruise or bleed easily, and may have less energy. Cells in hair roots and cells that line the digestive tract may be affected and patients may lose their hair and have other side effects, such as poor appetite, nausea and vomiting, or mouth sores. Usually, these side effects go away gradually during the recovery periods between treatments or after treatment is over.

FOLLOW-UP CARE

It is important for women who have had uterine cancer to have regular follow-up examinations after their treatment is over, in case the cancer comes back. Regular follow-up care ensures that any changes in health are discussed, and any recurrent cancer can be treated as soon as possible. Between follow-up appointments, women who have had uterine cancer should report any health problems as soon as they appear. Checkups may include a physical exam, a pelvic exam, a chest x-ray, and various laboratory tests.

The National Cancer Institute

The Blood

The average adult possesses a total quantity of about 10 pints of blood. The heart normally circulates all 10 pints once every minute when we're at rest—and up to four times a minute when we exercise.

The blood's duties are many. Its primary job is to supply all the cells in the body with nutrients harvested from the digestive system and oxygen drawn in through the lungs. Even as it completes this task, the blood becomes useful in another way, by picking up and taking away the cells' waste products. The carbon dioxide formed when cells burn oxygen is returned, via the bloodstream, to the tiny air sacs in the lungs, where it is then spirited away in an exhaled breath. Other toxins and chemical by-products are transported to the kidneys and liver, where they are filtered out and then excreted.

The blood also plays a crucial role in the immune system, and specific blood cells fight infection. When we are injured, bleeding helps wash dirt and microbes away from the site of the wound; then a complex mechanism prompts blood clotting and scab formation (to prevent us from losing too much blood) and initiates the healing process.

The circulatory system also carries hormones and other chemical messengers throughout the body to permit its remotest areas to communicate with each other and coordinate their functions. The blood helps regulate body temperature somewhat as well, by dissipating excess heat produced in the muscles—explaining the familiar flush we experience during vigorous activity. Conversely, when the air temperature is cold, blood moves away from the extremities and rushes toward the vital organs to keep them warm—which we notice as our fingertips and toes suffer the initial brunt of the chill.

About half of the blood is made up of blood cells; the other half is plasma, the fluid portion of the blood. There are three basic types of blood cells: red cells, white cells, and platelets.

The red cells (erythrocytes) are the most plentiful of all. These cells exchange fresh oxygen for the carbon dioxide exhaust. Red cells contain hemoglobin, a special iron-based protein that binds readily with oxygen when oxygen concentration is high, as it is in the lungs—but releases oxygen just as readily when oxygen concentration is low, as it is in body tissues.

The unique doughnutlike shape of the red blood cell is perfectly suited to its function. Its relatively great overall surface area allows maximal absorption of both oxygen and carbon dioxide gases, yet its thinness and small quotient of internal mass make the cell pliable enough to squeeze through minuscule blood vessels without rupturing. Abnormalities in red blood cells result in various types of anemia and other disorders.

The white cells (leukocytes) are broken down into several major types (granulocytes, monocytes, and lymphocytes), but all share a common purpose: to fight disease. Some of these cells literally seek out, engulf, and destroy invading bacteria. Other white cells produce antibodies, which form during a disease (such as measles or mononucleosis) and stay in the bloodstream long afterward to prevent a second attack. Sometimes the immune system goes awry, and forms antibodies against our own body cells. This process can result in autoimmune diseases such as rheumatoid arthritis.

Platelets (thrombocytes), the smallest of the blood elements, along with a number of clotting proteins in the blood, are responsible for the clotting mechanism. Clotting begins within seconds after a cut. Platelets move to the cut site, where they become sticky and clump together to form a plug in the injured blood vessel and minimize any blood loss.

But clots are not always a good thing; when they form in a major blood vessel, they can lead to heart attacks and strokes. So the system also has complex controls to prevent or dissolve unnecessary clots. A careful balance is essential. Abnormalities in the platelets or clotting proteins can result in the tendency to bleed too much (hemophilia, for example); when the balance is tipped the other way, dangerous clots are inclined to form (thrombosis).

Plasma is everything that's left over if you take away all the various cells. It is a yellowish liquid, 95 percent water, with a salt content closely approximating that of seawater. Adrift in the plasma are all of the blood cells, as well as proteins, hormones, sugars, minerals, and fats, including cholesterol.

Because blood interacts with almost every organ, diseases or malfunctions anywhere in the body are frequently reflected by changes in the blood. For this reason, blood tests are among the most fundamental and informative elements in making a medical diagnosis.

The most routine test, the complete blood count (CBC), determines the number of each type of blood cell in a given volume of blood, and then examines the cells for any abnormalities in structure. The hemoglobin or "hematocrit value" of a CBC measures the quantity of red blood cells; a "differential count" compares the relative numbers of the various white cells.

Mild degrees of anemia, in fact, usually produce few or no symptoms and are generally discovered only when a doctor obtains a complete blood count. Certain diseases have a direct and predictable effect on the chemical content of the blood. Diabetes, for example, is associated with elevated levels of glucose. Many types of liver disease, meanwhile, result in high levels of a compound called bilirubin.

The Editors

VITAMIN AND MINERAL DEFICIENCY ANEMIAS

People who are feeling fatigued, and believe the ads about "tired blood," might think that taking an iron supplement will cure iron deficiency anemia and pep them right up. In truth, however, most fatigue is not related to tired blood; most anemia comes on without any noticeable symptoms at all; and most anemia in older adults is not due to low iron intake, but is caused by slow intestinal bleeding.

Anemia is one of the most common disorders among older adults. It is usually not discovered by reporting symptoms to a doctor, but rather by the complete blood count the doctor periodically orders. Indeed, screening for anemia is one of the important reasons for doing a complete blood count.

Anemia is not a normal consequence of aging, as had been thought until recently. Nor is anemia itself a disease; it is instead a manifestation of any one of a number of different disorders that affect the red blood cells—ranging from iron deficiency anemia to the less common types, such as hemolytic and aplastic anemia. Each of the anemias has a different origin—and a different treatment. The focus of this section is on the three most common types, which originate in deficiencies of certain vitamins or minerals.

IRON DEFICIENCY ANEMIA
Iron deficiency anemia arises from too little iron in your body to make sufficient hemoglobin. Most of the blood cells, including the red blood cells that perform the crucial task of picking up oxygen in your lungs and taking it throughout your system, are produced in the marrow that lies within certain bones.

The principal component of red blood cells, the substance that enables them to transport oxygen, is a special protein, hemo-globin—and iron is a necessary component of hemoglobin. A decrease in the quality or quantity of hemoglobin, or in the number of red blood cells themselves, results in a reduced oxygen-carrying capacity in your blood—which is to say, in anemia (from the Greek, meaning "a lack of blood").

By far the most frequent cause of iron deficiency anemia in older adults is excessive blood loss, which takes iron from the body faster than it is replaced in the diet. This is usually the result of slow, persistent bleeding from any number of intestinal lesions—for example, an ulcer, polyps, or cancer.

The frequent use of aspirin, ibuprofen, or other nonsteroidal anti-inflammatory drugs (NSAIDs) can also result in chronic blood loss from irritation of the stomach lining. Bleeding from the intestines, when severe, generally shows up as black tarry stools, or even frankly bloody stools; most commonly, however, the bleeding is very slow and not readily apparent (so-called occult blood).

It is possible, too, that iron deficiency anemia can be caused by too little iron in your diet—though this is very unusual, except in menstruating women whose diets have a limited iron content. Most iron in red blood cells is recycled to make new red blood cells—and the amount of iron lost in the recycling process is minuscule (just 1 mg a day for men, 2 mg for menstruating women). Most diets easily compensate for the loss, except in those on severe weight-loss plans and impoverished people who have little variety of food sources. (Because your body absorbs only 10 percent of the iron you consume, you need to take in 10 mg of iron a day—an amount easily provided by a balanced diet of about 1,700 calories.)

Another possible cause of this type of anemia is an inability of the digestive system to absorb iron—most often because part of the stomach or intestine has been removed surgically. But this, too, is uncommon. Again, the most common cause of iron deficiency anemia is slow bleeding.

Not surprisingly, the symptoms of iron deficiency anemia—when and if they do appear—are paleness (because it is the pigmented red cells flowing near the skin that produce a pink complexion), weakness (because oxygen is required to use energy), and fatigue. In more severe cases, there can also be shortness of breath, heart palpitations, an increased heart rate, especially during

---

ANALGESICS AND ANEMIA

Both aspirin and the other nonsteroidal anti-inflammatory drugs (such as Motrin, Nalfon, Ponstel, and Naprosyn) share not only therapeutic effects—painkilling and reduction of inflammation in joints and muscles—but also a propensity toward some unwanted side effects. Chief among these is irritation of the lining of the stomach (gastritis). This effect is so common that evidence of some small amount of blood is found in the stool of as many as 70 percent of users. For this reason, these drugs are stopped for at least three days before the stool is checked for occult blood due to ulcers or tumors in the gastrointestinal tract.

To lessen stomach irritation, these medicines may be taken with food or an antacid (one containing magnesium and aluminum hydroxide is best). Unless your doctor has specifically told you to take aspirin and an NSAID together, it is best to avoid this combination, because it greatly increases the risk of irritation and possible bleeding. And be sure to tell your doctor if you are taking over-the-counter NSAIDs on a regular basis, as this could be very significant when trying to diagnose the origin of an iron deficiency anemia.

TAKING IRON SUPPLEMENTS

If your doctor prescribes iron supplements, ask your druggist for the cheapest generic available. Coated, time-release, or combination pills cost much more and may actually impede the absorption of iron.

• Take your iron pill with at least eight ounces of fluid.

• Take it between meals to maximize iron absorption; but if it causes stomach upset, take the pill with food or right after a meal.

• If you take iron in liquid form, mix it with water or fruit juice and drink it through a straw so that it doesn't stain your teeth. (If you do get stains, brush your teeth with baking soda or 3 percent hydrogen peroxide.)

• If you miss a dose, skip it; don't double-dose.

• Keep your medicine out of reach of children. As few as three or four adult iron tablets can cause serious poisoning in young children.

• Don't store iron tablets in a bathroom medicine chest; heat or moisture may cause the medicine to break down. Keep them in a cool, dry place.

• While you are taking iron, consume the following foods in only very small amounts, and then only an hour before or two hours after your iron tablet: tea, coffee, cheese, eggs, ice cream, and milk, because they decrease absorption; and whole-grain breads and cereals, because they are already iron-fortified.

• Check with your doctor if you have any of the more common side effects of iron supplements (constipation, diarrhea, heartburn), particularly if you experience nausea or vomiting.

• If you are taking a long-acting or enteric-coated iron tablet, such as Feosol or Fero-Gradumet, and your stools do not turn black, check with your doctor, because the tablets may not be breaking down properly. If your stools are black and tarry, and are accompanied by cramps, soreness, or sharp pains in the stomach, or red streaks in the stool, check with your doctor at once, because this may indicate gastrointestinal bleeding.

• Do not take iron supplements for more than six months without checking back with your doctor.

exertion (as the heart tries to compensate for the lack of oxygen-carrying hemoglobin by pumping out more blood), and even chest pains (not totally because the blood flow is impeded, as in coronary artery disease, but because the blood can't carry sufficient oxygen to the heart).

Certain nutritional anemias may cause a sore tongue or tiny cracks at the corners of your mouth.

But you should not, under any circumstances, attempt to treat yourself if you feel anemic. Adding iron-rich foods or multivitamins with iron to your diet, or taking Geritol, is almost certainly just a way of ignoring the problem. Taking iron supplements may not address the underlying condition (such as an ulcer or a cancer) that is causing the anemia.

VITAMIN B_{12} DEFICIENCY

Vitamin B_{12} deficiency, or pernicious anemia, most often occurs in older adults. Except among strict vegetarians, B_{12} deficiency is the result of an impaired ability of the digestive tract to absorb the B_{12} from your diet.

For some reason, the condition occurs more often in fair-haired older people of northern European descent.

Vitamin B_{12} is essential for the production of red blood cells; a deficiency leads to a decline in the production of red blood cells. Vitamin B_{12} is vital also to the maintenance of the nervous system, so a B_{12} deficiency produces not only the usual symptoms of anemia, but also leads to damage of the brain and spinal cord—which can show up in numbness and tingling in the hands and feet, a disturbed sense of balance with a change in walking gait, and mental disturbances such as confusion, personality changes, and depression. Because so much B_{12} is stored in the liver, a deficiency can take a long time to develop.

Having a close relative with pernicious anemia increases your risk of having it yourself. You ought to inform your physician and be certain to have the appropriate blood tests.

Although the disorder is called pernicious anemia because it used to be untreatable, today it can almost always be effectively treated.

Current treatment usually consists of a lifelong regimen of monthly B_{12} injections. Neither diet nor any oral supplement can help, because the underlying problem is nonabsorption of B_{12} from the gastrointestinal tract. If the deficiency is caught and treated promptly, you should recover completely.

FOLIC ACID DEFICIENCY

Folic acid deficiency is usually caused by an inadequate intake of folic acid, a vitamin mainly supplied by the fresh green leafy vegetables, mushrooms, lima beans, and kidney beans in your diet. The body cannot store folic acid, so a dietary deficiency will ordinarily show up in only a few weeks as anemia, because folic acid, like B_{12}, is essential for the production of red blood cells.

Folic acid deficiency may occur among older people who have a poor diet. It is particularly common in heavy alcohol drinkers.

This form of anemia is treated simply by taking folic acid tablets for a short period of time—followed by attention to including a range of green vegetables in your diet.

Treatment may be more complicated if the deficiency results from an inability to absorb folic acid from the digestive tract—though this is less common.

The Editors

SICKLE CELL ANEMIA

Sickle cell anemia is a worldwide health problem, affecting many races, countries, and ethnic groups. The World Health Organization estimates that each year more than 250,000 babies are born worldwide with this inherited blood cell disorder, which causes red blood cells to elongate and clog arteries. Chronic pain and life-threatening infections may result from the illness. About one in 400 African American newborns in the United States has sickle cell anemia, but the disease is also prevalent in many Spanish-speaking regions of the world, such as South America, Cuba, Central America, and among the Hispanic community in the United States. People in Mediterranean countries—Turkey, Greece,

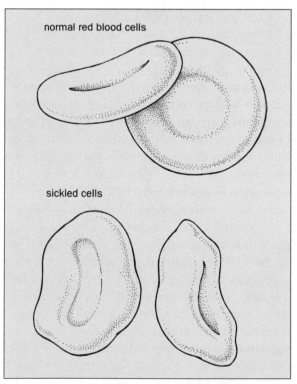

Sickle cell disease alters the shape of a red blood cell, so that it breaks down prematurely, functions inefficiently, and can clog tiny blood vessels.

and Italy—also have the illness. And many people, including one in 12 African Americans, carry the sickle cell trait—meaning they can pass the defect onto offspring, although their own health remains excellent.

CAUSES

What exactly causes sickle cell anemia and how did it spread to so many different parts of the world? The answer lies in a curious coincidence. It turns out that anyone who carries the inherited trait for sickle cell anemia, but does not have the actual illness, is protected against the severe form of malaria. So in countries that had a problem with malaria, children born with sickle cell trait survived. They grew up, had their own children, and passed the gene for sickle cell anemia on to these offspring. As populations migrated, the sickle cell trait and sickle cell anemia moved throughout the world.

One theory proposes that sickle cell anemia originated in Africa and, through the slave trade, spread to South America, North America, and Europe.

Another theory suggests that sickle cell anemia began in the Middle East and then spread from there.

Although we don't know for sure where sickle cell anemia began, scientists have identified four separate types of genetic mutations related to the illness, each associated with a different geographic area—Senegal, Benin, Central Africa, and the Middle East. This information excites geneticists and anthropologists because it allows them to trace the migration of populations depending on which sickle cell mutation they carry. And medically, identifying the type of mutation a person has can be critical to treatment, because the severity of disease appears to vary with the type of mutation.

To understand the causes of sickle cell anemia, we must focus attention on a special molecule found in red blood cells. That molecule, called hemoglobin, takes oxygen from the lungs and transports it to other parts of the body. Hemoglobin's oxygen-carrying ability is essential for living, but a structural defect in the pigmented molecule can wreak havoc in the blood cell.

Hemoglobin contains four chains, or strings, of amino acids—the compounds that make up proteins. Two of the amino acid chains are known as alpha chains, and two are called beta chains. In normal hemoglobin, the amino acid in the sixth position on the beta chains is glutamic acid. But in people with sickle cell anemia, that sixth position is occupied by another amino acid, valine, instead. This single amino acid substitution has some devastating consequences.

After releasing oxygen, hemoglobin molecules that contain the beta chain defect stick to one another instead of staying separate, forming long, rigid rods or tubules inside red blood cells. The rods cause the normally smooth, doughnut-shaped red blood cells to take on a sickle or curved shape and to lose their vital ability to deform and squeeze through tiny blood vessels. The sickled cells, which become stiff and sticky, clog small blood vessels, keeping tissue from receiving an adequate blood supply. Most of the problems associated with sickle cell anemia stem from this blockage.

SYMPTOMS

Pain caused by the blockage of sickled red blood is the most common symptom of sickle cell anemia, and it can occur unpredictably in any organ or joint of the body—wherever and whenever a blood clot develops. And as with any of the complications of the disease, the frequency and amount of pain vary widely. Some patients experience painful episodes only once a year; some may have as many as 15 to 20 episodes annually.

These painful, disruptive events can be so severe that the patient may require hospitalization for five to seven days to receive intravenous fluids and narcotic painkillers.

Recent studies have shown that the drug hydroxyurea can reduce the number and severity of these episodes in some patients.

The sickle cell clots can be life-threatening, depending on where they occur. For example, in the brain a clot may cause a stroke, leading to paralysis or death. Blood transfusions may be required every three to four weeks for an extended period to avoid recurrence of clots in the brain. Other clots, meanwhile, may damage such vital organs as the heart, kidney, lungs, liver, or eyes.

Complicating matters further, the pain associated with a clot can mimic symptoms of several other diseases, making sickle cell disease difficult to diagnose. Joint pain in sickle cell patients resembles that of arthritis, and pain in the intestines might be confused with appendicitis. A sickle-cell-induced clot in the skin can cause ulcers, a condition that may also cause the diagnosis to be diverted from the underlying sickle cell problem.

As patients get older, it becomes more difficult for the heart to function normally. Lung clots may also make them more prone to pneumonia or chronic lung disease. Gallstones are common in this illness and may require surgical removal.

Another particularly serious problem is the eyes. Many patients with sickle cell anemia have jaundice, causing their eyes to look yellow due to the rapid breakdown of red blood cells. But much more severe is damage to the retina, the onionskin-thin tissue that acts as the eye's version of photographic film. Containing thousands of tiny sensors that convert light into electrical information for the brain, the retina can severely deteriorate if it is not adequately nourished by the tiny arteries and veins that crisscross it. Blindness

may result from sickle cell blockage in the retina. Because of the seriousness of this complication, ophthalmologists should start examining children's eyes at the age of five.

As they mature, children with sickle cell anemia develop problems in the growth of their long bones, such as those in the spinal column or hip. Blood supply to the hip is barely adequate even in healthy people, so patients with sickle cell disease and its associated blockage can be especially vulnerable to hip problems. In severe cases, structural damage may require replacement with a prosthesis, or artificial device. Just as serious can be damage to the spinal column, which may compress and cause severe pain.

It's important to emphasize that not all patients have every complication, and that the severity of symptoms has wide variation. Sickle cell anemia can affect two brothers in dramatically different ways, even though they grew up in the same environment and have a similar genetic makeup.

One symptom that does affect most people who have the disease is the disorder for which the disease is named—anemia, or a lack of red blood cells.

Anemia occurs because sickled red blood cells last only 10 to 20 days in the bloodstream, rather than the normal 120-day lifetime. The sickled red blood cells are removed from circulation faster than the bone marrow can produce them.

GENETICS AND SICKLE CELL ANEMIA

There is a big distinction between someone with the sickle cell trait and someone who has the disease. To understand this bit of genetics, it's important to note that about 400 types of hemoglobin exist.

Because the gene for sickling disease is recessive, a child must inherit it from both parents in order to develop the full-blown illness. Similarly, if a child inherits sickled hemoglobin from one parent, and another type of hemoglobin, called hemoglobin C, from the other parent, that child develops a variation of sickle cell disease known as SC disease. (Some other variations of sickle cell anemia exist, depending on differences in the types of hemoglobin inherited from each parent.)

But if a child receives sickle hemoglobin from one parent and healthy hemoglobin from the other, that child has the sickle cell trait. That child does not develop sickled cells unless subjected to extreme environmental stress. The child then goes on to live a normal life. But that person does carry the sickle trait, meaning he or she has the ability to pass the sickle gene onto offspring.

SOME MISCONCEPTIONS

One in 12 African Americans in the United States has the sickle cell trait (not the disease), and many other races and nationalities also carry the genetic defect. In the past, many people with the trait felt they should not marry or have children, for fear the children might develop the disease. In fact, there were even laws passed in this country requiring African American couples to have a sickle cell test before they married. And if they did carry the trait, they were often counseled not to have children. This was never an acceptable approach. People who think they may carry the sickle trait may be tested for it if they wish. Professionals may give counseling if asked, but the ultimate decision to have children is up to the parents, as it is for any genetic disease.

There are several other misconceptions about sickle cell anemia. One is that the illness is contagious; most people now realize that this is not so.

Another misunderstanding is that sickle cell anemia patients rarely live past the age of 20; in fact, many people with the disease are in their forties, fifties, and sixties.

The Warren Grant Magnuson Clinical Center

CHAPTER 3

The Brain and Nervous System

It takes 100 billion neurons—amounting to about three pounds of matter—to comprise a human brain. A flow of electrical impulses across the neurons that make up the brain, the spinal cord, and the extensive network of nerves that branch out to the most remote places of the body is the basis of our talents and personality, our thoughts and emotions, our memories and dreams.

This continuous transmission of nerve impulses gives human behavior its vast complexity. The nervous system handles the vital primary tasks of regulating our metabolism, body temperature, and respiration—even as it also enables us to learn, remember, and draw sophisticated inferences about all that we experience.

Understanding the biological function of the components of the nervous system helps us understand our behavior. At the base of the brain is the brainstem, connecting the spinal cord to the brain. The spinal cord is a conduit for all nerve signals between the brain and body, and it handles a great many of the body's reflexes. The brainstem manages basic life-support—breathing, heart function, and sleep cycles. Above the brainstem at the back of the skull is the cerebellum. It controls coordination, balance, and posture.

Above the cerebellum is the group of structures known as the limbic system. This part of the brain, which we share in common with all other mammals, provides us with primal urges and powerful emotions crucial for self-preservation: rage, terror, hunger, and sexual desire. The limbic system's direct connections with some of the higher brain faculties allow us both to cogitate upon what we feel emotionally and to have emotional reactions to what we think about.

The four major components of the limbic system are the amygdala, the hippocampus, the hypothalamus, and the thalamus. The almond-shaped amygdala, which plays a role in the emotions, especially aggression, is the basic pathway into the limbic system for nerve impulses. The hippocampus is an information processor, matching new data against those already stored in the brain. It is therefore one of the structures absolutely critical in the process of ascribing meaning to the symbols and events of our lives. The hypothalamus, integral to our moods, regulates food intake, internal water balance, and reproductive cycles. It generally acts as a liaison between the brain and the rest of the body, initiating the release of at least seven different hormones to the pituitary (or master) gland, which in turn releases into the bloodstream other hormones that influence growth, aging, and all aspects of reproduction. Located near the center of the brain, the thalamus processes all of the senses except smell. It takes the incoming sensory signals and, like a switchboard, sends them to the appropriate region in the brain for interpretation.

Surrounding these evolutionarily older, more primitive, brain structures is the cerebrum, which in humans constitutes the largest portion of the brain. It's here that electrical nerve impulses are transformed into images,

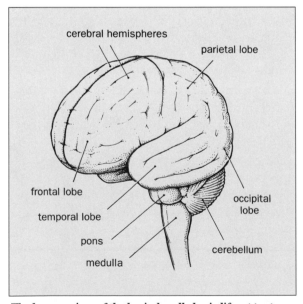

The lower regions of the brain handle basic life-support, while sophisticated interpretation of sensory data occurs in the lobes of the cerebral hemispheres.

symbols, and ideas. It's here that schemes, contraptions, sonnets, and melodies are invented. The outer surface of the cerebrum, known as the cortex, with its convoluted folds of gray matter, gives the brain its familiar appearance. The cortex is the seat of conscious thought, perception, and the integration of all sensory input.

A unique feature of the human brain is that the cerebral cortex is divided into two halves, or hemispheres, each with its own set of particular abilities. The right hemisphere specializes in matters of spatial relationships, color perception, visualization, and musical aptitude. For this, the right brain is often considered the creative, intuitive, or artistic side of the brain. The left brain is generally more adept at handling analytical tasks, such as mathematical calculation and logical reasoning. The left brain also has particular regions that seem to be dedicated to highly specific tasks, such as understanding words or generating speech (so it, too, is creative in its own right). The two hemispheres are connected by a thick neural cable known as the corpus callosum.

As we age, neurons die off at a rate of nearly 20 million per year. Surprisingly, this degeneration generally has no significant bearing on our "crystallized" intelligence—that is, our vocabulary, knowledge of specific details and general information, and the ability to comprehend abstract ideas. So our years of accumulated knowledge and experience do indeed confer a certain undeniable wisdom. Only "fluid" intelligence—or the amount of new information we're able to master at one time and the speed at which we process information—diminishes with normal aging. So we may know as much as we ever did, but it might take a bit longer to summon up information from the memory bank. Healthy people in their seventies have essentially the same rates of blood flow and oxygen consumption in their brains (about 20 percent of the body's total consumption, despite

the brain's fairly small size) as their 20-year-old counterparts; functional mental capacity is hardly altered throughout the course of adulthood.

Thus the onset of senility or general mental deterioration is in no way a natural or inevitable part of aging. It is true that certain areas of the nervous system fare better than others as neurons die off: In the cerebellum and brainstem region, little or no loss of neurons occurs with age, whereas the cortex—the thinking portion of the brain—can lose upwards of 50,000 neurons a day. Nature prepares us for this, however, by endowing us at birth with millions of extra or "redundant" neurons; as some die, others remain to preserve our memories and abilities. It's only in cases of head injury, side effects from drugs, diseases such as Alzheimer's or stroke, or degeneration due to malnutrition or alcoholism that the nervous system suffers damage and displays the more severe mental problems associated with aging.

The Editors

DEMENTIA

Dementia—more accurately, the dementias—are brain diseases that result in the progressive loss of mental faculties, often beginning with memory, learning, attention, and judgment. Though some types of dementia are curable, the most common dementing illnesses are not. In time, an unrelenting dementia will erode all aspects of thought, feeling, and behavior, and lead to death.

It is important to realize that demented persons are not insane in the sense of suffering a psychiatric disorder. They become—as the word dementia literally means—deprived of mind, deprived of the use of parts of the brain associated with a range of intellectual skills and activities unique to human beings.

Contrary to what many people think, dementing disorders are not the fate that awaits us all with aging. In the United States an estimated 5 percent of the population 65 or over is severely demented. Another 10 percent may be mildly to moderately impaired. That means that 85 percent of the elderly are not demented.

But there is an association of dementia with aging, and because Americans are living longer, the numbers affected will increase. There are now 2 million people in the United States 65 or over who are severely impaired intellectually.

Still another smaller group of adults succumbs to dementing illnesses earlier in life. Over half of these presenile dementias are due to Alzheimer's disease, a progressive dementia. Neurologists now agree that over half the dementias occurring among the elderly—disorders called senile dementia, or chronic organic brain syndrome—are actually cases of disease of the Alzheimer's type beginning at a later stage of life.

THE POWER OF WORDS

Words like "presenile," "senile," and "senility" help perpetuate the myth that aging means mental decline: The words are derived from a Latin root that simply means "to grow old." In Greek and Roman times people so dreaded the infirmities of old age that they regarded aging itself as a disease. Too many people today still hold such beliefs, and it is only as the proportion of older people in the population has risen—and become more vocal—that the myths are beginning to fade. Today neuroscientists know there are age-related changes in the brain, but the changes do not seriously affect mental vigor. Moreover, there are so many examples of intelligence and creativity among the elderly that the belief that getting old means getting senile is simply not true.

Negative feelings about aging, compounded with the fear and shame so often associated with brain disease, have made it difficult for laymen and health professionals to deal with problems posed by the dementias.

THE PSEUDODEMENTIAS

Neurologists seeing patients with suspected dementia work by a process of elimination: They review the roster of true dementing disorders as well as all the ailments that can masquerade as dementia ("pseudodementias").

Depression

High among the disorders that can simulate dementia are depression and manic-depression (see also Mental Health, page 455). Depressed individuals are frequently passive and unresponsive. They may appear confused, slow, and forgetful. In manic-depression, the individual may experience mood swings between depression and mania—the latter an excited state in which a person feels powerful and often acts recklessly or foolishly.

People experiencing a dementing illness may also act irrationally and appear excited. They may also be depressed—either as part of the disease process itself or as a reaction to their failing mental powers.

In sorting out depression from dementia, the physician may find that depressed individuals have had earlier bouts of depression along with symptoms of insomnia, fatigue, or loss of appetite. In contrast, a person in the early stages of dementia often singles out a memory problem, or difficulties in arithmetic, as the trouble. The onset of a progressive dementia like Alzheimer's disease is also likely to be slow and insidious, while depressions usually develop more quickly.

Sometimes an older person who appears passive, slow, or confused may have recently lost a spouse or close friend and is suffering what is called a reactive depression. It is not unusual for the mourner to seem distracted, speaking and acting as if the dead person were still alive, for example.

In other cases, a person who appears withdrawn or absent-minded may be reacting to the diminished circumstances of life, the loss of income and influence, for example. Loneliness and a disappointment with fate or with the state of society may be added burdens. Such a person's prevailing mood has been described as existential sadness—a mood that might benefit from sensitive human contact and rewarding activity, but not one that should be considered either mental or physical illness.

Drug Reactions

Rivaling depression as a major factor complicating the diagnosis of dementia are reactions to drugs. Often—especially in older adults—people are taking more than one drug for chronic conditions: water pills (diuretics) to control high blood pressure, sedatives for sleeplessness, tranquilizers for nerves—in addition to aspirin, laxatives, other over-the-counter drugs, and alcohol.

It is wise to assume that all drugs are powerful; all drugs have side effects, and most drugs interact: In combination, two or more drugs may be more powerful than each taken alone.

What makes drug use a particularly vexing problem in older people are age-related changes in metabolism. Both the liver and the kidneys may be less efficient in clearing the body of drugs, and along with a general slowing of metabolism, a drug may persist in the body longer than in a younger person. Often, too, the dosage appropriate for a 25-year-old is much too strong for a 60-year-old. Some physicians routinely wean a patient off all medications when confronted with mental symptoms.

Chemical Imbalances

The brain makes a high demand on nutrients, and poor eating habits or problems in food absorption can seriously affect the brain. Again the problems can be worse in older people who may be inactive, have little appetite, and often skimp on food. Interestingly, mental symptoms may appear before physical ones. Pernicious anemia, for example, is a blood disorder caused by impaired ability to use one of the B vitamins. In older people the first symptoms may be irritability or depression. Inadequate thyroid hormone can result in apathy, depression, or dementia. Hypoglycemia—a condition in which there is not enough sugar in the bloodstream—can give rise to confusion or personality change. Too little or too much sodium or calcium can also trigger disturbing mental changes. Tests can determine whether any of these imbalances are present.

Heart and Lung Problems

Just as the brain demands high-quality nutrition, it also requires a high level of oxygen. Chronic lung disease can lead to an oxygen shortage that can starve brain cells and lead to the symptoms of dementia. If the heart is not pumping efficiently, if there are disturbances in heart rhythm, malfunctioning heart valves, or other indications of heart disease, the brain may suffer.

All of these "pseudodementias" are treatable, and if the brain has not suffered permanent damage, the dementing symptoms should abate.

Other potentially reversible dementias may be caused by brain swelling (hydrocephalus), meningitis, brain tumor, head injury, certain hereditary disorders, chronic sleep deprivation, and poisoning by lead, mercury, or by exposure to carbon monoxide, some pesticides, and industrial pollutants. Chronic alcoholism can also seriously impair mental faculties, notably memory for recent events. Some investigators think that alcohol in itself may cause irreparable brain damage, but the memory deficit appears to be related to the chronic drinker's inadequate diet—specifically, thiamine (vitamin B_1) deficiency.

THE TRUE DEMENTIAS

Once the pseudodementias have been eliminated, the physician faced with a patient with failing mental powers will suspect circulatory problems or primary brain disease to be the cause.

Alzheimer's Disease and Infarct Dementia

Next to Alzheimer's disease (see next page), the leading cause of dementia in aging is obstruction to blood flow in the brain. Most commonly, a blood clot will clog a blood vessel, or a vessel may burst, hemorrhaging into a part of the brain. If a major vessel is involved, the symptoms are sudden, dramatic, and sometimes fatal—the consequences of a major stroke. A small stroke may go unnoticed, however, or result in specific symptoms—a slurring of speech, perhaps, or a numbness in one hand. The evidence of a brain blood vessel (cerebrovascular) accident shows up as a small mass of coagulating blood and dead tissue called an infarct. If the number of infarcts increases over time, the chances are that the individual will experience progressive mental and physical decline.

Multi-infarct dementia is now the preferred term for mental deterioration due to blood vessel disease in the brain. It replaces the old-fashioned and inaccurate "hardening of the arteries of the brain."

Multi-infarct dementia is now thought to account for between 12 and 20 percent of dementia in the elderly; another 16 to 20 percent of dementia patients have both infarcts and Alzheimer's disease.

It is usually not difficult to distinguish between the two most common dementias. Persons with infarct dementia often have a history of high blood pressure, vascular disease, or previous stroke. Infarcts are also the result of events that may occur months or years apart. Thus the dementia progresses in stepwise fashion in contrast to the steady decline seen in Alzheimer's disease. Since the infarct is usually limited to one part of the brain, the symptoms, too, are limited; they may affect only one side of the body or involve a specific faculty like language. Neurologists call these local or focal symptoms, as opposed to the global symptoms seen in Alzheimer's disease.

Other Causes of Progressive Dementia

The remaining causes of progressive dementia are less usual nervous system diseases. While each disorder alone affects a relatively small number of people, the group as a whole accounts for over a million patients with progressive and dementing brain disease in America today.

Multiple sclerosis. Among the better known neurological diseases is multiple sclerosis, a disorder characterized by destruction of the insulating material covering nerve fibers. Usually the disease progresses through a series of acute episodes and partial recoveries. In time, both mental and physical deterioration can occur.

Parkinson's disease. Tremor and difficulty in originating voluntary movements are the hallmarks of Parkinson's disease (see page 183), a disorder which strikes older adults. Drugs can relieve symptoms, but do not halt the progression of the disease. Symptoms of dementia may appear in severe or advanced cases.

Huntington's disease. Children with a parent who has Huntington's disease stand a 50 percent chance of inheriting this relentless dementing disease. Symptoms usually appear in early middle age and can include personality change, mental decline, psychotic symptoms, and a movement disturbance. Restlessness and facial tics may progress to severe uncontrollable flailing of head, limbs, and trunk. At the same time, mental capacity can deteriorate to dementia.

Pick's disease. Symptoms of Pick's disease are very similar to those of Alzheimer's disease, but the disease is associated with different changes in brain tissue.

Creutzfeldt-Jakob disease. Infectious agents are recognized as the culprits in a growing number of progressive dementias. In Creutzfeldt-Jakob disease, the infectious agent is an unusual virus that may lie dormant in the body for years (hence it is called a "slow" virus). When activated, the virus produces a rapidly progressive dementia along with muscle spasms and changes in gait.

Each of these "true" dementias has inspired new research into causes and cures. In each case, too, active voluntary organizations have mobilized efforts to educate the public and come to the aid of patients and families.

SENSITIVE CARING

From the moment of diagnosis of dementia to the end of life, patients and families are subjected to pressures and strains that rarely let up. If there is a genetic component, the effect of the doctor's pronouncement of the diagnosis can be even more devastating. Sons and daughters, sisters and brothers, fear they themselves may one day succumb to the same remorseless symptoms.

In conditions like Alzheimer's disease, it is often the spouse alone who is left to do the caring—at a time of life when he or she may be elderly and in diminished health. The role is truly exhausting: "It's like a 36-hour day," as one man described it.

More often than not, the husband or wife of a patient will have assumed the burden of responsibility before the patient was diagnosed, quietly covering up for mental failings. After the diagnosis is made, there may be a period in which the loyal spouse and other family members deny the severity of the symptoms. The patient is really not so bad, they say, not as bad as someone else with a similar disorder.

Increasingly, health care professionals are acknowledging that all dementing diseases are family afflictions; patients need family support and flexibility in care—at home, in the community, and finally, if necessary, in a hospital or nursing facility. The voluntary health organizations concerned with dementing disorders understand this, and through their programs of advice and information come to the psychological and practical aid of families. Often they catalogue community resources, offer nursing care tips, and direct families to programs designed for patients with chronic neurological disorders.

While it is important for patients with dementia to relearn old skills and to socialize, it is equally important that family members have time off—respite from around-the-clock nursing demands. Most families want to keep their ailing relatives at home as long as possible. But they need the support of community resources to provide respite facilities—places where a patient can go for brief stays. And they need practical guidance in caring for the patient at home.

Some excellent books have been published to help patients and families cope. Among them are a guide entitled *The 36-Hour Day,* published by the Johns Hopkins University Press, and a manual prepared by the Dementia Research Program group at Burke Rehabilitation Center.

The National Institute of Neurological Disorders and Stroke

ALZHEIMER'S DISEASE

"Alzheimer's disease" is the term used to describe a dementing disorder marked by certain brain changes, regardless of the age of onset. Alzheimer's disease is not a normal part of aging—it is not something that inevitably happens in later life. Rather, it is one of the dementing disorders, a group of brain diseases that lead to the loss of mental and physical functions. The disorder, whose cause is unknown, affects a small but significant percentage of older Americans.

A very small minority of Alzheimer's patients are under 50 years of age. Most are over 65. Alzheimer's disease is the exception, rather than the rule, in old age. Only about 5 to 6 percent of older people are afflicted by Alzheimer's disease or a related dementia.

Although Alzheimer's disease is not curable or reversible, there are ways to alleviate symptoms and suffering and to assist families. Not every person with this illness is better off in a nursing home. Many thousands of patients—especially those in the early stages of the disease—are cared for by their families.

Indeed, one of the most important aspects of medical management is family education and family support services. When, or whether, to transfer a patient to a nursing home is a decision that must be carefully determined by the family.

RISK FACTORS

The main risk factor for Alzheimer's disease is increased age. The rates of the disease increase markedly with advancing age, with 25 percent of people over 85 suffering from Alzheimer's or other severe dementia.

Some investigators, describing a family pattern of Alzheimer's disease, suggest that heredity may influence its development. A genetic basis has been identified through the discovery of several genetic markers on chromosomes 14 and 21 for a small subgroup of families in which the disease has frequently occurred at relatively early ages (beginning before age 50). Some evidence points to chromosome 19 as implicated in certain other families that have frequently had Alzheimer's disease develop at later ages.

At the same time, data indicate that the likelihood that a close relative (sibling, child, or parent) of an afflicted individual will develop Alzheimer's disease is low. In most cases, such an individual's risk is only slightly higher than that of someone in the general population, where the lifetime risk is below 1 percent. And, of course, many disorders have a genetic potential that is never expressed—that is, despite being at risk for a certain illness, one might go through life without ever developing any symptom of the disease. In other instances, a genetic potential for a certain disorder may be released only if it is triggered by other risk factors.

There have been a few reports of a possible association between serious head injuries and the later onset of Alzheimer's disease, but otherwise no other risk factors have been unequivocally identified for Alzheimer's disease.

GENERAL SYMPTOMS

The onset of Alzheimer's disease is usually very slow and gradual, seldom occurring before age 65. Over time, however, it follows a progressively more serious course. Among the symptoms that typically develop, none is unique to Alzheimer's disease at its various stages. It is therefore essential for suspicious changes to be thoroughly evaluated before they become inappropriately or negligently labeled Alzheimer's disease.

The Early Signs

Problems of memory, particularly recent or short-term memory, are common early in the course of the disease. For example, the individual may, on repeated occasions, forget to turn off the iron or may not recall which of the morning's medicines were taken. Mild personality changes, such as less spontaneity or a sense of apathy and a tendency to withdraw from social interactions, may occur early in the illness.

As the disease progresses, problems in abstract thinking or in intellectual functioning develop. The individual may begin to have trouble with figures when working on bills, with understanding what is being read, or with organizing the day's work. Further disturbances in behavior and appearance may also be seen at this point, such as agitation, irritability, quarrelsomeness, and diminishing ability to dress appropriately.

The Later Signs

Later in the course of the disorder, the affected individuals may become confused or disoriented about what month or year it is and be unable to describe accurately where they live or to name correctly a place being visited. Eventually they may wander, be unable to engage in conversation, seem inattentive and erratic in mood, appear uncooperative, lose bladder and bowel control, and, in extreme cases, become totally incapable of caring for themselves if the final stage is reached. Death then follows, perhaps from pneumonia or some other problem that occurs in severely deteriorated states of health.

The average course of the disease from onset to death is about six to eight years, but it may range from under two to over 20 years. Those who develop the disorder later in life may die from other illnesses (such as heart disease) before Alzheimer's disease reaches its final and most serious stage.

Living with the Symptoms

Though the changes just described represent the general range of symptoms for Alzheimer's disease, the specific problems, along with the rate and severity of decline, can vary considerably with different individuals. Indeed, most persons with Alzheimer's disease can function at a reasonable level and remain at home far into the course of the disorder. Moreover, throughout much of the course of the illness individuals maintain the capacity for giving and receiving love, for sharing warm interpersonal relationships, and for participating in a variety of meaningful activities with family and friends.

The reaction of an individual to the illness—his or her capacity to cope with it—also varies, depending on such factors as lifelong personality patterns and the nature and severity of stress in the immediate environment.

Depression, severe uneasiness, and paranoia or delusions may accompany or result from Alzheimer's disease, but they can often be alleviated by appropriate treatments. Although there is no cure for the disease, treatments are available to alleviate many of the symptoms that cause suffering.

DIAGNOSING ALZHEIMER'S DISEASE
Abnormal Brain Tissue Findings

Microscopic brain tissue changes have been described in Alzheimer's disease since Alois Alzheimer first reported them in 1906. These are the plaques and tangles—senile or neuritic plaques (degenerating nerve cells combined with a form of protein called amyloid) and neurofibrillary tangles (nerve cell malformations). The brains of Alzheimer's disease patients of all ages reveal these findings on autopsy examination.

Computed tomography (CT scan) changes become more evident as the disease progresses—not necessarily early on. Thus a CT scan that is performed in the first stages of the disease cannot in itself be used to make a definitive diagnosis of Alzheimer's disease; its value is in helping to establish whether certain disorders (some reversible) that mimic Alzheimer's disease are present. Later on, CT scans often reveal changes characteristic of Alzheimer's disease, namely an atrophied (shrunken) brain with widened sulci (tissue indentations) and enlarged cerebral ventricles (fluid-filled chambers).

Several new types of instrumentation are enabling researchers to learn even more about the brain. Both positron emission tomography (PET scan) and SPECT (single photon emission computed tomography) can map regional cerebral blood flow, metabolic activity, and distribution of specific receptors, as well as integrity of the blood-brain barrier. These procedures may reveal abnormalities characteristic of Alzheimer's disease. Another method, magnetic resonance imaging (MRI), probes the brain by examining the interaction of the magnetic properties of atoms with an external magnetic field. MRI provides both structural and chemical information and distinguishes moving blood from static brain tissue.

Clinical Features of Alzheimer's Disease

The clinical features of Alzheimer's disease, as opposed to the tissue changes, are threefold: (1) dementia—significant loss of intellectual abilities such as memory capacity, severe enough to interfere with social or occupational functioning; (2) insidious onset of symptoms—subtly progressive and irreversible course with documented deterioration over time; and (3) exclusion of all other specific causes of dementia by history, physical examination, laboratory tests, psychometric, and other studies.

Diagnosis by Exclusion

Based on these criteria, the clinical diagnosis of Alzheimer's disease has been referred to as "a diagnosis by exclusion," and one that can be made only in the face of clinical deterioration over time. There is no specific clinical test or finding that is unique to Alzheimer's disease. Hence, all disorders that can bring on similar symptoms must be systematically excluded or "ruled out." This explains why diagnostic workups of individuals where the question of Alzheimer's disease has been raised can be so frustrating to patient and family alike; they are not told that Alzheimer's disease has been specifically diagnosed, but that other possible diagnoses have been dismissed, leaving Alzheimer's disease as the likely diagnosis by the process of elimination.

Scientists hope to develop one day a specific test for Alzheimer's disease, based on a specific laboratory or genetic finding ("marker"). Some think that the results from genetic research may lead to a diagnostic marker for certain persons evaluated for Alzheimer's disease. Research has discovered a protein, called Alzheimer's disease associated protein (ADAP), in the autopsied brains of Alzheimer's patients. The protein, which seems to appear only in people with Alzheimer's, is mainly concentrated in the regions involved in memory function.

Researchers have found ADAP not only in brain tissue, but also in spinal fluid. If they can perfect a test to detect ADAP in the cerebrospinal fluid, or potentially even circulating in the blood, it may be possible to use this method of diagnosis on living patients.

Scientists are working at developing other tests or procedures that may someday identify living persons with the disorder, perhaps even early in its course before behavioral changes are evident. Still, a specific diagnostic marker for Alzheimer's disease is not yet available.

Meanwhile, Alzheimer's disease is the most overdiagnosed and misdiagnosed disorder of mental functioning in older adults. Part of the problem is that many other disorders show symptoms that resemble those of Alzheimer's disease. The crucial difference, though, is that many of these disorders—unlike Alzheimer's disease—may be stopped, reversed, or cured with appropriate treatment. But first they must be identified, not dismissed as Alzheimer's disease or senility.

Organic mental disorders. Conditions that affect the brain and result in intellectual, behavioral, and psychological dysfunction are referred to as "organic mental disorders." These disorders represent a broad grouping of diseases and include Alzheimer's disease. Organic mental disorders that can cause clinical problems like those of Alzheimer's disease, but might be reversible or controlled with proper diagnosis and treatment, include the following:

- *Side effects of medications.* Unusual reactions to medications, too much or too little of prescribed medications, combinations of medications which, when taken together, cause adverse side effects.
- *Substance abuse.* Abuse of legal and/or illegal drugs, alcohol abuse.
- *Metabolic disorders.* Thyroid problems, nutritional deficiencies, anemias, etc.
- *Circulatory disorders.* Heart problems, strokes, etc.
- *Neurological disorders.* Normal-pressure hydrocephalus, multiple sclerosis, etc.
- *Infections.* Especially viral or fungal infections of the brain.
- *Trauma.* Injuries to the head.
- *Toxic factors.* Carbon monoxide, methyl alcohol, etc.
- *Tumors.* Any type within the skull—whether originating or metastasizing there.

Other disorders. In addition to organic mental disorders resulting from these diverse causes, other forms of mental dysfunction or mental health problems can also be confused with Alzheimer's disease. For example, a severe form of depression, referred to as "pseudodementia," can cause problems with memory and concentration that initially may be indistinguishable from early symptoms of Alzheimer's disease. But pseudodementia, like depression in general, can be reversed. Other psychiatric problems can similarly masquerade as Alzheimer's disease, and, like depression, respond to treatment.

Of course, not all memory changes or complaints in later life signal Alzheimer's disease or mental disorder. Many memory changes are only temporary, such as those that occur with bereavement or any stressful situation that makes it difficult to concentrate. In fact, older people are often accused or accuse themselves of memory changes that are not really taking place. If a person in his thirties misplaces keys or a wallet, forgets the name of a neighbor, or calls one sibling by another's name, nobody gives it a second thought. But the same normal forgetfulness for people in their seventies may raise unjustifiable concern. On the other hand, serious memory difficulties should not be dismissed as an unavoidable part of normal aging.

Since rigorous studies on intelligence in later life show that healthy people who stay intellectually active maintain a sharp mind throughout the life cycle, noticeable decline in older adults that interferes with functioning should be clinically explored for an underlying problem.

Comprehensive Clinical Evaluation

Because of the many other disorders that can be confused with Alzheimer's disease, a comprehensive clinical evaluation is essential to arrive at a correct diagnosis of symptoms that look like those of Alzheimer's disease. Such an assessment should include at least three major components: (1) a thorough general medical workup, (2) a neurological examination, and (3) a psychiatric evaluation that may include psychological or psychometric testing. The family physician can be consulted regarding the best way to obtain the necessary examinations.

TREATMENT

Two critical crossroads reached in the approach to treatment for Alzheimer's disease were: (1) the recognition of Alzheimer's disease as a disorder distinct from the normal aging process; and (2) the realization that, in developing therapeutic and social interventions for a major illness or disability, the concept of care can be as important as the concept of cure.

Moreover, in addition to the symptoms of Alzheimer's disease mentioned earlier, other symptoms and aggravating factors may compound the problem. Patient, environmental,

NORMAL MEMORY CHANGES IN THE AGING BRAIN

As we age, we forget, or grope momentarily to recall—and then fear the possibility of Alzheimer's disease. And yet, there are many possible causes of forgetfulness and disorientation other than Alzheimer's. Some are relatively insignificant, and some are reversible.

Recent studies show that healthy older people are, in fact, only fractionally slower than healthy younger people in most tests of mental agility—and that the differences that do exist may have little or no practical importance. For example, it may take a 70-year-old man a quarter of a second longer, on average, than a 30-year-old man to identify a familiar object presented in a picture. Whether that slight lag is a result of deteriorating mental agility or a need to sort through a larger store of memories to locate the right answer, the importance of the delay is negligible for the majority of people.

Other tests have shown that while some of our mental abilities slow down with age, other mental abilities become enhanced. Being able to draw upon experience does improve judgment—we indeed tend to become wiser as we become older. And, although the brain is at its maximum weight (and contains its maximum number of neurons) at age 20, and thereafter gradually decreases, the intellect does not simply grow to its full splendor by the age of 20 and then begin inevitably to degenerate. Though older people have fewer brain cells than younger people, many of the younger people's brain cells are redundant; their loss over the years does not necessarily cause diminished brain function, because other cells take over for those that are lost. There is mounting evidence, too, that the brain retains its capacity for new growth in its nerve cells, as well as for new learning, as it ages.

In general, studies conducted by the National Institute on Aging have shown that 15 to 20 percent of older people have no detectable changes in mental function from youth to old age; the changes that are found in healthy people as they age are small. If you feel you are having trouble with your memory, you should consult your physician about it. For most of those over 50 who fail to do well on tests of mental agility, the impediment is not aging but illness, impairment due to the effects of alcohol, side effects of medications, or depression. Though none of these is benign, all are potentially reversible.

Tips to Improve Your Memory

The common causes of ordinary memory troubles include anxiety, fatigue, stress, grief, and mild depression. In addition, an illness, isolation, habitual inactivity, chronic illness that is preoccupying, limitations of vision or hearing, and excessive use of alcohol can all induce memory loss. Some of these factors might interfere with taking information in to begin with; others, with retaining or retrieving memories. Using your memory—reading, playing chess, doing crossword puzzles, playing bridge—will help keep your memory fit. And so will these specific tips:

• Make mental pictures of tasks, numbers, names, words, thoughts, or whatever it is that you want to remember.

• Talk about it: Working over material in a conversation helps implant it in your memory.

• Eliminate distractions, background noise, and other things competing for your attention when you are trying to take something in.

• Don't waste your attentiveness trying to retain things a mere piece of paper can retain. Keep lists and a daily calendar.

• Take occasional breaks to rest and refresh your mind, especially when you are trying to learn something new.

• Remember that it's okay to forget.

The Editors

and family stresses can converge to exaggerate patient dysfunction and family burden during the clinical course of Alzheimer's disease. Identifying these stresses and making appropriate changes can provide the foundation for more effective treatment and fewer everyday problems.

In the Alzheimer's disease patient, depression or delusions can aggravate dysfunction. These problems, which emerge during the course of the disorder in some individuals with Alzheimer's disease, compound memory impairment; they make the affected individual do worse than would be expected from the dementia alone—causing clinical conditions referred to as excess disability states. Depression by itself can mimic dementia, as in pseudodementia. When combined with dementia, depression exacts yet greater incapacity and suffering in the Alzheimer's disease patient.

Depression in the Alzheimer's patient can usually be lessened or relieved by treatment. Indeed, this highlights one of the truly extraordinary phenomena that can be observed in Alzheimer's disease: By alleviating an excess disability state, actual clinical improvement can result—even though the underlying pathological process is advancing. In other words, at a given point in time, the patient's symptoms can be reduced, suffering lowered, capacity to cope buttressed, with family burden eased as a further result. These are traditional goals of treatment for all illnesses.

The patient's immediate environment can similarly interfere with coping, adding to the level of impairment. Modifying the surroundings can reduce stresses imposed by environmental factors. There is the matter of safety, as in the need to protect the person from wandering toward a stairway and subsequently falling. There is the matter of lowering the individual's frustration level, such as by placing different cues in the immediate environment to combat memory loss and to reduce resulting stress and disorganization. There is the matter of finding the most protective but least restrictive setting for care, which at some point may involve a move away from home to a nursing home or other care facility well equipped to deal with those who have Alzheimer's disease.

Relieving Stress on the Family
Stress on the family can take a toll on patient and caregiver alike. Caregivers are usually family members—either spouses or children—and are preponderantly wives and daughters. As time passes and the burden mounts, it not only places the mental health of family caregivers at risk, it also diminishes their ability to provide care to the Alzheimer's disease patient. Hence, assistance to the family as a whole must be considered.

As the disease progresses, families experience increasing anxiety and pain at seeing unsettling changes in a loved one, and they commonly feel guilt over not being able to do enough. The prevalence of reactive depression among family members in this situation is disturbingly high—caregivers are chronically stressed and are much more likely to suffer from depression than the average person. If caregivers have been forced to retire from positions outside the home, they feel progressively more isolated and no longer productive members of society.

Support Through Interventions
The likelihood, intensity, and duration of depression among caregivers can all be lowered through available interventions. For example, to the extent that family members can offer emotional support to each other and perhaps seek professional consultation, they will be better prepared to help their loved one manage the illness and to recognize the limits of what they themselves can reasonably do.

Since the components of the problem vary, so too should the focus, nature, and sources of interventions. Interventions should focus on the patient's symptoms, the affected individual's everyday environment, and the family support system. Specific interventions can involve support from the family, the help of a homemaker or other aide in the home, employment of behavioral therapies, and the use of drugs.

The sources for interventions can range from family support groups such as those available through the Alzheimer's Association (AA), to professional consultations for the patient and family with a mental health specialist, to a variety of community programs such as day or respite care.

Although Alzheimer's disease cannot at present be cured, reversed, or stopped in its progression, much can be done to help both the patient and the family live through the course of the illness with greater dignity and less discomfort. Toward this goal, appropriate clinical interventions and community services should be vigorously sought.

The National Institute of Mental Health

CHRONIC PAIN

Rare is the person who has not experienced some beyond-belief episode of pain and misery. Mercifully, relief finally came. With treatment, or with the body's healing powers alone, you got better and the pain went away. Doctors call that kind of pain acute pain. It is a normal sensation triggered in the nervous system to alert you to possible injury and the need to take care of yourself.

Chronic pain is different. Chronic pain persists. Fiendishly, uselessly, pain signals keep firing in the nervous system for weeks, months, even years. There may have been an initial mishap—a sprained back, a serious infection—from which you've long since recovered. There may be an ongoing cause of pain—arthritis, cancer, ear infection. But some people suffer chronic pain in the absence of any past injury or evidence of body damage.

Whatever the matter may be, chronic pain is real, unremitting, and demoralizing.

THE TERRIBLE TRIAD

Pain of such proportions overwhelms all other symptoms and becomes the problem. People so afflicted often cannot work. Their appetite falls off. Physical activity of any kind is exhausting and may aggravate the pain. Soon the person becomes the victim of a vicious circle in which total preoccupation with pain leads to irritability and depression. The sufferer can't sleep at night and the next day's weariness compounds the problem—leading to more irritability, depression, and pain. Specialists call that unhappy state the "terrible triad" of suffering, sleeplessness, and sadness, a calamity that is as hard on the family as it is on the victim.

The urge to do something—anything—to stop the pain makes some patients drug dependent, drives others to undergo repeated operations or, worse, resort to questionable practitioners who promise quick and permanent "cures."

Many chronic pain conditions affect older adults. Arthritis, cancer, angina—the chest-binding, breath-catching spasms of pain associated with coronary artery disease—commonly take their greatest toll among the middle-aged and elderly. Tic douloureux (trigeminal neuralgia) is a recurrent, stabbing facial pain that is rare among young adults. But ask any resident of housing for retired persons if there are any tic sufferers around and you are certain to hear of cases. So the fact that Americans are living longer contributes to a widespread and growing concern about pain. Neuroscientists share that concern.

At a time when people are living longer and painful conditions abound, neuroscientists have made landmark discoveries that are leading to a better understanding of pain and more effective treatments.

SOUNDING THE PAIN ALARM

Part of the inspiration for the new groups has come from a deeper understanding of pain made possible by advances in research techniques. Not long ago neuroscientists debated whether pain was a separate sense at all, supplied with its own nerve cells and brain centers like the senses of hearing or taste or touch. Maybe people hurt, the scientists reasoned, because nerve endings sensitive to touch are pressed very hard. To some extent, that is true: Some nerve fibers in the skin will be stimulated by a painful pinch as well as a gentle touch. But neuroscientists now know that there are many small nerve cells with extremely fine nerve fibers that are excited exclusively by intense, potentially harmful stimulation. Scientists call the nerve cells nociceptors, from the word noxious, meaning physically harmful or destructive.

Some nociceptors sound off to several kinds of painful stimulation—a hammer blow that hits the thumb instead of a nail; a drop of acid; a flaming match. Other nociceptors are more selective. They are excited by a pinprick but ignore painful heat or chemical stimulation. It's as though nature had sprinkled the skin and insides with a variety of pain-sensitive cells, not only to report what kind of damage is occurring, but to make sure the message gets through on at least one channel.

BROADCASTING THE NEWS

That same dispersion of forces continues once pain messages reach the central nervous system. Suppose you touch a hot stove. Some incoming pain signals are immediately routed to nerve cells that signal muscles to contract, so you pull your hand back. That streamlined pathway is a reflex, one of many protective circuits wired into the nervous system at birth.

Meanwhile the message declaring that the stove has been touched travels along other pathways to higher centers in the brain. One path is an express route that reports the facts: where it hurts; how bad it is; whether the pain is sharp or burning. Other pain pathways plod along more slowly, the nerve fibers branching to make connections with many nerve cells (neurons) en route. Scientists think that these more meandering pathways act as warning systems alerting of impending damage and in other ways filling out the pain picture. All the pathways combined contribute to the emo-

tional impact of pain—whether the person feels frightened, anxious, angry, annoyed. Experts called those feelings the suffering component of pain.

Still other branches of the pain news network are alerting another major division of the nervous system, the autonomic nervous system. That division handles the body's vital functions like breathing, blood flow, pulse rate, digestion, and elimination.

Pain can sound a general alarm in the autonomic nervous system, causing the person to sweat or stop digesting food, increasing the pulse rate and blood pressure, dilating the pupils of the eye, and signaling the release of hormones like epinephrine (adrenaline). Epinephrine aids and abets all those responses, as well as triggering the release of sugar stored in the liver to provide an extra boost of energy in an emergency.

CENSORING THE NEWS

Obviously, not every source of pain creates a full-blown emergency with adrenaline-surging, sweat-pouring, pulse-racing responses. Moreover, observers are well aware of times and places when excruciating pain is ignored. Think of the quarterback's ability to finish a game oblivious of a torn ligament, or a fakir sitting on a bed of spikes. One of the foremost pioneers in pain research adds his own personal tale, too, of the time he landed a salmon after a long and hearty struggle, only then to discover the deep blood-dripping gash on his leg.

Acknowledging such events, neuroscientists have long suspected that there are built-in nervous system mechanisms that can block pain messages.

Now it seems that just as there is more than one way to spread the news of pain, there is more than one way to censor the news. These control systems involve pathways that come down from the brain to prevent pain signals from getting through.

THE GATE THEORY OF PAIN

Interestingly, a pair of Canadian and English investigators speculated that such pain-suppressing pathways must exist when they devised a new gate theory of pain in the mid-sixties. Their idea was that when pain signals first reach the nervous system, they excite activity in a group of small neurons that form a kind of pain pool. When the total activity of these neurons reaches a certain minimal level, a hypothetical gate opens up that allows the pain signals to be sent to higher brain centers. But nearby neurons in contact with the pain cells can suppress activity in the pain pool so that the gate stays closed. The gate-closing cells include large neurons that are stimulated by nonpainful touching or pressing of your skin. The gate could also be closed from above, by brain cells activating a descending pathway to block pain.

The theory explained such everyday behavior as scratching a scab, or rubbing a sprained ankle: the scratching and rubbing excite just those nerve cells sensitive to touch and pressure that can suppress the pain pool cells. The scientists conjectured that brain-based pain control systems were activated when people behaved heroically—ignoring pain in order to finish a football game, or to help a more severely wounded soldier on the battlefield.

The gate theory aroused both interest and controversy when it was first announced. Most important, it stimulated research to find the conjectured pathways and mechanisms. Pain studies got an added boost when investigators made the surprising discovery that the brain itself produces chemicals that can control pain.

The landmark discovery of the pain-suppressing chemicals came about because scientists in Aberdeen, Scotland, and at the Johns Hopkins University Hospital in Baltimore were curious about how morphine and other opium-derived painkillers, or analgesics, work.

For some time neuroscientists had known that chemicals were important in conducting nerve signals (small bursts of electric current) from cell to cell. In order for the signal from one cell to reach the next in line, the first cell secretes a chemical neurotransmitter from the tip of a long fiber that extends from the cell body. The transmitter molecules cross the gap separating the two cells and attach to special receptor sites on the neighboring cell surface. Some neurotransmitters excite the second cell—allowing it to generate an electrical signal. Others inhibit the second cell—preventing it from generating a signal.

When investigators in Scotland and at Johns Hopkins injected morphine into experimental animals, they found that the morphine molecules fitted snugly into receptors on certain brain and spinal cord neurons. Why, the scientists wondered, should the human brain—the product of millions of years of evolution—come equipped with receptors for a man-made drug? Perhaps there were naturally occurring brain chemicals that behaved exactly like morphine.

THE BRAIN'S OWN OPIATES

Both groups of scientists found not just one pain-suppressing chemical in the brain, but a whole family of such proteins. The Aberdeen investigators called the smaller members of the family enkephalins (meaning "in the head"). In time, the larger proteins were isolated and called endorphins, meaning "the morphine within." The term "endorphins" is now often used to describe the group as a whole.

The discovery of the endorphins lent weight to the general concept of the gate theory. Endorphins released from brain nerve cells might inhibit spinal cord pain cells through pathways descending from the brain to the spinal cord. Endorphins might also be activated when a person rubs or scratches itching skin or aching joints. Laboratory experiments subsequently confirmed that painful stimulation led to the release of endorphins from nerve cells. Some of these chemicals then turned up in cerebrospinal fluid, the liquid that circulates in the spinal cord and brain. Laced with endorphins, the fluid could bring a soothing balm to quiet nerve cells.

A NEW LOOK AT PAIN TREATMENTS

Further evidence that endorphins figure importantly in pain control comes from a new look at some of the oldest and newest pain treatments. The new look frequently involves the use of a drug that prevents endorphins and morphine from working. Injections of this drug, naloxone, can result in a return of pain that had been relieved by morphine and certain other treatments. But, interestingly, some pain treatments are not affected by naloxone: Their success in controlling pain apparently does not depend on endorphins. Thus nature has provided us with more than one means of achieving pain relief.

Acupuncture

Probably no other therapy for pain has stirred more controversy in recent years than acupuncture, the 2,000-year-old Chinese technique of inserting fine needles under the skin at selected points in the body. The needles are agitated by the practitioner to produce pain relief, which some individuals report lasts for hours, or even days. Does acupuncture really work? Opinion is divided. Many specialists agree that patients report benefit when the needles are placed near where it hurts, not at the body points indicated on traditional Chinese acupuncture charts. The case for acupuncture has been made by investigators who argue that local needling of the skin excites endorphin systems of pain control. Wiring the needles to stimulate nerve endings electrically (electroacupuncture) also activates endorphin systems, they believe. Further, some experiments have shown that there are higher levels of endorphins in cerebrospinal fluid following acupuncture.

Those same investigators note that naloxone injections can block pain relief produced by acupuncture. Others have not been able to repeat those findings. Skeptics also cite long-term studies of chronic pain patients that showed no lasting benefit from acupuncture treatments. Current opinion is that more controlled trials are needed to define which pain conditions might be helped by acupuncture and which patients are most likely to benefit.

Local Electrical Stimulation

Applying brief pulses of electricity to nerve endings under the skin, a procedure called transcutaneous electrical nerve stimulation (TENS) yields excellent pain relief in some chronic pain patients. The stimulation works best when applied to the skin near where the pain is felt and where other sensibilities like touch or pressure have not been damaged. Both the frequency and voltage of the electrical stimulation are important in obtaining pain relief.

Brain Stimulation

Another electrical method for controlling pain, especially the widespread and severe pain of advanced cancer, is through surgically implanted electrodes in the brain. The patient determines when and how much stimulation is needed by operating an external transmitter that beams electronic signals to a receiver under the skin that is connected to the electrodes. The brain sites where the electrodes are placed are areas known to be rich in opiate receptors and in endorphin-containing cells or fibers. Stimulation-produced analgesia (SPA) is a costly procedure that involves the risk of brain surgery. However, patients who have used this technique report that their pain seems to melt away. The pain relief is also remarkably specific: The other senses remain intact, and there is no mental confusion or cloudiness as with opiate drugs. The National Institute of Neurological Disorders and Stroke (NINDS) is currently supporting research on how SPA works and is also investigating problems of tolerance: Pain may return after repeated stimulation.

Placebo Effects

For years, doctors have known that a harmless sugar pill or an injection of salt water can make many a patient feel better—even after major surgery. The placebo effect, as it has been called, has been thought to be due to suggestion, distraction, the patient's optimism that something is being done, or the desire to please the doctor (placebo means "I will please" in Latin).

Now experiments suggest that the placebo effect may be neurochemical, and that people who respond to a placebo for pain relief—a remarkably consistent 35 percent in any experiment using placebos—are able to tap into their brain's endorphin systems. To evaluate it, two NINDS and NIDR (National Institute of Dental Research) supported investigators at the University of California at San Francisco designed an ingenious experiment. They asked adults scheduled for wisdom teeth removal to volunteer in a pain experiment. Following surgery, some patients were given morphine, some naloxone, and some a placebo. As expected, about one-third of those given the placebo reported pain relief. The investigators then gave these people naloxone. All reported a return of pain.

How people who benefit from placebos gain access to pain control systems in the brain is not known. Scientists cannot even predict whether someone who responds to a placebo in one situation will respond in another.

The San Francisco investigators suspect that stress may be a factor. Patients who are very anxious or under stress are more likely to react to a placebo for pain than those who are more calm, cool, and collected. But dental surgery itself may be sufficiently stressful

to trigger the release of endorphins—with or without the effects of placebo. For that reason, many specialists believe further studies are indicated to analyze the placebo effect.

As research continues to reveal the role of endorphins in the brain, neuroscientists have been able to draw more detailed brain maps of the areas and pathways important in pain perception and control. They have even found new members of the endorphin family: dynorphin, the newest endorphin, is reported to be 10 times more potent a painkiller than morphine.

At the same time, clinical investigators have tested chronic pain patients and found that they often have lower-than-normal levels of endorphins in their spinal fluid. If doctors could just boost their stores with man-made endorphins, perhaps the problems of chronic pain patients could be solved.

Not so easy. Some endorphins are quickly broken down after release from nerve cells. Other endorphins are longer lasting, but there are problems in manufacturing the compounds in quantity and getting them into the right places in the brain or spinal cord. In a few promising studies, clinical investigators have injected an endorphin called beta-endorphin under the membranes surrounding the spinal cord. Patients reported excellent pain relief lasting for many hours. Morphine compounds injected in the same area are similarly effective in producing long-lasting pain relief.

But spinal cord injections or other techniques designed to raise the level of endorphins circulating in the brain require surgery and hospitalization. And even if less drastic means of getting endorphins into the nervous system could be found, they are probably not the ideal answer to chronic pain. Endorphins are also involved in other nervous system activities such as controlling blood flow. Increasing the amount of endorphins might have undesirable effects on these other body activities. Endorphins also appear to share with morphine a potential for addiction or tolerance.

Meanwhile, chemists are synthesizing new analgesics and discovering painkilling virtues in drugs not normally prescribed for pain. Much of the drug research is aimed at developing nonnarcotic painkillers. The motivation for the research is not only to avoid introducing potentially addictive drugs on the market, but is based on the observation that narcotic drugs are simply not effective in treating a variety of chronic pain conditions. Developments in nondrug treatments are also progressing, ranging from new surgical techniques to physical and psychological therapies, including exercise, hypnosis, and biofeedback.

NEW AND OLD DRUGS FOR PAIN

When someone complains of headache or low back pain and the doctor says to take two aspirins every four hours and stay in bed, the patient may think the pain is being dismissed lightly. Not at all.

Aspirin

One of the most universally used medications, aspirin is an excellent painkiller. Scientists still cannot explain all the ways aspirin works, but they do know that it interferes with pain signals where they usually originate, at the nociceptive nerve endings outside the brain and spinal cord: peripheral nerves. Aspirin also inhibits the production of chemicals manufactured in the blood to promote blood clotting and wound healing: prostaglandins. Unfortunately, prostaglandins, released from cells at the site of injury, are pain-causing substances. They actually sensitize nerve endings, making them feel more pain. Along with increasing the blood supply to the area, the chemicals contribute to inflammation—the pain, heat, redness, and swelling of tissue damage.

Some investigators now think that the continued release of pain-causing substances in chronic pain conditions may lead to long-term nervous system changes in some patients that make them hypersensitive to pain. People suffering such hyperalgesia can cry out in pain at the gentlest touch, or even when a soft breeze blows over the affected area. In addition to the prostaglandins, blister fluid and certain insect and snake venoms also contain pain-causing substances. Presumably these chemicals alert the person to the need for care—a fine reaction in an emergency, but not in chronic pain.

Prescription Painkillers

There are several prescription drugs that usually can provide stronger pain relief than aspirin. These drugs include the opiate-related compounds codeine, propoxyphene (Darvon), morphine, and meperidine (Demerol). All these drugs have some potential for abuse, and may have unpleasant and even harmful side effects. In combination with other medications or alcohol, some can be dangerous. Used wisely, however, they are important recruits in the chemical fight against pain.

In the search for effective analgesics, physicians have discovered pain-relieving benefits from drugs not normally prescribed for pain. Certain antidepressants as well as antiepileptic drugs are used to treat several particularly severe pain conditions, notably the pain of shingles and of facial neuralgias like tic douloureux.

Antidepressants

Interestingly, pain patients who benefit from antidepressants report pain relief before any uplift in mood. Pain specialists think that the antidepressant works because it increases the supply of a naturally produced neurotransmitter, serotonin. (Doctors have long associated decreased amounts of serotonin with severe depression.) But now scientists have evidence that cells using serotonin are also an integral part of a pain-controlling pathway that starts with endorphin-rich nerve cells high up in the brain and ends with inhibition of pain-conducting nerve cells lower in the brain or spinal cord. Antidepressant drugs have been used successfully in treating the excruciating pain that can follow an attack of shingles.

Antiepileptic Drugs

Antiepileptic drugs have been used successfully in treating tic douloureux, the riveting attacks of facial pain that affect older adults. The rationale for the use of the antiepileptic drugs (principally carbamazepine—Tegretol) does not involve the endorphin system. It is based on the theory that a healthy nervous system depends on a proper balance of incoming and outgoing nerve signals. Tic and other facial pains or neuralgias are thought to result from damage to facial nerves. That means that the normal flow of messages to and from the brain is disturbed. The nervous system may react by becoming hypersensitive: It may create its own powerful discharge of nerve signals, as though screaming to the outside world, "Why aren't you contacting me?" Antiepileptic drugs—used to quiet the excessive brain discharges associated with epileptic seizures—quiet the distress signals associated with tic and may relieve pain that way.

PSYCHOLOGICAL METHODS

Psychological treatment for pain can range from psychoanalysis and other forms of psychotherapy to relaxation training, meditation, hypnosis, biofeedback, or behavior modification.

The philosophy common to all these varied psychological approaches is the belief that patients can do something on their own to control their pain.

That something may mean changing attitudes, feelings, or behaviors associated with pain, or understanding how unconscious forces and past events have contributed to the present painful predicament.

Psychotherapy

Freud was celebrated for demonstrating that for some individuals physical pain symbolizes real or imagined emotional hurts. He also noted that some individuals develop pain or paralysis as a form of self-punishment for what they consider to be past sins or bad behavior. Sometimes, too, pain may be a way of punishing others. This doesn't mean that the pain is any less real; it does mean that some pain patients may benefit from psychoanalysis or individual or group psychotherapy to gain insights into the meaning of their pain.

Relaxation and Meditation Therapies

These forms of training enable people to relax tense muscles, reduce anxiety, and alter mental state. Both physical and mental tension can make any pain worse, and in conditions such as headache or back pain, tension may be at the root of the problem. Meditation, which aims at producing a state of relaxed but alert awareness, is sometimes combined with therapies that encourage people to think of pain as something remote and apart from them. The methods promote a sense of detachment so that the patient thinks of the pain as confined to a particular body part over which he or she has marvelous control. The approach may be particularly helpful when pain is associated with fear and dread, as in cancer.

Hypnosis

No longer considered magic, hypnosis is a technique in which an individual's susceptibility to suggestion is heightened. Normal volunteers who prove to be excellent subjects for hypnosis often report a marked reduction or obliteration of experimentally induced pain, such as that produced by a mild electric shock. The hypnotic state does not lower the volunteer's heart rate, respiration, or other autonomic responses. These physical reactions show the expected increases normally associated with painful stimulation.

The role of hypnosis in treating chronic

pain patients is uncertain. Some studies have shown that 15 to 20 percent of hypnotizable patients with moderate to severe pain can achieve total relief with hypnosis. Other studies have reported that hypnosis reduces anxiety and depression. By lowering the burden of emotional suffering, pain may become more bearable.

Biofeedback

Some individuals can learn voluntary control over certain body activities if they are provided with information about how the system is working—how fast their heart is beating, how tense their head or neck muscles are, how cold their hands are. The information is usually supplied through visual or auditory cues that code the body activity in some obvious way—a louder sound meaning an increase in muscle tension, for example. How people use this biofeedback to learn control is not understood, but some masters of the art report that imagery helps: They may think of a warm tropical beach, for example, when they want to raise the temperature of their hands. Biofeedback may be a logical approach in pain conditions that involve tense muscles, like tension headache or low back pain. But results are mixed.

Behavior Modification

This psychological technique (sometimes called operant conditioning) is aimed at changing habits, behaviors, and attitudes that can develop in chronic pain patients. Some patients become dependent, anxious, and home-bound—if not bedridden. For some, too, chronic pain may be a welcome friend, relieving them of the boredom of a dull job or the burden of family responsibilities. These psychological rewards—sometimes combined with financial gains from compensation payments or insurance—work against improvements in the patient's condition, and can encourage increased drug dependency, repeated surgery, and multiple doctor and clinic visits.

There is no question that the patient feels pain. The hope of behavior modification is that pain relief can be obtained from a program aimed at changing the individual's lifestyle. The program begins with a complete assessment of the painful condition and a thorough explanation of how the program works. It is essential to enlist the full cooperation of both the patient and family members. The treatment is aimed at reducing pain medication and increasing mobility and independence through a graduated program of exercise, diet, and other activities. The patient is rewarded for positive efforts with praise and attention. Rewards are withheld when the patient retreats into negative attitudes or demanding and dependent behavior.

How effective are any of these psychological treatments? Are some superior to others? Who is most likely to benefit? Do the benefits last? The answers are not yet in hand. Patient selection and patient cooperation are all-important. Analysis of individuals who have improved dramatically with one or another of these approaches is helping to pinpoint what factors are likely to lead to successful treatment.

SURGERY TO RELIEVE PAIN

Surgery is often considered the court of last resort for pain: When all else fails, cut the nerve endings. Surgery can bring about instant, almost magical release from pain. But surgery may also destroy other sensations as well, or, inadvertently, become the source of new pain. Further, relief is not necessarily permanent. After six months or a year, pain may return.

The decision for surgery must always involve a careful weighing of the patient's condition and the outlook for the future. If surgery can mean the difference between a pain-wracked existence ending in death versus a pain-free time in which to compose one's life and see friends and family, then surgery is clearly a humane and compassionate choice.

145

There are a variety of operations to relieve pain. The most common is cordotomy: severing the nerve fibers on one or both sides of the spinal cord that travel the express routes to the brain. Cordotomy affects the sense of temperature as well as pain, because the fibers travel together in the express route.

Besides cordotomy, surgery within the brain or spinal cord to relieve pain includes severing connections at major junctions in pain pathways, such as at the places where pain fibers cross from one side of the cord to the other, or destroying parts of important relay stations in the brain like the thalamus, an egg-shaped cluster of nerve cells near the center of the brain.

In addition, surgeons sometimes can relieve pain by destroying nerve fibers or their parent cell bodies outside the brain or spinal cord. A case in point is the destruction of sympathetic nerves (a part of the autonomic nervous system) to relieve the severe pain that sometimes follows a penetrating wound from a sharp instrument or bullet.

When pain affects the upper extremities, or is widespread, the surgeon has fewer options and surgery may not be as effective. Still, skilled neurosurgeons have achieved excellent results with upper spinal cord or brain surgery to treat severe intractable pain. These procedures may employ chemicals or use heat or freezing treatments to destroy tissue, as well as the more traditional use of the scalpel.

Recently, Harvard Medical School surgeons reported success with a new brain operation called cingulotomy to relieve intractable pain in patients with severe psychiatric problems. The nerve fibers destroyed are part of a pathway important in emotions and motivation. The surgery appears to eliminate the discomfort and suffering the patient feels, but does not interfere with other mental faculties such as thinking and memory.

Prior to operating, physicians can often

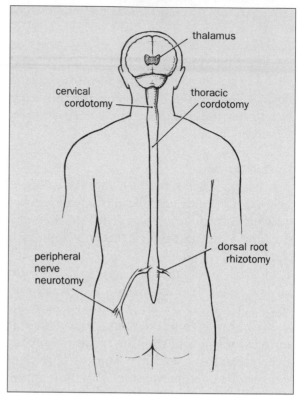

As a last resort for the relief of chronic pain, neurosurgeons can sever nerve fibers at various sites in the brain, along the spinal cord, or in peripheral nerves.

test the effectiveness of surgery by using anesthetic drugs to block nerves temporarily. In some chronic pain conditions—like the pain from a penetrating wound—these temporary blocks can in themselves be beneficial, promoting repair of nerve damage.

How do these current treatments apply to the more common chronic pain conditions? What follows is a brief survey of major pain disorders and the treatments most in use today.

THE MAJOR PAINS
Headache
Tension headache, involving continued contractions of head and neck muscles, is one of the most common forms of headache. The other common variety is the vascular headache, involving changes in the pressure

of blood vessels serving the head. Migraine headaches are of the vascular type, associated with throbbing pain on one side of the head. Genetic factors play a role in determining who will be a victim of migraine, but many other factors are important as well. A major difficulty in treating migraine headache is that changes occur throughout the course of the headache. Blood vessels may first constrict and then dilate. Changing levels of neurotransmitters have also been noted. While a number of drugs can relieve migraine pain, their usefulness often depends on when they are taken. Some are effective only if taken at the onset.

Drugs are also the most common treatment for tension headache, although attempts to use biofeedback to control muscle tension have had some success. Physical methods such as heat or cold applications often provide additional if only temporary relief.

Low Back Pain

The combination of aspirin, bed rest, and modest amounts of a muscle relaxant are usually prescribed for the first-time low back pain patient. At the initial examination, the physician will also note if the patient is overweight or works at an occupation such as truck-driving or a desk job that offers little opportunity for exercise.

Some authorities believe that low back pain is particularly prevalent in Western society because of the combination of overweight, bad posture (made worse if there is added weight up front), and infrequent exercise. Not surprisingly, then, when the patient begins to feel better, the suggestion is made to take off pounds and take on physical exercise. In some cases, a full neurological examination may be necessary, including an x-ray of the spinal cord called a myelogram, to see if there may be a ruptured disc or other source of pressure on the cord or nerve roots.

Sometimes x-rays will show a disc problem which can be helped by surgery. But neither the myelogram nor disc surgery is foolproof. Milder analgesics (aspirin or stronger non-narcotic medications) and electrical stimulation—using TENS or implanted brain electrodes—can be very effective. What is not effective is long-term use of the muscle-relaxant tranquilizers. Many specialists are convinced that chronic use of these drugs is detrimental to the back patient, adding to depression and increasing pain. Massage or manipulative therapy are used by some clinicians but, other than individual patient reports, their usefulness is still undocumented.

Cancer Pain

The pain of cancer can result from the pressure of a growing tumor or the infiltration of tumor cells into other organs. Or the pain can come about as the result of radiation or chemotherapy. These treatments can cause fluid accumulation and swelling (edema), irritate or destroy healthy tissue causing pain and inflammation, and possibly sensitize nerve endings.

Ideally, the treatment for cancer pain is to remove the cancerous tissue. When that is not possible, pain can be treated by any or all of the currently available therapies: electrical stimulation, psychological methods, surgery, and strong painkillers.

Arthritis Pain

"Arthritis" is a general descriptive term meaning an affliction of the joints. The two most common forms are osteoarthritis, which typically affects the fingers and may spread to important weight-bearing joints in the spine or hips, and rheumatoid arthritis, an inflammatory joint disease associated with swelling, congestion, and thickening of the soft tissue around joints. Recently, a distinguished panel of pain experts commenting on arthritis reported that "in all probability aspirin remains the most widely used . . . and important drug . . . although it may cause serious side effects."

PERIPHERAL NEUROPATHY

Peripheral neuropathy (or neuritis) is a deterioration in the function of the nerves that carry messages between the central nervous system and the extremities. It is caused by damage or irritation to the myelin sheaths that protect most nerves, or damage to the axons themselves (the conducting fibers of the nerve). Most commonly, the disorder is brought on by chronic excessive use of alcohol, metabolic disorders such as diabetes mellitus, in association with cancer, inflammatory disorders such as lupus, or by certain vitamin deficiencies. Quite often, a specific cause cannot be found, even after a thorough diagnostic evaluation. Peripheral neuropathy can affect sensory nerves to cause numbness, tingling, and pain, or motor nerves with loss of muscle strength and reflexes and muscle atrophy. People with peripheral neuropathy may describe unusual clumsiness or vague sensations. Because the onset is usually gradual, people with motor nerve damage often try to compensate by overusing other muscles; but, when the disorder is due to an infection or chronic alcohol intoxication, the onset is usually rapid. If the cause of the disorder can be identified and eliminated before nerve cells are irreversibly damaged, further progression of the neuropathy may be prevented. No specific therapeutic measures can repair the damage to nerve cells or reverse the loss of sensation, but pain can often be eliminated or alleviated with various medications.

The Editors

In the 1950s, the steroid drugs were introduced and hailed as lifesavers—important anti-inflammatory agents modeled after the body's own chemicals produced in the adrenal glands. But the long-term use of steroids has serious consequences, among them the lowering of resistance to infection, hemorrhaging, and facial puffiness—producing the so-called moon face.

Besides aspirin, current treatments for arthritis include several nonsteroid anti-inflammatory drugs (NSAIDs) like indomethacin and ibuprofen.

But these drugs, too, may have serious side effects. TENS and acupuncture have been tried with mixed results. In cases where tissue has been destroyed, surgery to replace a diseased joint with an artificial part has been very successful. The total hip replacement operation is an example.

Arthritis is best treated early, say the experts. A modest program of drugs combined with exercise can do much to restore full function and forestall long-term degenerative changes. Exercise in warm water is especially good because the water is both relaxing and provides buoyancy that makes exercises easier to perform. Physical treatments with warm or cold compresses are helpful sources of temporary pain relief.

Neurogenic Pain

The most difficult pains to treat are those that result from damage to the peripheral nerves or to the central nervous system itself. We have mentioned tic douloureux and shingles as examples of extraordinarily searing pain, along with several drugs that can help. In addition, tic sufferers can benefit from surgery to destroy the nerve cells that supply pain-sensation fibers to the face. Thermocoagulation—which uses heat supplied by an electrical current to destroy nerve cells—has the advantage that pain fibers are more sensitive to the treatment, resulting in less destruction of the other sensations (touch and temperature).

Sometimes specialists treating tic find that certain blood vessels in the brain lie near the group of nerve cells supplying sensory fibers to the face, exerting pressure that causes pain. The surgical insertion of a small sponge between the blood vessels and the nerve cells can relieve the pressure and eliminate pain.

Among other notoriously painful neurogenic disorders is pain from an amputated or paralyzed limb—so-called phantom pain—which affects up to 10 percent of amputees and paraplegia patients. Various combinations of antidepressants and weak narcotics like Darvon are sometimes effective. Surgery, too, is occasionally successful. Many experts now think that the electrical stimulating techniques hold the greatest promise for relieving these pains.

Psychogenic Pain

Some cases of pain are not due to past disease or injury, nor is there any detectable sign of damage inside or outside the nervous system. Such pain may benefit from any of the psychological pain therapies listed earlier. It is also possible that some new methods used to diagnose pain may be useful. One method gaining in popularity is thermography, which measures the temperature of surface tissue as a reflection of blood flow. A color-coded thermogram of a person with a headache or other painful condition often shows an altered blood supply to the painful area, appearing as a darker or lighter shade than the surrounding areas or the corresponding part on the other side of the body. Thus an abnormal thermogram in a patient who complains of pain in the absence of any other evidence may provide a valuable clue that can lead to a diagnosis and treatment.

WHERE TO GO FOR HELP

People with chronic pain have usually seen a family doctor and several other specialists as well. Eventually, they are referred to neurologists, orthopedists, or neurosurgeons. The patient/doctor relationship is extremely important in dealing with chronic pain. Both patients and family members should seek out knowledgeable specialists who neither dismiss nor indulge the patient—physicians who

understand full well how pain has come to dominate the patient's life and the lives of everyone else in the family.

Many specialists today refer chronic pain patients to pain clinics for treatment. Over 800 such clinics have opened their doors in the United States since a world leader in pain therapy established a pain clinic at the University of Washington in Seattle in 1960.

Pain clinics differ in their approaches. Generally speaking, clinics employ a group of specialists who review each patient's medical history and conduct further tests when necessary. If the applicant is admitted, the clinic staff designs a personal treatment program that may include individual and group psychotherapy, exercise, diet, ice massage for pain (especially before bedtime), electrical stimulation techniques, and the use of a variety of analgesic but nonnarcotic drugs. The aim is to reduce pain medication and so improve the patient's pain problem that, when he or she leaves the hospital, it is with the prospect of resuming more normal activities with a minimal requirement for analgesics and a positive self-image.

Contrary to what many people think, pain clinic patients are not malingerers or hypochondriacs. They are men and women of all ages, education, and social backgrounds, suffering a wide variety of painful conditions. Patients with low back pain are frequent, and so are people with the complications of diabetes, stroke, brain trauma, headache, arthritis, or any of the rarer pain conditions. The majority of patients participate for two or three weeks and usually report substantial improvement at discharge. One young man who had suffered a painful chest injury as a result of a factory accident said he literally felt taller after his pain clinic experience. Follow-up at three- and six-month intervals, and at lengthier intervals thereafter, is an essential part of the program, both to evaluate the long-term effectiveness of treatment and to initiate a further course of treatment or counseling if necessary.

The National Institute of Neurological Disorders and Stroke

HEADACHES

An estimated 40 million Americans experience chronic headaches. For at least half of these people, the problem is severe and sometimes disabling. It can also be costly: Headache sufferers make over 8 million visits a year to doctors' offices. Migraine victims alone lose over 64 million workdays because of headache pain.

WHY DOES IT HURT?

What hurts when you have a headache? Several areas of the head can hurt, including a network of nerves that extends over the scalp and certain nerves in the face, mouth, and throat. Also sensitive to pain, because they contain delicate nerve fibers, are the muscles of the head and blood vessels found along the surface and at the base of the brain.

The bones of the skull and tissues of the brain itself, however, never hurt, because they lack pain-sensitive nerve fibers.

The ends of these pain-sensitive nerves, called nociceptors, can be stimulated by stress, muscular tension, dilated blood vessels, and other triggers of headache. Once stimulated, a nociceptor sends a message up the length of the nerve fiber to the nerve cells in the brain, signaling that a part of the body hurts. The message is determined by the location of the nociceptor. A person who suddenly realizes "My toe hurts" is responding to nociceptors in the foot that have been stimulated by the stubbing of a toe.

A number of chemicals help transmit pain-related information to the brain. Some of these chemicals are natural painkilling proteins called endorphins, Greek for "the morphine within." One theory suggests that people who suffer from severe headache and other types of chronic pain have lower levels of endorphins than people who are generally pain free.

WHEN TO SEE A PHYSICIAN

Not all headaches require medical attention. Some result from missed meals or occasional muscle tension and are easily remedied. But some types of headache are signals of more serious disorders such as head injury and call for prompt medical care. These include:

- Sudden, severe headache
- Headache associated with convulsions
- Headache accompanied by confusion or loss of consciousness
- Headache following a blow on the head
- Headache associated with pain in the eye or ear
- Persistent headache in a person who was previously headache free
- Headache associated with fever
- Headache that interferes with normal life

A headache sufferer usually seeks help from a family practitioner. If the problem is not relieved by standard treatments, the patient may then be referred to a specialist— perhaps an internist or a neurologist. Additional referrals may be made to psychologists.

DIAGNOSING A HEADACHE

Diagnosing a headache is like playing Twenty Questions. Experts agree that a detailed question-and-answer session with a patient can often produce enough information for a diagnosis. Many types of headaches have clear-cut symptoms which fall into an easily recognizable pattern.

Patients may be asked: How often do you have headaches? Where is the pain? How long do the headaches last? When did you first develop headaches?

The patient's sleep habits and family and work situations may also be probed.

Most physicians will also obtain a full medical history from the patient, inquiring about past head trauma or surgery and about the use of medications.

A blood test may be ordered to screen for thyroid disease, anemia, or infections that might cause a headache.

X-rays may be taken to rule out the possibility of a brain tumor or blood clot.

A test called an electroencephalogram (EEG) may be given to measure brain activity. EEGs can indicate a malfunction in the brain, but they cannot usually pinpoint a problem that might be causing a headache.

A physician may suggest that a patient with unusual headaches undergo a computed tomography (CT) scan. The CT scan produces images of the brain that show variations in the density of different types of tissue. The scan enables the physician to distinguish, for example, between a bleeding blood vessel in the brain and a brain tumor.

The CT scan is an important diagnostic tool in cases of headache associated with brain lesions or other serious disease. Experts generally agree, however, that this sophisticated and expensive technology is not required to diagnose simple or periodic headache.

An eye exam is usually performed to check for weakness in the eye muscle or unequal pupil size. Both of these symptoms are evidence of an aneurysm—an abnormal ballooning of a blood vessel. A physician who suspects that a headache patient has an aneurysm may also order an angiogram. In this test, a special fluid which can be seen on an x-ray is injected into the patient and carried in the bloodstream to the brain to reveal any abnormalities in the blood vessels there.

Thermography, an experimental technique for diagnosing headache, promises to become a useful clinical tool. In thermography, an infrared camera converts skin temperature into a color picture or thermogram with different degrees of heat appearing as different colors. Skin temperature is affected primarily by blood flow. Research scientists have found that thermograms of headache patients show strikingly different heat patterns from those of people who never or rarely get headaches.

A physician analyzes the results of all these diagnostic tests along with a patient's medical history in order to arrive at a diagnosis.

Headaches are diagnosed as:

- Vascular
- Muscle contraction
- Traction
- Inflammatory

Vascular headaches—a group that includes the well-known migraine—are so named because they are thought to involve abnormal function of the brain's blood vessels or vascular system. Muscle-contraction headaches appear to involve the tightening or tensing of facial and neck muscles. Traction and inflammatory headaches are symptoms of other disorders, ranging from stroke to sinus infection. Some people have more than one type of headache.

MIGRAINE HEADACHES

The most common type of vascular headache is migraine. Migraine headaches are usually characterized by severe pain on one or both sides of the head, an upset stomach, and at times disturbed vision.

Symptoms of Migraine

Sensitivity to light is a standard symptom of the two most prevalent types of migraine-caused headache: classic and common. The major difference between the two types is the appearance of neurological symptoms 10 to

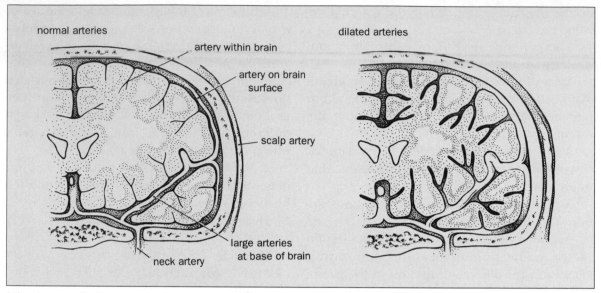

normal arteries

artery within brain

artery on brain surface

scalp artery

neck artery

dilated arteries

large arteries at base of brain

Migraines may begin as a spasm in arteries at the base of the brain, reducing its blood supply. The brain's arteries then dilate to meet its energy needs—but this action triggers a release of pain-causing chemicals.

30 minutes before a classic migraine attack. These symptoms are called an aura. The person may see flashing lights or zigzag lines, or may temporarily lose vision. Other classic symptoms include speech difficulty, weakness of an arm or leg, tingling of the face or hands, and confusion.

The pain of a classic migraine headache is described as intense, throbbing, or pounding and is felt in the forehead, temple, ear, jaw, or around the eye. Classic migraine starts on one side of the head but may eventually spread to the other side. An attack lasts one to two pain-wracked days.

The common migraine—a term that reflects the disorder's greater occurrence in the general population—is not preceded by an aura. But some people experience a variety of vague symptoms beforehand, including mental fuzziness, mood changes, fatigue, and unusual retention of fluids. During the headache phase of a common migraine, a person may have diarrhea and increased urination, as well as nausea and vomiting. Common migraine pain can last three or four days.

Both classic and common migraine can strike as often as several times a week, or as rarely as once every few years.

Both types can occur at any time. Some people, however, experience migraines at predictable times—near the days of menstruation or every Saturday morning after a stressful week of work.

The Migraine Process

Research scientists are unclear about the precise cause of migraine headaches. There seems to be general agreement, however, that a key element is blood flow changes in the brain. People who get migraine headaches appear to have blood vessels that overreact to various triggers.

Scientists have devised one theory of migraine that explains these blood flow changes and also certain biochemical changes that may be involved in the headache process. According to this theory, the nervous system responds to a trigger such as stress by creating a spasm in the nerve-rich arteries at the base of the brain. The spasm closes down or constricts several arteries supplying blood to the brain, including the scalp artery and the carotid or neck arteries.

As these arteries constrict, the flow of blood

to the brain is reduced. At the same time, blood-clotting particles called platelets clump together—a process which is believed to release a chemical called serotonin. Serotonin acts as a powerful constrictor of arteries, further reducing the blood supply to the brain.

Reduced blood flow decreases the brain's supply of oxygen. Symptoms signaling a headache, such as distorted vision or speech, may then result, similar to symptoms of stroke.

Reacting to the reduced oxygen supply, certain arteries within the brain open wider to meet the brain's energy needs. This widening or dilation spreads, finally affecting the neck and scalp arteries. The dilation of these arteries triggers the release of pain-producing substances called prostaglandins from various tissues and blood cells. Chemicals that cause inflammation and swelling, and substances that increase sensitivity to pain are also released. The circulation of these chemicals and the dilation of the scalp arteries stimulate the pain-sensitive nociceptors. The result, according to this theory: a throbbing pain in the head.

Women and Migraine

Although boys and girls seem to be equally affected by migraine, the condition is more common in adult women than in men. Both sexes may develop migraine in infancy, but most often the disorder begins between the ages of five and 35.

The relationship between female hormones and migraine is still unclear. Women may have menstrual migraine—headaches around the time of their menstrual period—which may disappear during pregnancy. Other women develop migraine for the first time when they are pregnant. Some are first affected after menopause.

The effect of oral contraceptives on headaches is perplexing. Scientists report that some migrainous women who take birth control pills experience more frequent and severe attacks. However, a small percentage of women have fewer and less severe migraine headaches when they take birth control pills. And normal women who do not suffer from headaches may develop migraines as a side effect when they use oral contraceptives. Investigators around the world are studying hormonal changes in migrainous women in the hope of identifying the specific ways these naturally occurring chemicals cause headaches.

Triggers of Headache

Many sufferers have a family history of migraine, but the exact hereditary nature of this condition is still unknown. People who get migraines are thought to have an inherited abnormality in the regulation of blood vessels.

"It's like a cocked gun with a hair trigger," explains one headache specialist. "A person is born with a potential for migraine and the headache is triggered by things that are really not so terrible."

These triggers include stress and other normal emotions, as well as biological and environmental conditions. Fatigue, glaring or flickering lights, the weather, and even certain foods can set off migraine. It may seem hard to believe that eating such seemingly harmless foods as yogurt, nuts, and lima beans can result in a painful migraine headache. However, some scientists believe that these foods and several others contain chemical substances such as tyramine which constrict arteries—the first step of the migraine process. Other scientists think foods cause headaches by setting off an allergic reaction in susceptible people.

Though a food-triggered migraine usually occurs soon after eating, other triggers may not cause immediate pain. Scientists report that people can develop migraine not only during a period of stress but also afterwards when their vascular systems are still reacting. The "preacher Monday morning headache" is named for those clergymen who get migraines a day after the stress of delivering a Sunday sermon. Migraines that wake people up in the middle of the night are also believed to result from a delayed reaction to stress.

Other Forms of Migraine

In addition to classic and common, migraine headache can take several other forms.

Hemiplegic migraine patients have temporary paralysis on one side of the body, a condition known as hemiplegia. Some people may experience vision problems and vertigo—a feeling that the world is spinning. These symptoms begin 10 to 90 minutes before the onset of headache pain.

Ophthalmoplegic migraine is characterized by pain around the eye and is associated with a droopy eyelid, double vision, and other sight problems.

Basilar artery migraine involves a disturbance of a major brain artery. Preheadache symptoms include vertigo, double vision, and poor muscular coordination. This type of migraine occurs primarily in adolescent and young adult women and is often associated with the menstrual cycle.

Benign exertional headache is brought on by running, lifting, coughing, sneezing, or bending. The headache begins at the onset of activity, and pain rarely lasts more than several minutes.

Status migrainosus is a rare and severe type of migraine that can last 72 hours or longer. The pain and nausea are so intense that people who have this type of headache must be hospitalized. The use of certain drugs can trigger status migrainosus. Neurologists report that many of their status migrainosus patients were depressed and anxious before they experienced headache attacks.

Headache-free migraine is characterized by such migraine symptoms as visual problems, nausea, vomiting, constipation, or diarrhea. Patients, however, do not experience head pain. Headache specialists have suggested that un-explained pain in a particular part of the body, fever, and dizziness could also be possible types of headache-free migraine.

Treating Migraine Headache

During the Stone Age, pieces of a headache sufferer's skull were cut away with flint instruments to relieve pain. Another unpleasant remedy used in the British Isles around the ninth century involved drinking "the juice of elderseed, cow's brain, and goat's dung dissolved in vinegar." Fortunately, today's headache patients are spared such drastic measures.

Drug therapy, biofeedback training, stress reduction, and elimination of certain foods from the diet are the most common methods of preventing and controlling migraine and other vascular headaches. Regular exercise, such as swimming or vigorous walking, can also reduce the frequency and severity of migraine headaches.

During a migraine headache, temporary relief can sometimes be obtained by using cold packs or by pressing on the bulging artery found in front of the ear on the painful side of the head.

Drug therapy. There are two ways to approach the treatment of migraine headache with drugs: prevent the attacks, or relieve symptoms after the headache occurs.

For infrequent migraine, drugs can be taken at the first sign of a headache in order to stop it or to at least ease the pain. People who get occasional mild migraine may benefit by taking aspirin or acetaminophen at the start of an attack. Aspirin raises a person's tolerance to pain and also discourages clumping of blood platelets. Small amounts of caffeine may be useful if taken in the early stages of migraine. But for most migraine sufferers who get moderate to severe headaches, and for all cluster patients, stronger drugs may be necessary to control the pain.

One of the most commonly used drugs for the relief of classic and common migraine symptoms is ergotamine tartrate, a vasoconstrictor which helps counteract the painful dilation stage of the headache. For optimal benefit, the drug is taken during the early stages of an attack.

If a migraine has been in progress for about an hour and has passed into the final throbbing stage, ergotamine tartrate will probably not help.

Because ergotamine tartrate can cause nausea and vomiting, it may be combined with antinausea drugs. Research scientists caution that ergotamine tartrate should not be taken in excess or by people who have angina pectoris, severe hypertension, or vascular, liver, or kidney disease. Patients who are unable to take ergotamine tartrate may benefit from other drugs that constrict dilated blood vessels or help reduce blood vessel inflammation.

For headaches that occur three or more times a month, preventive treatment is usually recommended. Drugs used to prevent classic and common migraine include methysergide maleate, which counteracts blood vessel constriction; propranolol, which stops blood vessel dilation; and amitriptyline, an antidepressant. In a study of propranolol, amitriptyline, and biofeedback conducted by the Houston Headache Clinic, scientists found that migraine patients improved most on a combination of propranolol and biofeedback. Patients who had mixed migraine and muscle-contraction headaches received the greatest benefit from a combination of propranolol, amitriptyline, and biofeedback.

Another recent study showed that propranolol may continue to prevent migraine headaches even after patients have stopped taking the drug. The scientists who conducted the study speculate that long-term therapy with propranolol may have a lasting effect on blood vessels, training them to react less than usual to the triggers of migraine.

Antidepressants called MAO inhibitors also prevent migraine. These drugs block an enzyme called monoamine oxidase, which normally helps nerve cells absorb the artery-constricting chemical serotonin.

MAO inhibitors can have potentially serious side effects—particularly if taken while ingesting foods or beverages that contain tyramine, a substance that constricts arteries.

Several new drugs for the prevention of migraine have been developed in recent years, including papaverine hydrochloride, which produces blood vessel dilation, and cyproheptadine, which counteracts serotonin.

Newer medications such as sumatriptan and related drugs may abort symptoms of a severe migraine if taken at the onset of the headache.

All these antimigraine drugs can have adverse side effects. But they are relatively safe when used carefully. To avoid long-term side effects of preventive medications, headache specialists advise patients to reduce the dosage of these drugs and then to stop taking them as soon as possible.

Biofeedback and relaxation training. Drug therapy for migraine is often combined with biofeedback and relaxation training. Biofeedback refers to a technique that can give people better control over such body function indicators as blood pressure, heart rate, temperature, muscle tension, and brain waves. Thermal biofeedback allows a patient to consciously raise hand temperature. Some patients who are able to increase hand temperature can reduce the number and intensity of migraines. The mechanism of this hand-warming effect is being studied by research scientists.

"To succeed in biofeedback," says one headache specialist, "you must be able to concentrate, and you must be motivated to get well."

A patient learning thermal biofeedback wears a device which transmits the temperature of an index finger or hand to a monitor. While the patient tries to warm his hands, the monitor provides feedback either on a gauge that shows the temperature reading or by emitting a sound or beep that increases in intensity as the temperature increases. The patient is not told how to raise hand temperature, but is given suggestions such as, "Imagine that your hands feel very warm and heavy." "I have a good imagination," says one headache sufferer who traded in her medication for thermal biofeedback. The technique decreased the number and severity of headaches she experienced.

In another type of biofeedback called electromyographic or EMG training, the patient learns to control muscle tension in the face, neck, and shoulders.

Either kind of biofeedback may be combined with relaxation training, during which patients learn to relax the mind and body.

Biofeedback can be practiced at home with a portable monitor. But the ultimate goal of treatment is to wean the patient from the machine. The patient can then use biofeedback anywhere at the first sign of a headache.

The antimigraine diet. Scientists estimate that a small percentage of migraine sufferers will benefit from a treatment program focused solely on eliminating headache-provoking foods and beverages.

Other migraine patients may be helped by a diet to prevent low blood sugar. Low blood sugar, or hypoglycemia, can cause dilation of the blood vessels in the head. This condition can occur after a period without food: overnight, for example, or when a meal is skipped. People who wake up in the morning with a headache may be reacting to the low blood sugar caused by the lack of food overnight.

Treatment for headaches caused by low blood sugar consists of scheduling smaller, more frequent meals for the patient. A special diet designed to stabilize the body's sugar-regulating system is sometimes recommended.

For the same reason, many specialists also recommend that migraine patients avoid oversleeping on weekends. Sleeping late can change the body's normal blood sugar level and lead to a headache.

OTHER VASCULAR HEADACHES
After migraine, the most common type of vascular headache is the toxic headache produced by fever. Pneumonia, measles, mumps, and tonsillitis are among the diseases that can cause severe toxic vascular headaches. Toxic headaches can also result from the presence of foreign chemicals in the body. Other kinds of vascular headaches include "clusters," which cause repeated episodes of intense pain, and headaches resulting from a rise in blood pressure.

Chemical Culprits
Repeated exposure to nitrite compounds can result in a dull, pounding headache that may be accompanied by a flushed face. Nitrite, which dilates blood vessels, is found in such products as heart medicine and dynamite, but is also used as a chemical to preserve meat. Hot dogs and other meats containing sodium nitrite can also cause headaches.

Eating foods prepared with monosodium glutamate (MSG) can result in headache. Soy sauce, meat tenderizer, and a variety of packaged foods contain this chemical which is touted as a flavor enhancer.

Vascular headache can also result from exposure to poisons, even common household varieties like insecticides, carbon tetrachloride, and lead. Anyone who has contact with lead batteries or lead-glazed pottery may develop headaches.

Artists and industrial workers may experience headaches after exposure to materials that contain chemical solvents. Solvents, like benzene, are found in turpentine, spray adhesives, rubber cement, and inks.

Drugs such as amphetamines can cause headaches as a side effect. Another type of drug-related headache occurs during withdrawal from long-term therapy with the antimigraine drug ergotamine tartrate.

Jokes are often made about alcohol hangovers, but the headache associated with "the morning after" is no laughing matter. Fortunately, there are several suggested remedies for the pain, including ergotamine tartrate. The hangover headache may also be reduced by taking honey, which speeds alcohol metabolism, or caffeine, a constrictor of dilated arteries. Caffeine can cause headaches as well as cure them. Heavy coffee drinkers often get headaches when they try to break the caffeine habit.

Cluster Headaches

Cluster headaches, named for their repeated occurrence in groups or clusters, begin as a minor pain around one eye, eventually spreading to that side of the face. The pain quickly intensifies, compelling the victim to pace the floor or rock in a chair. "You can't lie down, you're fidgety," explains a cluster patient. "The pain is unbearable." Other symptoms include a stuffed and runny nose and a droopy eyelid over a red and tearing eye.

Cluster headaches last between 30 and 45 minutes. But the relief people feel at the end of an attack is usually mixed with dread as they await a recurrence. Clusters can strike several times a day or night for several weeks or months. Then, mysteriously, they may disappear for months or years. Many people have cluster bouts during the spring and fall. At their worst, chronic cluster headaches can last continuously for years.

Cluster attacks can strike at any age but usually start between the ages of 20 and 40. Unlike migraine, cluster headaches are more common in men and do not run in families. Research scientists have observed certain physical similarities among people who experience cluster headache. The typical cluster patient is a tall, muscular man with a rugged facial appearance and a square, jutting, or dimpled chin. The texture of his coarse skin resembles an orange peel. Women who get clusters may also have this type of skin.

Studies of cluster patients show that they are likely to have hazel eyes and that they tend to be heavy smokers and drinkers. Paradoxically, both nicotine, which constricts arteries, and alcohol, which dilates them, trigger cluster headaches. The exact connection between these substances and cluster attacks is not known.

Despite a cluster headache's distinguishing characteristics, its relative infrequency and similarity to such disorders as sinusitis can lead to misdiagnosis. Some cluster patients have had tooth extractions, sinus surgery, or psychiatric treatment in a futile effort to cure their pain.

Research studies have turned up several clues as to the cause of cluster headache, but no answers. One clue is found in the thermograms of untreated cluster patients, which show a "cold spot" of reduced blood flow above the eye.

The sudden start and brief duration of cluster headaches can make them difficult to treat. By the time medicine is absorbed into the body, the attack is often over. However, research scientists have identified several effective drugs for these headaches. The antimigraine drug ergotamine tartrate can subdue a cluster, if taken at the first sign of an attack. Injections of dihydroergotamine, a form of ergotamine tartrate, are sometimes used to treat clusters.

Some cluster patients can prevent attacks by taking propranolol or methysergide. Investigators have also discovered that mild solutions of cocaine hydrochloride applied inside the nose can quickly stop cluster headaches in most patients. This treatment may work because it both blocks pain impulses and it constricts blood vessels.

Another option that works for some cluster patients is rapid inhalation of pure oxygen through a mask for five to 15 minutes. The oxygen seems to ease the pain of cluster headache by reducing blood flow to the brain.

In chronic cases of cluster headache, certain facial nerves may be surgically cut or destroyed to provide relief. These procedures have had limited success. Some cluster patients have had facial nerves cut only to have them regenerate years later.

Painful Pressure

Chronic high blood pressure can cause headache, as can rapid rises in blood pressure like those experienced during anger, vigorous exercise, or sexual excitement.

The severe "orgasmic headache" occurs right before orgasm and is believed to be a vascular type. Because sudden rupture of a cerebral blood vessel can also occur during orgasm, this type of headache should be promptly evaluated by a doctor.

MUSCLE-CONTRACTION HEADACHES

It's 5 p.m. and the boss has just demanded a 20-page briefing paper. Due date: tomorrow. The employee is angry and tired and the more he or she thinks about the assignment, the greater the tension. The teeth clench, the brow wrinkles, and soon a splitting tension headache results.

Tension headache is named not only for the role of stress in triggering the pain, but also for the contraction of neck, face, and scalp muscles brought on by stressful events. Tension headache is a severe but temporary form of muscle-contraction headache. The pain is mild to moderate and feels like pressure is being applied to the head or neck. The headache usually disappears after the period of stress is over. Ninety percent of all headaches are classified as tension/muscle-contraction headaches.

Chronic muscle-contraction headaches, by contrast, can last for weeks, months, and sometimes years. The pain of these headaches is often described as a tight band around the head or a feeling that the head and neck are in a cast. "It feels like somebody is tightening a giant vise around my head," says one patient. The pain is steady and is usually felt on both sides of the head. Chronic muscle-contraction headaches can cause a sore scalp—even combing one's hair can be painful.

Causes

Many scientists believe that the primary cause of the pain of muscle-contraction headache is sustained muscle tension. Other studies suggest that restricted blood flow may cause or contribute to the pain.

Occasionally, muscle-contraction headaches will be accompanied by nausea, vomiting, and blurred vision, but there is no preheadache syndrome as with migraine. Muscle-contraction headaches have not been linked to hormones or foods, as has migraine, nor is there a strong hereditary connection.

Research has shown that for many people, chronic muscle-contraction headaches are caused by depression and anxiety. These people tend to get their headaches in the early morning or evening when conflicts in the office or home are anticipated.

Emotional factors are not the only triggers of muscle-contraction headaches. Certain physical postures—such as holding one's chin down while reading—can lead to head and neck pain. So can prolonged writing under poor light, or holding a phone between the shoulder and ear, or even gum-chewing.

Other causes include more serious problems such as degenerative arthritis of the neck and temporomandibular joint dysfunction (TMD). TMD is a disorder of the joint between the temporal bone (above the ear) and the mandible or lower jaw bone. The disorder results from poor bite and jaw clenching.

Treatment

Treatment for muscle-contraction headache varies. The first consideration is to treat any specific disorder or disease that may be causing the headache. For example, arthritis of the neck is treated with anti-inflammatory medication, and TMD may be helped by corrective devices for the mouth and jaw.

Acute tension headaches not associated with a disease are treated with muscle relaxants and analgesics like aspirin and acetaminophen. Stronger analgesics, such as propoxyphene and codeine, are sometimes prescribed. As prolonged use of these drugs can lead to dependence, patients taking them should have periodic medical checkups and follow their physician's instructions carefully.

Nondrug therapy for chronic muscle-contraction headaches includes biofeedback, relaxation training, and counseling. A technique called cognitive restructuring teaches people to change their attitudes and responses to stress. Patients might be encouraged, for example, to imagine that they are coping successfully with a stressful situation. In progressive relaxation therapy, patients are taught to first tense and then relax individual muscle groups. Finally, the patient tries to relax his or her whole body. Many people imagine a peaceful scene—such as lying on the beach or by a beautiful lake. Passive relaxation does not involve tensing of muscles. Instead, patients are encouraged to focus on different muscles, suggesting that they relax. Some people might think to themselves, "Relax" or "My muscles feel warm."

People with chronic muscle-contraction headaches may also be helped by taking antidepressants or MAO inhibitors. Mixed muscle-contraction and migraine headaches are sometimes treated with barbiturate compounds, which slow down nerve function in the brain and spinal cord.

People who suffer infrequent muscle-contraction headaches may benefit from a hot shower or moist heat applied to the back of the neck. Cervical collars are sometimes recommended as an aid to good posture. Physical therapy, massage, and gentle exercise of the neck may also be helpful.

WHEN HEADACHE IS A WARNING

Like other types of pain, headaches can serve as warning signals of more serious disorders. This is particularly true for headaches caused by traction or inflammation.

Traction headaches can occur if the pain-sensitive parts of the head are pulled, stretched, or displaced, as, for example, when eye muscles are tensed in order to compensate for eyestrain. Headaches caused by inflammation include those related to meningitis, as well as those resulting from diseases of the sinuses, spine, neck, ears, and teeth. Ear and tooth infections and glaucoma can cause headaches. In oral and dental disorders, headache is experienced as pain throughout the entire head, including the face.

Traction and inflammatory headaches are treated by curing the underlying problem. This may involve surgery, antibiotics, or other drugs. Characteristics of the types of traction and inflammatory headaches vary by the disorder.

Brain Tumor

Brain tumors are diagnosed in about 11,000 people every year. As they grow, these tumors sometimes cause headache by pushing on the outer layer of nerve tissue that covers the brain or by pressing against pain-sensitive blood vessel walls. Headache resulting from a brain tumor may be periodic or continuous. Typically, it feels like a strong pressure is being applied to the head. The pain is relieved when the tumor is destroyed by surgery, radiation, or chemotherapy.

Stroke

Headache may accompany several conditions that can lead to stroke, including hypertension or high blood pressure, arteriosclerosis, and heart disease. Headaches are also associated with completed stroke, when brain cells die from lack of sufficient oxygen.

Many stroke-related headaches can be prevented by management of the patient's condition through diet, exercise, and medication.

Mild to moderate headaches are associated with transient ischemic attacks (TIAs), sometimes called "mini-strokes," which result from a temporary lack of blood supply to the brain. The head pain occurs near the clot or lesion that blocks blood flow.

The similarity between migraine and symptoms of TIA can cause problems in diagnosis. The rare person under age 40 who suffers a TIA may be misdiagnosed as having migraine; similarly, TIA-prone older patients who suffer migraine may be misdiagnosed as having stroke-related headaches.

Spinal Tap

About one-fourth of the people who undergo a lumbar puncture or spinal tap develop a headache. Many scientists believe these headaches result from leakage of the cerebrospinal fluid that flows through pain-sensitive membranes around the brain and down to the spinal cord. The fluid, they suggest, drains through the tiny hole created by the spinal tap needle, causing the membranes to rub painfully against the bony skull. Since headache pain occurs only when the patient stands up, the cure is to remain lying down until the headache runs its course—anywhere from a few hours to several days.

Head Trauma

Headaches may develop after a blow to the head, either immediately or months later. There is little relationship between the severity of the trauma and the intensity of headache pain. One cause of trauma headache is scar formation in the scalp. Another is ruptured blood vessels which result in an accumulation of blood called a hematoma. This mass of blood can displace brain tissue and cause headaches, as well as weakness, confusion, memory loss, and seizures. Hematomas can be drained in order to produce rapid relief of symptoms.

Arteritis and Meningitis

Arteritis, an inflammation of certain arteries in the head, primarily affects people over age 50. Symptoms include throbbing headache, fever, and loss of appetite. Some patients experience blurring or loss of vision. Prompt treatment with corticosteroid drugs helps to relieve symptoms.

Headaches are also caused by infections of meninges, the brain's outer covering, and phlebitis, a vein inflammation.

Trigeminal Neuralgia

Trigeminal neuralgia, or tic douloureux, results from a disorder of the trigeminal nerve. This nerve supplies the face, teeth, mouth, and nasal cavity with feeling and also enables the mouth muscles to chew. Symptoms are headache and intense facial pain that comes in short, excruciating jabs set off by the slightest touch to or movement of trigger points in the face or mouth. People with trigeminal neuralgia often fear brushing their teeth or chewing on the side of the mouth that is affected. Many trigeminal neuralgia patients are controlled with drugs, including carbamazepine. Patients who do not respond to drugs may be helped by surgery on the trigeminal nerve.

Sinus Infection

In a condition called acute sinusitis, a viral or bacterial infection of the upper respiratory tract spreads to the membrane that lines the sinus cavities. When one or all four of these cavities are filled with bacterial or viral fluid, they become inflamed, causing pain and sometimes headache. Treatment of acute sinusitis includes antibiotics, analgesics, and decongestants.

Chronic sinusitis may be caused by an allergy to such irritants as dust, ragweed, animal hair, and smoke. Research scientists dis-

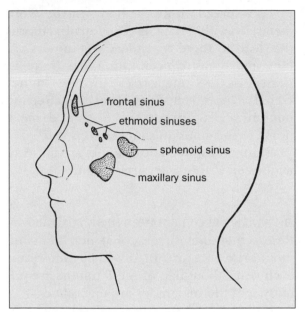

Acute sinusitis headaches can occur when one or more of the four sinus cavities fill with fluid resulting from bacterial or viral infections.

frontal sinus

ethmoid sinuses

sphenoid sinus

maxillary sinus

agree about whether chronic sinusitis triggers headache.

RESEARCH INTERVENES

Modern methods of diagnosis and treatment enable physicians and psychologists today to help about 90 percent of chronic headache patients, according to the director of a major U.S. headache clinic.

These methods are based on years of scientific research. New research should lead to even more advanced techniques of headache management.

The National Institute of
Neurological Disorders and Stroke

BRAIN AND SPINAL CORD TUMORS

Brain and spinal cord tumors are abnormal growths of tissue found inside the skull or the bony spinal column. The word "tumor" is used to describe both abnormal growths that are new (neoplasms) and those present at birth (congenital tumors). The following material will focus primarily on neoplasms.

No matter where they are located in the body, tumors are usually classified as benign (or noncancerous) if the cells that make up the growth are similar to other normal cells, grow relatively slowly, and are confined to one location. Tumors are called malignant (or cancerous) when the cells are very different from normal cells, grow relatively quickly, and can spread easily to other locations.

In most parts of the body, benign tumors are not particularly harmful. This is not necessarily true in the brain and spinal cord, which are the primary components of the central nervous system (CNS). Because the CNS is housed within rigid, bony quarters (that is, the skull and spinal column), any abnormal growth can place pressure on sensitive tissues and impair function.

In addition, any tumor located near vital brain structures or near sensitive spinal cord nerves can seriously threaten health. A benign tumor growing next to an important blood vessel in the brain does not have to grow very large before it can block blood flow. Or, if a benign tumor is found deep inside the brain, surgery to remove it may be very risky because of the chances of damaging vital brain centers. On the other hand, a tumor located near the brain's surface can often be removed surgically.

An important difference between malignant tumors in the CNS and those elsewhere in the body lies with their potential to spread. While malignant cells elsewhere in the body can easily seed tumors inside the brain and spinal cord, malignant CNS tumors rarely spread out to other body parts. Laboratory and clinical investigators are exploring such unusual characteristics of CNS tumors because these unique properties may suggest new strategies to prevent or treat them.

WHAT CAUSES THESE TUMORS?

When newly formed tumors begin within the brain or spinal cord, they are called primary tumors. Primary CNS tumors rarely grow from neurons—nerve cells that perform the nervous system's important functions—because once neurons are mature, they no longer divide and multiply.

Instead, most tumors are caused by out-of-control growth among cells that surround and support neurons. Primary CNS tumors—such as gliomas and meningiomas—are named by the types of cells they contain, their location, or both.

In a small number of individuals, primary tumors may result from specific genetic diseases—such as neurofibromatosis and tuberous sclerosis—or exposure to radiation or cancer-causing chemicals. Although smoking, alcohol consumption, and certain dietary habits are associated with some types of cancers, they have not been linked to primary brain and spinal cord tumors.

In fact, the cause of most primary brain and spinal cord tumors—and most cancers—remains a mystery. Scientists do not know exactly why and how cells in the nervous system or elsewhere in the body lose their normal identity as nerve, blood, skin, or other cell types and grow uncontrollably.

Researchers are looking for clues to this process with the goals of learning why and how cancer begins and developing new tools to stop it. Some of the possible causes under investigation include viruses and defective genes. Also, there is increasing interest in learning about the possible role played by environmental factors, such as chemicals and new technologies.

Metastatic tumors are caused by cancerous cells that shed from tumors in other parts of the body, travel through the bloodstream, burrow through the blood vessel walls, latch onto tissue, and spawn new tumors inside the brain or spinal cord.

For every four people who have cancer that has spread within the body, one develops metastasis within the CNS. The top two culprits that lead to these secondary CNS tumors are lung and breast cancer. Other, less frequent causes of CNS metastases include kidney (renal) cancer, lymphoma (a cancer affecting immune cells), prostate cancer, and melanoma (a form of skin cancer).

Brain and spinal cord tumors are not contagious or, at this time, preventable.

HOW MANY PEOPLE HAVE THESE TUMORS?

Research studies suggest that new brain tumors arise in more than 40,000 Americans each year. About half of these tumors are primary, and the remainder are metastatic.

Individuals of any age can develop a brain tumor. In fact, they are the second most common cause of cancer-related death in people up to the age of 35, with a slight peak in occurrence among children between the ages of six and nine. However, brain tumors are most common among middle-aged and older adults. People in their sixties face the highest risk—each year one of every 5,000 people in this age group develops a brain tumor.

Spinal cord tumors are less common than brain tumors. About 10,000 Americans develop primary or metastatic spinal cord tumors each year. Although spinal cord tumors affect people of all ages, they are most common in young and middle-aged adults.

WHAT ARE THE SYMPTOMS?

Brain and spinal cord tumors cause many diverse symptoms, which can make detection tricky. Whatever specific symptoms a patient has, the symptoms generally develop slowly and worsen over time.

Brain Tumors

A 3.5-pound wrinkled mass of tissue, the brain orchestrates behavior, movement, feeling, and sensation. It controls automatic functions

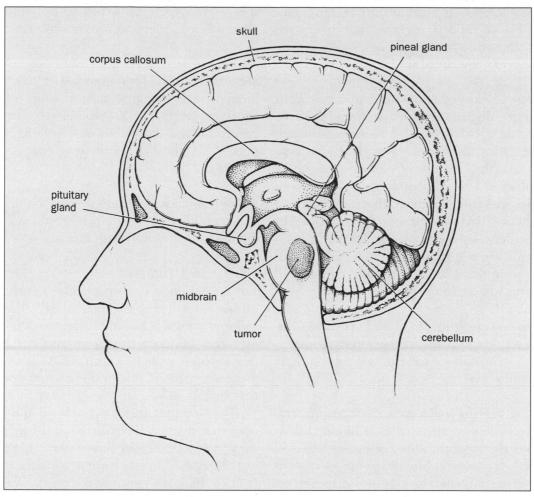

Surgery to remove this tumor in the midbrain would be a risky procedure, because the tumor is surrounded by vital brain centers. A tumor located nearer to the skull, however, might be removed with little noticeable damage to brain function.

like breathing and heartbeat. Many of these important functions are controlled by specialized brain areas. For example, the brain's left and right hemispheres jointly control hearing and vision; the front part of each hemisphere controls voluntary movements, like writing, for the opposite side of the body; and the brain stem is responsible for basic life-sustaining functions, including blood pressure, heartbeat, and breathing.

As a result, brain tumors can cause a bewildering array of symptoms depending on their size, type, and location. Certain symptoms are quite specific because they result from damage to particular brain areas. Other, more general symptoms are triggered by increased pressure within the skull as the tumor encroaches on the brain's limited space or blocks the flow of cerebrospinal fluid (fluid that bathes the brain and spinal cord). Some of the more common symptoms of a brain tumor include:

Headaches. More than half of people with brain tumors experience headaches. Because the skull cannot expand, the growing mass places pressure on pain-sensitive areas. The headaches recur, often at irregular periods, and can last several minutes or hours. They may worsen when coughing, changing posture, or straining. As the tumor grows, headaches often last longer, become more frequent, and grow more severe.

Seizures. The abnormal tissue found in a brain tumor can disrupt the normal flow of electricity through which brain cells communicate. The resulting bursts of electrical activity cause seizures with a variety of symptoms, such as convulsions, loss of consciousness, or loss of bladder control. Seizures that first start in adulthood (in a patient who has not been in an accident or had an illness that causes seizures) are a key warning sign of brain tumors. Sometimes seizures are the only sign of a slowly growing brain tumor.

Nausea and vomiting. Increased pressure within the skull can cause nausea and vomiting. These symptoms sometimes accompany headaches.

Vision or hearing problems. Increased intracranial pressure can also decrease blood flow in the eye and trigger swelling of the optic nerve, which in turn causes blurred vision, double vision, or partial visual loss. Tumors growing on or near sensory nerves often trigger visual or hearing disturbances, such as ringing or buzzing sounds, abnormal eye movements or crossed eyes, and partial or total loss of vision or hearing. Tumors that grow in the brain's occipital lobe, which interprets visual images, may also cause partial vision loss.

Behavioral and cognitive symptoms. Because they strike at the core of the individual's identity, changes in behavior and personality can be the most frightening and devastating symptoms of a brain tumor. These symptoms usually occur when the tumor is located in the brain's cerebral hemispheres, which are responsible, in part, for personality, communication, thinking, behavior, and other vital functions. Examples include problems with speech, language, thinking, and memory, or psychotic episodes and changes in personality.

Motor problems. When tumors affect brain areas responsible for command of body movement, they can cause motor symptoms, including weakness or paralysis, lack of coordination, or trouble with walking. Often muscle weakness or paralysis affects only one side of the body.

Balance problems. Brain tumors that disrupt the normal control of equilibrium can cause dizziness or difficulty with balance.

Spinal Cord Tumors

The spinal cord is, in part, like a living telephone cable. Lying protected inside the bony spine, it contains bundles of nerves that carry messages between the brain and the body's nerves, such as instructions from the brain to move an arm or information from the skin that signals pain.

A tumor that forms on or near the spinal cord can disrupt this communication. Often these tumors exert pressure on the spinal cord or the nerves that exit from it; sometimes, they restrict the cord's supply of blood. Common symptoms that result from this include:

Pain. Normally, the spinal cord carries important warnings about pain from the body's nerves to the brain. By putting pressure on the spinal cord, a tumor can trigger these circuits and cause pain that feels as if it is coming from various parts of the body. This pain is often constant, sometimes severe, and can have a burning or aching quality.

Sensory changes. Many people with spinal cord tumors suffer a loss of sensation. This usually takes the form of numbness and decreased skin sensitivity to temperature.

Motor problems. Since the nerves control the muscles, tumors that affect nerve communication can trigger a number of muscle-related symptoms. Early symptoms include muscle weakness, spasticity in which the muscles stay stiffly contracted, and impaired bladder and/or bowel control. If untreated, symptoms may worsen to include muscle wasting and paralysis. In addition, some people develop an abnormal walking rhythm known as ataxia.

The parts of the body affected by these symptoms vary with tumor location along the spinal cord. In general, symptoms strike body areas at the same level or at a level below that of the tumor. For example, a tumor midway along the spinal cord (in the thoracic spine) can cause pain that spreads over the chest in a girdle-shaped pattern and gets worse when the individual coughs, sneezes, or lies down. A tumor that grows in the top fourth of the spinal column (or cervical spine) can cause pain that seems to come from the neck or arms. And a tumor that grows in the lower spine (or lumbar spine) can trigger back or leg pain.

In some cases, one or more tumors extend over several sections of the spinal cord. This results in symptoms that are spread over various parts of the body. Sometimes sensory symptoms occur in a patchy, confusing pattern in which some parts of the body are unaffected even though they lie between affected areas.

Doctors divide spinal cord tumors into three major groups based on where they are found. Extradural tumors grow between the bony spinal canal and the tough membrane called dura mater that protects the spinal cord. Tumors inside the dura (intradural tumors) are further divided into those outside the spinal cord (extramedullary tumors) and those inside the spinal cord (intramedullary tumors).

DIAGNOSING CNS TUMORS

Research has made major strides in the ability to detect and diagnose CNS tumors. When a doctor suspects a brain or spinal cord tumor because of a patient's medical history and symptoms, he or she can turn to a number of specialized tests and techniques to confirm the diagnosis. However, the first test is often a traditional neurological exam. A neurological exam checks:

- *Eye movement, eye reflexes, and pupil reaction.* For example, the doctor can shine a pen light into the eye to see if the pupil contracts normally or ask the patient to follow a moving object, such as a finger.
- *Reflexes.* Tests like tapping below the knee with a rubber hammer help to identify changes in reflexes.
- *Hearing.* Using a tuning fork, the physician can check for changes in hearing.
- *Sensation.* The doctor can use something sharp like a pin to test the sense of touch.
- *Movement.* Problems with movement are often tested by asking the patient to move his or her tongue, head, or facial muscles—as in smiling—and to perform tasks with the arms and legs.
- *Balance and coordination.* Typical tests include maintaining balance with the eyes closed, walking heel-to-toe in a straight line, or touching the nose with the eyes closed.

The next step in diagnosing brain tumors often involves x-rays or special imaging techniques and laboratory tests that can detect the presence of a tumor and provide clues about its location and type.

Imaging and X-ray

Special imaging techniques developed through recent research, especially computed tomography (CT) and magnetic resonance imaging (MRI), have dramatically improved the diagnosis of CNS tumors in recent years. In many cases, these scans can detect the presence of a tumor even if it is less than half an inch across.

CT uses a sophisticated x-ray machine and a computer to create a detailed picture of the body's tissues and structures. Often doctors will inject a special dye into the patient before performing a CT scan. The dye, also called contrast material, makes it easier to see abnormal tissue. A CT scan often gives doctors a good idea of where the tumor is located in the brain or spinal cord and can sometimes help them determine the tumor's type. It can also help doctors detect swelling, bleeding, and other associated conditions. In addition, CT scans can help doctors check the results of treatment and watch for tumor recurrence.

MRI is a relatively new imaging technique that is rapidly gaining widespread use in diagnosing CNS tumors. This technique uses a magnetic field and radio waves, rather than x-rays, and can often distinguish more accurately between healthy and diseased tissue. MRI gives better pictures of tumors located near bone than CT, does not use radiation as CT does, and provides pictures from various angles that can enable doctors to construct a three-dimensional image of the tumor.

A third imaging technology called positron emission tomography (PET) provides a picture of brain activity rather than structure by measuring levels of injected glucose (sugar) that has been labelled with a radioactive tracer. Glucose is used by the brain for energy.

Detectors placed around the head can spot the labelled glucose, and a computer uses the pattern of glucose distribution to form an image of the brain. Since malignant tissue uses more glucose than normal, it shows up on the scan as brighter or lighter than surrounding tissue. Currently, PET is not widely used in tumor diagnosis, in part because the technique requires very elaborate, expensive equipment, including a cyclotron to create the radioactive glucose.

Although it is not widely used for diagnosis now that CT and MRI scans are possible, angiography continues to help doctors distinguish certain types of brain tumors and make decisions about surgery. In angiography, doctors inject dye into a major blood vessel, usu-

ally one of the large arteries in the neck. This dye deflects x-rays and makes it possible for doctors to see the network of blood vessels by taking a series of x-ray pictures as the dye flows through the brain. Since some tumors have a characteristic pattern of blood vessels and blood flow, the pictures can provide clues about the tumor's type. Information from angiography can also tell physicians if a tumor is located close to important, normal blood vessels that must be avoided during surgery.

Widespread use of CT and MRI has also largely displaced use of traditional x-rays for diagnosis of brain and spinal cord tumors, since x-rays do not provide very useful images of brain tissue. They are occasionally helpful when tumors cause changes in the skull or spinal cord or when they contain tiny deposits of bone-like material made of calcium.

Physicians may also use a specialized x-ray technique, called a myelogram, when diagnosing spinal cord tumors. In myelography, a special dye that absorbs x-rays is injected into the spinal cord. This dye outlines the spinal cord but will not pass through a tumor. The resulting x-ray picture shows a dark area or narrowing that reveals the tumor's location.

Laboratory Tests

Laboratory tests commonly used include the electroencephalogram (or EEG) and lumbar puncture, also known as the spinal tap. The EEG uses special patches placed on the scalp or fine needles placed in the brain to record electrical currents inside the brain. This recording can help the doctor see telltale patterns in the brain's electrical activity that suggest a brain tumor. Repeated EEG recordings can be particularly helpful in deciding if an abnormality in brain activity is getting worse.

In lumbar puncture, doctors obtain a small sample of cerebrospinal fluid. This fluid can be examined for abnormal cells or unusual levels of various compounds that suggest a brain or spinal cord tumor.

In the future, diagnosis of brain tumors

should grow more accurate as additional techniques—including new ways to image the CNS and advanced laboratory tests—are developed through basic laboratory studies and clinical research.

BIOPSY AND HOW IT IS USED

A biopsy is a surgical procedure in which a small sample of tissue is taken from the suspected tumor, often during surgery aimed at removing as much tumor as possible.

A biopsy gives doctors the clues they need to specifically diagnose the type of tumor. By examining the sample under a microscope, the pathologist—a physician who specializes in understanding how disease affects the body's tissues—can tell what kinds of cells are in a tumor. Pathologists also look carefully for certain changes that signal cancer. These signs include abnormal growths or changes in the cell membranes and telltale problems in the cell nuclei, which normally control cell characteristics and growth. For example, cancerous cells may grow small fingerlike projections on their normally smooth surface or have extra nuclei.

Using this information, the pathologist provides a diagnosis of the tumor type. The tumor may also be classified as benign or malignant and given a numbered score that reflects how malignant it is. This score can help doctors determine how to treat a tumor and predict the likely outcome, or prognosis, for the patient.

TREATMENT OF BRAIN AND SPINAL CORD TUMORS

The three most commonly used treatments—surgery, radiation, and chemotherapy—are largely the result of recent research. For some patients, doctors may suggest a new treatment still being tested. In any case, the doctor will recommend a treatment or a combination of treatments based on the tumor's location and type, any previous treatment the patient may have received, and the patient's medical history and general health.

Surgery

Surgery to remove as much tumor as possible is usually the first step in treating an accessible tumor—that is, a tumor that can be removed without unacceptable risk of neurological damage. Fortunately, research has led to advances in neurosurgery that make it possible for doctors to reach many tumors that were previously considered inaccessible.

These new techniques and tools equip neurosurgeons to operate in the tight, vulnerable confines of the CNS. Some recently developed approaches in use in the operating room include:

Microsurgery. In this widely used technique, the surgeon looks through a high-powered microscope to get a magnified view of the operating area. This makes it easier to see—and remove—tumor tissue while sparing surrounding healthy tissue.

Stereotactic procedures. In these procedures, a computer uses information from CT, MRI, or PET to create a three-dimensional map of the operation site. The computer uses the map to help the surgeon guide special, computer-assisted tools. This makes it possible for surgeons to approach certain difficult-to-reach tumors with greater precision. Many procedures can be performed using this approach, including biopsy, certain types of surgery, and planting radiation pellets in a tumor.

Lasers. Lasers release a beam of concentrated light energy that can destroy tissue. Lasers are occasionally helpful for tasks traditionally performed with a scalpel. For example, surgeons can use a laser to remove an entire tumor. Or, once most of a tumor is removed through surgery, they can destroy remaining tumor tissue with the laser's intense beam of energy.

Ultrasonic aspirators. Ultrasonic aspirators use sound waves to vibrate tumors and break them up. Like a vacuum, the aspirator then sucks up the tumor fragments.

Evoked potentials. Doctors use this test during surgery to determine the role of specific nerves and thus avoid damage. In this technique, small electrodes are used to stimulate a nerve so its electrical response, or evoked potential, can be measured.

Shunts. Shunts are flexible tubes used to reroute and drain fluid. Doctors sometimes insert a shunt into the brain when a tumor blocks the flow of cerebrospinal fluid and causes hydrocephalus. Shunting of the fluid can relieve headaches, nausea, and other symptoms caused by too much pressure inside the skull.

Surgery may be the beginning and end of treatment if the biopsy shows a benign tumor. If the tumor is malignant, however, doctors often recommend additional treatment following surgery, including radiation, chemotherapy, or experimental treatments. Sometimes, if a tumor is very large, radiation is used before surgery to reduce the tumor's size.

An inaccessible or inoperable tumor is one that cannot be removed surgically because of the risk of severe nervous system damage. These tumors are frequently located deep within the brain or near vital structures such as the brain stem—the part of the brain that controls many crucial functions including breathing and heart rate.

Malignant, multiple tumors may also be inoperable. Doctors treat most malignant, inaccessible, or inoperable CNS tumors with radiation and/or chemotherapy.

Among patients who have metastatic CNS tumors, doctors usually focus on treating the original cancer first. However, when a metastatic tumor causes serious disability or pain, doctors may recommend surgery or other treatments to reduce symptoms even if the original cancer has not been controlled.

Radiation Therapy

In radiation therapy, the tumor is bombarded with beams of energy that kill tumor cells. Traditional radiation therapy delivers radiation from outside the patient's body, usually begins a week or two after surgery, and continues for about six weeks. The dosage is fairly uniform throughout the treated areas, making it especially useful for tumors that are large or have infiltrated surrounding tissue.

However, when traditional radiation therapy is given to the brain, it may also cause damage to healthy tissue. Depending on the type of tumor, doctors may be able to choose a modified form of radiation therapy to help prevent this and to improve the effectiveness of treatment. Modifying therapy can be as simple as changing the dosage schedule and amount of radiation that a patient receives. For example, an approach called hyperfractionation uses smaller, more frequent doses.

Chemotherapy

Chemotherapy uses tumor-killing drugs that are given orally or injected into the bloodstream. Because not all tumors are vulnerable to the same anticancer drugs, doctors often use a combination of drugs for chemotherapy.

Chemotherapeutic drugs generally kill cells that are growing or dividing. This property makes them more deadly to malignant tissue, which contains a high proportion of growing and dividing cells, than to most normal cells. It also causes some of the side effects that can accompany chemotherapy—such as skin reactions, hair loss, or digestive problems—because a high proportion of these normal cell types are also growing and dividing at any given time.

The drugs most commonly used for CNS tumors are known by the initials BCNU (sometimes called carmustine) and CCNU (or lomustine). Research scientists are also testing

ON THE RESEARCH FRONT

• *Brachytherapy.* In brachytherapy, which is also known as interstitial radiation, doctors implant small, radioactive pellets directly into the tumor. The pellets may be left in permanently or for a few days, weeks, or months. This technique can deliver a large dose of radiation to the tumor while minimizing radiation of normal tissue. Through research, scientists thus far have found that brachytherapy is most useful for small tumors that are difficult to remove surgically. Research scientists continue to examine whether this technique can help patients with other tumor types as well.

• *Gamma knife.* The gamma knife, used for a procedure known technically as stereotactic gamma knife radiosurgery, combines precise stereotactic guidance and a sharply focused beam of radiation energy to deliver a single, precise dose of radiation. Despite its name, the gamma knife does not require a surgical incision. Investigators using this tool have found it can help them reach and treat some small tumors that are not accessible through surgery.

• *Gene therapy.* Gene therapy, an innovative approach to treating CNS cancer, is in the early stages of research in laboratories around the country. Genes are the blueprints the body's cells use to make proteins and other vital substances. In gene therapy, scientists insert a new gene into specific cells. In the case of gene therapy for brain tumors, this inserted gene could make the tumor cells sensitive to certain drugs, program the cancerous cells to self-destruct, or instruct them to manufacture substances that would slow their growth. Scientists are using tumor cells and animal models to learn how various genes, once introduced, hinder cancer growth and to identify the best methods for inserting new genes into tumor cells. Human trials are just beginning.

• *Oncogenes.* The body contains a number of genes that are important in normal cell growth and development. Changes in some of these genes—which might be triggered by such events as exposure to chemicals or radiation—can transform them into dangerous, cancer-causing oncogenes. A number of oncogenes have already been found, and scientists continue to look for more. They are also working to identify specific events that can create oncogenes and to learn if there may be ways to prevent oncogenes from forming or to impair oncogene function in cancerous cells.

Although many new approaches to treatment thus appear promising, it is important to remember that all potential therapies must stand the tests of well-designed, carefully controlled clinical trials and long-term follow-up of treated patients before any conclusions can be drawn about their safety or effectiveness.

Past research has led to improved tumor treatments and techniques, providing longer survival and richer lives for many CNS tumor patients. Current research promises to generate further improvements. In the years ahead, physicians and patients can look forward to new forms of therapy developed through an understanding of the unique traits of CNS tumors.

---

many promising drugs to learn if they can improve treatment for brain and spinal cord tumors and reduce side effects.

Other Drugs

Tumors, surgery, and radiation therapy can all result in swelling inside the CNS. Doctors may prescribe steroids for short or long periods to reduce this swelling. Examples of such drugs include dexamethasone, methylprednisolone, and prednisone.

WHERE TO GO FOR TREATMENT

Brain and spinal cord tumors are often difficult to diagnose, and surgery to remove them demands great skill. Experience, therefore, is probably the most important factor in choosing among physicians. Brain and spinal cord tumors are also relatively rare. Many physicians see only a few patients with CNS tumors each year. Others, however, have made treating brain and spinal cord tumors their specialty. Patients should consider how many patients a physician treats each year. Because many patients are understandably perplexed or frightened by a CNS tumor diagnosis, it is also important that they choose a physician who will answer questions and describe treatment options clearly and fully.

Patients should also learn what techniques and tools are available at the physician's hospital. Teaching hospitals affiliated with a medical college or university are more likely to be involved in research and, thus, have the equipment and specialists necessary to offer experimental treatments. Finally, if a patient is dissatisfied with a physician or a physician's recommendations, he or she may wish to seek another opinion.

CONCLUSION
Past research has led to improved tumor treatments and techniques, providing longer survival and richer lives for many CNS tumor patients. Current research promises to generate further improvements. In the years ahead, physicians and patients can look forward to new forms of therapy developed through an understanding of the unique traits of CNS tumors.

The National Institute of
Neurological Disorders and Stroke

DIZZINESS

Most of us can remember feeling dizzy—after a roller coaster ride, maybe, or when looking down from a tall building, or when, as children, we would step off a spinning merry-go-round. Even superbly conditioned astronauts have had temporary trouble with dizziness while in space. In these situations, dizziness arises naturally from unusual changes that disrupt our normal feeling of stability.

But dizziness can also be a sign that there is a disturbance or a disease in the system that helps people maintain balance. This system is coordinated by the brain, which reacts to nerve impulses from the ears, the eyes, the neck and limb muscles, and the joints of the arms and legs. If any of these areas fail to function normally or if the brain fails to coordinate the many nerve impulses it receives, a person may feel dizzy. The feeling of dizziness varies from person to person and, to some extent, according to its cause; it can include a feeling of unsteadiness, imbalance, or even spinning.

Disease-related dizziness, whether it takes the form of unsteadiness or spinning, is fairly common in the older population. Today, both older and younger people with serious dizziness problems can be helped by a variety of techniques—from medication to surgery to balancing exercises. Such techniques have been developed and improved by scientists studying dizziness.

A DELICATE BALANCING ACT
To understand what goes wrong when we feel dizzy, we need to know about the vestibular system by which we keep a sense of balance amid all our daily twisting and turning, starting and stopping, jumping, falling, rolling, and bending.

The Vestibular System
The vestibular system is located in the inner ear and contains the following structures: vestibular labyrinth, semicircular canals, vestibule, utricle, and saccule. These structures work in tandem with the vestibular areas of the brain to help us maintain balance.

The vestibular labyrinth is located behind the eardrum. The labyrinth's most striking feature is a group of three semicircular canals, or tubes, that arise from a common base. At the base of the canals is a rounded chamber called the vestibule. The three canals and the vestibule are hollow and contain a fluid called endolymph, which moves in response to head movement.

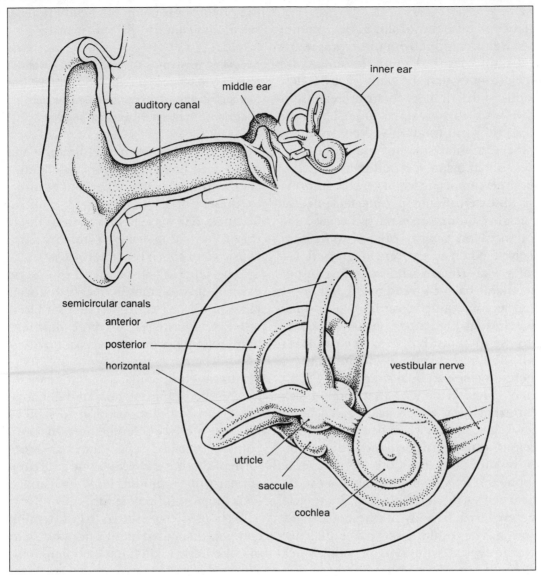

The semicircular canals and vestibule of the inner ear contain a fluid called endolymph that moves in response to head movement, triggering nerve signals to the brain that help maintain balance.

Within the vestibule and the semicircular canals are patches of special nerve cells called hair cells. Hair cells are also found in two fluid-filled sacs, the utricle and saccule, located within the vestibule. These cells are aptly named: rows of thin, flexible, hairlike fibers project from them into the endolymph.

Also located in the inner ear are tiny calcium stones called otoconia. When you move your head or stand up, the hair cells are bent by the weight of the otoconia or movement of the endolymph. The bending of the hair cells transmits an electrical signal about head movement to the brain. This signal travels from the inner ear to the brain along the eighth cranial nerve—the nerve involved in balance and hearing. The brain recognizes the signal as a particular movement of the head and is able to use this information to help maintain balance.

The Senses

The senses are also important in determining balance. Sensory input from the eyes as well as from the muscles and joints is sent to the brain, alerting us that the path we are following bends to the right or that our head is tilted as we bend to pick up a dime. The brain interprets this information—along with cues from the vestibular system—and adjusts the muscles so that balance is maintained.

Dizziness can occur when sensory information is distorted. Some people feel dizzy at great heights, for instance, partly because they cannot focus on nearby objects to stabilize themselves. When one is on the ground, it is normal to sway slightly while standing. A person maintains balance by adjusting the body's position to something close by. When someone is standing high up, objects are too far away to use to adjust balance. The result can be confusion, insecurity, and dizziness, which is sometimes resolved by sitting down.

Some scientists believe that motion sickness, a malady that affects sea, car, and even space travelers, occurs when the brain receives conflicting sensory information about the body's motion and position. For example, when someone reads while riding in a car, the inner ear senses the movement of the vehicle, but the eyes gaze steadily on the book that is not moving. The resulting sensory conflict may lead to the typical symptoms of motion sickness: dizziness, nausea, vomiting, and sweating.

Another form of dizziness occurs when we turn around in a circle quickly several times and then stop suddenly. Turning moves the endolymph. The moving endolymph tells us we are still rotating but our other senses say we've stopped. We feel dizzy.

DIAGNOSING THE PROBLEM

The dizziness one feels after spinning around in a circle usually goes away quickly and does not require a medical evaluation. But when symptoms appear to be caused by an underlying physical problem, the prudent person will see a physician for diagnostic tests.

According to a study supported by the National Institute of Neurological Disorders and Stroke (NINDS), a thorough examination can reveal the underlying cause of dizziness in about 90 percent of cases.

A person experiencing dizziness may first go to a general practitioner or family physician; between 5 and 10 percent of initial visits to these physicians involve a complaint of dizziness. The patient may then be referred either to an ear specialist (otologist) or a nervous system specialist (neurologist).

The patient will be asked to describe the exact nature of the dizziness, to give a complete history of its occurrence, and to list any other symptoms or medical problems. Patients give many descriptions of dizziness—depending to some extent on its cause. Common complaints are light-headedness, a feeling of impending faint, a hallucination of movement or motion, or a loss of balance without any strange feelings in the head. Some people also report they have vertigo—a form of dizziness in which one's surroundings appear to be spinning uncontrollably or one feels the sensation of spinning.

The physician will try to determine what components of a patient's nervous system are out of kilter, looking first for changes in blood pressure, heart rhythm, or vision. Sometimes dizziness is associated with an ear disorder. The patient may have loss of hearing, discomfort from loud sounds, or constant noise in the ear, a disorder known as tinnitus (see Hearing Loss and Aging, page 253). The physician will also look for other neurological symptoms: difficulty in swallowing or talking, for example, or double vision.

TESTS AND SCANS

After the initial history-taking and physical examination, the physician may deliberately try to make the patient feel dizzy. The patient may be asked to repeat actions or movements that generally cause dizziness: to walk in one direction and then turn quickly in the opposite direction, or to hyperventilate by breathing deeply for three minutes.

In another test, the patient sits upright on an examining table. The physician tilts the patient's head back and turns it partway to one side, then gently but quickly pushes the patient backward to a lying-down position.

The reaction to this procedure varies according to the cause of dizziness. Patients with benign positional vertigo may experience vertigo plus nystagmus: rapid, uncontrollable back-and-forth movements of the eyes.

Caloric test. One widely used procedure, called the caloric test, involves electronic monitoring of the patient's eye movements while one ear at a time is irrigated with warm water or warm air and then with cold water or cold air. This double stimulus causes the endolymph to move in a way similar to that produced by rotation of the head. If the labyrinth is working normally, nystagmus should result. A missing nystagmus reaction is a strong argument that the balance organs are not acting correctly.

NINDS-supported scientists at the Johns Hopkins University in Baltimore observed that not all patients can tolerate the traditional caloric test. Some become sick when the ear is irrigated with the standard amount of water or air before physicians can measure their eye movements. So the scientists are designing a method of conducting the test more gradually by slowly adjusting the amount of water or air reaching the inner ear. Their goal is to reduce patient discomfort while allowing the test to proceed.

Some patients who cannot tolerate the caloric test are given a rotatory test. In this procedure, the patient sits in a rotating chair, head tilted slightly forward. The chair spins rapidly in one direction, then stops abruptly. Depend-

ing on the cause of dizziness, the patient may experience vertigo after this rotation.

In one variation of this test, the chair is placed in a tent of striped cloth. As the chair rotates, electrodes record movements of the patient's eyes in response to the stripes. The physician evaluates these eye movements, a form of nystagmus, to determine if the patient has a disorder of the balance system.

Hearing test. Because disorders of balance are often accompanied by hearing loss, the physician may order a hearing test.

Brain-wave test. Hearing loss and associated dizziness could also be due to damaged nerve cells in the brainstem, where the hearing and balance nerve relays signals to the brain. To detect a malfunction, the physician may order a kind of computerized brain-wave study called a brainstem auditory evoked response test. In this procedure, electrodes are attached to several places on the surface of the patient's scalp and a sound is transmitted to the patient's ear. The electrodes then measure the time it takes the nerve signals generated by the sound to travel from the ear to the brainstem.

CT scan. If there is reason to suspect that the dizziness could stem from a tumor or cyst, the patient may undergo a computed tomography (CT) scan. In a CT scan, x-ray pictures are taken of the brain from several different angles. These images are then combined by a computer to give a detailed view that may reveal the damaging growth.

Psychological test. Sometimes anxiety and emotional upset cause a person to feel dizzy. Certain patients may be asked to take a psychological test, to try to find out whether the dizziness is caused or intensified by emotional stress.

The many tests administered by a physician will usually point to a cause for the patient's dizziness.

Disorders responsible for dizziness can be categorized as:

- *Peripheral vestibular disorders,* or those involving a disturbance in the labyrinth;
- *Central vestibular disorders,* or those resulting from a problem in the brain or its connecting nerves;
- *Systemic disorders,* or those originating in nerves or organs outside the head.

CONFUSED SIGNALS

When someone has vertigo but does not experience faintness or difficulty in walking, the cause is probably a peripheral vestibular disorder. In these conditions, nerve cells in the inner ear send confusing information about body movement to the brain.

Ménière's Disease

A well-known cause of vertigo is the peripheral vestibular disorder known as Ménière's disease. First identified in 1861 by Prosper Ménière, a French physician, the disease is thought to be caused by too much endolymph in the semicircular canals and vestibule. Some scientists think that the excess endolymph may affect the hair cells so that they do not work correctly. This explanation, however, is still under study.

The vertigo of Ménière's disease comes and goes without an apparent cause; it may be made worse by a change in position and reduced by being still.

In addition to vertigo, patients have hearing loss and tinnitus. Hearing loss is usually restricted at first to one ear and is often severe. Patients sometimes feel "fullness" or discomfort in the ear, and diagnostic testing may show unusual sensitivity to increasingly loud sounds. In 10 to 20 percent of patients, hearing loss and tinnitus eventually occur in the second ear.

Ménière's disease patients may undergo electronystagmography, an electrical recording of the caloric test, to determine if their labyrinth is working normally.

Attacks of Ménière's disease may occur several times a month or year and last from a few minutes to many hours. Some patients experience a spontaneous disappearance of symptoms while others may have attacks for years.

Treatment of Ménière's disease includes such drugs as meclizine hydrochloride and the tranquilizer diazepam to reduce the feeling of intense motion during vertigo. To control the buildup of endolymph, the patient may also take a diuretic, a drug that reduces fluid production. A low-salt diet—which reduces water retention—is claimed to be an effective treatment of Ménière's disease.

When these measures fail to help, surgery may be considered. In shunt surgery, part of the inner ear is drained to reestablish normal inner ear fluid or endolymph pressure. In another operation, called vestibular nerve section, surgeons expose and cut the vestibular part of the eighth nerve. Both vestibular nerve section and shunt surgery commonly relieve the dizziness of Ménière's disease without affecting hearing.

A more drastic operation, labyrinthectomy, involves total destruction of the inner ear. This procedure is usually successful in eliminating dizziness but causes total loss of hearing in the operated ear—an important consideration since the second ear may one day be affected.

Positional Vertigo

People with benign positional vertigo experience vertigo after a position change. One patient, named Barbara, noticed the first sign of this disorder one morning when she got up out of bed. She felt the room spinning. Frightened, she quickly returned to bed and lay down. After about 30 seconds the vertigo passed. Fearing a stroke, Barbara went to the emergency room of a hospital for a medical evaluation, which failed to show a problem. She had no symptoms for several days, then the problem returned. At this point, Barbara was referred to an otoneurologist, a physician who specializes in the ear and related parts of the nervous system.

Like Barbara, most patients with benign positional vertigo are extremely worried about their symptoms. But the patients usually feel less threatened once the disorder is diagnosed.

The cause of benign positional vertigo is not known, although some patients may recall an incident of head injury. The condition can strike at any adult age with attacks occurring periodically throughout a person's life.

In one type of treatment, the patient practices the position that provokes dizziness until the balance system eventually adapts. Rarely, a physician will prescribe medication to prevent attacks.

Vestibular Neuronitis

In this common vestibular disorder, the patient has severe vertigo. Jack experienced his first attack of this problem at 2 a.m. when he rolled over in bed and suddenly felt the room spinning violently. He started vomiting but couldn't stand up; finally, he managed to crawl to the bathroom. When he returned to bed, he lay very still—the only way to stop the vertigo. Three days later, he was able to walk without experiencing vertigo, but he still felt unsteady. Gradually, over the next several weeks, Jack's balance improved, but it was a year before he was entirely without symptoms.

Unlike Ménière's disease, vestibular neuronitis is not associated with hearing loss. Patients with vestibular neuronitis first experience an acute attack of severe vertigo lasting for hours or days, just as Jack did, with loss of balance sometimes lasting for weeks or months. About half of those who have a single attack have further episodes over a period of months to years.

The cause of vestibular neuronitis is uncertain. Since the first attack often occurs after a viral illness, some scientists believe the disorder is caused by a viral infection of the nerve.

Other Labyrinth Problems

Inner ear problems with resulting dizziness can also be caused by certain antibiotics used to fight life-threatening bacterial infections. Probably the best-known agent of this group is streptomycin. Problems usually arise when high doses of these drugs are taken for a long time, but some patients experience symptoms after short treatment with low doses, especially if they have impaired kidneys.

The first symptoms of damage to the inner ear caused by medication are usually hearing loss, tinnitus, or unsteadiness while walking. Stopping the antibiotic can usually halt further damage to the balance mechanism, but this is not always possible: The medicine may have to be continued to treat a life-threatening infection. Patients sometimes adapt to the inner ear damage that may occur after prolonged use of these antibiotics and recover their balance.

Balance can also be affected by a cholesteatoma, a clump of cells from the eardrum that grow into the middle ear and accumulate there. These growths are thought to result from repeated infections such as recurrent otitis media. If unchecked, a cholesteatoma can enlarge and threaten the inner ear. But if the growth is detected early, it can be surgically removed.

BRAIN AND NERVE DAMAGE

The vestibular nerve carries signals from the inner ear to the brainstem. If either the nerve or the brainstem is damaged, information about position and movement may be blocked or incorrectly processed, leading to dizziness.

Conditions in which dizziness results from damage to the brainstem or its associated nerves are referred to as "central causes of dizziness."

Acoustic Neuroma

One central cause of dizziness is a tumor called an acoustic neuroma. Although the most common sign of this growth is hearing loss followed by tinnitus, some patients also experience dizziness.

An acoustic neuroma usually occurs in the internal auditory canal, the bony channel through which the vestibular nerve passes as it leaves the inner ear. The growing tumor may press on the nerve, sending false messages about position and movement to the brain.

The hearing nerve running alongside the vestibular nerve can also be compressed by the acoustic neuroma, with resulting tinnitus and hearing loss. Or the tumor may press on other nearby nerves, producing numbness or weakness of the face. If the neuroma is allowed to grow, it will eventually reach the brain and may affect the function of other cranial nerves.

Computed tomography has revolutionized the detection of acoustic neuromas. If an early diagnosis is made, a surgeon can remove the tumor. The patient usually regains balance.

Stroke

Dizziness may be a sign of a "small stroke" or transient ischemic attack (TIA) in the brainstem. TIAs, which result from a temporary lack of blood supply to the brain, may also cause transient numbness, tingling, or weakness in a limb or on one side of the face. Other signs include temporary blindness and difficulty with speech. These symptoms are warning signs: One should see a physician immediately for treatment. If a TIA is ignored, a major stroke may follow.

SYSTEMIC DISEASES: UNDERLYING ILLNESS

Dizziness can be a symptom of diseases affecting body parts other than the brain and central nervous system. Systemic conditions like anemia or high blood pressure decrease oxygen supplies to the brain; a physician eliminates the resulting dizziness by treating the underlying systemic illness.

Damaged Sensory Nerves

We maintain balance by adjusting to information transmitted along sensory nerves from sensors in the eyes, muscles, and joints to the spinal cord or brain. When these sensory nerves are damaged by systemic disease, dizziness may result.

Multiple sensory deficits, a systemic disease, is believed by some physicians to be the chief cause of vaguely described dizziness in the aged population. In this disorder, several senses or sensory nerves are damaged. The result: faulty balance.

People with diabetes, which can damage nerves affecting vision and touch, may develop multiple sensory deficits. So can patients with arthritis or cataracts, both of which distort how sensory information reaches the brain.

The first step in treating multiple sensory deficits is to eliminate symptoms of specific disorders. Permanent contact lenses can improve vision in cataract patients, for example, and medication or surgery may ease pain and stiffness related to arthritis.

Symptoms of damaged sensory nerves may be relieved by a collar to eliminate extreme head motion, balancing exercises to help compensate for sensory losses, or a cane to aid balance. Some patients are helped by the drug methylphenidate, which can increase awareness of remaining sensations.

Systemic neurological disorders such as multiple sclerosis, Alzheimer's disease, Parkinson's disease, or Creutzfeldt-Jakob disease may also cause dizziness, primarily during walking. However, dizziness is rarely the sole symptom of these nervous system diseases.

Low Blood Pressure

One common systemic disease causing dizziness is postural or orthostatic hypotension. In this disease, the heart does not move the blood with enough force to supply the brain adequately.

Symptoms include sudden feelings of faintness, light-headedness, or dizziness when standing up quickly.

Because the muscles in aging blood vessels

are weak and the arteries inadequate in helping convey blood to the head, older people are particularly susceptible to this condition. Older persons who do not sit or lie down at the first sensation of dizziness may actually lose consciousness.

People who have undetected anemia or those who are taking diuretics to eliminate excess water from their body and reduce high blood pressure are also at risk of developing postural hypotension.

A physician can easily diagnose postural hypotension: The patient's blood pressure is measured before standing abruptly and immediately afterward. Treatment is designed to eliminate dizziness by reducing the patient's blood volume.

A Secondary Symptom

Dizziness may also be a secondary symptom in many other diseases. Faintness accompanied by occasional loss of consciousness can be due to low blood sugar, especially when the faint feeling persists after the patient lies down.

A common cause of mild dizziness—the kind described as light-headedness—is medicine. A number of major prescription drugs may produce light-headedness as a side effect.

Two types of drugs that can cause this problem are sedatives, which are taken to induce sleep, and tranquilizers, which are used to calm anxiety.

WHEN ANXIETY STRIKES

Tranquilizers may cause a type of dizziness referred to as light-headedness—but so may anxiety. Cynthia becomes light-headed under a variety of stressful circumstances. The light-headedness sometimes is accompanied by heart palpitations and panic. She can produce these symptoms at will by breathing rapidly and deeply for a few minutes.

Cynthia's light-headedness is due to hyper-ventilation: rapid, prolonged deep breathing or occasional deep sighing that upsets the oxygen and carbon dioxide balance in the blood. The episodes are typically brief and often associated with tingling and numbness in the fingers and around the mouth. Hyper-ventilation is triggered by anxiety or depression in about 60 percent of dizziness patients.

Once made aware of the source of the symptoms, a patient can avoid hyperventilation or abort attacks by breath-holding or breathing into a paper bag to restore a correct balance of oxygen and carbon dioxide. If hyperventilation is due to anxiety, psychological counseling may be recommended.

Some patients who report dizziness may be suffering from a psychiatric disorder. Generally these persons will say that they experience light-headedness or difficulty concentrating; they may also describe panic states when in crowded places. Tests of such patients reveal that the inner ear is working correctly. Treatment may include counseling.

The National Institute of
Neurological Disorders and Stroke

EPILEPSY

Convulsion, seizure, fit, falling sickness—the English language is rich in words that capture the stark drama of a severe epileptic attack. There are many forms of epilepsy, each with characteristic signs and symptoms.

FORMS OF EPILEPSY

The victim cries out, falls to the floor unconscious, the limbs twitch, saliva bubbles at the mouth. Bladder control may be lost. Within minutes the attack is over. The victim comes to, exhausted, dazed, embarrassed. That is the picture most people have in mind when they hear the word "epilepsy." But that type of seizure—the grand mal attack—is only one form of epilepsy.

Take Lisa, for example. She is an intelligent 15-year-old high school student with long dark hair and lashes to match. Lisa has suffered from absence seizures (sometimes called petit mal epilepsy) for some time. In an absence seizure, there is a momentary lapse in consciousness. Lisa is briefly "out of it." But there is no dramatic fall. Sometimes there may be purposeless movements—an arm jerk, for example—but in Lisa's case there is no noticeable symptom, not even the blink of an eye. Immediately following the seizure, Lisa can resume whatever she was doing. But her attacks happen so often—several hundred times a day—that she cannot concentrate in school and is in danger of failing her sophomore year. Moreover, she is so frightened and ashamed of the attacks that she won't tell her friends what is wrong.

In still a third form of the disorder, commonly called psychomotor epilepsy, the patient may laugh, talk strangely, walk around in circles, or make other automatic movements like lip-smacking or chewing. On rare occasions, the victim may strike out at walls or furniture as though angry or afraid. These attacks are also brief. Upon recovery, the individual will be confused and have no memory of what happened.

The strange symptoms and sometimes bizarre behavior of patients with epilepsy have contributed to age-old superstitions and prejudice. As long ago as 400 B.C., Hippocrates repeated the popular folklore that epilepsy was a visitation of the gods—a "sacred disease." He had the wisdom to question folklore, however. Hippocrates suspected that epilepsy was a disorder of the brain. And he was right.

Causes and Effects

Nowadays, scientists know that epilepsy is not a disease with a single cause. Rather, it is a set of symptoms associated with abnormal nerve cell activity in the brain.

Normally, each nerve cell (neuron) generates small bursts of electrical impulses. The impulses, moving from neuron to neuron, and communicating with the body's muscles, sense organs, and glands, underlie all human behavior—our thoughts, feelings, actions. The pattern of activity has been likened to tiny flashes of light flicking on and off in the brain, weaving a constantly changing pattern on an "enchanted loom."

In epilepsy the pattern of nerve cell activity is disturbed. Instead of small bursts of electrical impulses, a group of nerve cells fires a storm of strong bursts like a platoon of soldiers all firing at once. Moreover, the firing comes with machine-gun rapidity.

Whereas normal nerve cells generate electrical impulses up to 80 times a second, an epileptic neuron can fire impulses at rates of 500 times a second, disturbing the normal activity of the brain. If the abnormal activity is confined to only a part of the brain, the seizure is described as partial, and the area of the brain involved is called the epileptic focus. Partial seizures sometimes affect the temporal lobes at the sides of the brain near the ears. Nerve centers there are associated with speech and hearing and with emotions and memory. Disturbances in this part of the brain can account for the odd movements (automatisms) and behavior of psychomotor seizures.

In contrast, generalized seizures affect the whole brain, resulting in the unconsciousness, convulsions, and subsequent amnesia of a grand mal seizure. Similarly, seizures in absence epilepsy are generalized, with lapses of consciousness and occasional automatisms, but without convulsions. Sometimes what begins as a partial seizure can develop into a generalized seizure if the abnormal cell behavior spreads throughout the brain.

Classifications

The epilepsies are classified into subtypes within the broad categories of partial and generalized seizures. These divisions, and the more accurate descriptive terms neurologists prefer—"generalized tonic-clonic seizure" instead of grand mal; "absence" instead of petit mal; "complex partial seizure" instead of psychomotor seizure—mark important advances in understanding and controlling epilepsy. The more precise classifications of seizures enable physicians to devise better treatments. The good news is that seizures can be successfully controlled in over half the patients with epilepsy through daily medication with antiepileptic drugs.

History

The story of the ongoing conquest of epilepsy is closely bound up with the history of neurology. Epilepsy is the second most prevalent neurological disorder in the United States (following stroke). Over 2 million Americans have epilepsy: one out of 100 persons.

A century ago conditions were far worse. There were few treatments, and epileptic patients were regarded as undesirables whose condition might be contagious.

Many patients were placed in hospitals or institutions "for epileptics only." Faced with the challenge of so many suffering souls, pioneering neurologists of the nineteenth century turned their attention to the disorder and began the search for causes and cures that continues in the present.

DIAGNOSING EPILEPSY

Two steps are vital in screening and treating patients with suspected epilepsy. One, obvious but nontrivial, is a confirmation of the diagnosis. The second is a precise description of the pattern of seizures: their type or types, frequency, and duration.

Sometimes a child has a convulsion during the course of illness with high fever. Sometimes an adult has a seizure in reaction to anesthesia or a strong drug. Neither individual can

---

INTERNATIONAL CLASSIFICATION OF EPILEPTIC SEIZURES

Generalized Seizures
- **Tonic-clonic (grand mal)**
- **Absence (petit mal)**
- **Infantile spasms**
- **Other (myoclonic seizures, akinetic seizures, undetermined, etc.)**

Partial Seizures
- **Simple partial seizures (e.g., disturbances in movement only)**
- **Complex partial seizures (psychomotor, other)**
- **Secondarily generalized seizures**

---

be said to have epilepsy unless seizures recur in the absence of the original triggering event.

Sometimes patients with certain forms of mental illness show behavior that mimics a complex partial seizure. Other individuals with psychological problems may suffer seizures, even what appear to be generalized tonic-clonic attacks, but their brain cells show no abnormal activity. These "psychogenic" seizures indicate that the patient has serious problems such as the need for attention, dependency, or the avoidance of stress, but the condition is not epilepsy.

In making a diagnosis of epilepsy, physicians are guided by some general rules of thumb. Three-fourths of all patients with epilepsy have their first attacks before the age of 18. Usually a parent will bring a child to the family doctor and describe the symptoms, helpfully noting when seizures occur and how long they last. While this information is enormously useful, the most secure confirmation of the diagnosis can come only from observation of a seizure together with electrical recordings that show the abnormal brain cell activity. These recordings are the familiar wavy line tracings of the electroencephalogram (EEG) obtained from electrodes placed on the surface of the patient's head.

Many cases of epilepsy develop for no known reason. Sometimes the disorder runs in families, as in absence epilepsy, which always has its onset in children or young people. On the whole, however, genetic factors are considered to play a secondary role, as contributing or predisposing factors to epilepsy rather than a primary cause. Epilepsy can occur as a complication of infection, head injury, or other conditions affecting the brain. Epilepsy may also be associated with cerebral palsy, mental retardation, or rarer neurological conditions such as tuberous sclerosis. For these reasons the examining physician will always make an exhaustive search for underlying causes.

A CT scan—a computerized x-ray image of the brain—may show up a tumor or cyst, for example, or reveal excess fluid in the brain— hydrocephalus. If these conditions can be treated successfully, the seizures may stop. A lumbar puncture, in which cerebrospinal fluid is withdrawn from the spinal cord, may reveal the presence of infection or other abnormalities. In any case, a thorough medical history of the patient, including details of birth and the health of other family members, will be taken, and a battery of physical, mental, and neurological tests will be conducted.

The Unique Pattern

Every epileptic patient is unique in the symptoms, frequency, duration, and type (or types) of seizures he or she experiences. It is essential to describe the seizure pattern in detail because it is on that basis that the physician will determine treatment. Drugs used to treat epilepsy are selected according to the type of seizure the patient experiences. Other forms of treatment, such as surgery, may be appropriate for carefully selected patients with particular forms of epilepsy.

Some patients, particularly ones with complex partial seizures, experience a distinctive warning sign before a seizure, called an aura. The aura is itself a form of partial seizure, but

one in which the patient retains awareness. Sometimes the warning sign may be a peculiar odor, a feeling in the pit of the stomach, or a sound. One neurologist describes a patient who was an ardent racetrack gambler. The man invariably heard the roar of the crowd followed by the name of the favorite in the race just before falling unconscious. Another patient heard rock music. Because patients retain consciousness during the aura, they occasionally may be able to learn methods of warding off the more severe attack.

Drugs are the answer for the majority of patients whose seizures can be controlled. The sizable gains that have been made in recent years can be chalked up to the availability of more and better drugs administered in doses suited to the individual patient.

Taking the Seizure's Measure

In 1966, the National Institute of Neurological Disorders and Stroke (NINDS) began a research program of intensive long-term EEG monitoring of epilepsy patients. Electrodes placed on the patient's head transmit brain wave data to nearby recording equipment. At the same time a television camera provides both full-length and head views of the patient as he or she sits, lies, eats, or sleeps over the course of the day. The video image is displayed on a screen along with the brain wave recordings so that observers can simultaneously compare the EEG tracings with the patient's behavior. The recording sessions are six hours long and continue daily over a period of months.

Intensive monitoring has led to an extensive library of invaluable data on epilepsy and has paid off for many a patient whose seizures had been impossible to control. Often such patients experience seizures that are difficult to classify—a complex partial seizure that looks like an absence spell, for example, or vice versa. Interestingly, in some patients intensive monitoring shows up occasional abnormalities in the EEG between seizures. The technique also reveals that many epileptic patients experience psychogenic seizures some of the time. Sometimes, too, the EEG shows an epileptiform pattern but the patient shows no outward signs of a seizure.

Refinements in technology have made it possible to free the patient from the hospital setting and still conduct long-term EEG monitoring. The brain wave signals are detected by electrodes fitted into headgear that the patient wears. The signals are then amplified and converted to electronic signals stored on a tape recorder cassette that the patient also wears while moving about at home or work. Automated analysis of EEG data is also an improvement in technology, allowing reliable data to be derived from the recordings without an observer having to study the tapes hour after hour.

TREATMENT

Knowledge of the types of seizures a patient suffers paves the way for effective treatment.

Drugs

There are now 16 antiepileptic drugs on the market. Some work on several different types of seizure. Others, especially some of the new drugs, are suited to specific types of epilepsy.

The history of drugs in the treatment of epilepsy is a spotty one. The first effective antiepileptic drugs were bromides, introduced by an astute English physician, Sir Charles Locock, in 1857. He noted that the bromides had a sedative effect and seemed to reduce seizures in some patients. Over 50 years later came phenobarbital, introduced as a sedative in 1912. Phenobarbital and related compounds quickly proved superior to the bromides in controlling seizures, and side effects were less severe. Surprisingly, these early drugs were useful in treating the most severe form of epilepsy—grand mal—as well as partial seizures. They had no effect on absence epilepsy.

The next advances waited until the 1930s and 1940s, when the pharmaceutical industry began to grow rapidly and scientists developed ways of testing the anticonvulsant properties of drugs in experimental animals. Phenytoin (Dilantin) was introduced in 1938 and remains a drug of major importance in treating grand mal and partial seizures. Other drugs were introduced in the fifties and sixties, but by the late sixties and seventies there was a marked decline in new drug research. Amendments to the food and drug laws in 1962 required that new drugs had to be proven to be effective as well as safe. The new rules plus the opinion that the market for new antiepileptic drugs was too small to warrant the investment in time or money discouraged antiepileptic drug research as a commercial enterprise.

Tailoring the Dosage

Even when the neurologist is armed with an accurate picture of a patient's seizures, the drugs prescribed may not work. The seizures may be too varied and too frequent; the drugs may simply not help particular individuals; or side effects may be too toxic. Sometimes the problem is one of dosage, however, or of finding the right combination of drugs administered in the right proportion at the right time of day. For these reasons, patients with intractable seizures who undergo long-term EEG monitoring also have frequent blood samples taken to measure the amount of drug circulating in the bloodstream. At the beginning of the study, a patient may be weaned off all medication. Then drugs may be introduced gradually, increasing the amounts or changing the medication to arrive at the ideal treatment: dosages sufficient to control seizures with a minimum of side effects. Similar studies to devise the best medication program are highly recommended for all epilepsy patients.

Surgery

Surgery to remove an epileptic focus in the brain is sometimes successful in preventing seizures in patients whose epilepsy cannot be controlled by medications. In deciding which patients may benefit, surgeons will consider the location of the brain area involved and its importance in everyday behavior. Neurosurgeons will avoid operating in areas of the brain that will interfere with speech, language, hearing, or other major faculties.

Occasionally, surgery is performed to sever the connections between the two halves of the brain, the cerebral hemispheres. Such surgery can prevent the spread of abnormal discharges from one side of the brain to the other. Usually, such drastic surgery has little effect on behavior. Patients go about their normal activities as usual. It was only when research scientists began to set up experiments that deliberately studied what each half of the brain contributed to behavior that they discovered that the hemispheres were not like Siamese twins, identical in every way. While there is considerable similarity in structure, each hemisphere has special abilities and makes its own contribution to how a person sees, feels, or acts in the world. This is another instance of how concern for epilepsy has opened the door to new and fascinating discoveries about the nervous system.

Diet
In addition to drugs and surgery, treatment for epilepsy has also included special diets and new psychological approaches. Some years ago it was discovered that a diet rich in fats and low in carbohydrates led to a condition in the body called ketosis that benefits some epilepsy patients. Unfortunately, most people hate the diet. It makes them feel sick and they lose weight.

Biofeedback
One psychological approach to treating epilepsy involves training patients in methods that might allow them to control their brain waves. In the experimental technique called biofeedback, patients learn to correlate brain cell activity with visual images or sounds that are provided. They try to modify the sights or sounds and in this way alter the electrical activity in the brain. Biofeedback appears to help some patients, but how or why it does so remain tantalizing questions.

Recognizing the Patient's Multiple Needs
Sometimes people with epilepsy achieve complete control of seizures in the hospital only to have frequent seizures when they return home. The problem may be failure to take medication. Anticonvulsant medications are strong and can have unwanted side effects such as drowsiness, nausea, or other unpleasantness. One anticonvulsant drug has a tendency to increase appetite. Many patients gain weight when taking it—enough to discourage use of the drug.

When a patient is at home, there are other factors that may increase the chances of having seizures. The normal pressures of everyday living may create stresses that can trigger seizures. On the other hand, the patient who cannot drive a car or suffers occasional seizures at work may feel rejected, depressed, angry, or frustrated—often a combination of emotional states that can lower the threshold for seizures.

Recent findings about patients monitored at home point up the relations between mental states and seizure activity. In one study it was noted that patients with absence seizures tended to have more seizures at times when they were bored or idle, not when they were fully occupied or interested in some activity. Seizure activity also tended to increase during family discussions of their problem, or even when donning the headgear and cassette and thus being reminded of their condition.

Doctors and others who work closely with patients know that the problems the individual with epilepsy faces do not end with medication. The psychological, social, vocational, and emotional needs of patients—and those close to them—are equally important.

The National Institute of
Neurological Disorders and Stroke

PARKINSON'S DISEASE

Parkinson's disease may be one of the most baffling and complex of the neurological disorders. Its cause remains a mystery, but research in this area is active, with new and intriguing findings constantly being reported.

Parkinson's disease was first described in 1817 by James Parkinson, a British physician who published a paper on what he called "the shaking palsy." In this paper, he set forth the major symptoms of the disease that would later bear his name. For the next century and a half, scientists pursued the causes and treatment of the disease. They defined its range of symptoms, distribution among the population, and prospects for cure.

In the early 1960s, researchers identified a fundamental brain defect that is a hallmark of the disease: the loss of brain cells that produce a chemical—dopamine—that helps direct muscle activity. This discovery pointed to the first successful treatment for Parkinson's disease and suggested ways of devising new and even more effective therapies.

Society pays an enormous price for Parkinson's disease. According to the National Parkinson Foundation, each patient spends an average of $2,500 a year for medications. After factoring in office visits, Social Security payments, nursing home expenditures, and lost income, the total cost to the nation is estimated to exceed $5.6 billion annually.

WHAT IS PARKINSON'S DISEASE?

Parkinson's disease belongs to a group of conditions called motor system disorders. The four primary symptoms are tremor or trembling in the hands, arms, legs, jaw, and face; rigidity or stiffness of the limbs and trunk; bradykinesia or slowness of movement; and postural instability or impaired balance and coordination. As these symptoms become

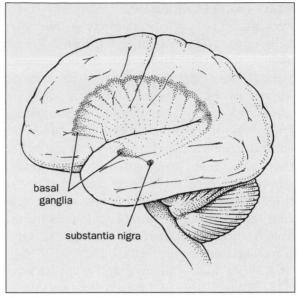

The loss of nerve cells from the brain's substantia nigra region is thought to be responsible for the symptoms of parkinsonism.

more pronounced, patients may have difficulty walking, talking, or completing other simple tasks.

The disease is both chronic, meaning it persists over a long period of time, and progressive, meaning its symptoms grow worse over time. It is not contagious nor is it usually inherited—that is, it does not pass directly from one family member or generation to the next.

Parkinson's disease is the most common form of parkinsonism, the name for a group of disorders with similar features (see Other Forms of Parkinsonism, page 187). These disorders share the four primary symptoms described above, and all are the result of the loss of dopamine-producing brain cells. Parkinson's disease is also called primary parkinsonism or idiopathic Parkinson's disease; "idiopathic" is a term describing a disorder for which no cause has yet been found. In the other forms of parkinsonism, either the cause is known or suspected, or the disorder occurs as a secondary effect of another, primary neurological disorder.

WHAT CAUSES THE DISEASE?

Parkinson's disease occurs when certain nerve cells, or neurons, in an area of the brain known as the substantia nigra die or become impaired. Normally, these neurons produce an important brain chemical known as dopamine. Dopamine is a chemical messenger responsible for transmitting signals between the substantia nigra and the next "relay station" of the brain, the corpus striatum, to produce smooth, purposeful muscle activity. Loss of dopamine causes the nerve cells of the striatum to fire out of control, leaving patients unable to direct or control their movements in a normal manner.

Studies have shown that Parkinson's patients have a loss of 80 percent or more of dopamine-producing cells in the substantia nigra. The cause of this cell death or impairment is not known, but significant findings by research scientists continue to yield fascinating new clues to the disease. One theory holds that free radicals—unstable and potentially damaging molecules generated by normal chemical reactions in the body—may contribute to nerve cell death, thereby leading to Parkinson's disease.

Free radicals are unstable because they lack one electron; in an attempt to replace this missing electron, free radicals react with neighboring molecules (especially metals such as iron), in a process called oxidation. Oxidation is thought to cause damage to tissues, including neurons.

Normally, free radical damage is kept under control by antioxidant chemicals that protect cells from this damage. Evidence that oxidative mechanisms may cause or contribute to Parkinson's disease includes the finding that patients with the disease have increased brain levels of iron, especially in the substantia nigra, and decreased levels of ferritin, which serves as a protective mechanism by chelating, or forming a ring around the iron, and isolating it.

Some scientists have suggested that Parkinson's disease may occur when either an external or an internal toxin selectively destroys dopaminergic neurons. An environmental risk factor such as exposure to pesticides or a toxin in the food supply is an example of the kind of external trigger that could hypothetically cause Parkinson's disease. The theory is based on the fact that there are a number of toxins, such as 1-methyl-4-phenyl-1,2,3,6-tetrahydropyridine (MPTP) and neuroleptic drugs, known to induce parkinsonian symptoms in humans. So far, however, no research has provided conclusive proof that a toxin is the cause.

A relatively new theory explores the role of genetic factors in the development of Parkinson's disease. Fifteen to twenty percent of Parkinson's patients have a close relative who has experienced parkinsonian symptoms (such as a tremor). After studies in animals showed that MPTP interferes with the function of mitochondria within nerve cells, investigators became interested in the possibility that impairment in mitochondrial DNA may be the cause of Parkinson's disease. Mitochondria are essential organelles found in all animal cells that convert the energy in food into fuel for the cells.

Yet another theory proposes that Parkinson's disease occurs when, for unknown reasons, the normal, age-related wearing away of dopamine-producing neurons accelerates in certain individuals. This theory is supported by the knowledge that loss of antioxidative protective mechanisms is associated with both Parkinson's disease and increasing age.

Many researchers believe that a combination of these four mechanisms—oxidative damage, environmental toxins, genetic predisposition, and accelerated aging—may ultimately be shown to cause the disease.

WHO GETS PARKINSON'S DISEASE?

About 50,000 Americans are diagnosed with Parkinson's disease each year, with more than half a million Americans affected at any one time. Getting an accurate count of the number of cases may be impossible however, because many people in the early stages of the disease assume their symptoms are the result of normal aging and do not seek help from a physician. Also, diagnosis is sometimes difficult and uncertain because other conditions may produce some of the symptoms of Parkinson's disease. People with Parkinson's disease may be told by their doctors that they have other disorders or, conversely, people with similar diseases may be initially diagnosed as having Parkinson's disease.

Parkinson's disease strikes men and women in almost equal numbers and it knows no social, economic, or geographic boundaries. Some studies show that African Americans and Asians are less likely than whites to develop Parkinson's disease. Scientists have not been able to explain this apparent lower incidence in certain populations.

Age, however, clearly correlates with the onset of symptoms. Parkinson's disease is a disease of late middle age, usually affecting people over age 50.

The average age of onset is 60 years. However, some physicians have reportedly noticed more cases of "early-onset" Parkinson's disease in the past several years, and some have estimated that 5 to 10 percent of patients are under the age of 40.

EARLY SYMPTOMS

Early symptoms of Parkinson's disease are subtle and occur gradually. Patients may be tired or notice a general malaise. Some may feel a little shaky or have difficulty getting out of a chair. They may notice that they speak too softly or that their handwriting looks cramped and spidery. They may lose track of a word or thought, or they may feel irritable or depressed for no apparent reason. This very early period may last a long time before the more classic and obvious symptoms appear.

Friends or family members may be the first to notice changes. They may see that the person's face lacks expression and animation (known as "masked face") or that the person remains in a certain position for a long time or does not move an arm or leg normally. Perhaps they see that the person seems stiff, unsteady, and unusually slow.

As the disease progresses, the shaking or tremor that affects the majority of Parkinson's patients may begin to interfere with daily activities. Patients may not be able to hold utensils steady or may find that the shaking makes reading a newspaper difficult. Parkinson's tremor may become worse when the patient is relaxed. A few seconds after the hands are rested on a table, for instance, the shaking is most pronounced. For most patients, tremor is usually the symptom that causes them to seek medical help.

MAJOR SYMPTOMS OF THE DISEASE

Parkinson's disease does not affect everyone the same way. In some people the disease progresses quickly; in others it does not. Although some people become severely disabled, others experience only minor motor disruptions. Tremor is the major symptom for some patients; for others tremor is only a minor complaint.

Tremor. The tremor associated with Parkinson's disease has a characteristic appearance. Typically, the tremor takes the form of a rhythmic back-and-forth motion of the thumb and forefinger at three to six beats per second. This is sometimes called "pill rolling." Tremor usually begins in a hand, although sometimes a foot or the jaw is affected first. It is most obvious when the hand is at rest or when a person is under stress. In three out of four patients, the tremor may affect only one part or side of the body, especially during the early stages of the disease. Later it may become more general. Tremor is rarely disabling and it usually disappears during sleep or improves with intentional movement.

Rigidity. Rigidity, or a resistance to movement, affects most parkinsonian patients. A major principle of body movement is that all muscles have an opposing muscle. Movement is possible not just because one muscle becomes more active, but because the opposing muscle relaxes. In Parkinson's disease, rigidity comes about when, in response to signals from the brain, the delicate balance of opposing muscles is disturbed. The muscles remain constantly tensed and contracted so that the person aches or feels stiff or weak. The rigidity becomes obvious when another person tries to move the patient's arm, which will move only in ratchetlike or short, jerky movements known as "cogwheel" rigidity.

Bradykinesia. Bradykinesia, or the slowing down and loss of spontaneous and automatic movement, is particularly frustrating because it is unpredictable. One moment the patient can move easily. The next moment he or she may need help. This may well be the most disabling and distressing symptom of the disease because the patient cannot rapidly perform routine movements. Activities once performed quickly and easily—such as washing or dressing—may take several hours.

Postural instability. Postural instability, or impaired balance and coordination, causes patients to develop a forward or backward lean and to fall easily. When bumped from the front or when starting to walk, patients with a backward lean have a tendency to step backwards, which is known as retropulsion. Postural instability can cause patients to have a stooped posture in which the head is bowed and the shoulders are drooped. As the disease progresses, walking may be affected. Patients may halt in mid-stride and "freeze" in place, possibly even toppling over. Or patients may walk with a series of quick, small steps as if hurrying forward to keep balance. This is known as festination.

OTHER SYMPTOMS

Various other symptoms accompany Parkinson's disease; some are minor, others are more bothersome. Many can be treated with appropriate medication or physical therapy. No one can predict which symptoms will affect an individual patient, and the intensity of the symptoms also varies from person to person. None of these symptoms is fatal, although swallowing problems can cause choking.

Depression. This is a common problem and may appear early in the course of the disease, even before other symptoms are noticed. Depression may not be severe, but it may be intensified by the drugs used to treat other symptoms of Parkinson's disease. Fortunately, depression can be successfully treated with antidepressant medications.

Emotional changes. Some people with Parkinson's disease become fearful and insecure. Perhaps they fear they cannot cope with new situations. They may not want to travel, go to parties, or socialize with friends. Some lose their motivation and become dependent on family members. Others may become irritable or uncharacteristically pessimistic. Memory loss and slow thinking may occur, although the ability to reason remains intact.

People with Parkinson's disease suffer from dementia. The exact incidence of dementia in Parkinson's patients is controversial, but a conservative estimate is that at least 15 percent of patients with Parkinson's disease will become demented.

Difficulty in swallowing and chewing. Muscles used in swallowing may work less efficiently in later stages of the disease. In these cases, food and saliva may collect in the mouth and back of the throat, which can result in choking or drooling. Medications can often alleviate these problems.

Speech changes. About half of all parkinsonian patients have problems with speech. They may speak too softly or in a monotone, hesitate before speaking, slur or repeat their words, or speak too fast. A speech therapist may be able to help patients reduce some of these problems.

Urinary problems or constipation. In some patients, bladder and bowel problems can occur due to the improper functioning of the autonomic nervous system, which is responsible for regulating smooth muscle activity. Some people may become incontinent while others have trouble urinating. In others, constipation may occur because the intestinal tract operates more slowly. Constipation can also be caused by inactivity, eating a poor diet, or drinking too little fluid. It can be a persistent problem and, in rare cases, can be serious enough to require hospitalization. Patients should not let constipation last for more than several days before taking steps to alleviate it.

Skin problems. In Parkinson's disease, it is common for the skin on the face to become very oily, particularly on the forehead and at the sides of the nose. The scalp may become oily too, resulting in dandruff. In other cases, the skin can become very dry. These problems are also the result of an improperly functioning autonomic nervous system. Standard treatments for skin problems help. Excessive sweating, another common symptom, is usually controllable with medications used for Parkinson's disease.

Sleep problems. These include difficulty staying asleep at night, restless sleep, nightmares and emotional dreams, and drowsiness during the day. It is unclear if these symptoms are related to the disease or to the medications used to treat Parkinson's disease. Patients should never take over-the-counter sleep aids without consulting their physicians.

OTHER FORMS OF PARKINSONISM

Postencephalitic parkinsonism. Just after the First World War, a viral disease, encephalitis lethargica, attacked almost 5 million people throughout the world, and then suddenly disappeared in the 1920s. Known as sleeping sickness in the United States, this disease killed one-third of its victims and in many others led to postencephalitic parkinsonism, a particularly severe form of movement disorder in which some patients developed, often years after the acute phase of the illness, disabling neurological disorders, including various forms of catatonia.

In 1973, neurologist Oliver Sacks published Awakenings, an account of his work in the late 1960s with surviving postencephalitic patients in a New York hospital. Using the then-experimental drug levodopa, Dr. Sacks was able to temporarily "awaken" these patients from their statue-like state. (A film by the same name was released in 1990.)

In rare cases, other viral infections, including western equine encephalomyelitis, eastern equine encephalomyelitis, and Japanese B encephalitis, can leave patients with parkinsonian symptoms.

Drug-induced parkinsonism. A reversible form of parkinsonism sometimes results from use of certain drugs—chlorpromazine and haloperidol, for example—prescribed for patients with psychiatric disorders. Some drugs used for stomach disorders (metoclopramide) and high blood pressure (reserpine) may also produce parkinsonian symptoms. Stopping the medication or lowering the dosage causes the symptoms to abate.

Arteriosclerotic parkinsonism. Sometimes known as pseudoparkinsonism, arteriosclerotic parkinsonism involves damage to brain vessels due to multiple small strokes. Tremor is rare in this type of parkinsonism, while dementia—the loss of mental skills and abilities—is common. Antiparkinsonian drugs are of little help to patients with this form of parkinsonism.

Toxin-induced parkinsonism. Some toxins—such as manganese dust, carbon disulfide, and carbon monoxide—can also cause parkinsonism. A chemical known as MPTP (l-methyl-4-phenyl-1,2,3,6-tetrahydropyridine) causes a permanent form of parkinsonism that closely resembles Parkinson's disease. Investigators discovered this reaction in the 1980s, when heroin addicts in California who had taken an illicit street drug contaminated with MPTP began to develop severe parkinsonism. This discovery, which demonstrated that a toxic substance could damage the brain and produce parkinsonian symptoms, caused a dramatic breakthrough in Parkinson's research: For the first time scientists were able to simulate Parkinson's disease in animals and conduct studies to increase understanding of the disease.

Parkinsonism accompanying other conditions. Parkinsonian symptoms may also appear in patients with other, clearly distinct neurological disorders such as Shy-Drager syndrome (also called multiple system atrophy), progressive supranuclear palsy, Wilson's disease, Huntington's disease, Hallervorden-Spatz syndrome, Alzheimer's disease, Creutzfeldt-Jakob disease, and post-traumatic encephalopathy.

DIAGNOSING PARKINSON'S DISEASE

Even for an experienced neurologist, making an accurate diagnosis in the early stages of Parkinson's disease can be difficult. There are, as yet, no sophisticated blood or laboratory tests available to diagnose the disease. The physician may need to observe the patient for some time until it is apparent that the tremor is consistently present and is joined by one or more of the other classic symptoms. Since other forms of parkinsonism have similar features but require different treatments, making a precise diagnosis as soon as possible is essential for starting a patient on proper medication.

TREATING THE DISEASE

At present, there is no cure for Parkinson's disease. But a variety of medications provide relief from the symptoms.

When recommending a course of treatment, the physician determines how much the symptoms disrupt the patient's life and then tailors therapy to the person's particular condition. Since no two patients will react the same way to a given drug, it may take time and patience to get the dose just right. Even then, symptoms may not be completely alleviated. In the early stages of Parkinson's disease, physicians often begin treatment with one or a combination of the less powerful drugs—such as the anticholinergics, amantadine, pramipexole, ropinirole, or tolcapone (see Other Medications for Managing Symptoms, page 190), saving the most powerful treatment, specifically levodopa, for the time when patients need it most.

Levodopa

Without doubt, the gold standard of present therapy is the drug levodopa (also called L-dopa). L-dopa (from the full name L-3,4-dihydroxyphenylalanine) is a simple chemical found naturally in plants and animals. Levodopa is the generic name used for this chemical when it is formulated for drug use in patients. Nerve cells can use levodopa to make dopamine and replenish the brain's dwindling supply. Dopamine itself cannot be given because it doesn't cross the blood-brain barrier, the elaborate meshwork of fine blood vessels and cells that filters blood reaching the brain. Usually, patients are given levodopa combined with carbidopa. When added to levodopa, carbidopa delays the conversion of levodopa into dopamine until it reaches the brain, preventing or diminishing some of the side effects that often accompany levodopa therapy. Carbidopa also reduces the amount of levodopa needed.

Levodopa's success in treating the major symptoms of Parkinson's disease is a triumph of modern medicine. First introduced in the 1960s, it delays the onset of debilitating symptoms and allows the majority of patients—who would otherwise be very disabled—to extend the period of time in which they can lead relatively normal, productive lives.

Although levodopa helps at least three-quarters of parkinsonian cases, not all symptoms respond equally to the drug. Bradykinesia and rigidity respond best, while tremor may be only marginally reduced. Problems with balance and other symptoms may not be alleviated at all.

People who have taken other medications before starting levodopa therapy may have to cut back or eliminate these drugs in order to feel the full benefit of levodopa. Once levodopa therapy starts, people often respond dramatically, but they may need to increase the dose gradually for maximum benefit.

Because a high-protein diet can interfere with the absorption of levodopa, some physicians recommend that patients taking the drug restrict protein consumption to the evening meal.

Levodopa is so effective that some people may forget they have Parkinson's disease. But levodopa is not a cure. Although it can diminish the symptoms, it does not replace lost nerve cells and does not stop the progression of the disease.

Side Effects of Levodopa

Although beneficial for thousands of patients, levodopa is not without its limitations and side effects. The most common side effects are nausea, vomiting, low blood pressure, involuntary movements, and restlessness. In rare cases, patients may become confused. The nausea and vomiting caused by levodopa are greatly reduced by the combination of levodopa and carbidopa, which enhances the effectiveness of a lower dose. A slow-release formulation of this product, which gives patients a longer lasting effect, is also available.

Dyskinesias, or involuntary movements such as twitching, nodding, and jerking, most commonly develop in people who are taking large doses of levodopa over an extended period. These movements may be either mild or severe and either very rapid or very slow. The only effective way to control these drug-induced movements is to lower the dose of levodopa or to use drugs that block dopamine, but these remedies usually cause the disease symptoms to reappear. Doctors and patients must work together closely to find a tolerable balance between the drug's benefits and side effects.

Other more troubling and distressing problems may occur with long-term levodopa use. Patients may begin to notice more pronounced symptoms before their first dose of medication in the morning, and they can feel when each dose begins to wear off (muscle spasms are a common effect). Symptoms gradually begin to return. The period of effectiveness from each dose may begin to shorten, called the wearing-off effect.

Another potential problem is referred to as the on-off effect—sudden, unpredictable changes in movement, from normal to parkinsonian movement and back again, possibly occurring several times during the day. These effects probably indicate that the patient's response to the drug is changing or that the disease is progressing.

One approach to alleviating these side effects is to take levodopa more often and in smaller amounts. Sometimes physicians instruct patients to stop levodopa for several days in an effort to improve the response to the drug and to manage the complications of long-term levodopa therapy. This controversial technique is known as a "drug holiday." Because of the possibility of serious complications, drug holidays should be attempted only under a physician's direct supervision, preferably in a hospital. Parkinson's disease patients should never stop taking levodopa without their physician's knowledge or consent because of the potentially serious side effects of rapidly withdrawing the drug.

OTHER MEDICATIONS FOR MANAGING SYMPTOMS

Levodopa is not a perfect drug. Fortunately, physicians have other treatment choices for particular symptoms or stages of the disease. Other therapies include the following:

Bromocriptine and pergolide. These two drugs mimic the role of dopamine in the brain, causing the neurons to react as they would to dopamine. They can be given alone or with levodopa and may be used in the early stages of the disease or started later to lengthen the duration of response to levodopa in patients experiencing wearing-off or on-off effects. They are generally less effective than levodopa in controlling rigidity and bradykinesia. Side effects may include paranoia, hallucinations, confusion, dyskinesias, nightmares, nausea, and vomiting.

Another class of drugs, which are being used more and more for initial therapy, in addition to anticholinergics or amantadine, include dopamine agonists such as pramipexole or ropinirole.

Selegiline. Also known as Deprenyl, selegiline has become a commonly used drug for Parkinson's disease. Recent studies supported by the National Institute of Neurological Dis-

orders and Stroke (NINDS) have shown that the drug delays the need for levodopa therapy by up to a year or more. When selegiline is given with levodopa, it appears to enhance and prolong the response to levodopa and thus may reduce wearing-off fluctuations. In studies with animals, selegiline has been shown to protect the dopamine-producing neurons from the toxic effects of MPTP. Selegiline inhibits the activity of the enzyme monoamine oxidase-B (MAO-B), the enzyme that metabolizes dopamine in the brain, delaying the breakdown of naturally occurring dopamine and of dopamine formed from levodopa. Dopamine then accumulates in the surviving nerve cells.

Tolcapone, the first in a new class of Parkinson's drugs called catechol-O-methyltransferase (COMT) inhibitors, is also being used to increase the effectiveness of levodopa. It is believed to increase blood levels of levodopa by blocking the action of COMT, one of the enzymes responsible for breaking down levodopa, before it reaches the brain.

Some physicians, but not all, favor starting all parkinsonian patients on selegiline because of its possible protective effect. Selegiline is an easy drug to take, although side effects may include nausea, orthostatic hypotension, or insomnia (when taken late in the day). Also, toxic reactions have occurred in some patients who took selegiline with fluoxetine (an antidepressant) and meperidine (used as a sedative and an analgesic).

Research scientists are still trying to answer questions about selegiline use: How long does the drug remain effective? Does long-term use have any adverse effects? Evaluation of the long-term effects will help determine its value for all stages of the disease.

Anticholinergics. These drugs were the main treatment for Parkinson's disease until the introduction of levodopa. Their benefit is limited, but they may help control tremor and rigidity. They are particularly helpful in reducing drug-induced parkinsonism. Anticholinergics appear to act by blocking the action of another brain chemical, acetylcholine, whose effects become more pronounced when dopamine levels drop. Only about half the patients who receive anticholinergics respond, usually for a brief period and with only a 30 percent improvement. Although not as effective as levodopa or bromocriptine, anticholinergics may have a therapeutic effect at any stage of the disease when taken with either of these drugs. Common side effects include dry mouth, constipation, urinary retention, hallucinations, memory loss, blurred vision, changes in mental activity, and confusion.

Amantadine. An antiviral drug, amantadine, helps reduce symptoms of Parkinson's disease. It is often used alone in the early stages of the disease or with an anticholinergic drug or levodopa. After several months amantadine's effectiveness wears off in a third to a half of the patients taking it, although effectiveness may return after a brief withdrawal from the drug. Amantadine has several side effects, including mottled skin, edema, confusion, blurred vision, and depression.

SURGERY TO TREAT
PARKINSON'S DISEASE
Treating Parkinson's disease with surgery was once a common practice. But after the discovery of levodopa, surgery was restricted to only a few cases. One of the procedures used, called cryothalamotomy, requires the surgical insertion of a supercooled metal tip of a probe into the thalamus (a "relay station" deep in the brain) to destroy the brain area that produces tremors. This and related procedures are coming back into favor for patients who have severe tremor or have the disease only on one

side of the body. Investigators have also revived interest in a surgical procedure called pallidotomy, in which a portion of the brain called the globus pallidus is lesioned. Some studies indicate that pallidotomy may improve symptoms of tremor, rigidity, and bradykinesia, possibly by interrupting the neural pathway between the globus pallidus and the striatum or thalamus. Further research on the value of surgically destroying these brain areas is currently being conducted.

The most recent innovation has been a move away from lesioning procedures (thalamotomy and pallidotomy) and toward the insertion of deep brain stimulators, which appear to work by "short-circuiting" impaired brain regions involved with Parkinson's disease. Thalamotomy and deep brain stimulation of the thalamus are used exclusively for tremor and do not help other aspects of Parkinson's disease. Pallidotomy and deep brain stimulation of the globus pallidus are used primarily for patients with treatment-related fluctuations and levodopa-induced involuntary movements, known as dyskinesias. The most recent surgical procedure is deep brain stimulation of the subthalamic nucleus, which appears to be helpful for reducing the amount of "off" time and therefore providing a more continuous, beneficial response to levodopa.

THE ROLE OF DIET AND
EXERCISE PROGRAMS
Diet. Eating a well-balanced, nutritious diet can be beneficial for anybody. But for preventing or curing Parkinson's disease, there does not seem to be any specific vitamin, mineral, or other nutrient that has any therapeutic value. A high protein diet, however, may limit levodopa's effectiveness.

Despite some early optimism, recent studies have shown that tocopherol (a form of vitamin E) does not delay Parkinson's disease. This conclusion came from a carefully conducted study supported by the NINDS called DATATOP (Deprenyl and Tocopherol Antioxidative Therapy for Parkinson's Disease) that examined, over five years, the effects of both Deprenyl (selegiline) and vitamin E on early Parkinson's disease. While Deprenyl was found to slow the early symptomatic progression of the disease and delay the need for levodopa, there was no evidence of therapeutic benefit from vitamin E.

Exercise. Because movements are affected in Parkinson's disease, exercising may help people improve their mobility. Some doctors prescribe physical therapy or muscle-strengthening exercises to tone muscles and to put underused and rigid muscles through a full range of motion.

Exercises will not stop disease progression, but they may improve body strength so that the person is less disabled. Exercises also improve balance (helping people with gait problems) and can strengthen certain muscles so that people can speak and swallow better.

Exercises can also improve the emotional well-being of parkinsonian patients by giving them a feeling of accomplishment. Although structured exercise programs help many patients, more general physical activities, such as walking, gardening, swimming, calisthenics, and using exercise machines, can also be beneficial.

THE BENEFITS OF SUPPORT GROUPS
One of the most demoralizing aspects of the disease is how completely the patient's world changes. The most basic daily routines may be affected—from socializing with friends and enjoying normal and congenial relationships with family members to earning a living and taking care of a home. Faced with a very different life, people need encouragement to remain as active and involved as possible. That's when support groups can be of particular

value to parkinsonian patients, their families, and their caregivers.

CAN PARKINSON'S BE PREDICTED OR PREVENTED?
As yet, there is no way to predict or prevent the disease. However, researchers are now looking for a biomarker—a biochemical abnormality that all patients with Parkinson's disease might share—that could be picked up by screening techniques or by a simple chemical test given to people who do not have any parkinsonian symptoms.

Positron emission tomography (PET) scanning may lead to important advances in our knowledge about Parkinson's disease. PET scans of the brain produce pictures of chemical changes as they occur in the living brain. Using PET, research scientists can study the brain's dopamine receptors (the sites on nerve cells that bind with dopamine) to determine if the loss of dopamine activity follows or precedes degeneration of the neurons that make this chemical. This information could help scientists better understand the disease process and may potentially lead to improved treatments.

The National Institute of
Neurological Disorders and Stroke

SHINGLES

When the itchy red spots of childhood chicken pox disappear and the child goes back to school, the battle with infection seems won. But for all too many of us this triumph of the body's immune system over a virus is only temporary. The virus has not been destroyed, but lies low, ready to strike again later in life. This second eruption of the chicken pox virus is the disease called shingles.

"I was having exams at college, and I got a

rash in a band around my waist. I first thought it was chicken pox, but I'd had that years before and instead of itching, this time the spots were very painful," recalls a young woman who had shingles in her twenties.

The young woman's memory was correct. She had had chicken pox as a child. You cannot develop shingles unless you have had an earlier bout of chicken pox. The woman was also typical in her symptoms: Shingles is often more painful than it is itchy. Her age was unusual, however. While young people do develop shingles, the disease most often strikes in later years. About 10 percent of normal adults can be expected to get shingles during their lifetime, usually after age 50. The incidence increases with age, so that shingles is 10 times more likely to occur in adults over 60 than in children under 10. The chances of developing shingles are greatest for individuals whose immune systems are weakened.

REVEALING SYMPTOMS

The first sign of shingles is often pain in or under the skin. The individual may also feel ill with fever or headache. After several days, a rash of small fluid-filled blisters appears on reddened skin.

The blisters, or lesions, are usually limited to a band spanning one side of the trunk or clustered on one side of the face. This striking pattern gives the disease its name: "Shingles" comes from "cingulum," the Latin word for belt or girdle. Similarly, the medical term for the disease, "zoster," is the Greek word for girdle.

More importantly, the distribution of the shingles spots is a telltale clue to where the chicken pox virus has been hiding for all the years following the initial infection. Scientists now know that the shingles lesions correspond to the area of skin supplied by one of the major nerves that exits from the brain or spinal cord.

The assumption is that the chicken pox viruses that weren't wiped out in the original

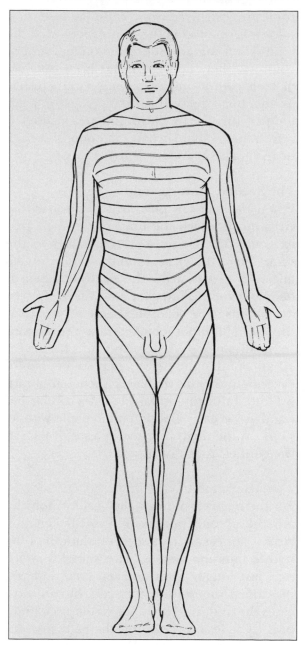

The lines mark the areas of skin served by individual brain or spinal nerves. When shingles strikes, the rash is confined to one of these narrow bands.

battle were able to leave the skin blisters and travel in the nervous system. There, the viruses settled down in an inactive form inside nerve cells (neurons) that lie in clusters adjacent to the spinal cord and brain. These neurons are called sensory cells because they relay information to the brain about what the body is sensing: whether the skin feels hot or cold, whether the person has been touched or feels pain. Comparable nerve cell clusters in the head relay information about pain, temperature, or touch in that area, as well as information about what someone is seeing, hearing, tasting, or smelling.

The Second Time Around

When the chicken pox virus reactivates, the virus moves down the long nerve fibers that extend from the sensory cell bodies to the skin. There the viruses multiply and the tell-tale rash erupts. Now the nervous system is deeply involved, however, and the symptoms are often more complex and severe than those of childhood chicken pox. People with "optical" shingles (where the virus has invaded an ophthalmic nerve) may suffer painful eye inflammations that leave them temporarily blind. Infections of facial nerves can lead to paralysis or excruciating pain. People with lesions on the torso may feel spasms of pain at the gentlest touch or breeze.

The Aftermath

For the majority of normally healthy individuals, the second bout with the chicken pox virus is almost always a second triumph of the body's immune system. The shingles attack may last longer than chicken pox, and you may need medication for pain, but in most cases the body has the inner resources to fight back. The lesions heal and the pain subsides within three to five weeks.

There are exceptions. Sometimes, particularly in older people, the pain and other symptoms persist long after the rash is healed. It is important to realize that these individuals no longer have shingles: Their infection is over. Instead, they are suffering a neurological disorder, the result of damage to the nervous system.

Investigators think that the virus attack has led to scarring or other lesions affecting the sensory cells and associated nerves. If the eye is involved, the damage from shingles can lead to blindness.

In other cases facial paralysis, headache, and persistent pain are the aftermath. Possibly because the nerve cells conveying pain sensations are hardest hit, or are exquisitely sensitized by the virus attack, pain is the principal complication of shingles. This pain, called postherpetic neuralgia, is among the most devastating known to mankind—the kind of pain that leads to insomnia, weight loss, depression, and that total preoccupation with unrelenting torment that characterizes the chronic pain sufferer.

Even in such severe cases, however, the paralysis, headaches, and pain generally subside, although it may take time. As one elderly sufferer recalls: "The worst thing was that the pain went on for months and months. Another bad part was reflecting on the 60 years since I had the chicken pox. Am I only a culture medium for viruses, for heaven's sake?"

Postherpetic neuralgia may be a nightmare, but it is not life-threatening. Doctors

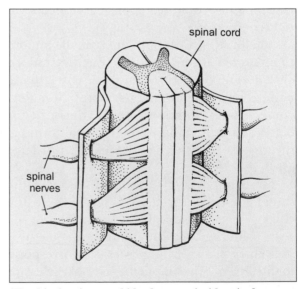

The shingles virus can hide, dormant, inside spinal nerves near the spinal cord or brain, then reactivate and travel along the nerve, out to the skin.

treating the pain currently employ a variety of medications. They generally avoid the powerful narcotic pain relievers in favor of newer nonaddictive but potent painkillers. Studies have also shown that some anticonvulsant drugs used to treat epilepsy, such as carbamazepine (Tegretol) are sometimes effective in relieving postherpetic neuralgia. Antidepressants can help, also. In addition to their effects on mood, the antidepressants appear to relieve pain. Some doctors report that patients occasionally benefit from some of the more controversial treatments for pain, such as acupuncture and electrical stimulation of nerve endings.

A threat to immunosuppressed patients. People with leukemia, Hodgkin's disease, or other cancers are often treated by drugs or radiation to destroy cancerous tissue. Unfortunately, these treatments also damage cells of the immune system that normally fight invading organisms. Patients with kidney or other organ diseases who receive organ transplants are also vulnerable to shingles. These patients are given drugs that suppress the immune system to prevent the body from rejecting the foreign tissue. Should any of these patients contract shingles, there is a real danger that the disease will spread throughout the body, reaching vital organs like the lungs. If unchecked, such disseminated shingles can lead to death from viral pneumonia or secondary bacterial infection.

THE LATENT VIRUS

The virus responsible for shingles and chicken pox belongs to the herpes group of viruses. The group includes the virus that causes cold sores, fever blisters, mononucleosis, and genital herpes—a sexually transmitted disease. Like the shingles-causing virus, many herpes viruses can take refuge in the nervous system after an individual has suffered an initial infection. The virus may remain latent for years,

ON CATCHING CHICKEN POX— BUT NOT CATCHING SHINGLES

Chicken pox is a highly contagious disease. Most of us catch it during childhood because the virus can be spread through air as well as through contact with the rash. The infection begins in the upper respiratory tract, where the virus reproduces over a period of 15 days or more (the incubation period). The virus then spreads to the bloodstream and migrates to the skin, giving rise to the familiar rash.

In contrast, you can't catch shingles. You must already have had a case of chicken pox and harbor the virus in your nervous system. When activated, the virus travels down nerves to your skin, causing the painful shingles rash. In shingles, the virus does not normally spread to the bloodstream or lungs, so the virus is not shed in air. Because the shingles rash contains active virus particles, however, a person who has never had chicken pox can contract chicken pox by exposure to the shingles rash.

then travel down nerve cell fibers to cause a renewed infection.

Scientists call the chicken pox/shingles-causing agent the VZ virus, short for varicella-zoster. "Varicella" is a Latin word meaning "little pox" to distinguish the virus from smallpox, the scourge that once disfigured or killed its victims. (The word "chicken" conveys the same idea of weakness or mildness as in "chicken-hearted.") Like many viruses, the varicella-zoster virus looks as though it were designed by a mathematician. It is a microscopic sphere encasing a 20-sided geometric figure called an icosahedron. Inside the icosahedron is the genetic material of the virus, deoxyribonucleic acid (DNA). When activated, the virus reproduces inside the nucleus of an infected cell. It acquires its spherical wrapping as it buds through the nuclear membrane.

As early as 1909, a German scientist suspected that the viruses causing chicken pox and shingles were one and the same. In the

1920s and 1930s, the case was strengthened. In an experiment, children were inoculated with fluid from the lesions of patients with shingles. Within two weeks about half the children came down with chicken pox. Finally, in 1958, detailed analyses of the viruses taken from patients with either chicken pox or shingles confirmed that the viruses were identical.

Note what that means: A person with shingles can communicate chicken pox to a susceptible individual. But the opposite is not true: A person with chicken pox cannot communicate shingles to someone else. You must already harbor the virus in your nervous system before shingles can develop. "It's a clever virus," notes a National Institute of Neurological Disorders and Stroke (NINDS) virologist. "It doesn't kill its host, but lives for a long time in a suppressed state. And it can reactivate, given the opportunity," he adds.

RESEARCH CHALLENGES

Shingles imposes two immediate challenges to medical research. The first is to develop drugs to fight the disease and to prevent complications. The second challenge is to understand the disease well enough to prevent it, especially in people known to be at high risk.

Developing Antiviral Drugs

Only recently have scientists succeeded in developing antiviral drugs. In 1975, there were virtually no virus-fighting drugs available. Progress has been impressive since then and now there are several antiviral agents in clinical use, with more on the way.

Understanding the Virus

The second major challenge to investigators is to protect susceptible patients from a shingles attack. To do that, scientists will need to know much more about the VZ virus, especially how it remains latent in the body for so long, and what induces it to become active again.

What keeps the VZ virus quiet during its long latency? Probably the immune system, scientists think. A healthy immune system protects against all kinds of diseases, but people with depressed immunity are vulnerable to many illnesses and have a high incidence of shingles. Even among normal individuals, temporary depression of the immune system because of stress, a cold, and even sunburn, may be associated with an attack of shingles.

Antibodies, one of the immune system's major defense mechanisms against infection, are not very helpful against shingles. Studies have shown that patients with shingles produce VZ antibodies: They just don't check the infection. Similarly, injections of antibody-rich blood serum do not prevent the dissemination of shingles in cancer patients or others whose immune systems are depressed. (This is in contrast to the protection conferred by the serum when given to newborns with chicken pox.)

The components of the immune system that do appear to combat shingles are two types of white blood cell: the T lymphocyte, and a scavenger cell called a macrophage. Scientists are trying to find ways of boosting the activity of these cells—especially in patients at high risk for severe or disseminated shingles.

The National Institute of
Neurological Disorders and Stroke

Dental and Oral Disorders

A healthy smile is a bonus at any age. Too often older people—especially those who wear dentures or false teeth—feel they no longer need dental checkups. Because the idea of preventive dental care dates back to the 1950s, many people over age 65 have not grown up with the idea of preventive care of the teeth.

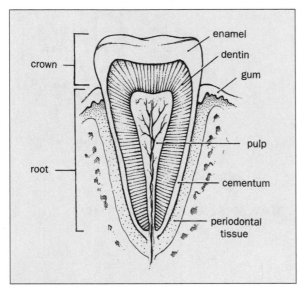

Each tooth consists of a crown and a root. Hard enamel surrounds the dentin, which in turn protects the softer pulp, containing nerves and blood vessels.

TOOTH DECAY

Tooth decay is not just a disease of children; it can continue throughout life as long as natural teeth are in the mouth. Tooth decay is caused by bacteria that normally live in the mouth. The bacteria stick to teeth and form a sticky, colorless film called dental plaque. The bacteria in plaque, which live on sugars, produce decay-causing acids that dissolve minerals in the tooth surfaces. In the presence of gum disease, tooth decay can develop on the exposed roots of the teeth.

Research has shown that adding fluoride to the water supply is the best and the least costly way to prevent tooth decay. Just as with children, fluoride is important for adult teeth. In addition to drinking fluoridated water, the use of fluoride toothpastes and mouth rinses can add protection. Fluoride mouth rinses are available in two different strengths, one for daily use, one for weekly use. Daily fluoride rinses can be bought without prescription. Your dentist or dental hygienist may give you regular fluoride treatments or prescribe a fluoride gel or mouth rinse for use at home.

The National Institute on Aging

PERIODONTAL DISEASE

Periodontal disease is a gradual and progressive destructive process that threatens the gums and other supporting structures of the teeth. In the most common form of periodontal disease—called gingivitis—the gums become inflamed and tend to bleed easily. Gingivitis can be controlled with thorough, frequent plaque removal, but if left untreated, it may progress to periodontitis, a more serious state of periodontal disease. In periodontitis, infected pockets may form between the teeth and the gums, and later the bone supporting the teeth may be destroyed. When this happens, perfectly healthy teeth become loosened and can ultimately be lost.

WHO IS AFFECTED BY PERIODONTAL DISEASE?
Everyone is susceptible. At least three out of four of us will probably have some periodontal destruction in our lifetime. A recent National Survey of Adult Oral Health revealed that 77 percent of employed adults aged 18 to 65 and 95 percent of the seniors surveyed had some periodontal attachment loss—a major sign of periodontal destruction.

WHAT CAUSES PERIODONTAL DISEASE?

Often periodontal disease results from poor oral hygiene. Masses of bacteria adhere to teeth and gums in a sticky film called dental plaque. Food particles, especially sweets, nourish the bacteria and cause them to secrete acids, enzymes, and other harmful substances that irritate soft tissues in the mouth and destroy bone. When plaque is not removed on a regular basis, the microbial attack is constant. Plaque can spread to hard-to-reach spots between the teeth and under the gums, making its removal difficult.

Other factors that can contribute to periodontal conditions include accumulated deposits of tartar or calculus, poor nutrition, hereditary lack of resistance, and imbalances in the body's system from various diseases—such as diabetes—or from pregnancy. Harmful habits such as using tobacco products and clenching and grinding the teeth can worsen periodontal disease.

Gingivitis

Gingivitis is an early stage of periodontal disease and is commonly seen in both youths and adults. The gums are aggravated by bacterial plaque and become inflamed—turning red and swelling around one or more of the teeth. Eventually, the redness and swelling become more pronounced, and the gums tend to bleed easily. Bleeding as a result of brushing or flossing is one of the earliest signs of gum disease. The gums may or may not be tender and sensitive, and there may be no warning initially that the disease is present. However, if gingivitis is not controlled, the inflammation can spread to underlying tissues that support the teeth. This causes a more severe condition called periodontitis, which involves bone destruction.

Periodontitis

Periodontitis is a more serious form of periodontal disease, which occurs in three phases: early, moderate, and advanced. In the early phase, accumulated plaque hardens and extends from the gum line down along the tooth root. The gums gradually pull away from the affected teeth, causing gaps or "pockets" to develop. In the moderate phase, gums are red and swollen and bleed easily. As the gums detach further, bacteria that collect

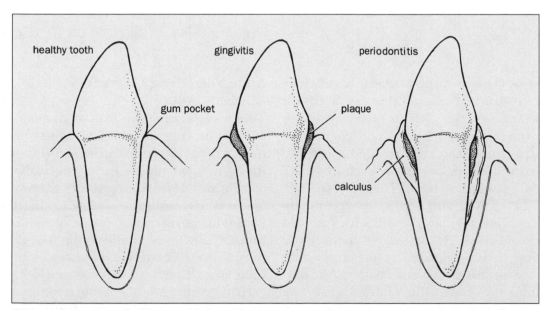

With gingivitis, plaque builds up and irritates the gums. As gum disease advances, gums gradually pull away from affected teeth, and underlying tissue and bone are destroyed (periodontitis).

COSMETIC DENTAL OPTIONS

Tobacco, coffee, tea, and foods such as berries can permanently stain tooth surfaces; antibiotics such as tetracycline, certain illnesses and injuries, and excessive fluoride can stain teeth internally. Commercially available tooth whiteners, such as Pearl Drops polish, are not the answer, as these tend to be abrasive.

However, there are dental techniques that can safely produce a brighter smile. The dentist will be able to diagnose and treat the problem. However, none of the services described below are inexpensive, and because they are primarily cosmetic, very few insurance policies will cover them.

• *Bleaching.* For teeth that are stained, bleaching may help. A simple, painless, in-office or at-home procedure, bleaching is the most thorough way to whiten teeth. The inside of the mouth is shielded with latex so that only the teeth are exposed, and a chemical bleaching agent is applied. A special light beam activates the process. Two to ten visits may be necessary to achieve desired results. Home bleaching with prescription products can be effective and less expensive. Side effects can include gum or tooth sensitivity.

• *Bonding.* For chips, cracks, or conspicuous gaps between the teeth, as well as severe stains, bonding may be the answer. An acid-etch solution is used to roughen the tooth surface and make it easier for the gluelike bonding agent to stick to the tooth. Over this, a malleable plastic resin is applied to reshape the tooth, fill in gaps or chips, or cover stains. Finally, the bonded surface is polished smooth. The procedure is usually performed in one visit. Bonding is fine for cosmetic reconstruction of teeth and can also be used for small fillings on front teeth, or, in some cases, even substitute for crowns on molars—but the materials used are never as strong as actual teeth, and therefore may require periodic replacement (usually about every five years).

• *Laminate Veneers.* Made of porcelain or a special resin, laminate veneers are thin shells affixed directly to the tooth. Impressions of the teeth are taken and the veneers are custom made to match the color and shape of the natural teeth. As with bonding, the tooth surface is first etched, followed by the application of a resin that holds the veneer in place.

• *Crowns.* When the structure of the tooth is weakened by previous fillings, veneers may not be the best choice. It may be better to cover the entire tooth with a metal and/or porcelain crown. The whole tooth is reduced in size, an impression is made, and a dental laboratory fabricates the crown, which is then cemented to the tooth.

The Editors

---

in the pockets produce toxins, which may begin to erode the underlying soft tissues and bone.

By the advanced stage of periodontal disease, the gums may have receded to expose tooth root surfaces, or deep pockets may have formed between the teeth. These pockets collect food particles and germs, which cause infection. They are likely to fill with pus and cause bad breath. At this stage of periodontitis, more than 50 percent of the supporting bone has disintegrated and many of the special fibers that fasten the teeth to bone have been destroyed. As a result, teeth loosen and may eventually fall out.

Acute Necrotizing Ulcerative Gingivitis (ANUG)

This is a less common form of gingivitis. Also called Vincent's infection or trench mouth, this bacterial infection causes painful sores on the gums and makes eating difficult. ANUG usually develops in times of severe stress. Smokers are more susceptible to the disease than nonsmokers. ANUG is one of the "opportunistic infections" that frequently strike AIDS patients. Dentists find that removal of the bacteria and dead tissues, good nutrition, rest, careful brushing and flossing, and sometimes treatment with an antibiotic usually manage to control this type of periodontal disease.

Because many of the symptoms of periodontal disease can occur without any discomfort, you might not be aware that it is developing. Your dentist can detect the disease in its early stages, so it is important to have regular checkups to prevent the unnecessary worsening of periodontal disease.

WHAT CAN BE DONE

Controlling bacteria is the key to prevention of periodontal disease. In its early stages, periodontal disease is completely reversible. Even when some disease has already developed, dentists find that many patients respond well to a plaque removal program. Within a week or so, the inflammation usually subsides, and the swollen gums shrink and grow firm. After a few weeks, loose teeth may become more stable. Although the active disease process can be stopped in a short time, tissues that have been lost will not grow back except in unusual circumstances. However, if you remove plaque regularly, you can usually avoid gum inflammation and the development of pockets.

Brushing is an important step in plaque removal. It should be done carefully, not too vigorously, with a soft nylon brush with rounded ends on its bristles.

Use dental floss to remove bacteria from between the teeth where most pockets begin, but be careful not to let the floss cut the gum tissue. Getting under the small collars of gum tissue around the teeth, especially at the back and between the teeth, takes time and care. Ask your dentist or dental hygienist to show you how to get at some of the harder-to-reach spots.

Occasionally you will want to check how well you are removing plaque. Because early bacterial film is colorless, a disclosing solution containing vegetable coloring may be applied to the teeth and gums. It will stain any remaining plaque and show you which areas you have missed. Just brush and floss these areas more carefully. Finally, rinse the mouth well.

Done at least daily, careful cleaning will help protect your teeth and gums from bacterial diseases. When you make your regular visits to the dentist, any calculus that may have accumulated can be removed, and a thorough oral examination will reveal spots requiring special attention. Your dentist can also check your gums to see if they bleed easily or if there has been any detachment of gum tissue from the teeth. An antimicrobial mouth rinse also may be prescribed to help control harmful bacteria in your mouth.

And even if you wear dentures, it is still important to observe proper cleaning techniques to protect your gums and dentures. (See Dentures and Dental Implants, pages 202-3.) *The National Institute of Dental Research*

DRY MOUTH (XEROSTOMIA)

Do you feel the need to moisten your mouth frequently? Does your mouth feel dry at mealtime? Do you have less saliva than you once did? Do you have difficulty swallowing? Do you have trouble eating dry foods such as crackers or toast? If you answer yes to these questions, you may be one of many people who suffer from dry mouth, or xerostomia.

Although xerostomia is not a disease in itself, it is a symptom of certain diseases. Dry mouth also is a common side effect of some medications and medical treatments. Most cases of dry mouth are caused by failure of the salivary glands to function properly. But some people have the sensation of a dry mouth even though their salivary glands are normal.

Dry mouth is a significant health problem because it can affect nutrition and psychological well-being, while also contributing to tooth decay and other mouth infections. Dry mouth also may signal more serious problems in the body. If you have a dry mouth, you should be seen by a dentist or physician to determine the cause of the symptom.

DENTURES AND DENTAL IMPLANTS

Dentures

Full or partial dentures are the rule rather than the exception for people over 60. Almost half of those in this age group have none of their natural teeth and many more are missing at least some. Because dentures are subject to many of the same problems as natural teeth, they need as much care.

Brushing and soaking are the mainstays of denture care. Not only do they keep your dentures looking good, but they also prevent the accumulation of plaque—a gummy film consisting of bacteria that is one of the main culprits in tooth and gum decay. Built-up plaque that remains on your dentures will be pressed directly against your mouth while you are wearing them, which can lead to sores, infections, pain, or even bone loss. Brushing actively removes most visible plaque and food debris. Soaking gets rid of plaque microorganisms that might still cling to your dentures after brushing; it also helps remove stains and reduces odors.

There is a plethora of commercial products available to help you with your denture care. However, you can substitute items that you probably already have at home for many of these products, and there are also some denture-care products that dentists do not advise using at all. Just what you choose to use is largely a matter of personal preference, but consult your dentist first to ask for any particular recommendations. Here's a basic rundown of what you will—and won't—need.

• *Brushes*. You can use a regular soft-bristled toothbrush, but special denture brushes are recommended, as their bristles are designed to mold to the shape of dentures. There are also special brushes for partial dentures that are designed to clean the clasps that attach to your natural teeth—a spot particularly prone to plaque buildup. Avoid stiff-bristled brushes; they can damage the plastic parts of dentures.

• *Cleansers*. Regular toothpaste won't do for cleaning your dentures; it's too abrasive and can damage the acrylic that most dentures are made of. Look for one of the special denture pastes that carries the approval seal of the American Dental Association's Council on Dental Materials, Instruments, and Equipment. However, plain hand soap, mild dishwashing liquid, or baking soda will also do a good job. Don't use a household cleaner or bleach.

• *Soaking solutions*. When your dentures aren't in your mouth, they should be soaking to keep them from drying out. Cool water will do the job (hot water can warp them), but for extra cleaning power you can buy a commercially prepared solution or make a solution yourself by mixing one tablespoon of vinegar with eight ounces of water. If you have any manual difficulties, such as arthritis, that make it hard to brush your dentures, it's particularly important that you use one of these cleaning solutions. Renew solution daily, because both the solution and the cup can be reservoirs for growth of microorganisms.

• *Adhesives*. Denture adhesives are widely marketed as the answer to loose dentures. Your dentures may feel loose when you first get them just because you're not

WHY IS SALIVA IMPORTANT?

Saliva has many important functions in the body. Each person needs saliva to:

• Limit the growth of bacteria that cause tooth decay and other oral infections
• Preserve teeth by bathing them with protective minerals that allow early cavities to remineralize and heal
• Lubricate the soft tissues lining the mouth to keep them pliable and make speaking and chewing easier
• Dissolve foods and allow us to experience their sweet, sour, salty, and bitter tastes
• Assist digestion by providing enzymes that break down food
• Lubricate food so that it can be easily swallowed
• Cleanse the teeth and soft tissues of food particles

WHAT CAUSES DRY MOUTH?

Changes in Salivary Gland Function

Dry mouth can be caused by changes in salivary gland function, brought on by the following situations.

used to them; this sensation should soon go away by itself. Dentures that gradually start to feel loose are usually a sign that the shape of the gum or supporting bone is undergoing changes, and that your dentures need to be relined or rebased.

Sometimes a small amount of powder-type adhesive is advisable to aid retention: Consult your dentist to determine when this is appropriate. Needing increasing amounts of adhesive is a sign of an ill-fitting denture. Aided by adhesives, long-term use of poorly fitted dentures can cause such severe mouth problems that it can even interfere with your ability to wear dentures at all.

• *Reliners and repair kits.* Avoid both of these do-it-yourself products. Most dentures periodically need to be relined or adjusted because of normal changes in your mouth. This takes sophisticated dental know-how, and trying to do it yourself can cause severe mouth problems. Likewise, let a dentist repair a cracked or chipped denture; self-repair kits can damage the denture, and some of the glues in these kits even contain chemicals that can harm your mouth as well as the dentures.

Just because you have dentures to care for—and have only some or none of your natural teeth—doesn't mean you can neglect caring for those teeth that remain, or your gums and other parts of your mouth. Every day, you should remove plaque from your mouth by brushing your gums, tongue, and the roof of your mouth with a soft-bristled brush (but not a denture brush), or rubbing them firmly with a piece of damp gauze. Brush and floss remaining teeth as recommended and get professional dental care at regular intervals.

Dental Implants

Now there may be an alternative to removable dentures and fixed bridges: dental implants.

Unlike replacements that rely on remaining natural teeth for support, a dental implant consists of a crown or bridge of metal or some other material fixed to the underlying bone. Once implanted, the teeth can't be removed by the wearer, who treats them like natural teeth and can reasonably expect them to last for a decade or more.

Dental implants can also be used to help stabilize and retain removable dentures. In this case, fewer implants are used, and dentures are fabricated to fit the gums and the implants.

Although more convenient, comfortable, and stable than dentures, dental implants are not an option for everybody. Any medical condition, such as diabetes, that might make healing difficult would rule out the surgical procedure.

The success of a dental implant depends on you as well as your dentist. Careful brushing and flossing to remove bacteria-laden plaque are vital to achieving and maintaining the seal between the gum tissue and the implant. You may need to use an antibacterial mouthwash and tiny brushes that fit in the gaps between your teeth as well.

The Editors

• **Medications.** Over 400 commonly used drugs list dry mouth as a side effect. The main culprits are the antihypertensives (for high blood pressure) and antidepressants. Both are prescribed for millions of Americans. Painkillers, tranquilizers, diuretics, and even over-the-counter antihistamines also can decrease saliva.

• **Cancer treatment.** Radiation therapy can permanently damage salivary glands if they are in the field of radiation. Chemotherapy can change the composition of saliva, creating a sensation of dry mouth.

• **Diseases.** Sjögren's syndrome is an autoimmune disorder whose symptoms include dry mouth and dry eyes. Some Sjögren's patients also have a connective tissue disorder, most commonly rheumatoid arthritis or systemic lupus erythematosus.

• **Other conditions.** Bone marrow transplants, endocrine disorders, nutritional deficiencies, anxiety, mental stress, and depression can cause a dry mouth.

Changes Not Related to Salivary Gland Function

Dry mouth can also be caused by certain changes not related to salivary glands, such as those that follow.

Nerve damage. Trauma to the head and neck area from surgery or wounds can damage the nerves that supply sensation to the mouth. While the salivary glands may be left intact, they cannot function normally without the nerves that signal them to produce saliva.

Altered perception. Conditions like Alzheimer's disease or stroke may change the ability to perceive oral sensations.

DOES AGING CAUSE DRY MOUTH?

Until recently dry mouth was regarded as a normal part of aging. Researchers now know that healthy older adults do not produce less saliva. When older people do experience dry mouth, it is because they suffer from diseases that cause the condition or they take medications that produce dry mouth as a side effect.

WHAT HAPPENS WHEN YOU HAVE DRY MOUTH?

Dry mouth caused by malfunctioning salivary glands is associated with changes in saliva. The flow of saliva can decrease. Or the composition of saliva can change.

Patients with dry mouth experience varying degrees of discomfort. Some people feel a dry or burning sensation in their mouth. A dry mouth may affect their ability to chew, taste, swallow, and speak. Changes in saliva also can affect oral and dental health. Severe cases of dry mouth can result in cracking of the lips, slits at the corners of the mouth, changes in the surface of the tongue, rampant tooth decay, ulceration of the mouth's linings, and infection.

IS RELIEF AVAILABLE?

There are a number of steps you can take to relieve the sense of dryness. The following suggestions will not correct the underlying cause of xerostomia, but may help you feel more comfortable.

- Take frequent sips of water or drinks without sugar. Pause often while speaking to sip some liquid. Avoid caffeine-containing coffee, tea, and soft drinks.
- Drink frequently while eating. This will make chewing and swallowing easier and may increase the taste of foods.
- Keep a glass of water by your bed for dryness during the night or upon awakening.
- Chew sugarless gum. The chewing may help produce more saliva.
- Eat sugarless mints or hard sugarless candies, but let them dissolve in your mouth. Cinnamon and mint are often the most effective.
- Place a small piece of lemon rind or a cherry pit in your mouth. The sucking action helps stimulate saliva.
- Avoid tobacco and alcohol.
- Avoid spicy, salty, and highly acidic foods that may irritate the mouth.
- Use a humidifier, particularly at night.
- Ask your dentist about using artificial salivas to help lubricate the mouth.
- An oral medication, pilocarpine, has recently been approved for treatment of dry mouth in Sjögren's syndrome. It has also been shown to be beneficial in reducing dry mouth associated with radiation therapy to head and neck tumors when prescribed during radiation treatments.

The National Institute of Dental Research

The Digestive System

OVERVIEW

The digestive system is a series of hollow organs joined in a long, twisting tube from the mouth to the anus. Inside this tube is a lining called the mucosa. In the mouth, stomach, and small intestine, the mucosa contains tiny glands that produce juices to help digest food.

There are also two solid digestive organs, the liver and the pancreas, which produce juices that reach the intestine through small tubes. In addition, parts of other organ systems (for instance, nerves and blood) play a major role in the digestive system.

When we eat such things as bread, meat, and vegetables, they are not in a form that the body can use as nourishment. Our food and drink must be changed into smaller molecules of nutrients before they can be absorbed

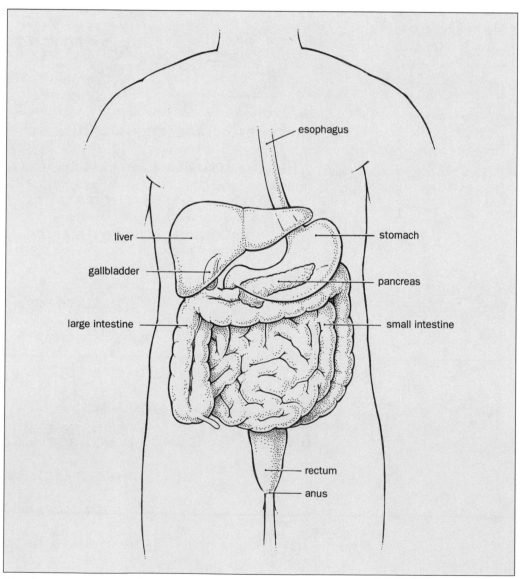

Digestion begins in the mouth and progresses through the esophagus, stomach, and intestines. The liver, gallbladder, and pancreas aid by contributing digestive enzymes.

into the blood and carried to cells throughout the body. Digestion is the process by which food and drink are broken down into their smallest parts so that the body can use them to build and nourish cells and to provide energy.

HOW FOOD IS DIGESTED

Digestion involves the mixing of food, its movement through the digestive tract, and chemical breakdown of the large molecules of food into smaller molecules. Digestion begins in the mouth, when we chew and swallow, and is completed in the small intestine. The chemical process varies somewhat for different kinds of food.

Movement of Food Through the System

The large, hollow organs of the digestive system contain muscle that enables their walls to move. The movement of organ walls can propel food and liquid and can also mix the contents within each organ. Typical movement of the esophagus, stomach, and intestine is called peristalsis. The action of peristalsis looks like an ocean wave moving through the muscle: The muscle of the organ produces a narrowing and then propels the narrowed portion slowly down the length of the organ. These waves of narrowing push the food and fluid in front of them through each hollow organ.

The first major muscle movement of digestion occurs when food or liquid is swallowed. Although we are able to start swallowing by choice, once the swallow begins, it becomes involuntary and proceeds under the control of the nerves.

The esophagus is the organ into which the swallowed food is pushed. It connects the throat above with the stomach below. At the junction of the esophagus and stomach, there is a ringlike valve closing the passage between the two organs. However, as the food approaches the closed ring, the surrounding muscles relax and allow the food to pass.

The food then enters the stomach, which has three mechanical tasks to do. First, the stomach must store the swallowed food and liquid. This requires the muscle of the upper part of the stomach to relax and accept large volumes of swallowed material. The second job is to mix up the food, liquid, and digestive juice produced by the stomach. The lower part of the stomach mixes these materials by its muscle action. The third task of the stomach is to empty its contents slowly into the small intestine.

Several factors affect emptying of the stomach, including the nature of the food (mainly its fat and protein content) and the degree of muscle action of the emptying stomach and the next organ to receive the stomach contents (the small intestine).

As the food is digested in the small intestine and dissolved into the juices from the pancreas, liver, and intestine, the contents of the intestine are mixed and pushed forward to allow further digestion.

Finally, all of the digested nutrients are absorbed through the intestinal walls. The waste products of this process include the undigested parts of the food, known as fiber, and the older cells that have been shed from the mucosa. These materials are propelled into the colon, where they remain, usually for a day or two, until the feces are expelled by a bowel movement.

Production of Digestive Juices

Glands of the digestive system are crucial to the process of digestion. They produce both the juices that break down the food and the hormones that help to control the process.

The glands that act first are in the mouth—the salivary glands. Saliva produced by these glands contains an enzyme that begins to digest the starch from food into smaller molecules.

The next set of digestive glands is in the stomach lining. They produce stomach acid and an enzyme that digests protein. One of the unsolved puzzles of the digestive system is why the acid juice of the stomach does not dissolve the tissue of the stomach itself. In most people, the stomach mucosa is able to resist the juice, although food and other tissues of the body cannot.

After the stomach empties the food and its juice into the small intestine, the juices of two other digestive organs mix with the food to continue the process of digestion. One of these organs is the pancreas. It produces a juice that contains a wide array of enzymes to break down the carbohydrates, fat, and protein in our food. Other enzymes active in the process come from glands in the wall of the intestine or are even a part of that wall.

The liver produces yet another digestive juice—bile. The bile is stored between meals in the gallbladder. At mealtime, it is squeezed out of the gallbladder into the bile ducts to reach the intestine and mix with the fat in our food. The bile acids dissolve the fat into the watery contents of the intestine, much like detergents in dishwater that dissolve grease from a frying pan. After the fat is dissolved, it is digested by enzymes from the pancreas and the lining of the intestine.

Absorption and Transport of Nutrients

Digested molecules of food, as well as water and minerals from the diet, are absorbed from the cavity of the upper small intestine. The absorbed materials cross the mucosa into the blood, mainly, and are carried off in the bloodstream to other parts of the body for storage or for further chemical change. As noted above, this part of the process varies with different types of nutrients.

Carbohydrates. An average American adult eats about half a pound of carbohydrate each day. Our most common and least costly foods contain mostly carbohydrate. Examples are bread, potatoes, pastries, candy, soft drinks, rice, spaghetti, fruits, and vegetables. Many of these foods contain both starch, which can

be digested, and fiber (sometimes called roughage), which the body cannot digest.

The digestible carbohydrates are broken into simpler molecules by enzymes in the saliva, in juice produced by the pancreas, and in the lining of the small intestine. Starch is digested in two steps: First, an enzyme in the saliva and pancreatic juice breaks the starch into molecules called maltose; then an enzyme in the lining of the small intestine (maltase) splits the maltose into glucose molecules that can be absorbed into the blood. Glucose is carried through the bloodstream to the liver, where it is stored or used to provide energy for the work of the body.

Table sugar is another carbohydrate that must be digested to be useful. An enzyme in the lining of the small intestine digests table sugar into glucose and fructose, each of which can be absorbed from the intestinal cavity into the blood. Milk contains yet another type of sugar, lactose, which is changed into absorbable molecules by an enzyme called lactase, also found in the intestinal lining.

Protein. Foods such as meat, eggs, and beans consist of giant molecules of protein that must be digested by enzymes before they can be used to build and repair body tissues. An enzyme in the juice of the stomach starts the digestion of swallowed protein. Further digestion of the protein is completed in the small intestine. Here, several enzymes from the pancreatic juice and the lining of the intestine carry out the breakdown of huge protein molecules into small molecules called amino acids. These small molecules can be absorbed from the hollow of the small intestine into the blood and then be carried to all parts of the body to build the walls and other parts of cells.

Fats. Fat molecules are a rich source of energy for the body. The first step in the digestion of a fat such as butter is to dissolve it into the watery content of the intestinal cavity. The bile acids produced by the liver act as natural detergents to dissolve fat in water and allow the enzymes to break the large fat molecules into smaller molecules, some of which are fatty acids and cholesterol. The bile acids combine with the fatty acids and cholesterol and help these molecules to move into the cells of the mucosa. In these cells the small molecules are formed back into large molecules, most of which pass into vessels (called lymphatics) near the intestine. These small vessels carry the re-formed fat to the veins of the chest, and the blood carries the fat to storage depots in different parts of the body.

Vitamins. Another vital part of our food that is absorbed from the small intestine is the class of chemicals we call vitamins. There are two different types of vitamins, classified by the fluid in which they can be dissolved: water-soluble vitamins (all the B vitamins and vitamin C) and fat-soluble vitamins (vitamins A, D, and K).

Water and salt. Most of the material absorbed from the cavity of the small intestine is water in which salt is dissolved. The salt and water come from the food and liquid we swallow and the juices secreted by the many digestive glands. In a healthy adult, more than a gallon of water containing over an ounce of salt is absorbed from the intestine every 24 hours.

HOW DIGESTION IS CONTROLLED
Hormone Regulators

A fascinating feature of the digestive system is that it contains its own regulators. The major hormones that control the functions of the digestive system are produced and released by cells in the mucosa of the stomach and small intestine. These hormones are released into the blood of the digestive tract, travel back to the heart and through the arteries, and return to the digestive system, where they stimulate the digestive juices and cause organ movement.

The hormones that control digestion are gastrin, secretin, and cholecystokinin (CCK).

- *Gastrin* causes the stomach to produce an acid for dissolving and digesting some foods. It is also necessary for the normal growth of the lining of the stomach, small intestine, and colon.
- *Secretin* causes the pancreas to send out a digestive juice that is rich in bicarbonate. It stimulates the stomach to produce pepsin, an enzyme that digests protein, and it also stimulates the liver to produce bile.
- *CCK* causes the pancreas to grow and to produce the enzymes of pancreatic juice, and it causes the gallbladder to empty.

Nerve Regulators

Two types of nerves help to control the action of the digestive system.

Extrinsic (outside) nerves come to the digestive organs from the unconscious part of the brain or from the spinal cord. They release a chemical called acetylcholine and another called adrenaline.

Acetylcholine causes the muscle of the digestive organs to squeeze with more force and increase the "push" of food and juice through the digestive tract. Acetylcholine also causes the stomach and pancreas to produce more digestive juice. Adrenaline relaxes the muscle of the stomach and intestine and decreases the flow of blood to these organs.

Even more important, though, are the intrinsic (inside) nerves, which make up a very dense network embedded in the walls of the esophagus, stomach, small intestine, and colon. The intrinsic nerves are triggered to act when the walls of the hollow organs are stretched by food. They release many different substances that speed up or delay the movement of food and the production of juices by the digestive organs.

The National Institute of Diabetes and Digestive and Kidney Diseases

GASTROESOPHAGEAL REFLUX DISEASE

Gastroesophageal reflux disease (GERD) is a digestive disorder that affects the lower esophageal sphincter (LES), the muscle connecting the esophagus with the stomach. Many people, including pregnant women, suffer from heartburn or acid indigestion caused by GERD. Doctors believe that some people suffer from GERD due to a condition called hiatal hernia. In most cases, heartburn can be relieved through diet and lifestyle changes; however, some people may require medication or surgery. This section provides information on GERD—its causes, symptoms, treatment, and long-term complications.

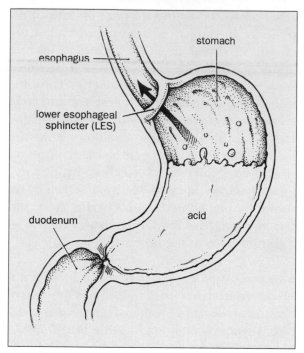

A weak lower esophageal sphincter (LES) or inappropriate relaxation of the LES allows stomach acid to escape into the esophagus, causing heartburn.

What is Gastroesophageal Reflux?

"Gastroesophageal" refers to the stomach and esophagus. "Reflux" means to flow back or return. Therefore, gastroesophageal reflux is the return of the stomach's contents back up into the esophagus.

In normal digestion, the LES opens to allow food to pass into the stomach and closes to prevent food and acidic stomach juices from flowing back into the esophagus. Gastroesophageal reflux occurs when the LES is weak or relaxes inappropriately, allowing the stomach's contents to flow up into the esophagus.

The severity of GERD depends on LES dysfunction as well as the type and amount of fluid brought up from the stomach and the neutralizing effect of saliva.

What Is the Role of Hiatal Hernia?

Some doctors believe a hiatal hernia may weaken the LES and cause reflux. Hiatal hernia occurs when the upper part of the stomach moves up into the chest through a small opening in the diaphragm (diaphragmatic hiatus). The diaphragm is the muscle separating the stomach from the chest. Recent studies show

that the opening in the diaphragm acts as an additional sphincter around the lower end of the esophagus. Studies also show that hiatal hernia results in retention of acid and other contents above this opening. These substances can reflux easily into the esophagus.

Coughing, vomiting, straining, or sudden physical exertion can cause increased pressure in the abdomen resulting in hiatal hernia. Obesity and pregnancy also contribute to this condition.

Many otherwise healthy people age 50 and over have a small hiatal hernia. Although considered a condition of middle age, hiatal hernias affect people of all ages.

Hiatal hernias usually do not require treatment. However, treatment may be necessary if the hernia is in danger of becoming strangulated (twisted in a way that cuts off blood supply, i.e., paraesophageal hernia) or is complicated by severe GERD or esophagitis (inflammation of the esophagus). The doctor may perform surgery to reduce the size of the hernia or to prevent strangulation.

What Other Factors Contribute to GERD?

Dietary and lifestyle choices may contribute to GERD. Certain foods and beverages, including chocolate, peppermint, fried or fatty foods, coffee, or alcoholic beverages, may weaken the LES causing reflux and heartburn. Studies show that cigarette smoking relaxes the LES. Obesity and pregnancy can also cause GERD.

What Does Heartburn Feel Like?

Heartburn, also called acid indigestion, is the most common symptom of GERD and usually feels like a burning chest pain beginning behind the breastbone and moving upward to the neck and throat. Many people say it feels like food is coming back into the mouth leaving an acid or bitter taste.

The burning, pressure, or pain of heartburn can last as long as two hours and is often worse after eating. Lying down or bending

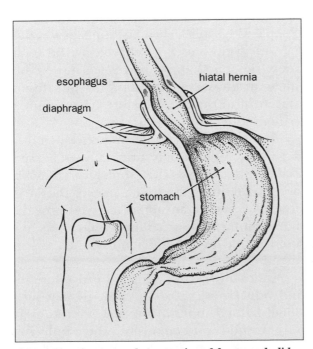

A hiatal hernia occurs when a portion of the stomach slides upward into the chest cavity, through the hiatus, or opening, of the diaphragm.

esophagus

diaphragm

hiatal hernia

stomach

TIPS TO CONTROL HEARTBURN

1. **Avoid foods and beverages that affect LES pressure or irritate the esophagus lining, including fried and fatty foods, peppermint, chocolate, alcohol, coffee, citrus fruit and juices, and tomato products.**
2. **Lose weight if overweight.**
3. **Stop smoking.**
4. **Elevate the head of the bed six inches.**
5. **Avoid lying down two to three hours after eating.**
6. **Take an antacid.**

---

over can also result in heartburn. Many people obtain relief by standing upright or by taking an antacid that clears acid out of the esophagus. Heartburn pain can be mistaken for the pain associated with heart disease or a heart attack, but there are differences. Exercise may aggravate pain resulting from heart disease, and rest may relieve the pain. Heartburn pain is less likely to be associated with physical activity.

How Common is Heartburn?

More than 60 million American adults experience GERD and heartburn at least once a month, and about 25 million adults suffer daily from heartburn. Twenty-five percent of pregnant women experience daily heartburn, and more than 50 percent have occasional distress. Recent studies show that GERD in infants and children is more common than previously recognized and may produce recurrent vomiting, coughing and other respiratory problems, or failure to thrive.

What Is the Treatment for GERD?

Doctors recommend lifestyle and dietary changes for most people with GERD. Treatment aims at decreasing the amount of reflux or reducing damage to the lining of the esophagus from refluxed materials.

Avoiding foods and beverages that can

weaken the LES is recommended. These foods include chocolate, peppermint, fatty foods, coffee, and alcoholic beverages. Foods and beverages that can irritate a damaged esophageal lining, such as citrus fruits and juices, tomato products, and pepper, should also be avoided.

Decreasing the size of portions at mealtime may also help control symptoms. Eating meals at least two to three hours before bedtime may lessen reflux by allowing the acid in the stomach to decrease and the stomach to empty partially. In addition, being overweight often worsens symptoms. Many overweight people find relief when they lose weight.

Cigarette smoking weakens the LES. Therefore, stopping smoking is important to reduce GERD symptoms.

Elevating the head of the bed on six-inch blocks or sleeping on a specially designed wedge reduces heartburn by allowing gravity to minimize reflux of stomach contents into the esophagus.

Take liquid antacids (Maalox or Mylanta II, for example) whenever heartburn occurs, especially after meals or at bedtime. Avoid Tums and Bisodol, because preparations containing calcium will increase the secretion of stomach acid.

Antacids taken regularly can neutralize acid in the esophagus and stomach and stop heartburn. Many people find that nonprescription antacids provide temporary or partial relief. An antacid combined with a foaming agent such as alginic acid helps some people. These compounds are believed to form a foam barrier on top of the stomach that prevents acid reflux from occurring.

Long-term use of antacids, however, can result in side effects, including diarrhea, altered calcium metabolism (a change in the way the body breaks down and uses calcium), and buildup of magnesium in the body. Too much magnesium can be serious for patients with kidney disease. If antacids are needed for more than three weeks, a doctor should be consulted.

For chronic reflux and heartburn, the doctor may prescribe medications to reduce acid in the stomach. These medicines include H_2-blockers, which inhibit acid secretion in the stomach. Currently, four H_2-blockers are available: cimetidine, famotidine, nizatidine, and ranitidine. Another type of drug, the proton pump (or acid pump) inhibitor omeprazole inhibits an enzyme (a protein in the acid-producing cells of the stomach) necessary for acid secretion. The acid pump inhibitor lansoprazole is currently under investigation as a new treatment for GERD.

Other approaches to therapy will increase the strength of the LES and quicken emptying of stomach contents with motility drugs that act on the upper gastrointestinal (GI) tract. These drugs include cisapride, bethanechol, and metoclopramide.

What If Symptoms Persist?
People with severe, chronic esophageal reflux or with symptoms not relieved by the treatment described above may need more complete diagnostic evaluation. Doctors use a variety of tests and procedures to examine a patient with chronic heartburn.

An upper GI series may be performed during the early phase of testing. This test is a special x-ray that shows the esophagus, stomach, and duodenum (the upper part of the small intestine). While an upper GI series provides limited information about possible reflux, it is used to rule out other diagnoses, such as peptic ulcers.

Endoscopy is an important procedure for individuals with chronic GERD. By placing a small lighted tube with a tiny video camera on the end (endoscope) into the esophagus, the doctor may see inflammation or irritation of the tissue lining the esophagus (esophagitis). If the findings of the endoscopy are abnormal or questionable, biopsy (removing a small sample of tissue) from the lining of the esophagus may be helpful.

The Bernstein test (dripping a mild acid through a tube placed in the mid-esophagus) is often performed. This test attempts to confirm that the symptoms result from acid in the esophagus. Esophageal manometric studies—pressure measurements of the esophagus—occasionally help identify critically low pressure in the LES or abnormalities in esophageal muscle contraction.

For patients in whom diagnosis is difficult, doctors may measure the acid levels inside the esophagus through pH testing. Testing pH monitors the acidity level of the esophagus and symptoms during meals, activity, and sleep. Newer techniques of long-term pH monitoring are improving diagnostic capability in this area.

Does GERD Require Surgery?

A small number of people with GERD may need surgery because of severe reflux and poor response to medical treatment. Fundoplication is a surgical procedure that increases pressure in the lower esophagus. However, surgery should not be considered until all other measures have been tried.

What Are the Complications of Long-Term GERD?

Sometimes GERD results in serious complications. Esophagitis can occur as a result of too much stomach acid in the esophagus. Esophagitis may cause esophageal bleeding or ulcers. In addition, a narrowing or stricture of the esophagus may occur from chronic scarring. Some people develop a condition known as Barrett's esophagus, which is severe damage to the skinlike lining of the esophagus. Doctors believe this condition may be a precursor to esophageal cancer.

Conclusion

Although GERD can limit daily activities and productivity, it is rarely life-threatening. With an understanding of the causes and proper treatment, most people will find relief.

The National Institute of Diabetes and Digestive and Kidney Diseases

H. PYLORI AND PEPTIC ULCER

During normal digestion, food moves from the mouth down the esophagus into the stomach. The stomach produces hydrochloric acid and an enzyme called pepsin to digest the food. From the stomach, food passes into the upper part of the small intestine, called the duodenum, where digestion and nutrient absorption continue.

An ulcer is a sore or lesion that forms in the lining of the stomach or duodenum where acid and pepsin are present. Ulcers in the

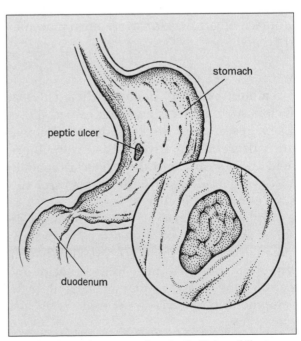

Peptic ulcers can occur anywhere in the lining of the stomach or duodenum. They may break through the lining, resulting in a perforated ulcer.

213

stomach are called gastric or stomach ulcers. Those in the duodenum are called duodenal ulcers. In general, ulcers in the stomach and duodenum are referred to as peptic ulcers. Ulcers rarely occur in the esophagus or in the first portion of the duodenum, the duodenal bulb.

WHO HAS ULCERS?

About 20 million Americans develop at least one ulcer during their lifetime. Each year:

- Ulcers affect about 4 million people.
- More than 40,000 people have surgery because of persistent symptoms or problems from ulcers.
- About 6,000 people die of ulcer-related complications.

Ulcers can develop at any age, but they are rare among teenagers and even more uncommon in children. Duodenal ulcers occur for the first time usually between the ages of 30 and 50. Stomach ulcers are more likely to develop in people over age 60. Duodenal ulcers occur more frequently in men than women; stomach ulcers develop more often in women than men.

WHAT CAUSES ULCERS?

For almost a century, doctors believed lifestyle factors such as stress and diet caused ulcers. Later, researchers discovered that an imbalance between digestive fluids (hydrochloric acid and pepsin) and the stomach's inability to defend itself against these powerful substances resulted in ulcers.

Today, research shows that most ulcers develop as a result of infection with bacteria called *Helicobacter pylori (H. pylori)*. While all three of these factors—lifestyle, acid and pepsin, and *H. pylori*—play a role in ulcer development, *H. pylori* is now considered the primary cause.

Lifestyle

While scientific evidence refutes the old belief that stress and diet cause ulcers, several lifestyle factors continue to be suspected of playing a role. These factors include cigarettes, foods and beverages containing caffeine or alcohol, and physical stress.

Smoking. Studies show that cigarette smoking increases one's chances of getting an ulcer. Smoking slows the healing of existing ulcers and also contributes to ulcer recurrence.

Caffeine. Coffee, tea, colas, and foods that contain caffeine seem to stimulate acid secretion in the stomach, aggravating the pain of an existing ulcer. However, the amount of acid secretion that occurs after drinking decaffeinated coffee is the same as that produced after drinking regular coffee. Thus, the stimulation of stomach acid cannot be attributed solely to caffeine.

Alcohol. Research has not found a link between alcohol consumption and peptic ulcers. However, ulcers are more common in people who have cirrhosis of the liver, a disease often linked to heavy alcohol consumption.

Stress. Although emotional stress is no longer thought to be a cause of ulcers, people with ulcers often report that emotional stress increases ulcer pain. Physical stress, however, increases the risk of developing ulcers, particularly in the stomach. For example, people with injuries such as severe burns and people undergoing major surgery often require rigorous treatment to prevent ulcers and ulcer complications.

Acid and pepsin. Researchers believe that the stomach's inability to defend itself against the powerful digestive fluids, acid and pepsin, contributes to ulcer formation. The stomach defends itself from these fluids in several ways. One way is by producing mucus—a lubricant-like coating that shields stomach tissues. Another way is by producing a chemical called bicarbonate. This chemical neutralizes and breaks down digestive fluids into substances less harmful to stomach tissue. Finally, blood circulation to the stomach lining, cell renewal, and cell repair also help protect the stomach.

Nonsteroidal anti-inflammatory drugs (NSAIDs) make the stomach vulnerable to the harmful effects of acid and pepsin. NSAIDs such as aspirin, ibuprofen, and naproxen sodium are present in many nonprescription medications used to treat fever, headaches, and minor aches and pains. These, as well as prescription NSAIDs used to treat a variety of arthritic conditions, interfere with the stomach's ability to produce mucus and bicarbonate and affect blood flow to the stomach and cell repair. They can all cause the stomach's defense mechanisms to fail, resulting in an increased chance of developing stomach ulcers. In most cases, these ulcers disappear once the person stops taking NSAIDs.

Helicobacter pylori

H. pylori is a spiral-shaped bacterium found in the stomach. Research shows that the bacteria (along with acid secretion) damage stomach and duodenal tissue, causing inflammation and ulcers. Scientists believe this damage occurs because of *H. pylori's* shape and characteristics.

H. pylori survives in the stomach because it produces the enzyme urease. Urease generates substances that neutralize the stomach's acid—enabling the bacteria to survive. Because of their shape and the way they move, the bacteria can penetrate the stomach's protective mucous lining. Here, they can produce substances that weaken the stomach's protective mucus and make the stomach cells more susceptible to the damaging effects of acid and pepsin.

The bacteria can also attach to stomach cells, further weakening the stomach's defensive mechanisms and producing local inflammation. For reasons not completely understood, *H. pylori* can also stimulate the stomach to produce more acid.

Excess stomach acid and other irritating factors can cause inflammation of the upper end of the duodenum, the duodenal bulb. In some people, over long periods of time, this inflammation results in production of stomachlike cells called duodenal gastric metaplasia. *H. pylori* then attacks these cells, causing further tissue damage and inflammation, which may result in an ulcer.

Within weeks of infection with *H. pylori*, most people develop gastritis—an inflammation of the stomach lining. However, most people will never have symptoms or problems related to the infection. Scientists do not yet know what is different in those people who develop *H. pylori*-related symptoms or ulcers. Perhaps, hereditary or environmental factors yet to be discovered cause some individuals to develop problems. Alternatively, symptoms and ulcers may result from infection with more virulent strains of bacteria. These unanswered questions are the subject of intensive scientific research.

Studies show that *H. pylori* infection in the United States varies with age, ethnic group, and socioeconomic class. The bacteria are more common in older adults, African Americans, Hispanics, and lower socioeconomic groups.

The *H. pylori* organism appears to spread through the fecal-oral route (when infected stool comes into contact with hands, food, or water). Most individuals seem to be infected during childhood, and their infection lasts a lifetime.

WHAT ARE THE SYMPTOMS OF ULCERS?

The most common ulcer symptom is a gnawing or burning pain in the abdomen between the breastbone and the naval. The pain often occurs between meals and in the early hours of the morning. It may last from a few minutes to a few hours and may be relieved by eating or by taking antacids.

Less common ulcer symptoms include nausea, vomiting, and loss of appetite and weight. Bleeding from ulcers may occur in the stomach and duodenum. Sometimes people are unaware that they have a bleeding ulcer, because blood loss is slow and blood may not be obvious in the stool. These people may feel tired and weak. If the bleeding is heavy, blood will appear in vomit or stool. Stool containing blood appears tarry or black.

HOW ARE ULCERS DIAGNOSED?

The NIH Consensus Panel emphasized the importance of adequately diagnosing ulcer disease and *H. pylori* before starting treatment. If the person has an NSAID-induced ulcer, treatment is quite different from the treatment for a person with an *H. pylori*-related ulcer. Also, a person's pain may be the result of nonulcer dyspepsia (persistent pain or discomfort in the upper abdomen, including burning, nausea, and bloating), and not at all related to ulcer disease. Currently, doctors have a number of options available for diagnosing ulcers, such as performing endoscopic and x-ray examinations, and for testing for *H. pylori*.

Locating and Monitoring Ulcers

Doctors may perform an upper GI series to diagnose ulcers. An upper GI series involves taking an x-ray of the esophagus, stomach, and duodenum to locate an ulcer. To make the ulcer visible on the x-ray image, the patient swallows a chalky liquid called barium.

An alternative diagnostic test is called an endoscopy. During this test, the patient is lightly sedated and the doctor inserts a small flexible instrument with a camera on the end through the mouth into the esophagus, stomach, and duodenum. With this procedure, the entire upper GI tract can be viewed. Ulcers or other conditions can be diagnosed and photographed, and tissue can be taken for biopsy, if necessary.

Once an ulcer is diagnosed and treatment begins, the doctor will usually monitor clinical progress. In the case of a stomach ulcer, the doctor may wish to document healing with repeat x-rays or endoscopy. Continued monitoring of a stomach ulcer is important because of the small chance that the ulcer may be cancerous.

Testing for *H. pylori*

Confirming the presence of *H. pylori* is important once the doctor has diagnosed an ulcer because elimination of the bacteria is likely to cure ulcer disease. Blood, breath, and stomach tissue tests may be performed to detect the presence of *H. pylori*. While some of the tests for *H. pylori* are not approved by the U.S. Food and Drug Administration (FDA), research shows these tests are highly accurate in detecting the bacteria. However, blood tests on occasion give false positive results, and the other tests may give false negative results in people who have recently taken antibiotics, omeprazole (Prilosec), or bismuth (Pepto-Bismol).

Blood tests. Blood tests such as the enzyme-linked immunosorbent assay (ELISA) and quick office-based tests identify and measure *H. pylori* antibodies. The body produces antibodies against *H. pylori* in an attempt to fight the bacteria. The advantages of blood tests are their low cost and availability to doctors The disadvantage is the possibility of false positive results in patients previously treated for ulcers because the levels of *H. pylori* antibodies fall slowly. Several blood tests have FDA approval.

Breath tests. Breath tests measure carbon dioxide in exhaled breath. Patients are given a substance called urea with carbon to drink. Bacteria break down this urea, and the carbon is absorbed into the bloodstream and lungs and exhaled in the breath. By collecting the breath, doctors can measure this carbon and determine whether *H. pylori* is present or absent. Urea breath tests are at least 90 percent accurate for diagnosing the bacteria and are particularly suitable for follow-up treatment to see if bacteria have been eradicated. These tests are awaiting FDA approval.

Tissue tests. If the doctor performs an endoscopy to diagnose an ulcer, tissue samples of the stomach can be obtained. The doctor may then perform one of several tests on the tissue. A rapid urease test detects the bacteria's enzyme urease. Histology involves visualizing the bacteria under the microscope. Culture involves specially processing the tissue and watching it for growth of *H. pylori* organisms.

HOW ARE ULCERS TREATED?
Lifestyle Changes
In the past, doctors advised people with ulcers to avoid spicy, fatty, or acidic foods. However, a bland diet is now known to be ineffective for treating or avoiding ulcers. No particular diet is helpful for most ulcer patients. People who find that certain foods cause irritation should discuss this problem with their doctor. Smoking has been shown to delay ulcer healing and has been linked to ulcer recurrence; therefore, persons with ulcers should not smoke.

Medicines
Doctors treat stomach and duodenal ulcers with several types of medicines, including H_2-blockers, acid pump inhibitors, and mucosal protective agents. When treating *H. pylori*, these medications are used in combination with antibiotics.

H_2-blockers. Currently, most doctors treat ulcers with acid-suppressing drugs known as H_2-blockers. These drugs reduce the amount of acid the stomach produces by blocking histamine, a powerful stimulant of acid secretion.

H_2-blockers reduce pain significantly after several weeks. For the first few days of treatment, doctors often recommend taking an antacid to relieve pain.

Initially, treatment with H_2-blockers lasts six to eight weeks. However, because ulcers recur in 50 to 80 percent of cases, many people must continue maintenance therapy for years. This may no longer be the case if *H. pylori* infection is treated. Most ulcers do not recur following successful eradication. Nizatidine (Axid) is approved for treatment of duodenal ulcers but is not yet approved for treatment of stomach ulcers. H_2-blockers that are approved to treat both stomach and duodenal ulcers are:

- Cimetidine (Tagamet)
- Ranitidine (Zantac)
- Famotidine (Pepcid)

Acid pump inhibitors. Like H_2-blockers, acid pump inhibitors modify the stomach's production of acid. However, acid pump inhibitors more completely block stomach acid production by stopping the stomach's acid pump—the final step of acid secretion. The FDA has approved use of omeprazole for short-term treatment of ulcer disease. Similar drugs, including lansoprazole, are currently being studied.

Mucosal protective medications. Mucosal protective medications protect the stomach's mucous lining from acid. Unlike H_2-blockers and acid pump inhibitors, protective agents do not inhibit the release of acid. These medications shield the stomach's mucous lining from the damage of acid. Two commonly prescribed protective agents are:

- Sucralfate (Carafate): This medication adheres to the ulcer, providing a protective barrier that allows the ulcer to heal and inhibits further damage by stomach acid. Sucralfate is approved for short-term treatment of duodenal ulcers and for maintenance treatment.
- Misoprostol (Cytotec): This synthetic prostaglandin, a substance naturally produced

by the body, protects the stomach lining by increasing mucus and bicarbonate production and by enhancing blood flow to the stomach. It is approved only for the prevention of NSAID-induced ulcers.

Two common nonprescription protective medications are:

- Antacids: Antacids can offer temporary relief from ulcer pain by neutralizing stomach acid. They may also have a mucosal protective role. Many brands of antacids are available without prescription.
- Bismuth subsalicylate: Bismuth subsalicylate has both a protective effect and an antibacterial effect against *H. pylori*.

Antibiotics. The discovery of the link between ulcers and *H. pylori* has resulted in a new treatment option. Now, in addition to treatment aimed at decreasing the production of stomach acid, doctors may prescribe antibiotics for patients with *H. pylori*. This treatment is a dramatic medical advance because eliminating *H. pylori* means the ulcer may now heal and most likely will not come back.

The most effective therapy, according to the NIH Panel, is a two-week, triple therapy. This regimen eradicates the bacteria and reduces the risk of ulcer recurrence in 90 percent of people with duodenal ulcers. People with stomach ulcers that are not associated with NSAIDs also benefit from bacterial eradication. While triple therapy is effective, it is sometimes difficult to follow because the patient must take three different medications four times each day for two weeks.

In addition, the treatment commonly causes side effects such as yeast infection in women, stomach upset, nausea, vomiting, bad taste, loose or dark bowel movements, and dizziness. The two-week, triple therapy combines two antibiotics, tetracycline (e.g., Achromycin or Sumycin) and metronidazole (e.g., Flagyl) with bismuth subsalicylate (Pepto-Bismol).

Some doctors may add an acid-suppressing drug to relieve ulcer pain and promote ulcer healing. In some cases, doctors may substitute amoxicillin (e.g., Amoxil or Trimox) for tetracycline or if they expect bacterial resistance to metronidazole, or other antibiotics such as clarithromycin (Biaxin).

As an alternative to triple therapy, several two-week, dual therapies are about 80 percent effective. Dual therapy is simpler for patients to follow and causes fewer side effects. A dual therapy might include an antibiotic, such as amoxicillin or clarithromycin, with omeprazole, a drug that stops the production of acid.

Again, an accurate diagnosis is important. Accurate diagnosis and appropriate treatment prevent people without ulcers from needless exposure to the side effects of antibiotics and should lessen the risk of bacteria developing resistance to antibiotics. Although all of the above antibiotics are sold in the United States, the FDA has not yet approved the use of antibiotics for treatment of *H. pylori* or ulcers. Doctors may choose to prescribe antibiotics to their ulcer patients as "off label" prescriptions as they do for many conditions.

WHEN IS SURGERY NEEDED?

In most cases, anti-ulcer medicines heal ulcers quickly and effectively. Eradication of *H. pylori* prevents most ulcers from recurring. However, people who do not respond to medication or who develop complications may require surgery. While surgery is usually successful in healing ulcers and preventing their recurrence and future complications, problems can sometimes result.

At present, standard open surgery is performed to treat ulcers. In the future, surgeons may use laparoscopic methods. A laparoscope is a long, tubelike instrument with a camera that allows the surgeon to operate through small incisions while watching a video monitor.

The common types of surgery for ulcers are described below:

Vagotomy. A vagotomy involves cutting the vagus nerve, a nerve that transmits messages from the brain to the stomach. Interrupting the messages sent through the vagus nerve reduces acid secretion. However, the surgery may also interfere with stomach emptying. The newest variation of the surgery involves cutting only parts of the nerve that control the acid-secreting cells of the stomach, thereby avoiding the parts that influence stomach emptying.

Antrectomy. Another surgical procedure is the antrectomy. This operation removes the lower part of the stomach (antrum), which produces a hormone that stimulates the stomach to secrete digestive juices. Sometimes a surgeon may also remove an adjacent part of the stomach that secretes pepsin and acid. A vagotomy is usually done in conjunction with an antrectomy.

Pyloroplasty. Pyloroplasty is another surgical procedure that may be performed along with a vagotomy. Pyloroplasty enlarges the opening into the duodenum and small intestine (pylorus), enabling contents to pass more freely from the stomach.

WHAT ARE THE COMPLICATIONS OF ULCERS?
People with ulcers may experience serious complications if they do not get treatment. The most common problems include bleeding, perforation of the organ walls, and narrowing and obstruction of digestive tract passages.

Bleeding. As an ulcer eats into the muscles of the stomach or duodenal wall, blood vessels may also be damaged, which causes bleeding. If the affected blood vessels are small, the blood may slowly seep into the digestive tract. Over a long period of time, a person may become anemic and feel weak, dizzy, or tired.

If a damaged blood vessel is large, bleed-

> **TYPICAL TWO-WEEK, DUAL THERAPY**
> • Amoxicillin two to four times a day, or clarithromycin three times a day
> • Omeprazole two times a day
>
> **TYPICAL TWO-WEEK, TRIPLE THERAPY**
> • Metronidazole four times a day
> • Tetracycline (or amoxicillin) four times a day
> • Bismuth subsalicylate four times a day

ing is dangerous and requires prompt medical attention. Symptoms include feeling weak and dizzy when standing, vomiting blood, or fainting. The stool may become a tarry black color from the blood.

Most bleeding ulcers can be treated endoscopically—the ulcer is located and the blood vessel is cauterized with a heating device or injected with material to stop bleeding. If endoscopic treatment is unsuccessful, surgery may be required.

Perforation. Sometimes an ulcer eats a hole in the wall of the stomach or duodenum. Bacteria and partially digested food can spill through the opening into the sterile abdominal cavity (peritoneum). This causes peritonitis, an inflammation of the abdominal cavity and wall. A perforated ulcer that can cause sudden, sharp, severe pain usually requires immediate hospitalization and surgery.

Narrowing and obstruction. Ulcers located at the end of the stomach where the duodenum is attached can cause swelling and scarring, which can narrow or close the intestinal opening. This obstruction can prevent food from leaving the stomach and entering the small intestine. As a result, a person may vomit the contents of the stomach. Endoscopic balloon dilation, a procedure that uses a balloon to force open a narrow passage, may be performed. If the dilation does not relieve the problem, then surgery may be necessary.

CONCLUSION

Although ulcers may cause discomfort, rarely are they life threatening. With an understanding of the causes and proper treatment, most people find relief. Eradication of *H. pylori* infection is a major medical advance that can permanently cure most peptic ulcer disease.

The National Institute of Diabetes and Digestive and Kidney Diseases

PANCREATITIS

The pancreas is a large gland behind the stomach and close to the duodenum. The pancreas secretes powerful digestive enzymes that enter the small intestine through a duct. These enzymes help in digesting fats, proteins, and carbohydrates. The pancreas also releases the hormones insulin and glucagon

Pancreatitis, or inflammation of the pancreas, activates the pancreas's own digestive enzymes, and the organ begins to attack itself.

into the bloodstream. These hormones play an important part in metabolizing sugar.

Pancreatitis is a rare disease in which the pancreas becomes inflamed. Damage to the gland occurs when digestive enzymes are activated and begin attacking the pancreas. In severe cases, there may be bleeding into the gland, serious tissue damage, infection, and cysts. Enzymes and toxins may enter the bloodstream and seriously injure organs, such as the heart, lungs, and kidneys.

There are two forms of pancreatitis. The acute form occurs suddenly and may be a severe, life-threatening illness with many complications. Usually, the patient recovers completely. If injury to the pancreas continues, such as when a patient persists in drinking alcohol, a chronic form of the disease may develop, bringing severe pain and reduced functioning of the pancreas that affects digestion and causes weight loss.

ACUTE PANCREATITIS

An estimated 50,000 to 80,000 cases of acute pancreatitis occur in the United States each year. This disease occurs when the pancreas suddenly becomes inflamed and then gets better. Some patients have more than one attack but recover fully after each one. Most cases of acute pancreatitis are caused either by alcohol abuse or by gallstones. Other causes may be use of prescribed drugs, trauma or surgery to the abdomen, or abnormalities of the pancreas or intestine. In rare cases, the disease may result from infections, such as mumps. In about 15 percent of cases, the cause is unknown.

Symptoms

Acute pancreatitis usually begins with pain in the upper abdomen that may last for a few days. The pain is often severe. It may be constant pain, just in the abdomen, or it may reach to the back and other areas. The pain may be sudden and intense, or it may begin as a mild pain that is aggravated by eating and slowly grows worse. The abdomen may be swollen and very tender. Other symptoms may include nausea, vomiting, fever, and an increased pulse rate. The person often feels and looks very sick.

About 20 percent of cases are severe. The patient may become dehydrated and have low blood pressure. Sometimes the patient's heart, lungs, or kidneys fail. In the most severe cases, bleeding can occur in the pancreas, leading to shock and sometimes death.

Diagnosis
During acute attacks, high levels of amylase (a digestive enzyme formed in the pancreas) are found in the blood. Changes also may occur in blood levels of calcium, magnesium, sodium, potassium, and bicarbonate. Patients may have high amounts of sugar and lipids (fats) in their blood too. These changes help the doctor diagnose pancreatitis. After the pancreas recovers, blood levels of these substances usually return to normal.

Treatment
The treatment a patient receives depends on how bad the attack is. Unless complications occur, acute pancreatitis usually gets better on its own, so treatment is supportive in most cases. Usually the patient goes into the hospital. The doctor prescribes fluids by vein to restore blood volume. The kidneys and lungs may be treated to prevent failure of those organs. Other problems, such as cysts in the pancreas, may need treatment too.

Sometimes a patient cannot control vomiting and needs to have a tube through the nose to the stomach to remove fluid and air. In mild cases, the patient may not have food for three or four days but is given fluids and pain relievers by vein. An acute attack usually lasts only a few days, unless the ducts are blocked by gallstones. In severe cases, the patient may be fed through the veins for three to six weeks while the pancreas slowly heals. Antibiotics may be given if signs of infection arise.

Surgery may be needed if complications such as infection, cysts, or bleeding occur. Attacks caused by gallstones may require removal of the gallbladder or surgery of the bile duct. Surgery is sometimes needed for the doctor to be able to exclude other abdominal problems that can simulate pancreatitis or to treat acute pancreatitis. When there is severe injury with death of tissue, an operation may be done to remove the dead tissue.

After all signs of acute pancreatitis are gone, the doctor will determine the cause and try to prevent future attacks. In some patients the cause of the attack is clear, but in others further tests need to be done.

What If the Patient Has Gallstones?
Ultrasound is used to detect gallstones and sometimes can provide the doctor with an idea of how severe the pancreatitis is. When gallstones are found, surgery is usually needed to remove them. When they are removed depends on how severe the pancreatitis is. If it is mild, the gallstones often can be removed within a week or so. In more severe cases, the patient may wait a month or more, until he improves, before the stones are removed. The CT (computed tomography) scan also may be used to find out what is happening in and around the pancreas and how severe the problem is. This is important information that the doctor needs to determine when to remove the gallstones.

After the gallstones are removed and inflammation subsides, the pancreas usually returns to normal. Before patients leave the hospital, they are advised not to drink alcohol and not to eat large meals.

CHRONIC PANCREATITIS
Chronic pancreatitis usually follows many years of alcohol abuse. It may develop after only one acute attack, especially if there is damage to the ducts of the pancreas. In the early stages, the doctor cannot always tell

whether the patient has acute or chronic disease. The symptoms may be the same. Damage to the pancreas from drinking alcohol may cause no symptoms for many years, and then the patient suddenly has an attack of pancreatitis. In more than 90 percent of adult patients, chronic pancreatitis appears to be caused by alcoholism. This is more common in men than women and often develops between 30 and 40 years of age. In other cases, pancreatitis may be inherited. Scientists do not know why the inherited form occurs. Patients with chronic pancreatitis tend to have three kinds of problems: pain, malabsorption of food leading to weight loss, or diabetes.

Some patients do not have any pain, but most do. Pain may be constant in the back and abdomen, and for some patients, the pain attacks are disabling. In some cases, the abdominal pain goes away as the condition advances. Doctors think this happens because pancreatic enzymes are no longer being made by the pancreas.

Patients with this disease often lose weight, even when their appetite and eating habits are normal. This occurs because the body does not secrete enough pancreatic enzymes to break down food, so nutrients are not absorbed normally. Poor digestion leads to loss of fat, protein, and sugar into the stool. Diabetes may also develop at this stage if the insulin-producing cells of the pancreas (islet cells) have been damaged.

Diagnosis

Diagnosis may be difficult but is aided by a number of new techniques. Pancreatic function tests help the physician decide if the pancreas still can make enough digestive enzymes. The doctor can see abnormalities in the pancreas using several techniques (ultrasonic imaging, endoscopic retrograde cholangiopancreatography [ERCP], and the CT scan). In more advanced stages of the disease, when diabetes and malabsorption (a problem due to lack of enzymes) occur, the doctor can use a number of blood, urine, and stool tests to help in the diagnosis of chronic pancreatitis and to monitor the progression of the disorder.

Treatment

The doctor treats chronic pancreatitis by relieving pain and managing the nutritional and metabolic problems. The patient can reduce the amount of fat and protein lost in stools by cutting back on dietary fat and taking pills containing pancreatic enzymes. This will result in better nutrition and weight gain. Sometimes insulin or other drugs must be given to control the patient's blood sugar.

In some cases, surgery is needed to relieve pain by draining an enlarged pancreatic duct. Sometimes part or most of the pancreas is removed in an attempt to relieve chronic pain.

Patients must stop drinking, adhere to their prescribed diets, and take the proper medications in order to have fewer and milder attacks.

The National Institute of Diabetes and
Digestive and Kidney Diseases

CIRRHOSIS OF THE LIVER

Many people think that cirrhosis is a disease. Cirrhosis is really what happens to the liver as a result of disease. The liver weighs about three pounds and is the largest organ in the body. It is located in the upper right side of the abdomen. When chronic diseases cause the liver to become permanently injured and scarred, the condition is called cirrhosis.

The scar tissue that forms in cirrhosis harms the structure of the liver, blocking the flow of blood through the organ. The loss of normal liver tissue slows the processing of nutrients, hormones, drugs, and toxins by the liver. Also slowed is production of proteins and other substances made by the liver.

Cirrhosis is the seventh leading cause of

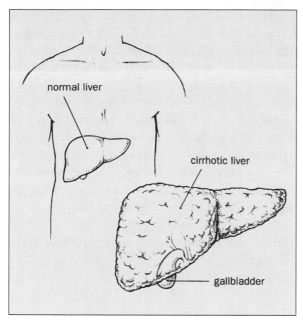

In a cirrhotic liver, healthy cells die and are replaced by scar tissue. Initially, the liver enlarges; in end-stage cirrhosis, the liver shrivels.

the liver and in other organs, such as the pancreas, skin, intestinal lining, heart, and endocrine glands.

If a person's bile duct becomes blocked, this also may cause cirrhosis. The bile ducts carry bile formed in the liver to the intestines, where the bile helps in the digestion of fat.

Alterations in the immune system can cause inflammation, scarring, and blockage of the larger bile ducts, a condition called primary sclerosing cholangitis. A type of biliary cirrhosis may occur after a patient has gallbladder surgery in which the bile ducts are injured or tied off.

Other, less common, causes of cirrhosis are severe reactions to prescribed drugs, prolonged exposure to environmental toxins, and repeated bouts of heart failure with liver congestion.

death by disease. About 25,000 people die from cirrhosis each year. There also is a great toll in terms of human suffering, hospital costs, and work loss by people with cirrhosis.

CAUSES

Cirrhosis has many causes. In the United States, chronic alcoholism is the most common cause. Cirrhosis also may result from chronic viral hepatitis (types B, C, and D). Liver injury that results in cirrhosis also may be caused by a number of inherited diseases such as cystic fibrosis, alpha-l antitrypsin deficiency, hemochromatosis, Wilson's disease, galactosemia, and glycogen storage diseases.

Two inherited disorders result in the abnormal storage of metals in the liver, leading to tissue damage and cirrhosis. People with Wilson's disease store too much copper in their livers, brains, kidneys, and in the corneas of their eyes. In another disorder, known as hemochromatosis, too much iron is absorbed, and the excess iron is deposited in

SYMPTOMS

People with cirrhosis often have few symptoms at first. The two major problems that eventually cause symptoms are loss of functioning liver cells and distortion of the liver caused by scarring. The person may experience fatigue, weakness, and exhaustion. Loss of appetite is usual, often with nausea and weight loss.

As liver function declines, less protein is made by the organ. For example, less of the protein albumin is made, which results in water accumulating in the legs (edema) or abdomen (ascites). A decrease in proteins needed for blood clotting makes it easy for the person to bruise or to bleed.

In the later stages of cirrhosis, jaundice (yellow skin) may occur, caused by the buildup of bile pigment that is passed by the liver into the intestines. Some people with cirrhosis experience intense itching due to bile products that are deposited in the skin. Gallstones often form in persons with cirrhosis because not enough bile reaches the gallbladder.

The liver of a person with cirrhosis also has

trouble removing toxins, which may build up in the blood. These toxins can dull mental function and lead to personality changes and even coma (encephalopathy). Early signs of toxin accumulation in the brain may include neglect of personal appearance, unresponsiveness, forgetfulness, trouble concentrating, or changes in sleeping habits.

Drugs taken are usually filtered out by the liver, and this cleansing process also is slowed down by cirrhosis. The liver does not remove the drugs from the blood at the usual rate, so the drugs act longer than expected, building up in the body. People with cirrhosis often are very sensitive to medications and their side effects.

A serious problem for people with cirrhosis is pressure on blood vessels that flow through the liver. Normally, blood from the intestines and spleen is pumped to the liver through the portal vein. But in cirrhosis, this normal flow of blood is slowed, building pressure in the portal vein (portal hypertension). This blocks the normal flow of blood, causing the spleen to enlarge. So blood from the intestines tries to find a way around the liver through new vessels.

Some of these new blood vessels become quite large and are called "varices." These vessels may form in the stomach and esophagus (the tube that connects the mouth with the stomach). They have thin walls and carry high pressure. There is great danger that they may break, causing a serious bleeding problem in the upper stomach or esophagus. If this happens, the patient's life is in danger, and the doctor must act quickly to stop the bleeding.

DIAGNOSIS

The doctor often can diagnose cirrhosis from the patient's symptoms and from laboratory tests. During a physical exam, for instance, the doctor could notice a change in how the liver feels or how large it is. If the doctor suspects cirrhosis, blood tests will be given. The purpose of these tests is to find out if liver disease is present. In some cases, other tests that take pictures of the liver are performed, such as the computed tomography (CT) scan, ultrasound, and the radioisotope liver/spleen scan.

The doctor may decide to confirm the diagnosis by putting a needle through the skin (biopsy) to take a sample of tissue from the liver. In some cases, cirrhosis is diagnosed during surgery when the doctor is able to see the entire liver. The liver also can be inspected through a laparoscope, a viewing device that is inserted through a tiny incision made in the abdomen.

TREATMENT

Treatment of cirrhosis is aimed at stopping or delaying its progress, minimizing the damage to liver cells, and reducing complications. In alcoholic cirrhosis, for instance, the person must stop drinking alcohol to halt progression of the disease. If a person has hepatitis, the doctor may administer steroids or antiviral drugs to reduce liver cell injury.

Medications may be given to control the symptoms of cirrhosis, such as itching. Edema and ascites (fluid retention) are treated by reducing salt in the diet. Drugs called diuretics are used to remove excess fluid and to prevent edema from recurring. Diet and drug therapies can help to improve the altered mental function that cirrhosis can cause. For instance, decreasing dietary protein results in less toxin formation in the digestive tract. Laxatives such as lactulose may be given to help absorb toxins and speed their removal from the intestines.

The two main problems in cirrhosis are liver failure, when liver cells just stop working, and the bleeding caused by portal hypertension. The doctor may prescribe blood pressure medication, such as a beta-blocker, to treat the portal hypertension. If the patient bleeds from the varices of the stomach or esophagus, the doctor can inject these veins with a sclerosing agent administered through a flexible tube (endoscope) that is inserted through the mouth and esophagus. In critical cases, the patient may be given a liver transplant or another surgery (such as a portacaval shunt) that is sometimes used to relieve the pressure in the portal vein and varices.

Patients with cirrhosis often live healthy lives for many years. Even when complications develop, they can be treated. Many patients with cirrhosis have undergone successful liver transplantation.

The National Institute of Diabetes and Digestive and Kidney Diseases

VIRAL HEPATITIS

Viral hepatitis is the most common of the serious contagious diseases caused by several viruses that attack the liver. About 70,000 cases are reported to the Centers for Disease Control each year, but this represents only a fraction of the cases occurring in this country.

Hepatitis means inflammation of the liver, usually producing swelling and tenderness and sometimes permanent damage to the liver. Hepatitis may also be caused by nonviral substances such as alcohol, chemicals, and drugs. These types of hepatitis are known respectively as alcoholic, toxic, and drug-induced hepatitis.

TYPES OF VIRAL HEPATITIS
At least five types of viral hepatitis are currently known, each caused by a different identified virus.

- *Hepatitis A,* formerly called infectious hepatitis, is most common in children in developing countries, but is being seen more frequently in adults in the western world.

- *Hepatitis B,* formerly called serum hepatitis, is the most serious form of hepatitis, with over 300 million carriers in the world and an estimated 1.2 million in the U.S.
- *Hepatitis C,* formerly called non-A, non-B hepatitis, is now the most common cause of hepatitis after blood transfusion. More than 3.9 million Americans are carriers of the virus.
- *Hepatitis D,* formerly called delta hepatitis, is found mainly in intravenous drug users who are carriers of the hepatitis B virus, which is necessary for the hepatitis D virus to spread.
- *Hepatitis E,* formerly called enteric or epidemic non-A, non-B hepatitis, resembles hepatitis A, but is caused by a different virus commonly found in the Indian Ocean area, Africa, and underdeveloped countries.
- *Other viruses,* especially members of the herpes virus family, including the cold sore virus, chicken pox virus, infectious mononucleosis virus, and others, can affect the liver as well as other organs they infect. This is particularly true when the immune system is impaired.

HOW THE INFECTION IS SPREAD
Hepatitis A and E viruses are excreted or shed in feces. Direct contact with an infected person's feces or indirect fecal contamination of food, the water supply, raw shellfish, hands, and utensils may result in sufficient amounts of virus entering the mouth to cause infections.

Hepatitis B is spread from mother to child at birth or soon after birth, through sexual contact, blood transfusions, or contaminated needles. Almost one-third of the cases may result from unknown sources in the general population. In families, the virus can be spread from adults to children.

Hepatitis C is spread directly from one person

to another via blood or contaminated needles. While sexual transmission and mother-to-child spread may occur, the transmission of this disease is not clearly understood.

Hepatitis D is spread mainly by contaminated needles and blood. Hepatitis D infects only individuals infected with hepatitis B and may be transmitted by carriers of hepatitis D and B.

SYMPTOMS

The most common symptoms are fatigue, mild fever, muscle or joint aches, nausea, vomiting, loss of appetite, vague abdominal pain, and sometimes diarrhea.

Many cases go undiagnosed because the symptoms are suggestive of a flulike illness or may be very mild or absent.

A minority of patients notice dark urine and light-colored stools, followed by jaundice in which the skin and whites of the eyes appear yellow. (Most individuals with viral hepatitis do not develop jaundice.) Itching of the skin may be present. With the onset of jaundice, other symptoms tend to subside. Some people may lose five to 10 pounds during the illness.

QUESTIONS FREQUENTLY ASKED

Can I get hepatitis again? Yes, because there are five or more hepatitis viruses, you can acquire different ones at different times. You will not be infected by the same virus as each produces its own immunity after the virus disappears. However, sometimes the viruses of B, C, and D hepatitis remain in the body forever. They can cause flare-ups of hepatitis that look like new disease.

What is a carrier and how can I tell if I am one? A carrier is a person who has hepatitis B, C, or D in his or her blood even after all symptoms (except fatigue) have disappeared. Because the virus is present in the blood, it can be transmitted to others. Hepatitis A does not have a chronic carrier state. The hepatitis B carrier can be recognized by a simple and specific blood test. Some of the carriers are contagious and others are not; this too can be determined by a simple blood test. Tests for the hepatitis C carrier have been developed. Prior to transfusion, all blood is now tested for abnormality of the liver function and for hepatitis B and C viruses. These tests have reduced the rate of the post-transfusion hepatitis C from 8 to 10 percent to 0.5 percent. Blood banks notify donors if they have found such abnormalities. Hepatitis D can be detected by a simple blood test for antibody to the virus and by a positive test for hepatitis B; both must be positive to be sure that the hepatitis D virus is present. Testing for hepatitis E is being developed but is not yet available.

What should I do if I have been exposed to or suspect that I have hepatitis? Consult a physician, who will examine you and order blood tests to confirm the diagnosis, identify the specific type of hepatitis, and advise about diet and activity. Any contacts should be notified about the infection and the need for immune globulin and vaccination for hepatitis A and B.

Should I see a specialist if I have hepatitis? Most physicians can care for a patient with an ordinary case of viral hepatitis. However, referral to a specialist in diseases of the liver (hepatologist, gastroenterologist) may be necessary if the disease appears to be unusually severe or complications are recognized.

Is hospitalization necessary? In most cases, no. Some patients are hospitalized if neither liquids nor food can be tolerated or if the disease is unusually severe or complications arise.

Are there medications for viral hepatitis? Interferon alpha-2b produces a remission of the disease in 35 percent of those with chronic hepatitis B and 25 percent of those infected with chronic hepatitis C. Only 10 percent of hepatitis B cases are cleared of the virus.

Ribavirin, in combination with interferon, improves the response to treatment.

If I take medicine for other purposes, can I continue to do so? Medications taken regularly should be reviewed by a physician and a decision made regarding their continuation. Because the liver plays a key role in processing drugs and this function may be impaired in the patient with hepatitis, medications are usually withheld unless they are essential for the treatment of other problems.

Can I exercise while I have hepatitis? Vigorous exercise during the acute stage of the disease should be discouraged. Light or moderate exercise may be undertaken as symptoms subside.

Must I stay in bed? Restriction to bed is not necessary for patients with viral hepatitis. A good general rule is: "If you feel well, get up, but if you do not, take it easy."

How great is the risk of hepatitis to me and my family? Infection within the family can occur with hepatitis A, B, or E. Prompt diagnosis and appropriate precautions with immune globulin or vaccination for hepatitis A and B are important for those who are exposed.

Do I need a special diet or vitamins? A nutritious, well-balanced diet with additional calorie-rich fluids (fruit juices) is normally sufficient during the illness. Since many patients describe a reduction in appetite and an increase in nausea as the day progresses, a hearty breakfast is often the best tolerated meal of the day. Small snacks between meals are encouraged if large meals cause prob-

lems. Vitamin supplements have no clear value if a balanced diet can be eaten.

Must I give up alcohol? All alcoholic beverages should be avoided during the acute phase of the disease since metabolism of the alcohol stresses the already sick liver. (Modest alcohol consumption later in the convalescent phase or after recovery is not harmful.)

Should I avoid sexual activity? Sexual activity does not seem to affect the disease or recovery. However, your partner may be at risk of acquiring the infection, especially of hepatitis B.

Do dishes and clothing of the patient need special care? Hot water and soap or detergent is sufficient for cleaning dishes or clothing of patients with hepatitis A or E. Special care must be taken if anything has blood on it when the patient has hepatitis B or C. Dishes, utensils, and clothing do not harbor the hepatitis B or C virus.

Can I prepare meals? If you have hepatitis A or E, you should not prepare meals or handle food to be eaten by others. However, you were especially contagious before the symptoms of hepatitis were recognized, and you may have already transmitted the infection or exposed others unknowingly.

If you have hepatitis B, C, or D, limitations on food handling are not necessary.

How long does the illness last? The onset is often abrupt and recovery occurs in a few weeks to a month or two. The contagious period lasts two to three weeks. With hepatitis B, the onset is more gradual and the course is longer. Over 90 to 95 percent of adult patients recover within six months, while 5 to 10 percent either develop chronic hepatitis or become carriers. The onset of hepatitis C is often not recognized and the disease becomes apparent months to years after infection. More than half of the patients who are infected by blood transfusions will develop chronic hepatitis with fluctuating symptoms and laboratory test results. Hepatitis D coinfection with hepatitis B acts as though it were very serious hepatitis B, but recovery after a few months is usual. Hepatitis D concurrent infection in a hepatitis B carrier looks like a flare-up of hepatitis B and symptoms may become lifelong. The symptoms of hepatitis E are like those of hepatitis A, although the period of illness may be as long as several months.

How long should I continue to see a doctor? You should continue to see your doctor until blood tests indicate the illness is clearly over. Abnormalities in the blood tests that persist beyond six months must be carefully evaluated, since they may indicate the development of chronic infections.

What are the complications of hepatitis? Fortunately, most people recover completely from hepatitis A, B, D, and E. Mild flare-ups may occur over a period of several months. Each flare-up is usually less severe than the initial attack, and a relapse does not necessarily indicate that complete recovery will not take place.

About 70 to 80 deaths are caused by hepatitis A each year. The mortality rate of hepatitis D and B is higher than for hepatitis B alone. Not enough is yet known of hepatitis E.

About 5 to 10 percent of patients with hepatitis B and more than 80 percent of patients with hepatitis C develop chronic liver disease, which may be mild and slowly progressive, or may be serious and rapidly lead to cirrhosis. The terms "chronic persistent" and "chronic aggressive" have been used for these two varieties, but we now know that the degree of activity varies with time and in different places in the liver at the same time. Cirrhosis is the final state of scarring which develops in chronic hepatitis. To determine how much scarring is present or how rapidly it may be progressing, a liver biopsy is usually necessary. Predicting who will develop chronic liver dis-

ease is not possible at the time of acute hepatitis. Identification of those at risk and methods to prevent these consequences are the subjects of ongoing research.

Is the spread of hepatitis preventable? Adequate sanitation and good personal hygiene will reduce the spread of hepatitis A and E. Water should be boiled prior to its use if any question of safety exists. Similarly, in areas where sanitation is questionable, food should be cooked well and fruits peeled. Washing hands with medicated soap, cleaning utensils, bedding, and clothing with soap and water is necessary for those involved in treating patients, especially in the first weeks of illness.

Those planning to travel to areas where hepatitis A is widespread are advised to take immune globulin or to be vaccinated before leaving. Protection with the immune globulin is effective for two to six months, and the vaccine for at least a year.

To prevent spread of hepatitis B, avoid exposure to infectious blood or body fluids. Do not have intimate contact, share razors, scissors, nail files, toothbrushes, or needles. If any risk is present, you should receive immune globulin and vaccine as soon as possible.

Blood banks are hard at work to insure the safety of the blood supply. Hepatitis B or C from transfusion is rare. Sharing needles with anyone should be avoided. Dentists, doctors, nurses, laboratory technicians, and others who may draw blood, perform surgical procedures, or handle sharp instruments used on hepatitis patients or carriers must be informed so that adequate precautions can be taken.

Family members and other intimate contacts must be advised to seek medical advice about immune globulin shots or vaccination.

Are there vaccines and can the disease be prevented? A vaccine for hepatitis A is given in two doses, the second six to 12 months after the first.

The vaccine for hepatitis B is derived from yeast and has replaced the plasma-derived vaccine in the U.S. It is safe and effective in preventing infection if started within a few days of exposure. The normal vaccination schedule used in the United States is two injections a month apart followed by a third injection six months after the first one. Hepatitis B immune globulin may also prevent infection after exposure, but it must be given within 48 hours to be useful. Since both vaccination and immune globulin are expensive, rapid confirmation of the diagnosis of hepatitis B is needed. Hepatitis D is prevented by preventing hepatitis B. No vaccine or immune globulin is yet available for hepatitis C or E.

Does hepatitis cause cancer? A high incidence of liver cancer is found in some African and Asian countries where there are many hepatitis B carriers and appears to be related to the chronic hepatitis B carrier state. Research on this relationship is being actively pursued.

The number of cases of liver cancer in patients with chronic hepatitis C is increasing, but whether the cancer rate will ever be as high as with hepatitis B is unknown. About 15 percent of hepatitis B carriers in the Orient are at risk of developing liver cancer, but the rate seems to be considerably lower in the United States.

Is hepatitis related to AIDS? Any relation between AIDS and hepatitis is coincidental. Male homosexuals and intravenous drug users who are at high risk for infection with the human immunodeficiency virus (HIV), the cause of AIDS, are at equally high risk for infection with the hepatitis B virus.

ADVANCES IN RESEARCH
Tremendous advances through research have been made in the field of viral hepatitis within the past decade. These all have followed iden-tification of the specific viruses that cause diseases and will result in development of vaccines that eventually will prevent the one million new cases of viral hepatitis occurring in children and adults each year in the United States.

Vaccination eventually will lead to the prevention of liver cancer found in chronic carriers of some of the viruses.

Recent research has discovered a laboratory method of detecting hepatitis C. This will lead to further reductions in hepatitis after blood transfusions. It will also enable better monitoring of treatment.

Research is also being carried out on drugs that have the potential for eradicating some of these viruses and for improving treament of chronic hepatitis.

The American Liver Foundation

GALLSTONES

This year, over one million people in the United States will discover that they have gallstones. They will join an estimated 20 million Americans, approximately 10 percent of the population, who have gallstones. Gallstones form within the gallbladder. Cholecystectomy, the surgical removal of the gallbladder, is the most common surgical procedure performed in the United States. Approximately 500,000 persons will undergo surgery to remove their gallbladder this year simply because of gallstones.

Who Is at Risk to Develop Gallstones?
People with certain characteristics have been associated with the development of gallstone disease. These include:

• People who are overweight
• Older persons
• Pregnant women
• Women who use hormone contraceptives and postmenopausal hormones

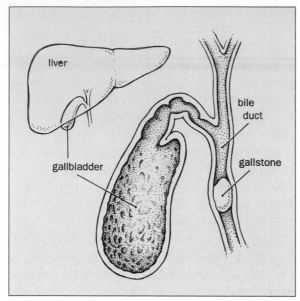

Gallstones may remain in the gallbladder or pass painlessly through the bile duct. Problems generally occur only when stones get trapped in the bile duct.

- Persons with a family history of gallstones
- Persons of Native American ancestry
- Persons with diseases of the small intestine
- Persons who have recently lost weight

The three most important risk factors for developing gallstone disease are body weight, increasing age, and being female. The risk of developing gallstones in obese persons is three to sevenfold greater than for persons of normal weight. Women are more likely to develop gallstones than men. Approximately 12 percent of all women, but only 8 percent of men, have gallstones. The risk of gallstones increases with age for men and women. By age 60, nearly 10 percent of men and over 20 percent of women have gallstones.

Rapid weight reduction has also been associated with the development of gallstones. However, several studies now demonstrate that it is not the actual weight loss which causes gallstones to form. Why gallstones form during weight loss is unclear.

We are just beginning to understand answers to questions, such as what causes gallstones to form and the relative roles of the liver and gallbladder in gallstone formation. Although many risk factors for developing gallstones have been identified, we still do not understand why some persons with many of these risk factors do not develop gallstones while others do. Researchers are working on answers to these questions.

What Is the Gallbladder and What Does It Do?
The gallbladder is a small pear-shaped organ that averages three to six inches in length. It lies underneath the liver in the upper right side of the abdomen. It is connected to the liver and small intestine by small tubes called bile ducts. Bile, a greenish-brown fluid, is utilized by the body to digest fatty foods and assists in the absorption of certain vitamins and minerals. The gallbladder serves as a reservoir for bile. Between meals, bile accumulates and is concentrated within this organ. During meals, the gallbladder contracts and empties bile into the intestine to assist in digestion.

What Are Gallstones and How Are They Formed?
Gallstones are lumps of solid material that form within the gallbladder. There are two major types of gallstones:

- *Cholesterol gallstones* are composed mainly of cholesterol which is made in the liver. These account for nearly 80 percent of all cases of gallstones in the United States.
- *Pigment gallstones* are composed of calcium salts, bilirubin, and other material. They account for the remaining 20 percent of gallstones in this country.

Excess cholesterol is removed from the blood by the liver and is then secreted into bile. When bile contains too much cholesterol, small crystals form in bile and they fall to the bottom of the gallbladder. This is like adding too much sugar to coffee and finding sugar at the bottom of the cup. Cholesterol crystals fuse together in the gallbladder to form stones of varying sizes.

Pigment gallstones are formed by the secretion of excess bile pigments and bilirubin into bile. The excess pigments and bilirubin form crystals in the gallbladder.

Gallstones vary in size. They may be as small as tiny specks, or as large as a small ball. The vast majority measure less than 20 mm, about one inch, across. Over time gallstones may grow in size or numbers. However, many gallstones remain the same size for years.

Gallbladder sludge occurs when multiple crystals of cholesterol and bilirubin pigments accumulate within the gallbladder but do not fuse together to form a gallstone. Gallbladder sludge typically occurs with fasting and resolves spontaneously. In some but not all persons, gallbladder sludge can develop into gallstones. In the majority of cases, gallbladder sludge is asymptomatic. However, sludge may cause symptoms identical to those attributed to gallstones.

How Often Do Gallstones Cause Problems?
Approximately 80 percent of all gallstones are completely asymptomatic and "silent." These stones cause no problems and there is no need for treatment. Once symptoms arise, not only do they persist but they increase in frequency. The chance that a "silent" gallstone will become symptomatic is 2 percent for each year. The longer gallstones are present, the more likely it is that they could cause symptoms. However, it will take approximately 25 years for the majority of persons with asymptomatic gallstones to develop symptoms. When symptoms occur in the elderly, they can be more difficult to treat, especially if the person has other medical problems.

What Are the Signs and Symptoms of Gallstone Disease?
Symptoms of gallbladder disease occur when gallstones irritate the gallbladder. The most common symptoms associated with gallstone disease include:

- Severe and intermittent pain in the right upper abdomen. This pain can also spread to the chest, shoulders, or back. Sometimes this pain may be mistaken for a heart attack.
- Chronic indigestion and nausea.

In addition to these symptoms, gallstones can also cause more serious complications. These occur when stones are expelled from the gallbladder during contraction and become lodged within bile ducts. This can lead to infection and obstruction of these ducts. When this occurs it is called acute cholecystitis (if the infection is within the gallbladder) or cholangitis (if the infection is within the bile ducts). Occasionally gallstones may block the bile duct at the entrance to the pancreas and intestine, causing pancreatitis (inflammation of the pancreas).

Gallstones are the most common cause of acute pancreatitis. If gallstones block the bile ducts for many years, then liver damage occurs, leading to liver failure. In rare cases, large gallstones may move into the small intestine and cause obstruction near the junction of the small and large intestine.

The most common symptoms associated with these complications include the following:

- Severe and steady pain in the right upper abdomen that does not resolve on its own
- Fever and chills
- Severe nausea with vomiting
- Severe pain in the middle of the abdomen and back
- Jaundice, a yellow discoloration of the skin and eyes

How Are Gallstones Identified?
Nearly all gallstones can be easily identified by an ultrasound examination. This is a simple and painless procedure in which sound waves

are utilized to create pictures of the gallbladder, bile ducts, and its contents. This test is highly sensitive for identifying either gallstones or sludge within the gallbladder.

If gallstones are suspected within the bile ducts, then more specific and complicated testing may need to be performed. The most common test to evaluate bile ducts is called ERCP (endoscopic retrograde cholangiopancreatography). This involves swallowing a small flexible tube through which a physician looks. The tube is then passed through the stomach and into the small intestine where the bile duct enters. Dye is then injected into the bile ducts, and x-rays are taken.

If it is impossible to perform the ERCP, then a PTC (percutaneous transhepatic cholangiogram) can be done. In this test, a very thin needle is passed through the abdomen into the bile ducts, dye is injected, and an x-ray is taken.

How Can Gallstones Be Treated?

Surgery. The gallbladder is an important organ but is not essential for life. Many patients with gallstones or its complications have their gallbladders surgically removed safely. Until recently this was performed by "open" surgery, where the surgeon makes a large abdominal incision. Now the preferred surgical technique is to remove the gallbladder through a half-inch incision using a pencil-thin microscope, a tiny video camera, and long, thin instruments that are inserted through other tiny incisions.

This procedure is called laparoscopic cholecystectomy. It is used in 80 percent of the gallbladder removals because it is relatively safe, reduces the hospital stay to a day or two, is less painful, and allows the patient to return to work or normal activity in a short time. A medical committee of the National Institutes of Health said the laparoscopic technique is used in 400,000 of the 500,000 gallbladder removals performed annually.

The risk of surgically removing the gall-

bladder increases with the patient's age and when the patient has other medical illnesses. When the gallbladder is removed, bile flows directly from the liver into the small intestine. For most patients, this has little to no effect on digestion. However, some patients may continue to have symptoms of gas, intermittent pain, bloating, and nausea.

Medication. An oral medication, ursodiol, dissolves cholesterol gallstones and is a safe alternative to gallbladder surgery. Ursodiol is a natural bile salt that reduces the amount of cholesterol the liver secretes into bile. The time required to dissolve is directly related to the size of the stone. Multiple small stones dissolve more easily than a single large stone. On average, the time required to dissolve gallstones is approximately six months. Symptoms, however, resolve in the majority of patients soon after starting this medication.

Ursodiol is rarely utilized and often works poorly. A major problem with ursodiol treatment is the high incidence of recurrent stones, up to 70 percent, especially in elderly patients. It is used mostly in patients who are too ill to tolerate surgery.

Other Treatments. The following techniques are considered experimental and are available only on a limited basis.

Shock-wave lithotripsy is a technique that utilizes sound waves to crush and fragment stones into small pieces. The pieces are then dissolved by the oral medication ursodiol. This technique is best utilized for persons with a single large gallstone.

Contact dissolution involves inserting a needle through the abdomen into the gallbladder and instilling an agent that rapidly dissolves the stones. Utilizing this technique, most gallstones can be dissolved in hours. The needle is then removed.

Only a small proportion of patients are good candidates for shock-wave lithotripsy. Moreover, the cost-effectiveness of this treatment has been questioned.

Can Gallstones Be Prevented?

Recent studies have suggested that persons at highest risk for gallstone formation, obese persons undergoing weight reduction, can virtually eliminate their risk for developing gallstones by taking the oral medication urso-diol. Prevention of gallstone formation with ursodiol in persons with other risk factors has not been investigated.

The American Liver Foundation

CROHN'S DISEASE

Inflammatory bowel disease (IBD) is a group of chronic disorders that cause inflammation or ulceration in the small and large intestines. Most often IBD is classified as ulcerative colitis or Crohn's disease but may be referred to as colitis, enteritis, ileitis, and proctitis.

Ulcerative colitis causes ulceration and inflammation of the inner lining of the colon and rectum, while Crohn's disease is an inflammation that extends into the deeper layers of the intestinal wall. Ulcerative colitis and Crohn's disease cause similar symptoms that often resemble other conditions such as irritable bowel syndrome (spastic colitis). The correct diagnosis may take some time.

Crohn's disease usually involves the small intestine, most often the lower part (the ileum). In some cases, both the small and large intestine (colon or bowel) are affected. In other cases, only the colon is involved. Sometimes inflammation also may affect the mouth, esophagus, stomach, duodenum, appendix, or anus. Crohn's disease is a chronic condition and may recur at various times over

a lifetime. Some people have long periods of remission, sometimes for years, when they are free of symptoms. There is no way to predict when a remission may occur or when symptoms will return.

What Are the Symptoms?

The most common symptoms of Crohn's disease are abdominal pain, often in the lower right area, and diarrhea. There also may be rectal bleeding, weight loss, and fever. Bleeding may be serious and persistent, leading to anemia (low red blood cell count). Children may suffer delayed development and stunted growth.

What Causes Crohn's Disease and Who Gets It?

There are many theories about what causes Crohn's disease, but none has been proven. One theory is that some agent, perhaps a virus or a bacterium, affects the body's immune system to trigger an inflammatory reaction in the intestinal wall. Although there is a lot of evidence that patients with this disease have abnormalities of the immune system, doctors do not know whether the immune problems are a cause or a result of the disease. Doctors believe, however, that there is little proof that Crohn's disease is caused by emotional distress or by an unhappy childhood.

Crohn's disease affects males and females equally and appears to run in some families. About 20 percent of people with Crohn's disease have a blood relative with some form of inflammatory bowel disease, most often a brother or sister and sometimes a parent or child.

How Is Crohn's Disease Diagnosed?

If you have experienced chronic abdominal pain, diarrhea, fever, weight loss, rectal bleeding, and anemia, the doctor will examine you for signs of Crohn's disease. The doctor will take a history and give you a thorough physical exam. This exam will include blood tests to find out if you are anemic as a result of blood loss, or if there is an increased number of white blood cells, suggesting an inflammatory process in your body. Examination of a stool sample can tell the doctor if there is blood loss, or if an infection by a parasite or bacteria is causing the symptoms.

The doctor may look inside your rectum and colon through a flexible tube (endoscope) that is inserted through the anus. During the exam, the doctor may take a sample of tissue (biopsy) from the lining of the colon to look at under the microscope.

Later, you also may receive x-ray examinations of the digestive tract to determine the nature and extent of disease. These exams may include an upper gastrointestinal (GI) series, a small intestinal study, and a barium enema intestinal x-ray. These procedures are done by putting the barium, a chalky solution, into the upper or lower intestines. The barium shows up white on x-ray film, revealing inflammation or ulceration and other abnormalities in the intestine.

If you have Crohn's disease, you may need medical care for a long time. Your doctor also will want to test you regularly.

What Is the Treatment?

Several drugs are helpful in controlling Crohn's disease, but at this time there is no cure. The usual goals of therapy are to correct nutritional deficiencies; to control inflammation; and to relieve abdominal pain, diarrhea, and rectal bleeding.

Abdominal cramps and diarrhea may be helped by drugs such as loperamide or codeine once inflammation subsides. The drug sulfasalazine often lessens the inflammation, especially in the colon. This drug can be used for as long as needed, and it can be used along with other drugs. Side effects such as nausea, vomiting, weight loss, heartburn, diarrhea, and headache occur in a small percentage of cases. Patients who do not do well on sulfasalazine often do very well on related drugs known as mesalamine or 5-ASA agents.

More serious cases may require steroid drugs, antibiotics, or drugs that affect the body's immune system, such as azathioprine or 6-mercaptopurine (6-MP).

Can Diet Control Crohn's Disease?

No special diet has been proven effective for preventing or treating this disease. Some people find their symptoms are made worse by milk, alcohol, hot spices, or fiber. But there are no hard and fast rules for most people. Follow a good nutritious diet and try to avoid any foods that seem to make your symptoms worse. Large doses of vitamins are useless and may even cause harmful side effects.

The doctor may recommend nutritional supplements, especially for children with growth retardation. Special high-calorie liquid formulas are sometimes used for this purpose.

A small number of patients may need periods of feeding by vein. This can help patients who temporarily need extra nutrition, those whose bowels need to rest, or those whose bowels cannot absorb enough nourishment from food taken by mouth.

What Are the Complications of Crohn's Disease?

The most common complication is blockage (obstruction) of the intestine. Blockage occurs because the disease tends to thicken the bowel wall with swelling and fibrous scar tissue, narrowing the passage. Crohn's disease also may cause deep ulcer tracts that burrow all the way through the bowel wall into surrounding tissues, into adjacent segments of intestine, into other nearby organs such as the urinary bladder or vagina, or into the skin. These tunnels are called fistulas. They are a common complication and often are associated with pockets of infection or abscesses (infected areas of pus). The areas around the anus and rectum often are involved. Sometimes fistulas can be treated with medicine, but in many cases they must be treated surgically.

Crohn's disease also can lead to complications that affect other parts of the body. These systemic complications include various forms of arthritis, skin problems, inflammation in the eyes or mouth, kidney stones, gallstones, or other diseases of the liver and biliary system. Some of these problems respond to the same treatment as the bowel symptoms, but others must be treated separately.

Is Surgery Often Necessary?

Crohn's disease can be helped by surgery, but it cannot be cured by surgery. The inflammation tends to return in areas of the intestine next to the area that has been removed. Many Crohn's disease patients require surgery, either to relieve chronic symptoms of active disease that does not respond to medical therapy or to correct complications such as intestinal blockage, perforation, abscess, or bleeding. Drainage of abscesses or resection (removal of a section of bowel) due to blockage are common surgical procedures.

Sometimes the diseased section of bowel is removed. In this operation, the bowel is cut above and below the diseased area and reconnected. Infrequently, some people must have their entire colon removed (colectomy) and an ileostomy created.

In an ileostomy, a small opening is made in the front of the abdominal wall, and the tip of the lower small intestine (ileum) is brought to the skin's surface. This opening, called a stoma, is about the size of a quarter or a 50-cent piece. It usually is located in the right lower part of the abdomen in the area of the beltline. A bag is worn over the opening to collect waste, and the patient empties the bag periodically. The majority of patients go on to live normal, active lives with an ostomy.

The fact that Crohn's disease often recurs after surgery makes it very important for the patient and doctor to consider carefully the benefits and risks of surgery compared with other treatments. Remember, most people with this disease continue to lead useful and productive lives. Between periods of disease activity, patients may feel quite well and be free of symptoms. Even though there may be long-term needs for medicine and even periods of hospitalization, most patients are able to hold productive jobs, marry, raise families, and function successfully at home and in society.

The National Institute of Diabetes and Digestive and Kidney Diseases

ULCERATIVE COLITIS

Inflammatory bowel disease (IBD) is a group of chronic disorders that cause inflammation or ulceration in the small and large intestines. Most often IBD is classified as ulcerative colitis or Crohn's disease but may be referred to as colitis, enteritis, ileitis, and proctitis.

Ulcerative colitis causes ulceration and inflammation of the inner lining of the colon and rectum, while Crohn's disease is an inflammation that extends into the deeper layers of the intestinal wall. Crohn's disease also may affect other parts of the digestive tract, including the mouth, esophagus, stomach, and small intestine. Ulcerative colitis and Crohn's disease cause similar symptoms that often resemble other conditions, such as irritable bowel syndrome (spastic colitis). The correct diagnosis may take some time.

In ulcerative colitis, the inner lining of the large intestine (colon or bowel) and rectum becomes inflamed. The inflammation usually begins in the rectum and lower (sigmoid) intestine and spreads upward to the entire colon. The inflammation causes the colon to empty frequently, resulting in diarrhea. As cells on the surface of the lining of the colon die and slough off, ulcers (tiny open sores) form, causing pus, mucus, and bleeding.

Ulcerative colitis occurs most often in people ages 15 to 40, although children and older people sometimes develop the disease. Ulcerative colitis affects males and females equally and appears to run in some families.

What Are the Symptoms of Ulcerative Colitis?

The most common symptoms of ulcerative colitis are abdominal pain and bloody diarrhea. Patients also may experience fatigue, weight loss, loss of appetite, rectal bleeding, and loss of body fluids and nutrients. Severe bleeding can lead to anemia. Sometimes patients also have skin lesions, joint pain, inflammation of the eyes, or liver disorders. No one knows for sure why problems outside the bowel are linked with colitis. Scientists think these complications may occur when the immune system triggers inflammation in other parts of the body. These disorders are usually mild and go away when the colitis is treated.

What Causes Ulcerative Colitis?

The cause of ulcerative colitis is not known, and currently there is no cure, except through surgical removal of the colon. Many theories about what causes ulcerative colitis exist, but none has been proven. The current leading theory suggests that some agent, possibly a virus or an atypical bacterium, interacts with the body's immune system to trigger an inflammatory reaction in the intestinal wall.

Although much scientific evidence shows that people with ulcerative colitis have abnormalities of the immune system, doctors do not know whether these abnormalities are a cause or result of the disease. Doctors believe, however, that there is little proof that ulcerative colitis is caused by emotional distress or sensitivity to certain foods or food products or is the result of an unhappy childhood.

How Is Ulcerative Colitis Diagnosed?

If you have symptoms that suggest ulcerative colitis, the doctor will look inside your rectum and colon through a flexible tube (endoscope) inserted through the anus. During the exam, the doctor may take a sample of tissue (biopsy) from the lining of the colon to view under the microscope. You also may receive a barium enema x-ray of the colon to determine the nature and extent of disease. This procedure involves putting a chalky solution (barium) into the colon. The barium shows up white on x-ray film, revealing growths and other abnormalities in the colon.

The doctor will give you a thorough physical exam, including blood tests to see if you are anemic (as a result of blood loss), or if your white blood cell count is elevated (a sign of inflammation). Examination of a stool sample can tell the doctor if an infection, such as by amoebae or bacteria, is causing the symptoms.

If you have ulcerative colitis, you may need medical care for some time. Your doctor also will want to see you regularly.

How Serious Is This Disease?

About half of patients have only mild symptoms. Others suffer frequent fever, bloody diarrhea, nausea, and severe abdominal cramps. Only in rare cases, when complications occur, is the disease fatal. There may be remissions—periods when the symptoms go away—that last for months or even years. However, most patients' symptoms eventually return. This changing pattern of the disease can make it hard for the doctor to tell when treatment has helped.

What Is the Treatment?

While no special diet for ulcerative colitis is given, patients may be able to control mild symptoms simply by avoiding foods that seem to upset their intestine. In some cases, the doctor may advise avoiding highly seasoned foods or milk sugar (lactose) for a while. When treatment is necessary, it must be tailored for each case, since what may help one patient may not help another. The patient also should be given needed emotional and psychological support.

Patients with either mild or severe colitis are usually treated with the drug sulfasalazine.

This drug can be used for as long as needed, and it can be used along with other drugs. Side effects such as nausea, vomiting, weight loss, heartburn, diarrhea, and headache occur in a small percentage of cases. Patients who do not do well on sulfasalazine often do well on related drugs known as 5-ASA agents.

In some cases, patients with severe disease, or those who cannot take sulfasalazine-type drugs, are given adrenal steroids (drugs that help control inflammation and affect the immune system) such as prednisone or hydrocortisone. All of these drugs can be used in oral, enema, or suppository forms. Other drugs may be given to relax the patient or to relieve pain, diarrhea, or infection.

Patients with ulcerative colitis occasionally have symptoms severe enough to require hospitalization. In these cases, the doctor will try to correct malnutrition and to stop diarrhea and loss of blood, fluids, and mineral salts. To accomplish this, the patient may need a special diet, feeding through a vein, medications, or, sometimes, surgery.

The risk of colon cancer is greater than normal in patients with widespread ulcerative colitis. The risk may be as high as 32 times the normal rate in patients whose entire colon is involved, especially if the colitis exists for many years. However, if only the rectum and lower colon are involved, the risk of cancer is not higher than normal.

Sometimes precancerous changes occur in the cells lining the colon. These changes in the cells are called "dysplasia." If the doctor finds evidence of dysplasia through endoscopic exam and biopsy, it means the patient is more likely to develop cancer. Patients with dysplasia, or whose colitis affects the entire colon, should receive regular follow-up exams, which may involve colonoscopy (examination of the entire colon using a flexible endoscope) and biopsies.

About 25 to 40 percent of ulcerative colitis patients eventually require surgery for removal of the colon because of massive bleeding, chronic debilitating illness, perforation of the colon, or risk of cancer. Sometimes the doctor will recommend removing the colon when medical treatment fails or the side effects of steroids or other drugs threaten the patient's health. Patients have several surgical options, each of which has advantages and disadvantages. The surgeon and patient must decide on the best individual option.

The most common surgery is the proctocolectomy, the removal of the entire colon and rectum, with ileostomy, creation of a small opening in the abdominal wall where the tip of the lower small intestine, the ileum, is brought to the skin's surface to allow drainage of waste. The opening (stoma) is about the size of a quarter and is usually located in the right lower corner of the abdomen in the area of the beltline. A pouch is worn over the opening to collect waste and the patient empties the pouch periodically.

The proctocolectomy with continent ileostomy is an alternative to the standard ileostomy. In this operation, the surgeon creates a pouch out of the ileum inside the wall of the lower abdomen. The patient is able to empty the pouch by inserting a tube through a small, leak-proof opening in his or her side. Creation of this natural valve eliminates the need for an external appliance. However, the patient must wear an external pouch for the first few months after the operation.

Sometimes an operation that avoids the use of a pouch can be performed. In the ileoanal anastomosis ("pull-through operation"), the diseased portion of the colon is removed and the outer muscles of the rectum are preserved. The surgeon attaches the ileum inside the rectum, forming a pouch, or reservoir, that holds the waste.

This allows the patient to pass stool through the anus in a normal manner, although the bowel movements may be more frequent and watery than usual.

The decision about which surgery to have

is made according to each patient's needs, expectations, and lifestyle. People who are faced with this decision should remember that getting as much information as possible is important. Talk to a doctor, to nurses who work with patients who have had colon surgery (enterostomal therapists), and to other patients. In addition, read pamphlets and books, such as those available from the Crohn's & Colitis Foundation of America, before deciding.

Most people with ulcerative colitis will never need to have surgery. If surgery ever does become necessary, however, they may find comfort in knowing that after the surgery, the colitis is cured and most people go on to live normal, active lives.

The National Institute of Diabetes and Digestive and Kidney Diseases

IRRITABLE BOWEL SYNDROME

Irritable bowel syndrome (IBS) is a common disorder of the intestines that leads to crampy pain, gassiness, bloating, and changes in bowel habits. Some people with IBS have constipation (difficult or infrequent bowel movements); others have diarrhea (frequent loose stools, often with an urgent need to move the bowels); and some people experience both. Sometimes the person with IBS has a crampy urge to move the bowels but cannot do so.

Through the years, IBS has been called by many names—colitis, mucous colitis, spastic colon, spastic bowel, and functional bowel disease. Most of these terms are inaccurate. Colitis, for instance, means inflammation of the large intestine (colon). IBS, however, does not cause inflammation and should not be confused with ulcerative colitis, which is a more serious disorder.

The cause of IBS is not known, and as yet there is no cure. Doctors call it a functional disorder because there is no sign of disease when the colon is examined. IBS causes a great deal of discomfort and distress, but it does not cause permanent harm to the intestines and does not lead to intestinal bleeding of the bowel or to a serious disease such as cancer.

Often IBS is just a mild annoyance, but for some people it can be disabling. They may be afraid to go to social events, to go out to a job, or to travel even short distances. Most people with IBS, however, are able to control their symptoms through diet, stress management, and sometimes with medications prescribed by their physicians.

What Causes IBS?

The colon, which is about six feet long, connects the small intestine with the rectum and anus. The major function of the colon is to absorb water and salts from digestive products that enter from the small intestine. Two quarts of liquid matter enter the colon from the small intestine each day. This material may remain there for several days until most of the fluid and salts are absorbed into the body. The stool then passes through the colon by a pattern of movements to the left side of the colon, where it is stored until a bowel movement occurs.

Colon motility (contraction of intestinal muscles and movement of its contents) is controlled by nerves and hormones and by electrical activity in the colon muscle. The electrical activity serves as a "pacemaker" similar to the mechanism that controls heart function. Movements of the colon propel the contents slowly back and forth but mainly toward the rectum. A few times each day, strong muscle contractions move down the colon pushing fecal material ahead of them. Some of these strong contractions result in a bowel movement.

Because doctors have been unable to find an organic cause, IBS often has been thought to be caused by emotional conflict or stress. While stress may worsen IBS symptoms, research suggests that other factors also are important. Researchers have found that the colon muscle of a person with IBS begins to spasm after only mild stimulation. The person with IBS seems to have a colon that is more sensitive and reactive than usual, so it responds strongly to stimuli that would not bother most people.

Ordinary events such as eating and distention from gas or other material in the colon can cause an overreaction in the person with IBS. Certain medicines and foods may trigger spasms in some people. Sometimes the spasm delays the passage of stool, leading to constipation. Chocolate, milk products, or large amounts of alcohol are frequent offenders. Caffeine causes loose stools in many people, but it is more likely to affect those with IBS. Researchers also have found that women with IBS may have more symptoms during their menstrual periods, suggesting that reproductive hormones can increase IBS symptoms.

What Are the Symptoms of IBS?

If you are concerned about IBS, it is important to realize that normal bowel function varies from person to person. Normal bowel movements range from as many as three stools a day to as few as three a week. A normal movement is one that is formed but not hard, contains no blood, and is passed without cramps or pain.

People with IBS, on the other hand, usually have crampy abdominal pain with painful constipation or diarrhea. In some people, constipation and diarrhea alternate. Sometimes people with IBS pass mucus with their bowel movements. Bleeding, fever, weight loss, and persistent severe pain are not symptoms of IBS but may indicate other problems.

How Is IBS Diagnosed?

IBS usually is diagnosed after doctors exclude more serious organic diseases. The doctor will take a complete medical history that includes a careful description of symptoms. A physical examination and laboratory tests will be done. A stool sample will be tested for evidence of bleeding. The doctor also may do diagnostic procedures such as x-rays or endoscopy (viewing the colon through a flexible tube inserted through the anus) to find out if there is organic disease.

How Do Diet and Stress Affect IBS?

The potential for abnormal function of the colon is always present in people with IBS, but a trigger also must be present to cause symptoms. The most likely culprits seem to be diet and emotional stress. Many people report that their symptoms occur following a meal or when they are under stress. No one is sure why this happens, but scientists have some clues.

Eating causes contractions of the colon. Normally, this response may cause an urge to have a bowel movement within 30 to 60 minutes after a meal. In people with IBS, the urge may come sooner with cramps and diarrhea.

The strength of the response is often related to the number of calories in a meal, and especially the amount of fat in a meal. Fat in any form (animal or vegetable) is a strong stimulus of colonic contractions after a meal. Many foods contain fat, especially meats of all kinds, poultry skin, whole milk, cream, cheese, butter, vegetable oil, margarine, shortening, avocados, and whipped toppings.

Stress also stimulates colonic spasm in people with IBS. This process is not completely understood, but scientists point out that the colon is controlled partly by the nervous system. Mental health counseling and stress reduction (relaxation training) can help relieve the symptoms of IBS. However, doctors are quick to note that this does not mean IBS is the result of a personality disorder. IBS is at least partly a disorder of colon motility.

How Does a Good Diet Help IBS?

For many people, eating a proper diet lessens IBS symptoms. Before changing your diet, it is a good idea to keep a journal noting which foods seem to cause distress. Discuss your findings with your doctor. You also may want to consult a registered dietitian, who can help you make changes in your diet. For instance, if dairy products cause your symptoms to flare up, you can try eating less of those foods. Yogurt might be tolerated better because it contains organisms that supply lactase, the enzyme needed to digest lactose, the sugar found in milk products. Because dairy products are an important source of calcium and other nutrients that your body needs, be sure to get adequate nutrients in the foods that you substitute.

Dietary fiber may lessen IBS symptoms in many cases. Whole grain breads and cereals, beans, fruits, and vegetables are good sources of fiber. Consult your doctor before using an over-the-counter fiber supplement. High-fiber diets keep the colon mildly distended, which may help to prevent spasms from developing. Some forms of fiber also keep water in the stools, thereby preventing hard stools that are difficult to pass. Doctors usually recommend that you eat just enough fiber so that you have soft, easily passed, painless bowel movements. High-fiber diets may cause gas and bloating, but within a few weeks, these symptoms often go away as your body adjusts to the diet.

Large meals can cause cramping and diarrhea in people with IBS. Symptoms may be eased if you eat smaller meals more often or just eat smaller portions. This should help, especially if your meals are low in fat and high in carbohydrates such as pasta, rice, whole-grain breads and cereals, fruits, and vegetables.

Can Medicines Relieve IBS Symptoms?

There is no standard way of treating IBS. Your doctor may prescribe fiber supplements or occasional laxatives if you are constipated. Some doctors prescribe antispasmodic drugs or tranquilizers, which may relieve symptoms. Antidepressant drugs also are used sometimes in patients who are depressed.

The major concerns with drug therapy in IBS are the potential for drug dependency and the effects the disorder can have on lifestyle. In an effort to control their bowels or reduce stress, some people become dependent on laxatives or tranquilizers. If this happens, doctors try to withdraw the drugs slowly.

Is IBS Linked to More Serious Problems?

IBS has not been shown to lead to any serious, organic diseases. No link has been established between IBS and inflammatory bowel diseases such as Crohn's disease or ulcerative colitis. IBS does not lead to cancer. Some patients have a more severe form of IBS, and the fear of pain and diarrhea may cause them to withdraw from normal activities. In such cases, doctors may recommend mental health counseling.

The National Institute of Diabetes and Digestive and Kidney Diseases

DIVERTICULOSIS AND DIVERTICULITIS

Many people have in their colons small pouches that bulge outward through weak spots. These pouches, known as diverticula, are about the size of large peas. The condition of having diverticula is called diverticulosis. When the pouches become infected or inflamed, the condition is called diverticulitis. Diverticulosis and diverticulitis are also called diverticular disease.

SYMPTOMS

Most people with diverticulosis do not have any discomfort or symptoms. They may never know they have the condition. However, symptoms may include mild cramps, bloating, and constipation. Other diseases such as irritable bowel syndrome and stomach ulcers cause similar problems, so these symptoms do not always mean a person has diverticulosis. The most common symptom of diverticulitis is abdominal pain. The most common sign is tenderness around the left side of the lower abdomen. If infection is the cause, fever, nausea, vomiting, chills, cramping, and constipation may occur as well. The severity of symptoms depends on the extent of the infection and complications.

Diverticulitis can lead to complications such as infections, perforations or tears, blockages, or bleeding. These complications always require treatment to prevent them from progressing and causing serious illness.

Bleeding from diverticula is a rare complication. When diverticula bleed, blood may appear in the toilet or in your stool. Bleeding can be severe, but it may stop by itself and not require treatment. Doctors believe bleeding diverticula are caused by a small blood vessel in a diverticulum that weakens and finally bursts. If you have bleeding from the rectum, you should see your doctor. If the bleeding does not stop, surgery may be necessary.

The infection causing diverticulitis often clears up after a few days of treatment with antibiotics. If the condition gets worse, an abscess may form in the colon. An abscess is an infect-

ed area with pus that may cause swelling and destroy tissue. Sometimes the infected diverticula may develop small holes, called perforations. These perforations allow pus to leak out of the colon into the abdominal area. If the abscess is small and remains in the colon, it may clear up after treatment with antibiotics. If the abscess does not clear up with antibiotics, the doctor may need to drain it. To drain the abscess, the doctor uses a needle and a small tube called a catheter. The doctor inserts the needle through the skin and drains the fluid through the catheter. This procedure is called "percutaneous catheter drainage." Sometimes surgery is needed to clean the abscess and, if necessary, remove part of the colon.

A large abscess can become a serious problem if the infection leaks out and contaminates areas outside the colon. Infection that spreads into the abdominal cavity is called peritonitis. Peritonitis requires immediate surgery to clean the abdominal cavity and remove the damaged part of the colon. Without surgery, peritonitis can be fatal.

A fistula is an abnormal connection of tissue between two organs or between an organ and

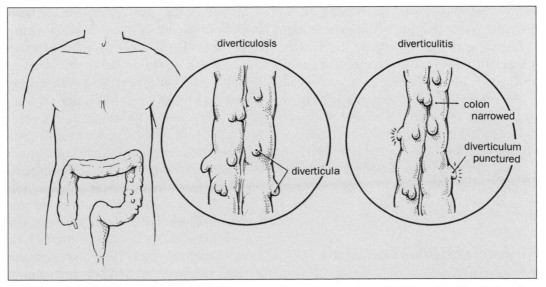

In diverticulosis, small pouches (diverticula) form in weakened areas in the wall of the colon. Should these become infected or inflamed (diverticulitis), serious problems can set in.

the skin. When damaged tissues come into contact with each other during infection, they sometimes stick together. If they heal that way, a fistula forms. When diverticulitis-related infection spreads outside the colon, the colon's tissue may stick to nearby tissues. The most common organs involved are the urinary bladder, small intestine, and skin. The most common type of fistula occurs between the bladder and the colon. It affects men more than women. This type of fistula can result in a severe, long-lasting infection of the urinary tract. The problem can be corrected with surgery.

The scarring caused by infection may cause partial or total blockage of the large intestine. When this happens, the colon is unable to move bowel contents normally. When the obstruction totally blocks the intestine, emergency surgery is necessary. Partial blockage is not an emergency, so the surgery to correct it can be planned.

DIAGNOSIS

To diagnose diverticular disease, the doctor asks about medical history, does a physical exam, and may perform one or more diagnostic tests. Because most people do not have symptoms, diverticulosis is often found through tests ordered for another ailment. When taking a medical history, the doctor may ask about bowel habits, symptoms, pain, diet, and medications. The physical exam usually involves a digital rectal exam. To perform this test, the doctor inserts a gloved, lubricated finger into the rectum to detect tenderness, blockage, or blood. The doctor may check stool for signs of bleeding and test blood for signs of infection. The doctor may also order x-rays or other tests.

HOW COMMON ARE THESE DISORDERS?

About half of all Americans age 60 to 80, and almost everyone over age 80, have diverticulosis. But among those who are found to have diverticula, only about 10 to 25 percent develop diverticulitis.

WHAT CAUSES DIVERTICULA TO FORM?

Doctors believe a low-fiber diet is the main cause of diverticular disease. Fiber is the part of fruits, vegetables, and grains that the body cannot digest. Some fiber dissolves easily in water (soluble fiber). It takes on a soft, jellylike texture in the intestines. Some fiber passes almost unchanged through the intestines (insoluble fiber). Both kinds of fiber help make stools soft and easy to pass. Fiber also prevents constipation. Constipation makes the muscles strain to move stool that is too hard. It is the main cause of increased pressure in the colon. The excess pressure causes the weak spots in the colon to bulge out and become diverticula. Diverticulitis occurs when diverticula become infected or inflamed. Doctors are not certain what causes the infection. It may begin when stool or bacteria are caught in the diverticula. An attack of diverticulitis can develop suddenly and without warning.

TREATMENT

A high-fiber diet and, occasionally, mild pain medications will help relieve symptoms in most cases. Until recently, many doctors suggested avoiding foods with small seeds such as tomatoes or strawberries because they believed that particles could lodge in the diverticula and cause inflammation. However, this is now a controversial point and no evidence supports this recommendation. Treatment for diverticulitis focuses on clearing up the infection and inflammation, resting the colon, and preventing or minimizing complications. An attack of diverticulitis without complications may respond to antibiotics within a few days if treated early. To help the colon rest, the doctor may recommend bed rest and a liquid diet, along with a pain reliever or a drug such as propantheline to control muscle spasms in the colon. An acute attack with severe pain or severe infection may require a hospital stay. Most acute cases of diverticulitis are treated with antibiotics and a liquid diet. The antibiotics are given by injection into a vein. In some cases, however, surgery may be necessary.

SURGERY

If attacks are severe or frequent, the doctor may advise surgery. The surgeon opens the abdomen and removes the affected part of the colon. The remaining sections of the colon are rejoined. This type of surgery, called colon resection, aims to keep attacks from coming back and to prevent complications. The doctor may also recommend surgery for complications of a fistula or intestinal obstruction. If antibiotics do not correct the attack, emergency surgery may be required. Other reasons for emergency surgery include a large abscess, perforation, peritonitis, or continued bleeding. Emergency surgery usually involves two operations. The first surgery will clear the infected abdominal cavity and remove part of the colon. Because of infection and sometimes obstruction, it is not safe to rejoin the colon during the first operation. The surgeon creates a temporary hole, or stoma, in the abdomen during the first operation. The end of the colon is connected to the hole, a procedure called a colostomy, to allow normal eating and bowel movement. The stool goes into a bag attached to the opening in the abdomen. In the second operation, the surgeon rejoins the ends of the colon.

The National Institute of Diabetes and Digestive and Kidney Diseases

CONSTIPATION

Constipation is passage of small amounts of hard, dry bowel movements, usually fewer than three times a week. People who are constipated may find it difficult and painful to have a bowel movement. Other symptoms of constipation include feeling bloated, uncomfortable, and sluggish.

Many people think they are constipated when, in fact, their bowel movements are regular. For example, some people believe they are constipated, or irregular, if they do not have a bowel movement every day. However, there is no right number of daily or weekly bowel movements. Normal may be three times a day or three times a week depending on the person. In addition, some people naturally have firmer stools than others.

At one time or another almost everyone gets constipated. Poor diet and lack of exercise are usually the causes. In most cases, con-

ORAL LAXATIVES

• Bulk-forming laxatives are generally considered the safest but can interfere with absorption of some medicines. These laxatives, also known as fiber supplements, are taken with water. They absorb water in the intestine and make the stool softer. Bulk laxatives include psyllium (Metamucil), methylcellulose (Citrucel), and bran (in food and supplements).

• Stimulants cause rhythmic muscular contractions in the small or large intestine. Products include phenolphthalein (Correctol, Ex-Lax), bisacodyl (Dulcolax), castor oil (Purge, Neoloid), and senna (Senokot, Fletcher's Castoria).

• Stool softeners provide moisture to the stool and prevent dehydration. These laxatives often are recommended after childbirth or surgery. Products include those with docusate (Colace, Dialose, and Surfak).

• Lubricants grease the stool enabling it to move through the intestine more easily. Mineral oil is the most commonly used lubricant.

• Saline laxatives, or osmotics, act like a sponge to draw water into the colon for easier passage of stool. Laxatives in this group include milk of magnesia, citrate of magnesia, lactulose, and Epsom salts.

stipation is temporary and not serious. Understanding causes, prevention, and treatment will help most people find relief.

WHO GETS CONSTIPATED?

According to the 1991 National Health Interview Survey, about 4.5 million people in the United States say they are constipated most or all of the time. Those reporting constipation most often are women, children, and adults age 65 and over. Pregnant women also complain of constipation, and it is a common problem following childbirth or surgery.

Constipation is the most common gastrointestinal complaint in the United States, resulting in about 2 million annual visits to the doctor. However, most people treat themselves without seeking medical help, as is evident from the $725 million Americans spend on laxatives each year.

CAUSES

To understand constipation, it helps to know how the colon (large intestine) works. As food moves through it, the colon absorbs water while forming waste products, or stool. Muscle contractions in the colon push the stool toward the rectum. By the time stool reaches the rectum, it is solid because most of the water has been absorbed.

The hard and dry stools of constipation occur when the colon absorbs too much water. This happens because the colon's muscle contractions are slow or sluggish, causing the stool to move through the colon too slowly.

- *Poor diet.* The most common cause of constipation is a diet high in animal fats (meats, dairy products, eggs), but low in fiber (vegetables, fruits, whole grains). Fiber—soluble and insoluble—is the part of fruits, vegetables, and grains that the body cannot digest. Soluble fiber dissolves easily in water and takes on a soft, gel-like texture in the intestines. Insoluble fiber passes almost unchanged through the intestines. The bulk and soft texture of fiber help prevent hard, dry stools that are difficult to pass.

- *Not enough liquids.* Liquids like water and juice add fluid to the colon and bulk to stools, making bowel movements softer and easier to pass. People who have problems with constipation should drink enough of these liquids every day, about eight 8-ounce glasses. Other liquids, like coffee and soft drinks, that contain caffeine seem to have a dehydrating effect.

- *Irritable bowel syndrome (IBS).* Some people with IBS, also known as spastic colon, have spasms in the colon that affect bowel movements. Constipation and diarrhea often alternate, and abdominal cramping, gassiness, and bloating are other common complaints. Although IBS can produce lifelong symptoms, it is not a life-threatening condition. It often worsens with stress, but there is no specific cause or anything unusual that the doctor can see in the colon.

- *Poor bowel habits.* A person can initiate a cycle of constipation by ignoring the urge to have a bowel movement. Some people do this to avoid using public toilets, others because they are too busy. After a period of time, a person may stop feeling the urge. This leads to progressive constipation.

- *Laxative abuse.* Laxatives usually are not necessary and can be habit-forming. The colon begins to rely on laxatives to bring on bowel movements. Over time, laxatives can damage nerve cells in the colon and interfere with the colon's natural ability to contract. For the same reason, regular use of enemas can also lead to a loss of normal bowel function.

- *Changes in life or routine.* During pregnancy, women may be constipated because of hormonal changes or because the heavy uterus compresses the intestine. Aging may also affect bowel regularity because a slower metabolism results in less intestinal activity and muscle tone. In addition, people often become constipated when traveling because their normal diet and daily routines are disrupted.

- **Lack of exercise.** Lack of exercise can lead to constipation, although doctors do not know precisely why. For example, constipation often occurs after an accident or during an illness when one must stay in bed and cannot exercise.
- **Specific diseases.** Many disorders that affect the body tissues, such as scleroderma, amyloidosis, or lupus; certain neurological or muscular disorders, such as multiple sclerosis, Parkinson's disease, spinal cord injuries, and stroke; and some metabolic and endocrine conditions, such as diabetes or hyperthyroidism, can cause constipation.
- **Mechanical compression.** Scarring, inflammation around diverticula, tumors, and cancer can produce mechanical compression of the intestines and can result in constipation.
- **Medications.** Pain medications (especially narcotics), antacids that contain aluminum, antispasmodics, antidepressants, iron supplements, diuretics, and anticonvulsants for epilepsy can slow passage of bowel movements.

CAUSES OF CONSTIPATION IN OLDER PEOPLE
Older people are much more likely than younger people to report problems with constipation. Poor diet, insufficient intake of fluids, lack of exercise, the use of certain drugs to treat other conditions, and poor bowel habits can all result in constipation. Experts agree, however, that too often older people become overly concerned with having a bowel movement.

Diet and dietary habits can play a role in developing constipation. Lack of interest in eating—a problem common to many single or widowed older people—may lead to heavy use of convenience foods, which tend to be low in fiber. In addition, loss of teeth may force older people to choose soft, processed foods, which also tend to be low in fiber.

Older people sometimes cut back on fluids, especially if they are not eating regular or balanced meals. Water and other fluids add bulk to stools, making bowel movements softer and easier to pass.

Prolonged bed rest, for example, after an accident or during an illness, and lack of exercise may contribute to constipation. Also, drugs prescribed for other conditions (for example, certain antidepressants, antacids containing aluminum or calcium, antihistamines, diuretics, and antiparkinsonism drugs) can produce constipation in some people.

The preoccupation with bowel movements sometimes leads older people to depend heavily on laxatives. This is not only unnecessary, but it can be habit-forming. The bowel begins to rely on laxatives to bring on defecation and, over time, the natural mechanisms fail to work without the help of drugs. Habitual use of enemas also can lead to a loss of normal function.

DIAGNOSTIC TESTS
Most people do not need extensive testing and can be treated with changes in diet and exercise. The doctor may ask a patient to describe his or her constipation, including duration of symptoms, frequency of bowel movements, consistency of stools, presence of blood in the stool, and toilet habits (how often and where one has bowel movements). A physical exam may include a digital rectal exam with a gloved, lubricated finger to evaluate the tone of the muscle that closes off the anus (anal sphincter) and to detect tenderness, obstruction, or blood. In some cases, blood and thyroid tests may be necessary.

Extensive testing usually is reserved for people with severe symptoms, for those with sudden changes in number and consistency of bowel movements or blood in the stool, and for older adults. Because of an increased risk of colorectal cancer in older adults, the doctor may use these tests to rule out a diagnosis of cancer: a sigmoidoscopy may help detect problems in the rectum and lower colon. In this procedure, which can be done in the doctor's office, the doctor inserts a flexible, lighted instrument through the anus to examine the rectum and lower intestine. The doctor may perform a colonoscopy to inspect the entire colon. In colonoscopy, an instrument similar to the sigmoidoscope, but longer and able to follow the twists and turns of the intestine, is used. A barium enema x-ray will provide similar information. If bleeding is present, a double-contrast barium enema is preferred. Other highly specialized techniques are available for measuring pressures and movements within the colon and its sphincter muscles, but these are used only in unusual cases.

IS CONSTIPATION SERIOUS?

Sometimes constipation can lead to complications. These complications include hemorrhoids caused by straining to have a bowel movement or anal fissures (tears in the skin around the anus) caused when hard stool stretches the sphincter muscle. As a result, rectal bleeding may occur that appears as bright red streaks on the surface of the stool. Treatment for hemorrhoids may include warm tub baths, ice packs, and application of a cream to the affected area. Treatment for anal fissure may include stretching the sphincter muscle or surgical removal of tissue or skin in the affected area.

Sometimes straining causes a small amount of intestinal lining to push out from the anal opening. This condition is known as rectal prolapse and may lead to secretion of mucus from the anus. Usually, eliminating the cause of the prolapse such as straining or coughing is the only treatment necessary. Severe or chronic prolapse requires surgery to strengthen and tighten the anal sphincter muscle or to repair the prolapsed lining.

Constipation may also cause hard stool to pack the intestine and rectum so tightly that the normal pushing action of the colon is not enough to expel the stool. This condition, called fecal impaction, occurs most often in children and older adults. An impaction can be softened with mineral oil taken by mouth and an enema. After softening the impaction, the doctor may break up and remove part of the hardened stool by inserting one or two fingers in the anus.

TREATMENT

Although treatment depends on the cause, severity, and duration, in most cases dietary and lifestyle changes will help relieve symptoms and help prevent constipation.

A diet with enough fiber (20 to 35 grams each day) helps form soft, bulky stool. A doctor or dietitian can help plan an appropriate diet. High-fiber foods include beans; whole grains and bran cereals; fresh fruits; and vegetables such as asparagus, brussels sprouts, cabbage, and carrots. For people prone to constipation, limiting foods that have little or no fiber such as ice cream, cheese, meat, and processed foods is also important.

Other changes that can help treat and prevent constipation include drinking enough water and other liquids such as fruit and vegetable juices and clear soup, engaging in daily exercise, and reserving enough time to have a bowel movement. In addition, the urge to have a bowel movement should not be ignored.

Most people who are mildly constipated do not need laxatives. However, for those who have made lifestyle changes and are still constipated, doctors may recommend laxatives or enemas for a limited time. These treatments can help retrain a chronically sluggish bowel. For children, short-term treatment with laxatives, along with retraining to establish regular bowel habits, also helps prevent constipation. A doctor should determine when a patient needs a laxative and which form is best. Laxatives taken by mouth are available in liquid, tablet, gum, powder, and granule forms. They work in various ways (see box on page 243). People dependent upon laxatives need to slowly stop using the medications. A doctor can assist in this process. In most people, this restores the colon's natural ability to contract.

Treatment may be directed at a specific cause. For example, the doctor may recommend discontinuing medication or performing surgery to correct an anorectal problem such as rectal prolapse.

People with chronic constipation caused by anorectal dysfunction can use biofeedback to retrain the muscles that control release of bowel movements. Biofeedback involves using a sensor to monitor muscle activity that at the same time can be displayed on a computer screen allowing for an accurate assessment of body functions. A health-care professional uses this information to help the patient learn how to use these muscles.

Surgical removal of the colon may be an option for people with severe symptoms caused by colonic inertia. However, the benefits of this surgery must be weighed against possible complications, which include abdominal pain and diarrhea.

The National Institute of Diabetes and Digestive and Kidney Diseases

DIARRHEA

"The trots," which goes by many other names, polite and impolite, is not funny. Fortunately, it's usually a self-limited ailment—that is, it gets better in a day or two by itself. Diarrhea is the result of the loss of too much water with the stool.

Normally, fluids in the digestive tract are mostly reabsorbed through the inner lining of the intestines and colon, so that fecal matter solidifies as it travels onward. If something interferes with the effectiveness of that process, you'll pass excess fluid as you defecate. (This is why severe diarrhea dehydrates you—and dehydration is its most serious result.)

Drugs for diarrhea work by decreasing water in the stool one of three ways: slowing intestinal motility, increasing reabsorption of fluid through the intestinal lining, or decreasing the amount of material secreted by the intestine.

Diarrhea can have many different causes; most are not particularly dangerous, but a few must be taken seriously.

"NONSPECIFIC" DIARRHEA

The most common kind by far, nonspecific diarrhea, appears and disappears so fast that the cause (generally viruses or bacteria) never gets definitively diagnosed, hence the term nonspecific. "Stomach flu" or the "bug that's going around" are terms commonly applied to nonspecific diarrhea.

Symptoms are frequent: watery bowel movements, excess gas, and stomach cramps.

If you have appointments to keep and work to do, you may want to take something. Since most of the standard drugstore remedies won't help, your best bet may be Imodium (the brand name for loperamide). Formerly available by prescription only, liquid Imodium A-D is now approved for over-the-counter (OTC) sale.

Altering your diet temporarily may help. Avoid milk and dairy products, alcohol, and caffeine. Drink lots of water, juices, broth, and other clear liquids to make up for fluid loss.

Whether you take medicine or not, diarrhea lasting more than 48 hours, fever above 101°F, severe cramping, blood in your stool, or light-headedness or dizziness (indicating dehydration) are signals to see a doctor. Frequently recurring diarrhea may be a symptom of more serious bowel disorders and needs prompt medical attention.

TRAVELER'S DIARRHEA

Sometimes dubbed "Montezuma's Revenge," traveler's diarrhea strikes after eating or drinking something contaminated with *E. coli* or other types of fecal bacteria. It can be serious and debilitating.

MEDICATION-INDUCED DIARRHEA

If you've just started a new medication, don't rule it out as a cause of sudden diarrhea. Certain antibiotics, heart drugs, and high blood pressure medications can cause diarrhea. So can many over-the-counter drugs, such as antacids with magnesium (Maalox, for example), and of course, laxatives. So can large amounts of sorbitol, xylitol, and mannitol (sweeteners used in vitamins, diet foods, and sugar-free chewing gum). Stop using any product you suspect, unless it's a prescription drug. In that case, consult your doctor as soon as possible.

The Editors

HEMORRHOIDS

Hemorrhoids are swollen but normally present blood vessels in and around the anus and lower rectum that stretch under pressure, similar to varicose veins in the legs. The increased pressure and swelling may result from straining to move the bowel. Other contributing factors include pregnancy, heredity, aging, and chronic constipation or diarrhea. Hemorrhoids are either inside the anus (internal) or under the skin around the anus (external).

What Are the Symptoms?

Many anorectal problems, including fissures, fistulae, abscesses, or irritation and itching (pruritus ani), have similar symptoms and are incorrectly referred to as hemorrhoids. Hemorrhoids usually are not dangerous or life threatening. In most cases, hemorrhoidal symptoms will go away within a few days.

Although many people have hemorrhoids, not all experience symptoms. The most common symptom of internal hemorrhoids is bright red blood covering the stool, on toilet paper, or in the toilet bowl. However, an internal hemorrhoid may protrude through the anus outside the body, becoming irritated and painful. This is known as a protruding hemorrhoid. Symptoms of external hemorrhoids may include painful swelling or a hard lump around the anus that results when a blood clot forms. This condition is known as a thrombosed external hemorrhoid.

In addition, excessive straining, rubbing, or cleaning around the anus may cause irritation with bleeding and/or itching, which may produce a vicious cycle of symptoms. Draining mucus may also cause itching.

How Common Are Hemorrhoids?

Hemorrhoids are very common in men and women. About half of the population have hemorrhoids by age 50. Hemorrhoids are also common among pregnant women. The pressure of the fetus in the abdomen, as well as hormonal changes, cause the hemorrhoidal vessels to enlarge. These vessels are also placed under severe pressure during childbirth. For most women, however, hemorrhoids caused by pregnancy are a temporary problem.

How Are Hemorrhoids Diagnosed?

A thorough evaluation and proper diagnosis by the doctor is important any time bleeding from the rectum or blood in the stool lasts more than a couple of days. Bleeding may also be a symptom of other digestive diseases, including colorectal cancer.

The doctor will examine the anus and rectum to look for swollen blood vessels that indicate hemorrhoids and will also perform a digital rectal exam with a gloved, lubricated finger to feel for abnormalities.

Closer evaluation of the rectum for hemorrhoids requires an exam with an anoscope, a hollow, lighted tube useful for viewing internal hemorrhoids, or a proctoscope, useful for more completely examining the entire rectum.

To rule out other causes of gastrointestinal bleeding, the doctor may examine the rectum and lower colon (sigmoid) with sigmoidoscopy or the entire colon with colonoscopy. Sigmoidoscopy and colonoscopy are diagnostic procedures that also involve the use of lighted, flexible tubes inserted through the rectum.

What Is the Treatment?

Medical treatment of hemorrhoids initially is aimed at relieving symptoms. Measures to reduce symptoms include: warm tub or sitz baths several times a day in plain, warm water for about 10 minutes; ice packs to help reduce swelling; application of a hemorrhoidal cream or suppository to the affected area for a limited time.

Prevention of the recurrence of hemorrhoids is aimed at changing conditions associated with the pressure and straining of constipation. Doctors will often recommend increasing fiber and fluids in the diet. Eating the right amount of fiber and drinking six to eight glasses of fluid (not alcohol) result in softer, bulkier stools. A softer stool makes emptying the bowels easier and lessens the pressure on hemorrhoids caused by straining. Eliminating straining also helps prevent the hemorrhoids from protruding.

Good sources of fiber are fruits, vegetables, and whole grains. In addition, doctors may suggest a bulk stool softener or a fiber supplement such as psyllium (Metamucil) or methylcellulose (Citrucel).

In some cases, hemorrhoids must be treated surgically. These methods are used to shrink and destroy the hemorrhoidal tissue and are performed under anesthesia. The doctor will perform the surgery during an office or hospital visit.

A number of surgical methods may be used to remove or reduce the size of internal hemorrhoids. These techniques include:

• ***Rubber band ligation.*** A rubber band is

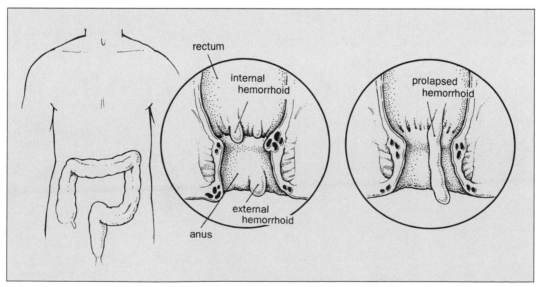

Internal hemorrhoids occur in the veins of the rectum; external hemorrhoids, in veins of the anus. A prolapsed hemorrhoid results when an internal hemorrhoid protrudes outward, through the anus.

placed around the base of the hemorrhoid inside the rectum. The band cuts off circulation, and the hemorrhoid withers away within a few days.

- *Sclerotherapy*. A chemical solution is injected around the blood vessel to shrink the hemorrhoid.

Techniques used to treat both internal and external hemorrhoids include:

- *Electrical or laser heat (laser coagulation) or infrared light (infrared photo coagulation)*. Both techniques use special devices to burn hemorrhoidal tissue.
- *Hemorrhoidectomy*. Occasionally, extensive or severe internal or external hemorrhoids may require removal by surgery known as hemorrhoidectomy. This is the best method for permanent removal of hemorrhoids.

How Are Hemorrhoids Prevented?
The best way to prevent hemorrhoids is to keep stools soft so they pass easily, thus decreasing pressure and straining, and to empty bowels as soon as possible after the urge occurs. Exercise, including walking, and increased fiber in the diet help reduce constipation and straining by producing stools that are softer and easier to pass. In addition, a person should not sit on the toilet for a long period of time.

The National Institute of Diabetes and Digestive and Kidney Diseases

The Ears, Nose, and Throat

In medicine, the ears, nose, and throat are traditionally treated as a single, integrated system. This is because all three parts overlap in terms of function, structure, surface coverings, and nerve supply. A disorder in any one of the areas may manifest in the other two. So often, for example, a cold that starts off as only a runny nose leads to an earache or a sore throat. Or perhaps you're on an airplane, and the change in altitude creates an uncomfortable sensation of pressure in your ears. You discover that a simple swallow—opening up the throat—is all it takes to clear the discomfort in your ears.

The specialty dealing with the ears, nose, and throat—and how they are interrelated—is called otolaryngology; the specialist (usually a surgeon) is called an otolaryngologist or, more simply, an ENT (for ear, nose, and throat) doctor.

THE EARS

Each ear is divided into three distinct sections: outer, middle, and inner ear.

The outer ear consists of the visible, external folds of cartilage and the canal that leads into the middle ear. If you lost the external cartilage due to an accident, your hearing would not be affected very much. This portion of the ear—the shape of which is unique to each individual and does not change throughout life—is only a rudimentary funnel for sound. It offers some physical protection, but in its absence, sounds still reach the eardrum through the canal of the outer ear. This canal is lined with short hairs and thousands of wax-generating glands. The wax and hair help to stop dust, dirt, small insects—anything that might infiltrate the ear—from reaching the middle ear. The outer ear also modifies the air that reaches the deeper parts of the ear, so that the ear's internal temperature and humidity levels are nearly always constant, regardless of the climate outside.

The middle ear begins where the outer ear ends: at the eardrum, or tympanic membrane.

Also in the middle ear are the three smallest bones in the body: the hammer (malleus), the anvil (incus), and the stirrup (stapes). These bones amplify and conduct sound signals to the inner ear.

The inner ear consists of two essential parts: the cochlea and the semicircular canals. The cochlea converts sounds into electrical nerve impulses which can then be sent, via the auditory nerve, to the brain, where they are interpreted. The semicircular canals are responsible for maintaining our sense of balance. The inner ear, containing as many circuits as a city telephone system, is one of the most complex and delicate parts of the body. Fortunately—situated deep within the hard skull and surrounded by a fluid cushion—the inner ear is also one of the best-protected parts of the body.

THE NOSE

The nose provides critical information about our immediate surroundings: warning us of a fire while it is still only smoldering; letting us know when it's time to throw out the leftovers that could result in food poisoning; or simply adding to our appreciation of a garden in full bloom. The sense of taste, in fact, is deeply reliant upon the sense of smell. When the olfactory senses fail (as occurs with a bad cold), you lose about 80 percent of your ability to discern flavors.

In addition to olfaction, the nose is the main conduit for respiration, and it filters the approximately 500 cubic feet of air we breathe every day. The hairs that line the nostrils block airborne pollen, dust, or grit from getting into the lungs; when such particles are especially irritating, the sneeze reflex is triggered, ejecting the offending matter at speeds upwards of 200 miles per hour. The membranes that line the nasal passages secrete mucus that continually cleans and lubricates the region. Not only does mucus physically surround foreign material, but it contains a substance called lysozyme that chemically destroys bacteria. The nose also warms and humidifies air coming into the lungs.

Beyond these functions, your nose also gives your voice extra richness and resonance, without which you'd sound as if you were always "holding your nose" when you talk. The four sets of sinus cavities are simply air-filled spaces within certain bones of the face. The sinuses allow these bones to be lighter in weight and they too give the voice resonance. Each of the sinuses is lined with a mucous membrane that is integrally connected to the mucous membranes of the throat and, in particular, the nose.

THE THROAT

The throat (pharynx) is the passageway that brings food and drink to the digestive system, as well as air to and from the lungs. It also conducts air through the vocal cords (larynx), allowing us to speak and sing.

The approximately five-inch-long pharynx, a muscular tube lined with a mucous membrane, has the crucial task of handling traffic flow between its two divisions: the trachea (windpipe) and the esophagus (food passage). Without constant automatic regulation, food would enter the lungs and air would enter the stomach. But when we swallow, a small flap of skin called the epiglottis acts as a safety valve, closing over the top of the larynx to seal off the windpipe. Muscles at the top of the throat help push food down along the esophagus. At the end of the swallow, the epiglottis relaxes again so that breathing can resume.

Sometimes—usually when we're eating too fast or are talking or laughing as we eat—the process doesn't work quite right and food may get stuck at the entrance of the windpipe. Typically, this will trigger powerful choking and coughing to dislodge the blockage. If not, the more aggressive Heimlich maneuver might be necessary.   *The Editors*

HEARING LOSS AND AGING

It is easy to take good hearing for granted. For people with hearing impairments, words in a conversation may be misunderstood, musical notes might be missed, and a ringing doorbell may go unanswered. Hearing impairment ranges from having difficulty understanding words or hearing certain sounds to total deafness.

Because of fear, misinformation, or vanity, some people will not admit to themselves or anyone else that they have a hearing problem. It has been estimated, however, that about 30 percent of adults age 65 through 74 and about 50 percent of those age 75 through 79 suffer some degree of hearing loss. In the United States alone, more than 28 million older people are hearing impaired.

If ignored and untreated, hearing problems can grow worse, hindering communication with others, limiting social activities, and reducing the choices of leisure time activities. People with hearing impairments often withdraw socially to avoid the frustration and embarrassment of not being able to understand what is being said. In addition, hearing-impaired people may become suspicious of relatives and friends who "mumble" or "don't speak up."

Hearing loss may cause an older person to be wrongly labeled as "confused," "unresponsive," or "uncooperative." At times a person's feeling of powerlessness and frustration in trying to communicate with others results in depression and withdrawal.

Older people today more often demand greater satisfaction from life, but those with hearing impairments can find the quality of their lives reduced. Fortunately, help is available in the form of treatment with medicines, special training, a hearing aid or an alternate listening device, and surgery.

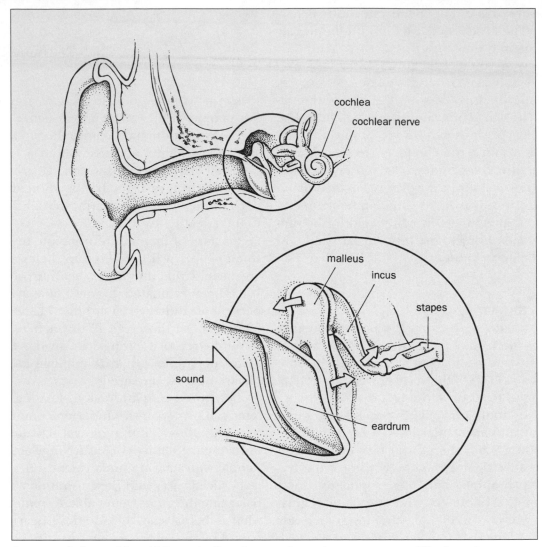

As we age, the bones of the middle ear (malleus, incus, and stapes) may move more stiffly, the eardrum may thicken, and conduction problems in the cochlea may occur—all leading to hearing loss.

SOME COMMON SIGNS OF HEARING IMPAIRMENT

- Words are difficult to understand.
- Another person's speech sounds slurred or mumbled, worsening when there is background noise.
- Speech can be hard or impossible to understand, depending on the kind of hearing impairment.
- Certain sounds are overly loud or annoying.
- A hissing or ringing background noise may be heard constantly or the sound may be interrupted.
- TV shows, concerts, or social gatherings are less enjoyable because much goes unheard.

DIAGNOSIS OF HEARING PROBLEMS

If you have trouble hearing, see your doctor for treatment or a referral to an ear specialist. By ignoring the problem, you may be overlooking a serious medical condition. Hearing impairments may be caused by exposure to very loud noises over a long period of time, viral infections, vascular disorders (such as heart conditions or stroke), head injuries, tumors, heredity, certain medications, or age-related changes in the ear.

In some cases, the diagnosis and treatment of a hearing problem may take place in the family doctor's office. More complicated cases may require the help of specialists known as otologists, otolaryngologists, or otorhinolaryngologists—all of whom are trained to perform surgery on the ear. These specialists are doctors of medicine or doctors of osteopathy with extensive training in ear problems. They will take a medical history, ask about problems affecting family members, conduct a thorough exam, and order any needed tests.

An audiologist is another health professional who is trained to identify and measure hearing loss and to help with rehabilitation. However, audiologists do not prescribe drugs or perform surgery. To measure hearing they use a device that produces sounds of different pitches and loudness (an audiometer), as well as other electronic devices. These hearing measurements test a person's ability to understand speech. The tests are painless and can in a short time locate a hearing problem, allowing the doctor to recommend a course of treatment.

TYPES OF HEARING LOSS

Conductive hearing loss occurs in some older people. It involves the blocking of sounds that are carried from the eardrum (tympanic membrane) to the inner ear. This may be caused by ear wax in the ear canal, fluid in the middle ear, or abnormal bone growth or infection in the middle ear.

Sensorineural hearing loss involves damage to parts of the inner ear or auditory nerve. When sensorineural hearing loss occurs in older people, it is called presbycusis. Changes in the delicate workings of the inner ear lead to difficulties understanding speech and possibly an intolerance for loud sounds, but not total deafness. Thus, "Don't shout—I'm not deaf!" is often said by older people with this type of hearing impairment.

Every year after age 50 we are likely to lose some of our hearing ability. The decline is so gradual that by age 60 or 70 as many as 25 percent of older people are noticeably hearing impaired. Just as the graying of hair occurs at different rates, presbycusis may develop differently from person to person.

Although presbycusis is usually attributed to aging, it does not affect everyone. Environmental noise, certain medicines, improper diet, and genetic makeup may all contribute to the severity of the hearing impairment. The condition is permanent, but there is much a person can do to function well.

Central auditory dysfunction is a third type of hearing loss that occurs in older people, although it is quite rare even in this age group. It is caused by damage to the nerve centers within the brain. Sound levels are not affected, but understanding language usually is. The causes include extended illness with a high fever, head injuries, vascular problems, or tumors. A central auditory dysfunction cannot be treated medically or surgically; but for some, special training by an audiologist or speech pathologist can help.

TREATMENT

Examination and test results from the family doctor, ear specialist, and audiologist will determine the best treatment for a specific hearing problem. In some cases, medical treatment such as cleansing the ear canal to remove ear wax or surgery may restore some or all hearing ability.

At other times a hearing aid may be recommended. A hearing aid is a small device designed to make sounds louder and clearer. Before you can buy a hearing aid, you must either obtain a written statement from your doctor (saying that your hearing impairment has been medically evaluated and that you might benefit from a hearing aid) or sign a waiver stating that you do not desire medical evaluation.

Many hearing aids are on the market, each offering different kinds of help for different problems. Professional advice is needed regarding the design, model, and brand of the hearing aid best for you. This advice, which is part of your hearing aid evaluation, is given by the audiologist who considers your hearing level, your understanding of speech in each ear, your ability to handle the aid and its controls, and your concern about appearance and comfort.

Remember that you are buying a product and specific services, including any necessary adjustments, counseling in the use of the aid, maintenance, and repairs throughout the warranty period. Before deciding where to buy your aid, consider the quality of service as well as the quality of the product.

Buy an aid with only those features you need. The most costly hearing aid may not be the best for you, and the one selling for less may offer more satisfaction. Also, be aware that the controls for many of the special features are tiny and may be difficult to adjust. Practice will make operating the aid easier. Your hearing aid dealer (usually called a dispenser) should have the patience and skill to help you through the adjustment period. It is a good idea to take advantage of his or her help, since it often takes at least a month to become comfortable with a new hearing aid.

People with certain types of hearing impairments may need special help. Speech-reading allows people to receive visual cues from lip movements as well as facial expressions, body posture and gestures, and the environment. Auditory training may include hearing aid orientation, but it is also designed to help hearing-impaired persons identify and better handle their specific communication problems. Both speech-reading and auditory training can reduce the handicapping effects of the hearing loss. If needed, counseling is also available so that people with hearing impairments can understand their communication abilities and limitations while maintaining a positive image.

Profound hearing impairment may prevent significant benefit with hearing aids. In such cases, a cochlean implant can often offer substantial benefit in hearing speech.

IF YOU HAVE PROBLEMS HEARING

If you suspect there may be a problem with your hearing, visit your doctor as soon as possible. Medicare will pay for the doctor's exam and hearing tests that are ordered by the doctor. Medicare will not pay for the hearing aid.

- Ask your doctor to explain the cause of your hearing problem and if you should see a specialist.
- Don't hesitate to ask people to repeat what they have just said.
- Try to reduce background noise (stereo, television, or radio).
- Tell people that you have a hearing problem and what they can do to make communication easier.

IF YOU KNOW SOMEONE WITH
A HEARING PROBLEM

- Speak at your normal rate but not too rapidly. Do not overarticulate. This distorts the sounds of speech and makes visual cues more difficult to interpret. Shouting will not make the message any clearer and may distort it.
- Speak to the person at a distance of three to six feet. Position yourself near good light so that your lip movements, facial expressions, and gestures may be seen clearly. Wait until you are visible to the hearing-impaired person before speaking. Avoid chewing, eating,

or covering your mouth while speaking.

- Never speak directly into the person's ear. This prevents the listener from making use of visual cues.
- If the listener does not understand what was said, rephrase the idea in short, simple sentences.
- Arrange living rooms or meeting rooms so that no one is more than six feet apart and all are completely visible. In meetings or group activities where there is a speaker presenting information, ask the speaker to use the public address system.
- Treat the hearing-impaired person with respect. Include the person in all discussions about him or her. This helps relieve the feelings of isolation common in hearing-impaired people.

FOR MORE INFORMATION

If you would like further information about hearing problems, contact the organizations listed below. Please be sure to state clearly what type of information you would like to receive.

The American Academy of Otolaryngology, Head and Neck Surgery, Inc., is a professional society of medical doctors specializing in diseases of the ear, nose, and throat. They can provide information on hearing, balance, and other disorders affecting the ear, nose, and throat. Write to 1 Prince Street, Alexandria, VA 22314.

The American Speech-Language-Hearing Association and the National Association of Hearing and Speech Action can both answer questions and mail information on hearing aids or hearing loss and communication problems in older people. They can also provide a list of certified audiologists and speech language pathologists. Write to the American Speech-Language-Hearing Association at 10801 Rockville Pike, Dept. AP, Rockville, MD 20852; or call the National Association of Hearing & Speech Action at (800) 638-8255.

Self-Help for Hard of Hearing People, Inc., is a national self-help organization for those who are hard of hearing. SHHH can help with information on coping with a hearing loss and new hearing aids and technology, and they publish *Hearing Loss* (formerly the *Shhh Journal*) bimonthly. Write to SHHH, 7800 Wisconsin Avenue, Bethesda, MD 20892.

The National Information Center on Deafness at Gallaudet University provides information on all areas related to deafness and hearing loss, including educational programs, vocational training, sign language programs, law, technology, and barrier-free design. Write to the NICD, 800 Florida Avenue, NE., Washington, DC 20002.

The National Institute on Deafness and Other Communication Disorders at the National Institutes of Health provides information on research on hearing, balance, smell, taste, voice, speech, and language. Write to the NIDCD, Building 31, Room 1B62, Bethesda, MD 20892. Their National Information Clearinghouse also provides information to health professionals, patients, industry, and the public. Write to the NIDCD Clearinghouse, P.O. Box 37777, Washington, DC 20013-7777.   *National Institute on Aging*

SINUSITIS

Every year over one and a half billion dollars worth of sinus medicine is purchased in America for the symptoms of sinus disease (i.e., stuffy nose, congestion, headache, and nasal drainage). Everyone has sinuses, which begin as pea-size pouches extending outward from the inside of the nose into the bones of the face and skull. They expand and grow through childhood into young adulthood. They are air pockets, cavities that are lined with the same kind of membranes that line the nose, and they are connected to the inside of the nose through small openings about the size of a pencil lead.

257

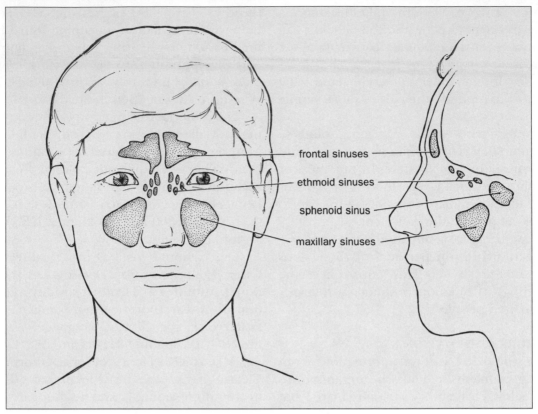

frontal sinuses

ethmoid sinuses

sphenoid sinus

maxillary sinuses

There are four sets of sinus cavities. The maxillary sinuses—the largest—account for most sinus problems in adults. Pain occurs when the thin drainage channels become blocked.

WHAT DO SINUSES DO?

Sinuses are part of the nasal air and membrane system that produces mucus. Normally, the nose and sinuses produce between a pint and a quart of mucus and secretions per day. This mucus passes into and through the nose, sweeping and washing the membranes, picking up dust particles, bacteria, and other air pollutants along the way. The mucus then flows backward into the throat where it is swallowed, down into the stomach where acids destroy any dangerous bacteria. Most people do not notice this mucus flow because it is just a normal bodily function.

WHAT IS POSTNASAL DRIP?

When the nasal passages are irritated by allergies, air pollution, smoke, or viral infections

(such as a cold), then the nose and sinus membranes secrete more than the normal amount of mucus. This will be a clear, watery, and profuse mucus that is supposed to wash away the irritation or allergy. This is the most common type of postnasal drip. Another form of postnasal drip is mucus that is thick and sticky. This occurs when the air is too dry and the nose membranes cannot produce enough moisture to put into the mucus for it to flow easily. Bacterial infections also produce a thick, sticky mucus with pus in it, turning it a yellow or green color.

WHAT IS SINUSITIS?

The suffix "-itis" is a medical term for infection or inflammation, so sinusitis is an infection or inflammation of the sinuses. A typical case of acute sinusitis begins with a cold or flu or an allergy attack that causes swelling of the nasal membranes and increased watery mucus production. The membranes can become so swollen that the tiny openings from the sinuses become blocked. When mucus and air cannot flow easily between the nose and sinuses, abnormal pressures occur in the sinuses, and mucus can build up in them. This creates a pressure-pain in the forehead or face, between and behind the eyes, or in the cheeks and upper teeth, depending on which sinuses are involved.

A blocked sinus cavity filled with mucus becomes a fine place for bacteria to grow. When a person's cold lasts more than the typical week or so, and when the mucus turns yellow-green or develops a bad odor or taste, then a bacterial infection has probably taken over. The pressure and pain in the face and forehead can be quite severe in acute bacterial sinusitis. Chronic sinusitis occurs when the sinus opening is blocked for an extended period. Headaches are less prominent in chronic sinusitis, but congestion and unpleasant nasal secretions usually persist. Also, fleshy growths known as polyps can develop as an exaggerated form of inflammatory swelling of the membranes.

Some cases of sinusitis are brought on by infections in the upper teeth that extend into the sinuses.

IS SINUSITIS DANGEROUS?
Most cases of sinusitis respond promptly to medical treatment and are not serious. It should be noted, however, that an infection that is in the sinus is also very close to the eye and to the brain. But extension of a sinus infection to the eye or brain is rare.

Furthermore, it is not healthy for the lungs to have infected mucus dripping down from infected sinuses. Bronchitis, chronic cough, and asthma are often aggravated, or even brought on, by sinusitis.

WHAT IS A SINUS HEADACHE?
A headache in the face, cheeks, forehead, or around the eyes that comes on during a cold, or when the nose is congested and runny or filled with mucus, is probably a sinus headache: one caused by sinus infection.

Another kind of sinus headache is the one that occurs in the sinus areas during descent (landing) in an airplane, especially if you have a cold or active allergy (this is called a vacuum headache).

Unfortunately, there are many other causes of headaches that can be confused with sinusitis. For example, migraine and other forms of vascular or tension headaches also give pain in the forehead and around the eyes, and they may even cause a slight stuffy-runny nose. But they are more likely to come and go away in a day or so without a physician's treatment, whereas sinusitis usually produces a headache that lasts for days or weeks until it is treated with antibiotics.

Furthermore, intermittent headaches that cause nausea and vomiting are more typical of a migraine-type headache than sinusitis.

Severe, frequent, or prolonged headaches require a visit to a physician for diagnosis and treatment. (See also Headaches, page 150.)

WHO GETS SINUS TROUBLE?
Actually, anyone can catch a sinus infection, but certain groups of people, such as the following, are more likely to develop sinusitis.
- *People with allergies.* An allergy attack, like a cold, causes swelling in the nasal membranes that will block the sinus openings, obstruct the mucus drainage, and predispose to infection.
- *People with deformities of the nose* that impair good breathing and proper drainage. Examples are a crooked nose or a deviated septum (the structure between the nostrils that divides the inside of the nose into right and left sides).

- *People who are frequently exposed to infection.* Schoolteachers and health workers are especially susceptible.
- *People who smoke.* Tobacco smoke, nicotine, and other pollutants impair the natural resistance to infection.

WHAT WILL A DOCTOR DO FOR YOUR SINUSES?

Your physician will ask you questions about your breathing, the nature of your nasal mucus, and the circumstances (time of day or seasons) that give you symptoms. Be prepared to explain your headaches: when and how often they occur; how long they last; and if they are associated with nausea, vomiting, vision changes, or nasal congestion. An otolaryngologist—head and neck surgeon—is the kind of physician who will carefully examine your ears, nose, mouth, teeth, and throat with particular attention to the appearance of your nasal membranes and secretions. He or she will check for deformities of your nose that impair breathing and for tenderness over your sinuses. X-rays of your sinuses might be needed.

Treatment will depend on the diagnosis that your physician establishes. Infections may require either antibiotics or surgery or sometimes both. Acute sinusitis most likely will improve on medication, but chronic sinusitis more often requires surgery. If your symptoms are due to allergy, migraine, or some other disease that mimics sinusitis, your doctor will have alternative treatment plans.

WHAT CAN YOU DO FOR YOUR OWN SINUSES?

Manage your allergies if you have them. Use a humidifier when you have a cold and sleep with the head of your bed elevated. This promotes sinus drainage. Decongestants can also be helpful, but they contain chemicals that act like adrenaline and are dangerous for persons with high blood pressure, irregular heart rhythms, heart disease, or glaucoma. They are also like stimulants that can produce sleeplessness. You should consult your physician before you use these medications.

Avoid air pollutants that irritate the nose, especially tobacco smoke.

Live by good health practices that include a balanced diet and regular exercise.

Minimize exposure to persons with known infections, if possible, and practice sanitary health habits when you must be around them (such as hand washing and avoidance of shared towels, napkins, and eating utensils).

A large variety of nonprescription medications are sold as sinus remedies, but it is folly to try them before a proper diagnosis is established. The best advice you can ever get, of course, is that given to you by your physician, who evaluates your own special symptoms and examines your nose and sinuses.

The American Academy of Otolaryngology— Head and Neck Surgery

SMELL AND TASTE DISORDERS

Smell and taste problems can have a big impact on our lives. Because these senses contribute substantially to our enjoyment of life, our desire to eat and be social, smell and taste disorders can be serious. When they are impaired, life loses some zest; we eat poorly, socialize less, and as a result, feel worse. Many older people experience this problem.

Smell and taste also warn us about dangers, such as fire, poisonous fumes, and spoiled food. Certain jobs require that these senses be accurate. One study estimates that more than 200,000 people visit a doctor with smell and taste disorders every year, but many more cases go unreported.

Loss of the sense of smell may be a sign of sinus disease, growths in the nasal passages, or, in rare circumstances, brain tumors.

HOW DO SMELL AND TASTE WORK?

Smell and taste belong to our chemical sensing system, or chemosensation. The complicated processes of smelling and tasting begin when molecules released by the substances around us stimulate special nerve cells in the nose, mouth, or throat. These cells transmit messages to the brain, where specific smells or tastes are identified.

Olfactory (smell nerve) cells are stimulated by the odors around us—the fragrance from a rose, the smell of bread baking. These nerve cells are found in a tiny patch of tissue high up in the nose, and they connect directly to the brain.

Taste cells react to food or drink mixed with saliva and are clustered in the taste buds of the mouth and throat. Many of the small bumps that can be seen on the tongue contain taste buds. These surface cells send taste information to nearby nerve fibers, which send messages to the brain.

Cells governing our senses of taste and smell are the only cells in the nervous system that are replaced when they become old or damaged. Scientists are examining this phenomenon while studying ways to replace other damaged nerve cells.

A third chemosensory mechanism, called the common chemical sense, contributes to our senses of smell and taste. In this system, thousands of free nerve endings—especially on the moist surfaces of the eyes, nose, mouth, and throat—identify sensations like the sting of ammonia, the coolness of menthol, and the heat of chili peppers.

We can commonly identify four basic taste sensations: sweet, sour, bitter, and salty. Certain combinations of these tastes—along with texture, temperature, odor, and the sensations from the common chemical sense—produce a flavor. It is flavor that lets us know whether we are eating peanuts or caviar.

Many flavors are recognized mainly through the sense of smell. If you hold your nose while eating chocolate, for example, you will have trouble identifying the chocolate flavor—even though you can distinguish the food's sweetness or bitterness. This is because the familiar flavor of chocolate is sensed largely by odor. So is the well-known flavor of coffee. This is why a person who wishes to fully savor a delicious flavor (i.e., an expert chef testing his own creation) will exhale through his nose after each swallow.

CAUSES OF SMELL AND TASTE DISORDERS

The predominant problem is a natural decline in smelling ability that typically occurs after age 60. Scientists have found that the sense of smell is most accurate between the ages of 30 and 60 years. It begins to decline after age 60, and a large proportion of elderly persons have lost their smelling ability. Women of all ages are generally more accurate than men in identifying odors.

Some people are born with a poor sense of smell or taste, but most patients develop them after an injury or illness. Upper respiratory infections are blamed for some losses, and injury to the head can also cause smell or taste problems.

Loss of smell and taste may result from polyps in the nasal or sinus cavities, hormonal disturbances, or dental problems. They can also be caused by prolonged exposure to certain chemicals such as insecticides and by some medicines.

Tobacco smoking is the most concentrated form of pollution that most people will ever be exposed to. It certainly impairs a person's ability to identify odors and diminishes the sense of taste.

Many patients who receive radiation therapy for cancers of the head and neck later complain of lost smell and taste. They can also be lost in the course of some diseases of the nervous system.

Patients who have lost their larynx or voice box commonly complain of poor ability to smell and taste. This emphasizes the contribution of air flow through the nose for these two functions.

DIAGNOSIS

The extent of loss of smell or taste can be tested with a measurement of the lowest concentration of a chemical that a person can accurately detect and recognize. A patient may also be asked to compare the smells or tastes of different chemicals, the intensities of smells or tastes of different chemicals, or how the intensities of smells or tastes grow when a chemical's concentration is increased.

Scientists have developed an easily administered scratch-and-sniff test to evaluate the sense of smell. A person scratches pieces of treated paper to release different odors, sniffs them, and tries to identify each odor from a list of possibilities.

In taste testing, the patient reacts to different chemical concentrations. This may involve a simple sip-spit-and-rinse test, or chemicals may be applied directly to specific areas of the tongue.

TREATMENT

Sometimes a medication causes a smell or taste disorder, and improvement occurs when that medicine is stopped or changed.

Although certain medications can cause chemosensory problems, others—particularly antiallergy drugs—seem to improve the senses of taste and smell.

Some patients—notably those with serious respiratory infections or seasonal allergies—regain their smell or taste simply by waiting for their illness to run its course.

In many cases, nasal obstructions such as polyps can be removed to restore air flow to the receptor area and can correct the loss of smell and taste. Occasionally, chemosenses return to normal just as spontaneously as they disappeared.

WHAT YOU CAN DO

If you experience a smell or taste problem, try to identify and record the circumstances surrounding it. When did you first become aware of it? Did you have a cold or flu then? Did you have a head injury? Were you exposed to air pollutants, pollens, danders, or dust to which you might be allergic? Is this a recurring problem? Does it come in any special season, like hay-fever time?

Bring all this information with you when you visit a physician who deals with diseases of the nose and throat. Also be prepared to tell him about your general health and any medications you are taking. Proper diagnosis by a trained professional can provide reassurance that your illness is not imaginary. You may even be surprised by the results. For example, what you may think is a taste problem could actually be a smell problem, because much of what you think you taste you really smell.

Diagnosis may also lead to treatment of an underlying cause for the disturbance.

Many types of smell and taste disorders are reversible, but if yours is not, it is important for you to remember that you are not alone. Thousands of other patients have faced the same situation.

The American Academy of Otolaryngology—
Head and Neck Surgery

SORE THROAT

Sore throat is one of the most common medical complaints. As many as one out of every 10

Americans develops a strep throat every year, and 40 million adults will see a doctor for it.

CAUSES

Sore throat is one symptom of an array of different medical disorders.

Infections cause the majority of sore throats, and these are the sore throats that are contagious. Infections are caused by either viruses (such as the flu, the common cold, or mononucleosis) or bacteria (such as strep, mycoplasma, or hemophilus).

The most important difference between viruses and bacteria is that bacteria respond well to antibiotic treatment, but viruses do not.

Viruses

Most viral sore throats accompany the flu or a cold. When a stuffy-runny nose, sneezing, and generalized aches and pains accompany the sore throat, it is probably caused by one of the hundreds of known viruses. These are highly contagious and cause epidemics in a community, especially in the winter. The body cures itself of a viral infection by building antibodies that destroy the virus, a process that takes about a week.

Sore throats accompany other viral infections such as measles, chicken pox, whooping cough, and croup. Canker sores and fever blisters in the throat also can be very painful.

Infectious mononucleosis. One special viral infection takes much longer than a week to be cured: infectious mononucleosis or "mono." This virus lodges in the lymph system, causing massive enlargement of the tonsils (with white patches on their surface) and swollen glands in the neck, armpits, and groin. It creates a severely sore throat, sometimes causes serious difficulties breathing, and can affect the liver, leading to jaundice (yellow skin and eyes). It also causes extreme fatigue that can last six weeks or more.

Because mono can be transmitted by saliva, it has been nicknamed the "kissing disease." However, it can also be transmitted from mouth to hand or from hand to mouth or by the sharing of towels and eating utensils.

Bacteria

Strep throat is an infection caused by a particular strain of streptococcus bacteria. This infection can also cause damage to the heart valves (rheumatic fever) and kidneys (nephritis). Streptococcal infections can also cause scarlet fever, tonsillitis, pneumonia, sinusitis, and ear infections.

Because of these possible complications, a strep throat should be treated with an antibiotic. Strep infections usually cause a longer-lasting sore throat than a cold or the flu. But strep is not always easy to detect by examination, and a throat culture may be needed.

A newly developed strep test detects a streptococcal infection in about 15 minutes, instead of the 24 hours or more required for a culture to grow. These tests, when positive, cause the physician to prescribe antibiotics.

However, strep tests and cultures might not detect a number of other bacteria that can also cause severe sore throats that deserve antibiotic treatment. For example, severe and chronic cases of tonsillitis or tonsillar abscess may be culture negative; similarly, negative cultures are seen with diphtheria, and infections from oral sexual contacts will escape detection with strep culture tests.

Tonsillitis is an infection of the lumpy tissues on each side of the throat toward the back of the tongue. In the first two to three years of childhood, these tissues catch infections, sampling the child's environment to help develop his immunities (antibodies). Healthy tonsils do not remain infected, however, and frequent sore throats from tonsillitis suggest the infection is not fully eliminated between episodes. A recent study has shown that patients who suffer from frequently recurrent episodes of tonsillitis (such as three to four episodes each year for several years) were healthier after their tonsils were surgically removed.

Infections in the nose and sinuses can also cause sore throats because mucus from the nose drains down into the throat and carries the infection with it.

Epiglottitis. The most dangerous throat infection is epiglottitis, caused by bacteria that infect a portion of the larynx (voice box) and cause swelling that closes the airway. This infection is an emergency condition that requires prompt medical attention. Suspect it when swallowing is extremely painful (causing drooling), when speech is muffled, and when breathing becomes difficult. A strep culture may miss this infection and be negative.

Allergy

Hay fever and allergy sufferers can get an irritated throat during an allergy attack the same way they get a stuffy, itchy nose, sneezing, and postnasal drip. The same pollens and molds that irritate the nose when they are inhaled also may irritate the throat. People allergic to cat and dog danders can suffer an irritated throat when they are around such animals. A very common allergy is house dust, and it is a special problem in the winter when a heating system blows dust throughout the house.

Irritation

Dry heat. During the cold winter months, dry heat may create a recurring, mild sore throat with a parched feeling, especially in the mornings. This often responds to humidification of bedroom air and increased liquid intake. Patients with a chronic stuffy nose, causing mouth breathing, also suffer with a dry throat. These patients need examination and treatment of the nose.

Regurgitation of stomach acids. An occasional cause of morning sore throat is regurgitation of stomach acids up into the back of the throat where they are extremely irritating. This can be avoided if you tilt your bed frame so that the head is elevated four to six inches higher than the foot. You should also avoid eating and drinking for one to two hours before retiring. You might find antacids helpful. If these fail, see your doctor.

Industrial pollutants and chemicals in the air can irritate the nose and throat, but by far the most common and pervasive air pollutant is tobacco smoke. It cannot be tolerated by many persons who are either allergic or oversensitive to its contents. Other irritants include smokeless tobacco, alcoholic beverages, and spicy foods.

Voice strain. A person who strains the voice (yelling at a sports event, for example) gets a sore throat not only from muscle strain, but also from the rough treatment of the throat membranes. Well-trained, experienced public speakers and singers learn not to abuse their throats and voices in this way. They produce loud voices by taking deep breaths and using their chest and abdominal muscles more than their throat muscles.

Tumors

Tumors of the throat, tongue, and larynx (voice box) are usually (but not always) associated with the long-time use of tobacco and alcohol. A sore throat and difficult swallowing—sometimes with pain radiating to the ear—may be symptoms of such a tumor. More often the sore throat is so mild or so chronic that it is hardly noticed. Other important symptoms include hoarseness, a lump in the neck, unexplained weight loss, and/or spitting up blood in the saliva or phlegm.

The diagnosis will require examination by a physician with special training in diseases of the ears, nose, throat, head, and neck. Special mirrors or telescopic instruments will be used to see the suspicious areas of the throat.

HOW YOU CAN TREAT A MILD SORE THROAT

A mild sore throat associated with cold or flu symptoms can be made more comfortable with the following remedies:

- Increase your liquid intake (warm tea with honey is a favorite home remedy)
- Use a steamer or humidifier in your bedroom
- Gargle with warm salt water several times daily: one-quarter teaspoon salt to one-half cup water
- Take mild pain relievers such as acetaminophen (Tylenol, Datril), ibuprofen (Advil), or others
- Take nonprescription throat lozenges

WHEN TO SEEK A DOCTOR'S TREATMENT

Whenever a sore throat is severe, persists longer than the usual five-to-seven-day duration of a cold or flu, and is not associated with an avoidable allergy or irritation, you should seek medical attention.

The following signs and symptoms should alert you to see your physician:

- Severe and prolonged sore throat
- Difficulty breathing
- Difficulty swallowing
- Difficulty opening the mouth
- Joint pains
- Earache
- Rash
- Fever (over 101°F)
- Blood in saliva or phlegm
- Frequently recurring sore throat
- Lump in the neck
- Hoarseness lasting over two weeks

Antibiotics

Antibiotics are drugs that kill or impair bacteria. Penicillin or erythromycin are prescribed when the physician suspects streptococcal or other bacterial infection that will respond to them. However, a number of bacterial throat infections do not respond to penicillin, but require other categories of antibiotics. Antibiotics do not cure viral infections, but viruses do lower the patient's resistance to bacterial infections. When such a combined infection occurs, antibiotics may be needed.

When an antibiotic is prescribed, it should be taken—as the physician directs—for the full course (usually 10 days). Otherwise, the infection will probably be suppressed rather than eliminated, and it can return, in some cases producing a more intense infection.

Throat Culture

A strep culture tests only for the presence of streptococcal infections. Many other infections, both bacterial and viral, will yield negative cultures and sometimes so does a streptococcal infection. Therefore, when your culture is negative, your physician will base the treatment on the severity of your symptoms and the appearance of your throat. Do not discontinue your medications unless your physician instructs you to do so.

Should Other Family Members Be Treated or Cultured?

When strep throat is proven by test or culture, many experts advise treating other family members, because streptococcal infections are so highly contagious. Others recommend treating only those with sore throats and culturing the others. So be sure you tell your physician how other family members are feeling. Practice good sanitary habits. Avoid close physical contact and the sharing of napkins, towels, and utensils with the infected person. Hand washing makes good sense.

The American Academy of Otolaryngology— Head and Neck Surgery

265

The Endocrine System

The endocrine system is a complex network of glands that secrete hormones, which travel through the bloodstream to regulate the function of nearly all the organs and tissues of the body. The glands that make up the endocrine system (pituitary, thyroid, parathyroid, adrenal, islet cells of the pancreas, and ovaries or testes) secrete hormones to regulate growth, sexual function, the body's fluid and salt balance, glucose metabolism, and a wide array of other functions.

Because of the complex interactions among various hormones—and between the endocrine system and the nervous system—many facets of the endocrine system are not fully understood. What is clear is that the minuscule amounts of hormones in the bloodstream ordinarily work so smoothly that they go unnoticed; but when the system malfunctions— usually when too much or too little of a particular hormone is secreted, or when an organ or tissue does not respond to the hormone efficiently—the results can be dramatic and even fatal. For example, malfunctions of the pituitary gland in a child can produce a giant or a dwarf. And diabetes results from a malfunction of the pancreas, which secretes insulin to regulate the conversion of sugar into energy, or from an inability of the body to respond to the insulin that is secreted.

The Editors

DIABETES MELLITUS

Diabetes is a disease that affects the way the body uses food. It causes sugar levels in the blood to be too high.

Normally, during digestion, the body changes sugars, starches, and other foods into a form of sugar called glucose. Then the blood carries this glucose to cells throughout the body. There, with the help of insulin (a hormone), glucose is changed into quick energy for immediate use by the cells or is stored for future needs. (Insulin is made in the beta cells of the pancreas, a small organ that lies behind the stomach.) This process of turning food into energy is crucial, because the body depends on food for every action, from pumping blood and thinking to running and jumping.

In diabetes, something goes wrong with the normal process of turning food into energy. Food is changed into glucose readily enough, but there is a problem with insulin. In one type of diabetes, the pancreas cannot make insulin. In another type, the body makes some insulin but either makes too little or has trouble using the insulin (or both). When insulin is absent or ineffective, the glucose in the bloodstream cannot be used by the cells to make energy. Instead, glucose collects in the blood, eventually leading to the high sugar levels that are the hallmark of untreated diabetes.

Types of Diabetes

The two main types of diabetes are insulin-dependent and noninsulin-dependent.

Insulin-dependent (type 1) diabetes used to be called juvenile-onset diabetes because it occurs most often in children and young adults. But the name was changed after doctors realized it could occur at any age. In this form of diabetes, the pancreas stops making insulin or makes only a tiny amount. Insulin is necessary to life, so the hormone must be injected every day.

Noninsulin-dependent (type 2) diabetes used to be called maturity-onset diabetes because it occurs most often in adults. In noninsulin-dependent diabetes, the pancreas produces some insulin, but it is not used effectively.

There are other kinds of diabetes, but these are less common.

Gestational diabetes is high blood sugar that first occurs during pregnancy. It usually disappears after the birth of the baby, although nearly 50 percent of these women develop diabetes (usually noninsulin-dependent) within five to 10 years.

Secondary diabetes is the type caused by damage to the pancreas from chemicals, certain medicines, or diseases of the pancreas (such as cancer) or other glands.

Impaired glucose tolerance used to be called latent, chemical, or borderline diabetes but is no longer considered to be a form of diabetes. The blood sugar of the people who have this diagnosis falls between normal and diabetic levels. People with impaired glucose tolerance have an increased risk of developing diabetes.

The Warning Signs
The following symptoms are typical. However, some people with type 2 diabetes have symptoms so mild that they go unnoticed.

- *Type 1 symptoms* (usually occur suddenly): frequent urination; excessive thirst; extreme hunger; extreme weight loss; irritability; weakness and fatigue; nausea and vomiting.
- *Type 2 symptoms* (usually occur less suddenly): any of the type 1 symptoms; recurring or hard-to-heal skin, gum, or bladder infections; drowsiness; blurred vision; tingling or numbness in hands or feet; itching.

Causes
The causes of diabetes are still a mystery. But researchers believe that the tendency for diabetes is present at birth.

In type 1 diabetes, any of several different viral infections and a process called autoimmunity are believed to trigger diabetes. In the autoimmune process, the body's defense system attacks its own cells: in type 1 diabetes, the insulin-producing beta cells in the pancreas. Note: Although viruses may help

to cause some cases of type 1 diabetes, diabetes itself is not catching.

In people prone to type 2 diabetes, being overweight can cause diabetes, because excess fat prevents insulin from working properly.

Prevention and Treatment
So far, type 1 diabetes cannot be prevented, although researchers are working on many promising approaches. Type 2 diabetes can often be prevented by maintaining normal body weight and keeping physically fit throughout life. A major aim of treatment is to control blood sugar levels, which means keeping them in the normal range.

Research has shown that strict control of blood sugar levels can dramatically prevent or delay three long-term diabetes complications, retinopathy, nephropathy, and peripheral neuropathy.

Type 1 diabetes is treated with daily insulin injections, regular exercise, and a balanced meal plan that limits sugar. Your meal plan will be tailored to your individual needs and is likely to include three meals and two or three snacks a day. You will generally have to eat these meals and snacks at set times each day to properly balance insulin, which is also given at fixed times. (Insulin lowers blood sugar, and food raises it. To control diabetes, you need to balance these effects.)

Type 2 diabetes is treated with an individualized diet plan that restricts calories. If you are overweight, you need to slim down. Treatment also includes restricting sugar and following an exercise plan. These steps should improve your body's ability to use its insulin. If diet and exercise alone do not control blood sugar, prescribed pills or insulin may be needed. They do not take the place of diet and exercise, however.

Oral medications for type 2 diabetes include drugs that increase insulin secretion by the pancreas (sulfonylureas and repaglinide), drugs that increase the effectiveness of insulin action (metformin and thiazolinediones), and one that slows the absorption of sugar from the intestine (acarbose).

Testing

Two types of tests are used to monitor blood sugar levels: blood tests and urine tests. Blood tests, done by pricking the finger for a drop of blood, are recommended by most doctors because they give the exact amount of blood sugar at any given moment.

Tests that measure ketones in the urine are also important. Ketones are acids that collect in the blood and urine when the body uses fat (instead of glucose) for energy.

Another important test, done by a doctor every three to six months, is a glycohemoglobin test. This measures the average blood sugar level over the past 30 to 60 days.

Problems to Handle Promptly

Hypoglycemia, low blood sugar, is sometimes called an insulin reaction or insulin shock. It can occur suddenly in people using insulin if too little food is eaten, if a meal is delayed, or if extra exercise is done. It is less common in people whose diabetes is treated with pills, but it can occur. Low blood sugar must be treated quickly, with sugar or sugary foods because, untreated, hypoglycemia can lead to unconsciousness.

The typical symptoms include feeling cold, clammy, nervous, shaky, weak, or very hungry. Some people become pale, get headaches, or act strangely. If a person becomes unconscious, glucagon, a hormone (available by prescription) that raises blood sugar, must be injected.

Hyperglycemia, or high blood sugar, occurs when too much food is eaten or not enough insulin is taken. Illness and emotional stress can also cause high blood sugar. The warning signs are large amounts of sugar in the urine and blood. You may also urinate often, be very thirsty, and feel nauseated. Treat high blood sugar with the help of your doctor.

Ketoacidosis, or diabetic coma, may accompany high blood sugar. It develops when insulin and blood sugar are so out of balance that ketones accumulate in the blood. High levels of ketones are poisonous. Fortunately, ketoacidosis, which develops over several hours or days, can usually be avoided if diabetes is brought under control at the first signs of high blood sugar or ketones in the urine. (Call the doctor for instructions.) In addition to high blood and urine sugar tests and high ketone levels, the symptoms include dry mouth, great thirst, loss of appetite, excessive urination, dry and flushed skin, labored breathing, fruity-smelling breath, and possibly vomiting, abdominal pain, and unconsciousness. Ketoacidosis is most likely to occur in people with type 1 diabetes.

Anyone with diabetes should wear a medical ID necklace or bracelet stating the type of treatment they use, in case of emergencies.

Long-Term Health Problems

Diabetic complications are usually caused by changes in the blood vessels and nerves. Unfortunately, they can include eye and kidney disease, heart attack, numbness or pain in the legs, foot infections leading to gangrene, and stroke. Fortunately, however, treatments continue to improve. Also, many researchers now believe that keeping blood sugar levels tightly controlled from the moment of diagnosis can help to prevent complications.

INSULIN-DEPENDENT DIABETES

Insulin-dependent diabetes is a disease that affects the way your body uses food. Insulin-dependent diabetes is also called type 1 diabetes or insulin-dependent diabetes mellitus (IDDM, for short).

Type 1 diabetes starts when your body stops making insulin or makes only a tiny amount. Your body needs insulin to use food for energy. Without insulin, your body cannot control blood levels of sugar. And without insulin, you would die. So people with type 1 diabetes give themselves at least one shot of insulin every day.

Type 1 diabetes usually strikes children and young adults. But it can occur at any age. It used to be called juvenile-onset diabetes. About one million Americans have this type of diabetes. That is about 10 percent of all Americans with diabetes.

Why Insulin Must Be Injected
You must inject insulin under the skin—in the fat—for it to work. You cannot take insulin in a pill. The juices in your stomach would destroy the insulin before it could work. Scientists are looking for new ways to give insulin. But today, shots are the only method.

Symptoms of Type 1 Diabetes
Type 1 diabetes often appears suddenly, and you should watch for the following symptoms:

- Frequent urination
- Extreme hunger
- Extreme thirst
- Extreme weight loss
- Weakness and tiredness
- Feeling edgy and having mood changes
- Feeling sick to your stomach and vomiting

Causes
We do not know exactly what causes diabetes. We do know that people inherit a tendency to get diabetes. But not all people who have this tendency will get the disease. Other things such as illnesses must also come into play for diabetes to begin.

Diabetes is not like a cold. Your friends and family cannot catch it from you.

Living with Type 1 Diabetes
People with type 1 diabetes can live happy, healthy lives. The key is to follow your diabetes treatment plan. The goal of this plan is to keep your blood sugar level as close to normal as possible (good blood sugar control). Your treatment plan will probably include:

Insulin, which lowers blood sugar. Your health-care practitioner will prescribe how much and when to take insulin and what kinds.

Food, which raises blood sugar. Most people with type I diabetes have a meal plan. A registered dietitian makes a plan for you. It tells you how much food you can eat and when to eat it. Most people have three meals and at least two snacks every day. Your meal plan can have foods you enjoy.

Exercise, which lowers blood sugar. Like insulin, exercise also helps your body to use blood sugar. So exercise will probably be prescribed for you. Your health-care practitioner can help you fit exercise safely into your daily routine.

Blood and urine testing. Testing your blood lets you know if your blood sugar level is high, low, or near normal. The tests are simple. You prick your finger to get a drop of blood. A nurse-educator can teach you how to do this test and use the test results.

You may need to test your urine for ketones. Ketones in the urine may mean that your diabetes is not under good control. A nurse-educator can teach you how to test ketones.

Problems
Type 1 diabetes can cause problems that you should be prepared for. There are three key problems.

Hypoglycemia, or low blood sugar; sometimes called an insulin reaction. This occurs when your blood sugar drops too low. You correct this problem by eating some sugar—such as three glucose tablets, one-half cup of fruit juice, or five or six pieces of hard candy. Your health-care practitioner will teach you the signs of hypoglycemia and show you how to treat it.

Hyperglycemia, or high blood sugar. This occurs when your blood sugar is too high. It can be a sign that diabetes is not well controlled. Your health-care practitioner will explain the signs and symptoms and the best way to treat hyperglycemia.

Ketoacidosis, or diabetic coma. This is very serious. Discuss its signs with your health-care practitioner.

NONINSULIN-DEPENDENT DIABETES

Noninsulin-dependent diabetes is a disease that affects the way your body uses food. Noninsulin-dependent diabetes is also called type 2 diabetes or noninsulin-dependent diabetes mellitus (NIDDM, for short).

Type 2 diabetes used to be called maturity-onset diabetes because most people who get it are over 40. The most common type of diabetes, it affects about 11 million Americans. Nine out of 10 cases of diabetes are type 2. Most of the people who get type 2 diabetes are overweight.

When you have type 2 diabetes, your body does not make enough insulin. Or your body still makes insulin but can't use it. Without enough insulin, your body cannot move blood sugar into the cells. Sugar builds up in the bloodstream. High blood levels of sugar can cause problems.

Medical experts do not know the exact cause of type 2 diabetes. They do know type 2 diabetes runs in families. A person can inherit a tendency to get type 2 diabetes. But it usually takes another factor such as obesity to bring on the disease.

Signs and Symptoms of Type 2 Diabetes

Type 2 diabetes often develops slowly. Most people who get it have increased thirst and an increased need to urinate. Many also feel edgy, tired, and sick to their stomach. Some people have an increased appetite, but they lose weight. Other signs and symptoms include the following:

- Repeated or hard-to-heal infections of the skin, gums, vagina, or bladder
- Blurred vision
- Tingling or loss of feeling in the hands or feet
- Dry, itchy skin

These symptoms can be so mild that you don't notice them. Older people may confuse these symptoms with signs of aging and may not go to their health-care practitioner. Half of all Americans who have diabetes may not know it.

Living with Type 2 Diabetes

People with diabetes can live happy, healthy lives. The key is to follow a diabetes treatment plan. The goal of this plan is to keep blood sugar levels as close to normal as possible (good blood sugar control).

Your first step is to see your health-care practitioner. He or she will prescribe a daily treatment plan. The plan should include a healthy diet and regular exercise. You can often control type 2 diabetes with diet and exercise alone. But some people also need medicine—either diabetes pills or insulin shots. Many people find their diabetes gets better when they follow their treatment plan.

For people who have type 2 diabetes, losing weight is important. Losing weight helps some overweight people to bring their blood sugars into the normal range. People who have a tendency to get type 2 diabetes can avoid it by losing weight or not becoming overweight. (The health-care practitioner may allow some people who are overweight to stop their medication—if they lose weight and follow a good meal plan.)

Your health-care practitioner may also want you to test your blood sugar levels regularly. Testing will let you know if your diabetes is in control. Be sure to ask how to do these tests.

You can help control your diabetes if you follow your physician's treatment plan and eat a healthy diet, control your weight, exercise regularly, have regular checkups, and do not smoke.

HYPERGLYCEMIA
"Hyperglycemia" is the technical term for high blood sugar. High blood sugar happens when the body has too little insulin, or when the body can't use insulin properly.

A number of things can cause hyperglycemia. For example, if you have type 1 (insulin-dependent) diabetes, you may not have given yourself enough insulin. If you have type 2 (noninsulin-dependent) diabetes, your body may have enough insulin, but is not as effective as it should be. Or the problem could be that you ate more than planned or exercised less than planned. The stress of an illness, such as a cold or flu, could also be the cause. Other stresses, such as family conflicts, could also cause hyperglycemia.

Symptoms
The symptoms of hyperglycemia include frequent urination and increased thirst.

Blood Sugar Levels
Part of keeping your diabetes in control is testing your blood sugar often. Ask your doctor how often you should test and what your blood sugar levels should be.

Testing your blood and then treating high blood sugar early will help you avoid the other symptoms of hyperglycemia.

Hyperglycemia is defined as a blood sugar level above

120 milligrams per deciliter (mg/dl) of blood. Moderate degrees of hyperglycemia (that is, 120 to 220 mg/dl) need to be carefully monitored, but may not require immediate treatment.

It's important to treat hyperglycemia as soon as you detect it. If you fail to treat hyperglycemia, a condition called ketoacidosis (diabetic coma) could occur. Ketoacidosis develops when your body doesn't have enough insulin. Without insulin, your body can't use glucose for fuel. So, your body breaks down fats to use for energy.

When your body breaks down fats, waste products called ketones are produced. Your body cannot tolerate large amounts of ketones and will try to get rid of them through the urine. Unfortunately, the body cannot release all the ketones and they build up in your blood. This can lead to ketoacidosis. Ketoacidosis is life-threatening and needs immediate treatment. Symptoms include shortness of breath, breath that smells fruity, nausea and vomiting, and a very dry mouth. Talk to your doctor about how to handle this condition.

Treatment
Oftentimes, you can lower your blood sugar level by exercising. However, if your blood sugar is above 240 mg/dl, check your urine for ketones. If you have ketones, do not exercise. Exercising when ketones are present may make your blood sugar level go even higher. You'll need to work with your doctor to find the safest way for you to lower your blood sugar level.

Cutting down on the amount of food you eat might also help. Work with your dietitian to make changes in your meal plan. If exercise and changes in your diet don't work, your doctor may change the amount of your medication or insulin, or the times of when you take it.

Prevention
Your best bet is to practice good diabetes con-

trol. The trick is learning to detect and treat hyperglycemia early—before it can get worse.

HYPOGLYCEMIA

"Hypoglycemia" is the technical term for low blood sugar. It is often called an insulin reaction. An insulin reaction can be caused by a number of things. You may have taken too much insulin, eaten too little food or not eaten on time, or exercised too much.

Symptoms

The symptoms of hypoglycemia include the following:

- Shakiness
- Dizziness
- Sweating
- Hunger
- Headache
- Pale skin color
- Sudden moodiness or behavior changes, such as crying for no apparent reason
- Clumsy or jerky movements
- Difficulty paying attention or confusion
- Tingling sensations around the mouth

Blood Sugar Levels

Part of keeping diabetes in control is testing your blood sugar often. Ask your doctor how often you should test and what your blood sugar levels should be. The results from testing your blood will tell you when your blood sugar is low and that you need to treat it. You should test your blood sugar level according to the schedule you work out with your doctor. More importantly, though, you should test your blood whenever you feel an insulin reaction coming on. After you test and see that your blood sugar level is low, you should treat this condition quickly.

If you feel a reaction coming on but cannot test, it's best to treat the reaction rather than wait. Remember this simple rule: When in doubt, treat.

Treatment

The quickest way to raise your blood sugar is with some form of sugar, such as three glucose tablets (you can buy these at the drug store), one-half cup of fruit juice, or five or six pieces of hard candy. Ask your health-care practitioner or dietitian to list foods that you can use to treat an insulin reaction. And then, be sure you always have at least one type of sugar with you.

Once you have tested your blood and treated your reaction, wait 15 or 20 minutes and test your blood again. If your blood sugar is still low and your symptoms don't go away, repeat the treatment. After you feel better, be sure to eat your regular meals and snacks as planned to keep your blood sugar level up.

It's important to treat hypoglycemia quickly because it can get worse and you could pass out. If you pass out, you will need immediate treatment, such as an injection of glucagon or emergency treatment in a hospital.

Glucagon raises blood sugar. It is injected like insulin. Ask your doctor to prescribe it for you and tell you how to use it. You need to tell people around you (such as family members and co-workers) how and when to inject glucagon should you ever need it. If glucagon is not available, you should be taken to the nearest hospital emergency room for treatment. If you need immediate medical assistance or an ambulance, someone should call the emergency number in your area (such as 911) for help. It's a good idea to post emergency numbers by the telephone.

If you pass out, people should inject glucagon and call for emergency help. They should not inject insulin, give you food or fluids, or put their hands in your mouth.

Prevention

Good diabetes control is the best way we know

to prevent hypoglycemia. The trick is to learn to recognize the symptoms of an insulin reaction. This way, you can treat low blood sugar before it gets worse.

BLOOD TESTING

Blood testing is one of the main tools you have to keep your diabetes in control. Testing lets you know what your blood sugar level is at any one time.

This information will help you decide what adjustments to make in your diabetes control plan. For example: After exercising, you feel shaky and sweaty. Do you feel this way because you've exercised, or because your blood sugar is low? If your blood test shows that your glucose is low, then you know you need to eat a fast-acting sugar. If your blood test is normal, then you know you are shaky and sweaty because you exercised. Then you won't eat anything extra, which could cause your blood sugar to be high later.

How to Test Your Blood

There are two ways you can test your blood. In both tests, you first need to prick your finger with a special needle called a lancet to get a drop of blood. You then place the drop of blood on a test strip. The steps you follow to do your blood test will depend on what brand of test strip you use or what brand of meter you use. Ask your doctor or nurse-educator to explain the testing process that you need to follow.

In one method, you wait for the test strip to change colors. (The glucose in your blood causes the change.) You then match the color of the strip to a color chart, which is usually on the test strip container. The colors represent ranges of glucose levels, such as 60 to 90. If your test strip color matches 60, then your blood sugar is 60. If it falls between the 60 and 90 color, then it is recorded as 75.

In the second method, you place the test strip in a blood glucose meter. A meter is a small computerized machine that reads your test strip. Your blood glucose level is printed on a digital screen (like that on a pocket calculator).

Meters may provide more accurate blood glucose readings than matching the test strip colors to a chart. This is because the meter gives you an exact number so you don't have to guess at the number. It is important that you follow the test directions exactly. Not following the test directions may give you false results.

Recording the Results

Be sure to write down your blood test results. These records will help you and your doctor make adjustments in your diabetes control plan. If your blood glucose levels are frequently higher or lower than normal, you should contact your doctor.

Getting in the habit of testing may be hard at first. But as you get used to it, you'll find that blood testing makes keeping your diabetes in control a lot easier.

KETOACIDOSIS

Ketoacidosis is a serious condition that can lead to diabetic coma and even death. Ketoacidosis may happen to people with insulin-dependent (type 1) diabetes.

Ketoacidosis does not occur in people with noninsulin-dependent (type 2) diabetes. But some people—especially older people—with type 2 diabetes may experience a different serious condition. It's called hyperosmolar non-ketotic coma.

Ketoacidosis means dangerously high levels of ketones. Ketones are acids that build up in the blood. They appear in the urine when your body doesn't have enough insulin. Ketones can poison the body. They are a warning sign that your diabetes is out of control or that you are getting sick.

Treatment usually takes place in the hospital. But you can help prevent ketoacidosis by learning to recognize the warning signs and testing your urine and blood regularly.

HYPEROSMOLAR NONKETOTIC COMA

People with type 2 diabetes are at risk for hyperosmolar nonketotic coma (HNKC)—a change in body chemistry that can occur when there is a progressive rise in blood sugar coupled with an inability to drink enough water to keep up with the dramatic loss of fluid that accompanies the excretion of excessive sugar through the kidneys. The condition is usually brought on by the stress of another illness. Commonly, for example, an elderly person with diabetes may suffer a stroke, or come down with pneumonia, which both elevates blood sugar and makes it difficult to maintain an adequate fluid intake. The patient experiences no nausea or vomiting or other symptom that might alert him to the need for medical help, and thus simply slips into a coma. For this reason, it is crucial for those with even a moderate degree of diabetes to drink a generous amount of water during any illness. *The Editors*

Warning Signs

Ketoacidosis usually develops slowly. But when vomiting occurs, this life-threatening condition can develop in a few hours. The first symptoms are:

- Thirst or a very dry mouth
- Frequent urination
- High blood sugar levels
- High levels of ketones in the urine

Later symptoms include:

- Constantly feeling tired
- Dry or flushed skin
- Nausea, vomiting, or abdominal pain (Vomiting can be caused by many illnesses, not just ketoacidosis. If vomiting continues for more than two hours, contact your health-care practitioner.)
- A hard time breathing (short, deep breaths)
- Fruity odor on breath
- A hard time paying attention, or confusion

Ketoacidosis is dangerous and serious. If you have any of the above symptoms, contact your health-care practitioner immediately, or go to the nearest emergency room of your local hospital.

Detecting Ketones

A simple urine test can detect ketones. Urine testing is very easy. You use a test strip, like a blood-testing strip, and watch what color it becomes when wet with urine. The color will mean trace (very small), small, moderate, or large amounts of ketones, as shown on the test strip container. Some test strip containers use pluses (+) to show level of ketones.

Your health-care practitioner can show you how to test for ketones. Different brands have different procedures, so always read the directions. Many experts advise to check your urine for ketones when your blood sugar is more than 240 mg/dl.

When you are ill (when you have a cold or the flu, for example), test for ketones every four to six hours. And test every four to six hours when your blood sugar is more than 240 mg/dl.

Also, test for ketones when you have any symptoms of ketoacidosis.

Higher-Than-Normal Ketone Levels

If your health-care practitioner has not told you what levels of ketones are dangerous, then call when you find moderate amounts after more than one test. Often, your health-care practitioner can tell you what to do over the phone. Call your health-care practitioner at once if:

- Urine tests show large amounts of ketones
- Urine tests show large amounts of ketones and your blood sugar level is high
- You have vomited more than twice in four hours and your urine tests show large amounts of ketones

Do not exercise when your urine tests show ketones and your blood sugar is high. High levels of ketones and high blood sugars can mean your diabetes is out of control. Check with your health-care practitioner about how to handle this situation.

Causes of Ketoacidosis

Ketones mean your body is burning fat to get energy. Moderate or large amounts of ketones in your urine are dangerous. They upset the chemical balance of the blood.

Commonly, the flu, a cold, or other infections may sometimes bring on ketoacidosis.

The following are three basic reasons for moderate or large amounts of ketones in the urine.

Not getting enough insulin. Maybe you did not inject enough insulin. Or your body could need more insulin than usual because of illness. If there is not enough insulin, your body begins to break down body fat for energy.

Not enough food. When people are sick, they often do not feel like eating. Then, high ketones may result. High ketones may also occur when someone misses a meal.

An insulin reaction (low blood sugar). When blood sugar levels fall too low, the body must use fat to get energy. If testing shows high ketones in the morning, the person may have had an insulin reaction while asleep.

DIABETES COMPLICATIONS: AN OVERVIEW

Diabetes complications are medical problems that occur more often in people with diabetes than in people without diabetes. Changes in the blood vessels or the nerves are often the causes of diabetes complications.

Diabetes can cause two types of complications: Acute

complications can occur anytime blood sugar levels are high; other, chronic complications, like vascular disease, develop after many years of diabetes.

Vascular disease. Some people with diabetes may be at greater risk for changes in large blood vessels. This complication is called vascular disease. It starts when the linings of the blood vessels get thicker. Then, blood has a hard time flowing through the narrowed vessel. As a result, the blood cannot carry nutrients to your body's many organs. Heart disease or stroke can result.

Small blood vessel disease. Damage to small blood vessels can occur in the eyes and the kidneys of people with diabetes. At first, there may be no outward symptoms. But damage to blood vessels can lead to blindness and kidney disease.

Nerve damage, or neuropathy. Most often, nerve damage affects the feet and legs. Serious problems can occur in people who have nerve and blood vessel damage in the legs or feet. These people may not feel a blister or a small cut on the foot. The blister or cut may become infected, which may sometimes lead to amputation.

People with diabetes are especially susceptible to bacterial and fungal infections of many sorts—including skin infections, urinary tract infections, vaginitis, mouth infections such as thrush and gum disease, and infections of wounds. Moreover, infections significantly increase the need for insulin. As a result, anyone with diabetes should be alert to treating even minor cuts and blisters so they do not develop into major complications.

Who Gets Diabetes Complications?

No one can tell who will have diabetes complications. But experts think that keeping blood sugar levels close to normal helps to prevent or delay trouble.

High levels of sugar in the blood over time (poorly controlled diabetes) may speed the onset of complications.

Good control of blood sugar may help delay some complications.

Some people try hard to control their blood sugars. But they still may have a complication. Experts aren't sure why this happens. But even if you do have complications, there is hope. So be sure to see your health-care practitioner regularly.

What You Can Do to Avoid Diabetes Complications

First, get regular checkups. You may not know that you have a complication. But your health-care practitioner can spot trouble long before symptoms appear. Finding problems early is the best way to keep complications from getting serious.

Keep your appointments with your health-care practitioner—even if you are feeling fine. This includes your eye doctor and any other specialists you may need to see.

Also be aware of the following warning signs of trouble:

- Vision problems (blurriness, spots)
- Tiredness or pale skin color
- Obesity (more than 20 pounds overweight)
- Numbness or tingling feelings in hands or feet
- Repeated infections or slow healing of wounds
- Chest pain
- Vaginal itching
- Constant headaches (this may be a symptom of high blood pressure)

If you have one or more of these symptoms, be sure to let your health-care practitioner know.

And practice good diabetes control. Taking care of your health makes medical sense.

- Keep blood sugar levels close to normal (control diabetes).
- Control your weight.
- Eat a healthy, well-balanced diet.
- Get regular exercise.
- Have regular checkups.
- Check your feet every day for minor cuts or blisters. Show them to your health-care practitioner.
- Do not smoke.

If you have high blood pressure or high blood cholesterol, follow the medical advice you have been given.

HEART AND BLOOD VESSEL COMPLICATIONS

People with diabetes are more likely to have heart disease—and have it at an earlier age—than people without diabetes. That's because diabetes may damage blood vessels.

Blood vessels bring blood to the organs and cells of our body. There are two kinds of blood vessels: large vessels and small vessels. Large vessels carry blood from the heart to the organs, such as the liver or kidneys. Small blood vessels carry blood to the body's cells. Diabetes may lead to damage of both large blood vessels and small blood vessels.

Large Blood Vessels

Sometimes, large blood vessels of the heart or legs become blocked or damaged. When this happens, heart disease or leg problems can result.

The heart. When blood vessels of the heart become blocked or damaged, the heart does not get enough blood. Heart disease can result. This is called cardiovascular disease or coronary (heart) disease.

All people with diabetes are at increased risk for heart disease. Your risk is even greater if you have high

blood pressure, high cholesterol levels, and/or you smoke. Lowering blood pressure, controlling cholesterol levels, and stopping smoking are all proven to reduce the risk of heart disease and strokes in people with diabetes.

The warning signs of heart disease are chest pain, shortness of breath, swollen ankles, and/or irregular heartbeat. If you have any of these symptoms, talk with your health-care practitioner.

The legs. Blood vessels in the legs can also be blocked or damaged. This is called peripheral arterial disease.

You may feel weak and have pain and cramping in the legs when walking, but not when standing or sitting. Other symptoms include cold feet and loss of hair on the feet or legs. Your feet may become red when they dangle (for example, when you are sitting on a table and your feet hang over the edge). Your health-care practitioner can check for symptoms during your regular office visit. Be sure to tell your health-care practitioner if you have any of these problems.

The brain. People who have diabetes are also at increased risk for stroke. Many have hypertension, a major risk factor for stroke. Atherosclerosis occurs at an earlier age among people with diabetes than among others, and advances more rapidly, even in the face of good control of blood sugar levels.

Roughly two-thirds of all strokes are caused by a blood clot that completely blocks an artery that has already been narrowed by atherosclerotic plaque.

The symptoms of a stroke usually occur within minutes or hours of the event, although they can sometimes progress over several days. Some strokes cause symptoms that are scarcely noticeable. Others, depending on their location and severity, may cause headache, dizziness and disorientation, vomiting, burning or tingling sensations, some disturbance in your visual field, slurred speech or a loss of speech, difficulty swallowing, and paralysis. If paralysis occurs, most often one side of the body is affected, but sometimes only an arm or a leg. Severe strokes may cause loss of consciousness, coma, or death—or, among survivors, enduring physical or mental handicaps.

Small Blood Vessels
Diabetes can affect the small blood vessels in the eyes and kidneys of some people with the condition.

The eyes. Blood from a broken or leaky blood vessel can affect vision and can even lead to blindness.

You may notice sudden changes in vision, such as blurriness, dark spots, or loss of some vision. Or you may not know that small blood vessels in the eye have been damaged. That's why it's important to go regularly to your health-care practitioner. Report any changes in your sight. Don't take chances with your eyes. If you do have a serious problem, early treatment and good care could save your sight.

The kidneys. Small blood vessels in the kidneys can be blocked or damaged. This can lead to kidney disease. Damage to the kidneys usually happens slowly, without symptoms, over many years.

It's hard for you to know when blood vessels in your kidneys have been damaged. At first, the damage may be very small. That's why it's important to visit your health-care practitioner. He or she can check for symptoms of kidney damage during your regular office visits.

EYE COMPLICATIONS
All people with diabetes need to know that the disease can harm their eyesight. If you have di-

abetes, you must see your eye doctor regularly. Many eye problems are minor and can be easily treated. But some eye problems may be serious and might lead to blindness.

Report any changes in your sight to your doctor. Don't take chances with your eyes! If you do have a serious problem, early treatment and good care could save your sight.

Causes of Eye Problems in People with Diabetes

Experts do not know exactly how diabetes harms the eyes. They also can't predict who will have problems and who will not. But many experts think that high blood sugar levels over time (poorly controlled diabetes) can cause the small blood vessels in the eye to weaken, become leaky, or burst.

Diabetic Retinopathy

Diabetic retinopathy affects the retina of the eye. The retina is the area inside the eyeball that records images of objects and sends information about these images to the brain. There are two types of retinopathy.

Background retinopathy is more common. Background retinopathy occurs in about half of all people with diabetes after they have had diabetes for 10 to 15 years. This kind of retinopathy is often mild and does not affect vision. If retinopathy gets worse, the retina may swell. This is called macular edema. Macular edema does affect vision. It is a common cause of decreased vision in people with diabetes. If found early enough, macular edema can be treated. Background retinopathy may develop into the second, more serious type, called proliferative retinopathy.

Proliferative retinopathy. This type of retinopathy can cause blindness. But most people with diabetes never have this disease. It affects the fluid-filled center of the eye, called the vitreous. Tiny blood vessels grow and push into the vitreous. They may break and the retina may swell, or they can cause bleeding. This may lead to blindness.

Treatment

An operation called vitrectomy can help restore sight for people who have bleeding in the vitreous. And laser surgery has been helpful in slowing the development of proliferative retinopathy. Laser surgery can prevent further bleeding and is proven effective at reducing visual loss in patients with macular edema.

But the key to preventing eye damage is regular checkups with your eye doctor. Retinopathy comes quietly. At first, you may not know that you have the disease. An eye exam is the best way to find retinopathy early. Then laser treatments can begin to control the disease.

Maintaining tight control of blood sugar levels, a good diet, and good eye care may all help prevent retinopathy. Background retinopathy may simply require better diabetes control.

Also, make sure your blood pressure is not too high. People with diabetes and high blood pressure can have a lot more problems. Avoid too much salt and heavy lifting.

Other Types of Eye Problems

A common eye problem related to diabetes is blurred vision. People with noninsulin-dependent (type 2) diabetes or insulin-dependent (type 1) diabetes may have blurry vision when their diabetes is out of control. When diabetes is brought under control, the blurriness often goes away.

People with diabetes may get cataracts earlier than people without diabetes. Cataract is when the lens of the eye becomes cloudy. Most often, cataracts can be removed with outpatient surgery.

Glaucoma is more common in people with diabetes. Glaucoma means the pressure inside the eye is increased. Your eye doctor will check for glaucoma at your regular visits. If you have glaucoma, your eye doctor will advise treatment.

KIDNEY COMPLICATONS

Kidneys help to keep us alive. They remove harmful wastes and chemicals from the blood. These wastes leave the body in urine. Each kidney is made up of tiny blood vessels that act as filters. When these filters work well, they help keep waste products in our blood at a low level.

Kidney disease called diabetic nephropathy develops over several years. Over time, high blood sugar levels may cause blood vessel changes in some people with diabetes. These changes can harm the tiny vessels in the kidneys. Then the filters cannot remove wastes from the blood.

Who Is at Risk?

Most people who have kidney disease from diabetes have had diabetes for at least 10 to 15 years. The disease comes on so slowly that many people do not know they have it. The first sign of kidney disease is the presence of small amounts of protein, termed microabuminaria, in the urine. If you have protein in the urine, you may need more tests to check for kidney damage.

Other symptoms of kidney problems are swelling of the feet and ankles, feeling tired, and pale skin color.

Normal aging also can affect your kidneys. Adults with diabetes need to have more tests for kidney disease than younger people.

High blood pressure and frequent urinary tract infections can also affect the kidneys. If you have diabetes and either of these conditions, your health-care practitioner should check how your kidneys are working.

Treatment

If your health-care practitioner finds kidney damage, he or she will make changes in your treatment plan. Lowering blood pressure, cutting salt intake, and better controlling your blood sugar levels may help to slow the progress of kidney disease. Stopping smoking also helps.

Making certain to lower blood pressure is essential to slowing the progress of kidney disease. There is growing evidence, too, that reducing your dietary intake of protein helps to slow the progression of kidney damage. Research has also shown that a class of drugs, ACE inhibitors, slow the progression of kidney disease.

If kidney failure occurs, you will need to have treatments using an artificial kidney. This is called kidney dialysis, or hemodialysis. In one kind of dialysis, blood passes from the body through a dialysis machine. Then the clean blood returns to the body. Another kind of kidney dialysis sends fluids to the stomach area. The special fluid removes wastes from the blood. This is called peritoneal dialysis. (See also Dialysis, page 360.)

Kidney transplants may free some people from kidney dialysis. But transplant surgery does have some risk. Also, some people may not be a candidate for a transplant because of age or other health problems.

NERVE COMPLICATONS

Neuropathy is damage to the nerves. Both people with insulin-dependent (type 1) and noninsulin-dependent (type 2) diabetes can get neuropathy. Neuropathy affects nerves that connect the spinal cord to muscles, skin, blood vessels, and organs. Although neuropathy can affect many parts of the body, it most often affects the feet and the legs.

The longer you have had diabetes, the higher your risk for getting neuropathy. Young people do not usually have it. But people who get diabetes as adults may have neuropathy soon after diagnosis.

Symptoms

The most common symptoms of neuropathy are numbness, tingling, weakness, burning, or pain. These sensations often start in the fingers or toes and move up the arms or legs.

The pain is usually worse at night. It may ease in the morning.

Symptoms of neuropathy depend on which nerves are affected. If the nerves of the leg muscles are affected, the result may be difficulty walking. Damage to other nerves may result in frequent diarrhea or constipation, difficult urination, bladder infections, impotence, or poor balance.

Dangers of Neuropathy

Neuropathy can cause numbness or loss of feeling. You may not feel pain, heat, cold, or pressure. This can be dangerous. You might feel no pain when the feet are injured, frozen, or burned. Or a stone in the shoe could cause a blister or ulcer. This could lead to serious foot problems.

Infections can be very serious in people with diabetes. So even minor problems, such as a blister on a heel, need prompt attention.

People with diabetes may also have poor circulation from narrowed blood vessels. Poor circulation and the numbness of neuropathy can be especially dangerous. An injury you don't notice may cause infection, gangrene, or even amputation.

Treatment

Today there are no cures for neuropathy. But health-care practitioners may prescribe drugs to treat pain, depression, and the loss of sleep that neuropathy often brings. Good diabetes control seems to be the best bet in controlling symptoms of neuropathy.

If you have neuropathy, your health-care practitioner may refer you to a podiatrist (a foot specialist). A podiatrist can help with nail problems, foot infections, calluses, ulcers, and other problems you may have with your feet.

Losing excess weight may also help. And there is hope for the future. New drugs are being tested for the treatment of neuropathy.

COMPLICATIONS: IMPOTENCE

Impotence means that a man's penis doesn't get or stay hard enough for sex. He can't have or keep an erection. (See also Erectile Dysfunction, page 422.)

Men with diabetes become impotent more often than other men. But not all men with diabetes become impotent. Even if you have diabetes and become impotent, it does not mean that diabetes is the cause.

Causes

There are many causes of impotence. Some causes, such as diabetes, can be physical. But there are also many psychological causes. Men with diabetes may become impotent from psychological causes, too.

In impotence caused by diabetes, the nerves that cause an erection may be damaged. Impotence can be one symptom of nerve damage.

Another cause of impotence in men with diabetes is called penile artery blockage. This occurs when blood vessels in the penis are damaged.

Some medications can cause impotence. For example, drugs prescribed for colds, stomachaches, ulcers, depression, high blood pressure, epilepsy, and pain all may cause impotence. (But do not stop taking any medicine unless your health-care practitioner agrees.) Injury, illness, lack of male hormones (such as testosterone), and alcoholism are also causes of impotence.

Impotence can be related to feelings. Feelings of fear, anxiety, or anger may cause impotence. In fact, some men who have had a heart attack become impotent—not because of the heart attack, but because they are afraid of having another heart attack during sex. (A heart attack during sex does not often happen.)

Tiredness and stress can also be causes of impotence.

Treatment

See section on Erectile Dysfunction, page 422.

Prevention

Sometimes the fear that they will become impotent causes men with diabetes to become impotent. If you are afraid of impotence, talk with your health-care practitioner.

Experts agree that keeping your blood sugar levels near normal is the best way to avoid any diabetes complication. This includes nerve or blood vessel problems that can cause impotence.

Avoid heavy drinking and do not smoke. Alcoholism itself may cause impotence. And smoking may cause problems with blood flow. So if you smoke, stop.

Remember: Impotence does not mean an end to your sex life. You can still enjoy sex.

FOOT CARE

Some people with diabetes may have nerve damage and/or poor circulation in the legs and feet. They may not feel a little cut or a blister. Later, the cut or blister could become infected, leading to gangrene. If not treated, amputation is sometimes needed to save the rest of the foot or leg.

If you have any cut, scrape, or break in the skin of your foot, keep the area clean and dry. Use adhesive tape bandages with care. When you pull off the tape, do not tear the skin. If you notice redness or heat from a cut or blister, tell your health-care practitioner immediately.

Diabetes can also cause changes in the skin of your feet. At times your feet may become very dry. The skin may peel and crack. Proper treatment for dry, scaly feet is easy. After bathing, dry your feet. Rub on a thin coating of petroleum jelly or hand cream. Do not put the jellies or creams between your toes.

People with diabetes—like anyone else—can suffer from common foot problems, such as ingrown toenails or plantar warts. You should make an appointment with your health-care practitioner or podiatrist if you have any of the following foot problems:

- *Ingrown toenails.* Your toe can be red, tender, painful, and swollen.
- *Plantar warts.* These are viral infections on the sole of the foot. They can be painful. Your health-care practitioner can treat these.
- *Puncture wounds* (stepping on a nail, for example). These are always serious and should be treated quickly.

Protecting Your Feet

You can take steps to protect your feet. Follow these tips for good foot care.

- Visit your health-care practitioner regularly. Be sure that your feet are examined at each visit. Taking off your shoes and socks is a good reminder to your health-care practitioner.
- Wash your feet every day. Dry them carefully, especially between the toes.
- Check your feet and between your toes daily. Look for blisters, cuts, and scratches.
- If you have a foot infection, report it quickly to your health-care practitioner.
- Before you put your shoes on, check for pebbles or other objects inside the shoe that could hurt your feet.
- Before bathing, use your finger or elbow—not your feet—to check the temperature of the water.
- Be careful with hot water bottles, heating pads, or electric blankets. Burns may occur without your feeling them.
- Never walk barefoot.
- Do not cut corns and calluses yourself. Let your health-care practitioner cut them.
- Be careful when you trim your toenails. Cut nails straight across.
- Wear shoes that fit your feet and that feel comfortable.
- Change your socks every day. Socks or nylons should be even and smooth. Socks that are mended or bumpy can put extra pressure on feet.

• If your feet become numb or start to burn or tingle, be sure to check with your health-care practitioner.

NUTRITION

Nutrition means eating well-balanced meals. Nutrition, along with exercise and medications (insulin or oral diabetes pills), is important for good diabetes control.

People with diabetes have the same nutritional needs as anyone else. Regular, well-balanced meals may help to improve their overall health. Eating healthy foods in the right amounts and keeping weight under control may help diabetes management.

The following dietary tips offer good general guidelines for a diet if you have diabetes, but every person with diabetes needs a specific meal plan tailored to his or her individual needs by a diabetes specialist or dietitian.

Which Foods Are Healthy?

No single food will supply all the nutrients your body needs, so good nutrition means eating a variety of foods.

Food is divided into four main groups: (1) fruits and vegetables (oranges, apples, bananas, carrots, and spinach); (2) whole grains, cereals, and bread (wheat, rice, oats, bran, and barley); (3) dairy products (whole or skim milk, cream, and yogurt); and (4) meats, fish, poultry, eggs, dried beans, and nuts. It's important to eat foods from each group every day. By doing that, you will make sure that your body has all the nutrients it needs.

The main nutrients in food are carbohydrates, proteins, fats, vitamins, and minerals. Nutrients help your body work right.

Carbohydrates give you energy. Healthy choices are dried beans, peas, and lentils; whole grain breads, cereals, and crackers; and fruits and vegetables.

Protein is necessary for growth and provides a good back-up supply of energy.

Healthy choices include lean meats and low-fat dairy products.

Foods high in fiber are healthy, too. Fiber comes from plants and may help to lower blood sugar and blood fat levels. Foods high in fiber include bran cereals, cooked beans and peas, whole grain bread, fruits, and vegetables.

Which Foods Are Unhealthy?

Fat is a nutrient, and you need some fat in your diet. But too much fat isn't good for anyone. And it can be very harmful to people with diabetes.

Too much fat or cholesterol may increase the chances of heart disease and/or atherosclerosis. People with diabetes have a greater risk of developing these diseases than those without diabetes. So, it is very important that you limit the fat in your diet.

Fat is found in many foods. Red meat, dairy products (whole milk, cream, cheese, and ice cream), egg yolks, butter, salad dressings, vegetable oils, and many desserts are high in fat. To cut down on fat and cholesterol:

• Choose lean cuts of meat; remove extra fat.
• Eat more fish and poultry (without the skin).
• Use diet margarine instead of butter.
• Drink low-fat or skim milk.
• Limit the number of eggs you eat to three or four a week and choose liver only now and then.

Too much salt may worsen high blood pressure. Many foods contain salt. Sometimes you can taste it (as in pickles or bacon). But there is also "hidden" salt in many foods, such as cheeses, salad dressings, and canned soups. When using salt or fat, remember: A little goes a long way.

People with diabetes should eat less sugar. Foods high in sugar include desserts such as frosted cake and pie, sugary breakfast foods, table sugar, honey, and syrup. One can of regular soft drink has nine teaspoons of sugar.

Finally, good advice is to stay away from alcohol. If you like an alcoholic drink now and then, ask your dietitian for advice.

Setting Up a Meal Plan

You and your dietitian should work together to design a meal plan that's right for you and includes foods that you enjoy. A diabetes meal plan is a guide that tells you how much and what kinds of food you can choose to eat at meals and snack times. A good meal plan should fit in with your schedule and eating habits. The right meal plan will also help keep your weight where it should be. Whether you need to lose weight, gain weight, or stay where you are, your meal plan can help.

EXERCISE

Exercise, along with good nutrition and medications (insulin or oral diabetes pills), is important for good diabetes control.

Exercise benefits everyone. It is especially good for people with diabetes. Exercise can be almost any activity you enjoy: walking, bicycling, swimming, jogging, hiking, tennis, or golf.

Exercise usually lowers blood sugar. That helps your body utilize its food supply better. Also, exercise may help insulin work better. And, if you are overweight, exercise—plus careful attention to diet—can help take off extra pounds.

Exercise is important in many other ways. It improves the flow of blood through the small blood vessels and increases your heart's pumping power. The right exercise program may make you look and feel better.

Your health-care practitioner can help you decide what kinds of exercise—and how much exercise—are best suited to your needs. If your blood sugar control is poor, do not exercise. Get medical advice first. If you have retinopathy (diabetic eye disease) or blood vessel problems, see your health-care practitioner before you start exercising.

Exercise has value only if it's done regularly.

People with diabetes should exercise at least several days a week.

Exercise and Type 1 Diabetes

Before starting any exercise program, check with your health-care practitioner. Your activity must be planned to fit in with your meal plan and with the action times and amounts of your insulin.

If you're exercising more than one hour after eating, it's a good idea to eat before you start. As a rule, a high-carbohydrate snack, such as six ounces of fruit juice or one-half a plain bagel, is good before mild to moderate exercise (walking, bicycling, or golf).

If you plan on doing heavier exercise (such as aerobics, running, squash, or handball), you may need to eat a little more, such as half of a meat sandwich and a cup of low-fat milk.

It's always a good idea to check your blood sugar level before you start exercising. If you are low (under 70 mg/dl), you will need a snack to avoid having low blood sugar while you exercise. This would cause an insulin reaction. A reaction might make you feel sweaty, dizzy, or confused. An insulin reaction can occur while you exercise or several hours, even up to 12 hours, later. If you feel one coming on while exercising, stop. Immediately have one-half cup of orange juice or nondiet soft drink or three glucose tablets. You need to treat an insulin reaction as soon as you feel it coming on. Do not wait, otherwise it could become worse. When you exercise, you should bring along some raisins or hard candy to eat, just in case. They will raise your blood sugar level.

If you play a team sport such as baseball or basketball, you should let someone know you have diabetes and teach them how to help you, if needed. If you like running or cycling, do it with a friend or family member. If you can't find anyone to go with you, let someone know where you are going and when you will be back.

With regular exercise, you will need to test your blood sugar more often.

Exercise and Type 2 Diabetes

Almost nine out of 10 people with type 2 diabetes are overweight. Most often, they are also past age 40. In many cases, type 2 diabetes can be controlled through diet and exercise alone. For these reasons, exercise is a very important part of the control plan for those with type 2 diabetes.

Exercise burns calories, which your body would otherwise store as extra weight. And because exercise also helps lower blood sugar levels, exercise can help you better control your diabetes.

Starting an Exercise Program

The first step is to check with your health-care practitioner. Together, you can decide how much and which kinds of exercise are best suited for you.

SICK-DAY CARE

The common cold, the flu, and other illnesses can present special problems when you have diabetes. The physical stress of illness can raise blood sugar. And loss of appetite or vomiting can affect diabetes control.

You may not be able to prevent catching a cold. But you can help prevent a minor illness from becoming a big problem by being prepared—before you become sick.

How Do You Prepare for an Illness?

You need to have a sick-day plan of action. Your health-care practitioner can help you make up the plan. It should include instructions for the following:

- When to call the health-care practitioner
- Blood sugar and urine ketone testing
- Foods and fluids to take during your illness
- Medication changes

Remember: Only your health-care practitioner knows when to change your insulin, diabetes pills, or diet.

When Do You Call the Health-Care Practitioner?

You should call the health-care practitioner if you have:

- An illness that does not improve after one or two days
- Diarrhea or vomiting for over six hours
- Moderate to large amounts of ketones in the urine
- High blood sugar readings (Your sick-day plan should list the exact limits.)
- Sleepiness that is not normal for you
- Doubt about what you need to do for the illness
- Stomach or chest pain, difficulty breathing, or a very dry mouth (If you have any of these symptoms, call your health-care practitioner immediately.)

Should You Test More Often?

When you first think that you are sick, test your blood sugar. Be prepared to follow your sick-day plan. You should also test your urine for ketones.

People with type 1 diabetes should check blood sugar and urine ketones every four hours. Some people may need to check more often.

People with type 2 diabetes should check blood sugar at least four times a day (usually before each meal and at bedtime). They should check for urine ketones if the blood sugar is more than 240 mg/dl.

Should You Stop Taking Diabetes Medication?

No. Do not stop taking your insulin or diabetes pills. Even if you cannot eat, your body needs the medication that's been prescribed for you.

If you take insulin, take your usual dose. You may need to take more rapid-acting (regular) insulin. Check with your health-care practitioner.

If you take diabetes pills, take them if you can. Sometimes on sick days, you may need to take insulin. Check with your health-care practitioner.

How Do You Stick to a Meal Plan?

Sometimes during illness, sticking to your meal plan is a problem. When you are sick, you may not feel like eating. You may find it hard to eat some foods on your regular meal plan. That's why you need a list of foods and liquids for sick days.

Drinking plenty of fluids during sick days is important. There is no set rule for how much extra fluid to drink. About four to six ounces every 30 to 60 minutes is reasonable. These extra fluids should not have calories— for example, drink water, diet soft drinks, or tea without sugar.

Eating is important, too. If you can't eat your regular foods, replace them with sugar-containing liquids or soft foods. For example, one-half cup apple juice, one-half cup orange juice, one-half cup fruit-flavored yogurt, or six crackers are good choices.

If you are so sick that you keep throwing up fluids, call your health-care practitioner immediately.

Can Sick-Day Medications Affect Diabetes?

Yes. If you are sick, you may be taking drugs other than those for diabetes alone. Many cough syrups and cough drops have sugar. Some cold remedies may raise your blood sugar. Be sure to read the labels on any nonprescription drugs you use. Before you use a nonprescription drug, check with your health-care practitioner or pharmacist. They can help you choose safe nonprescription medications.

The American Diabetes Association

OBESITY

Obesity is one of the most written about, most discussed, and least understood public health problems facing our nation. An enormous amount of misinformation, myth, and unsuccessful medical management surrounds this serious medical problem.

CAUSES

At the simplest level, obesity is the result of eating more calories in food than required by the body. Many potential causes for this exist, and therefore physicians think of this disorder not as a single disease but as several different conditions that have the symptom of overweight in common. In most cases the underlying cause of obesity in a given individual is unknown. Physicians are able to identify the specific cause in less than 5 percent of the people who suffer from obesity.

Obesity is a common problem varying in degree from mild to severe. Although the exact prevalence of obesity in the population is not known, the most recent survey showed that one-third of adult Americans are overweight. There is evidence that the incidence of obesity may be increasing.

Several factors appear to influence the prevalence of obesity in the American population. While excess body weight can affect people of all ages, obesity increases in prevalence with increasing age, peaking in middle age. Obesity is common throughout all segments of our society, but it appears to have a particular relationship to socioeconomic status. The lower the socioeconomic status, the greater the prevalence of obesity. Similarly, as the level of education decreases, the prevalence of obesity increases. Obesity among African Americans in this country, particularly among African American women, appears to be greater in proportion to population than obesity among Caucasians. These socioeconomic trends, however, do not apply to individuals at or below the poverty level; these individuals have a low incidence of obesity.

Genetic factors appear to be important in obesity, although their exact nature or role is not well understood at present. Obesity tends to run in families, a fact that reflects, at least in part, the genetic or hereditary basis for obesity. But, environmental, lifestyle factors such as attitudes and practices regarding eating, and physical activity also are important determinants of obesity. Thus, it is probable that both genetic and environmental factors contribute to the development and perpetuation of obesity, and it is often very difficult to separate these two factors in a given individual.

HEALTH CONSEQUENCES

Obesity is associated with serious and significant negative health consequences. For example, obesity appears to be associated with serious consequences for the quality and length of life.

In adults, the mortality rate for obese individuals exceeds the expected death rate for other individuals in that age group, especially for individuals who are more than 30 percent above standard body weight as defined by the Metropolitan Life Insurance Company's 1959 height-weight table. Individuals who are overweight by less than 30 percent are also at increased risk for mortality.

A person does not need to be massively overweight to face an increased risk of death; even a moderate or mild degree of overweight can increase the risk of mortality at each age group.

In large part, this appears to be related to the fact that the obese individual is prone to a greater variety of serious and life-threatening diseases than is the nonobese person.

Diabetes Mellitus

The obese individual runs a greater risk of developing diabetes mellitus than the nonobese person. The chance of developing diabetes may be two or three times greater for the obese person. The health consequences of diabetes are so serious and widespread that public health experts view the increase in obesity with alarm.

The risk of diabetes is especially high with the accumulation of excess fat in the abdomen. Abdominal obesity can be defined by measuring the circumference of the abdomen with a tape measure: a circumference greater than 40 inches in a man or greater than 35 inches in women.

Researchers do not fully understand the mechanism whereby obesity increases the risk of developing diabetes. Information from several laboratories, in this country and abroad, suggests that obesity somehow interferes with the action of insulin. In addition, in some obese individuals there appears to be a decreased ability of the pancreas to secrete sufficient amounts of insulin into the blood. As a consequence of insufficient insulin action, the body's regulation of glucose (sugar) metabolism may be abnormal and the blood glucose level may become elevated. A blood test, urinalysis, or glucose tolerance test can detect excessive amounts of glucose in the blood.

If the obese individual with diabetes and an abnormal glucose metabolism loses weight by losing body fat, insulin's ability to regulate glucose metabolism improves, the blood insulin level returns to or toward normal, and the blood glucose concentration decreases. Moreover, the symptoms of diabetes often disappear.

Heart Disease

The obese individual also runs an increased risk of developing a variety of cardiac diseases. The most serious of these conditions, atherosclerotic heart disease, can lead to heart attacks.

Obesity and associated poor insulin action commonly cause a collection of abnormalities that predispose to atherosclerosis: high triglycerides, low levels of HDL ("good") cholesterol, and high blood pressure. Weight loss often improves blood levels of triglycerides and HDL cholesterol as well as blood pressure.

Other Consequences

Obesity affects the individual in many other ways. It places severe stress on the internal organs, the musculoskeletal system, the digestive tract, and the psychological state of the obese person.

Obese individuals often find that they are outcasts in our society. They may encounter discrimination in employment as well as daily living situations. This treatment generates emotional stress, an important health consequence of obesity.

WHAT IS OBESITY?

Obesity is an excessive increase in body fat. In man and in animals, fat in the body is stored primarily in specific cells (adipose or fat cells) in the adipose (fat) tissue.

Microscopic examination shows that a fat cell is very different in appearance from other cells. Most cells contain a large amount of cytoplasm, with the cell nucleus near the center of the cell. Fat constitutes almost the entire area of the adipose cell, and the cytoplasm and nucleus are displaced. Thus, fat, in the form of triglyceride, is the major component of the adipose cell.

In the nonobese adult male, approximately 10 to 15 percent of the total body weight is fat. In the nonobese woman, fat may constitute up to 20 percent of total body weight. If fat comprises more than 20 percent of the total body weight, the individual is obese.

At the present time, there is no practical or simple way to determine the amount of a person's body weight that is fat. For this reason, people have developed alternative ways to assess obesity.

The most common index of obesity is body weight. Several standard tables exist that calculate recommended body weight in relation to height and body frame.

If an individual weighs more than the ideal or average weight for his or her age, height, and body frame, as shown in any of the standard tables, he or she is overweight. An individual who is more than 15 to 20 percent overweight is considered to be definitely obese. Obesity may also, and probably does, exist in individuals who are 5 to 15 percent over the ideal or average body weights shown in the standard tables.

There are difficulties, however, in determining obesity from any standard weight-height tables. For example, of two men with the same weight and height, one may be obese, and the other not. Both may weigh 225 pounds and be six feet tall; one man is an athlete and his weight is due to increased muscle mass, while the weight of the second man, in poor physical condition, is due to an increased amount of fat. Both of these men would be classified as overweight according to any of the standard tables, but only one is obese, because obesity is an increase in body fat and not an increase in muscle.

Another way to assess obesity is to determine the body mass index (BMI) as follows: Multiply weight in pounds by 704 and divide the result by the square of the height in inches. A BMI between 25 and 29.9 is considered overweight. Obesity is defined by a BMI of 30 or greater.

ADIPOSE TISSUE AND ENERGY

In man, the adipose tissue (fat) has a very important function; it serves as the principal

LOSING WEIGHT AND KEEPING IT OFF

The trick to weight loss is not so much how to lose the weight (many different diets will help achieve that), but how to keep it off. The 34 million overweight Americans, including close to a third of all those over 50, put themselves at increased risk for diabetes, heart disease, and even some forms of cancer. At any given time, about 25 percent of all men and half of all women are trying to lose weight—but most of them will subsequently regain what they lost. Not only is "rebound" weight gain demoralizing, it also can change metabolism so that losing regained weight becomes even more difficult. And, though losing weight lowers blood pressure and cholesterol levels, some studies have shown that rebound weight gain can more than offset these positive benefits.

A survey published in the *American Journal of Clinical Nutrition* examined differences between women who keep weight off and those who lose it and gain it back again. (Though the survey only included women, rebound weight gain is a problem for men as well.) The researchers interviewed 108 women, mostly middle-aged: 30 "maintainers" (women who were formerly obese, or more than 20 percent above desired weight, who had lost weight and kept it off); 44 "relapsers" (obese women who had lost weight but regained it); and 34 "controls" (women who had never been obese). All were asked about their weight history and childhood eating patterns; about their current eating patterns; if they felt supported by others in their weight-loss endeavors; if they drank alcohol or smoked; if they ate in response to emotional issues; if they had recently been under stress. The results showed sharp differences between maintainers and relapsers. The strategies used by the successful dieters, summarized as follows, are ex-

cellent guidelines for anyone wanting to keep excess weight off.

• *Exercise regularly.* Staying active was the primary difference between maintainers and relapsers. Close to 90 percent of maintainers and 82 percent of controls exercised regularly—at least three times a week for at least 30 minutes a session—to stay at their desired weight; only 36 percent of relapsers exercised regularly, and they exercised less frequently and strenuously.

• *Eat a healthful diet, but don't deprive yourself.* Maintainers ate an improved diet consisting of less fat and sugar and more fruits and vegetables, and they cooked in a more healthful way (restricting fried foods). However, they occasionally allowed themselves favorite foods so that they didn't feel deprived. Ultimately, they developed new eating habits. In contrast, relapsers resorted to appetite suppressants, fasting, or extremely restrictive diets for weight loss—all of these approaches enhance feelings of deprivation and do not foster eating habits that can be sustained for the long haul.

• *Feel good about your body.* Relapsers were, overall, unhappy with their bodies: More than 70 percent saw themselves as heavy or ugly. In contrast, 86 percent of maintainers and 94 percent of controls saw themselves as thin or of average weight.

• *Actively confront problems.* Most of the women were currently tackling a stressful or troubling issue, but the problem-solving methods differed between the groups. Relapsers were more likely to try to escape from dealing with problems by eating, sleeping more, or wishing the problem would go away. Maintainers and controls were more likely to seek social support from friends, or professional help, actively confront the problem, and try to solve it. *The Editors*

---

energy storage organ of the body. Energy is measured in calories. Adipose tissue is the caloric reservoir of the body.

Chemical energy—calories—originates in food ingested as nourishment. The digestive system enables the body to extract a portion of the chemical energy in the food, and to use

the calories for fuel. Only a portion of this energy, however, can be used by the body. Researchers estimate that the body uses roughly 40 percent of the potential chemical energy in foodstuffs as fuel for cells. The remaining energy is converted to heat and is lost from the body.

Foodstuffs are composed of carbohydrates, fats, and proteins; energy is extracted from all three nutrients.

This energy is used by the body for two purposes. First, it supports vital bodily functions such as respiration, the action of the heart muscle, synthesis and secretion of compounds, and maintenance and repair of tissues. These and other vital bodily functions require energy, the same as an automobile requires gasoline. A sufficient amount of energy (number of calories) must be supplied to the body for it to perform its vital functions; this energy is therefore essential for life. Excess calories are stored as fat in adipose cells. Generally, fat is stored as triglyceride in the adipose tissue for future use.

Second, energy is used by the body to perform physical activity. Performance of a given amount of activity requires a certain amount of energy be supplied to the body.

When the amount of energy provided by the calories in the ingested food is equal to the amount of energy needed by the body to perform all of its vital functions plus any additional physical activity, the individual is said to be in energy balance. In this situation, the person will maintain the amount of adipose tissue and body weight at a constant level. When the amount of energy provided by the calories in the ingested food is less than the amount of energy needed by the body, the individual is said to be in negative energy balance. In this situation, the adipose tissue will be broken down to provide the energy needed by the body, this tissue will decrease in size, and the individual will lose body weight. When energy intake in food is greater than the amount needed by the body, the person will increase the amount of adipose tissue, that is, will become fatter, and will increase in weight.

In an obese person the caloric intake is consistently greater than the amount the body needs to maintain its vital functions and to perform daily activities. The excess calories go to fat. Since the individual is in positive energy balance, the body weight increases and body fat increases, expanding the adipose tissue.

At rest, an adult man requires about 1,200 to 1,500 calories a day to maintain his vital functions. If the person is doing something other than lying at rest, such as working or walking, his energy requirements will rise. In order to maintain his body weight and energy balance, he will have to ingest perhaps 2,000 calories a day. If he does, his body weight remains stable, whereas if he ingests less, his body weight decreases. If he ingests more calories than he expends in his activities, the excess calories are converted to triglyceride and stored in the adipose tissue. Vigorous physical activity, such as exercise, will raise energy requirements even more and caloric requirements will increase. The same principles governing energy balance and body weight just described still apply, however.

The same principles apply to women, although the energy requirements of men and women do differ slightly. A woman at rest requires approximately 1,000 calories to 1,300 calories a day, on the average. When she is active she will require more calories to maintain her weight. Of course, if she ingests more than she needs, she will store the excess in adipose tissue and will gain fat and weight.

Energy requirements at rest and during activity will vary from person to person. People have different rates of basal metabolism; therefore people have slightly different caloric needs. In addition, some people's bodies are physiologically more efficient than others at extracting and utilizing the energy within foodstuffs. One must tailor a nutritional assessment and caloric intake plan to each person individually. Although there is at present no definitive or conclusive data to support the view that subtle differences in the ability to extract or utilize calories cause obesity, recent research may suggest that such differences might contribute to the development or perpetuation of the obese state in some individuals.

Recent studies have shown that adipose tissue produces a hormone-like substance called leptin, which acts on the brain to decrease food intake and increase exercise. The fact that obese people have high levels of leptin suggests that centers in their brain are insensitive to leptin action.

OPPORTUNITIES FOR CHANGE

Overeating seems to be endemic to the American adult population. Our society is oriented toward eating. Food advertisements are persuasive. Fast food restaurants and automats are everywhere; buildings contain canteens, often on every floor. Although it will be very difficult to effect, Americans will have to change their lifestyle—their beliefs, attitudes, and practices regarding eating and exercise—if they are to solve the problem of obesity.

Lack of exercise, the other major factor in adult obesity, applies to most men and women in our society. American adults tend to participate in physical activities as spectators rather than as participants. Again, only a fundamental change in lifestyle can alter the pattern.

The Warren Grant Magnuson Clinical Center

THYROID DISEASE AND AGE

Aging affects all of the systems of the body. Therefore, many diseases have different presentations, follow different patterns, and require different treatments when they affect older patients. Diseases of the thyroid gland are no exception. Thyroid problems occur in great frequency in patients over the age of 60. When they do occur, physicians often may find them difficult to diagnose. Even the patients themselves may not realize they are sick, and the courses of the illnesses and their outcomes frequently differ from those in younger patients.

HYPERTHYROIDISM

Hyperthyroidism is common among elderly individuals. In many cases, the symptoms are typical and include nervousness, palpitations, sweating, tremors, and weight loss. However, often the most striking characteristic of hyperthyroidism in older patients is the paucity of symptoms which they describe. They frequently do not have enlarged thyroids and do not complain of nervousness or heat intolerance. Rather than the usual picture of weight loss despite an increased appetite, older patients may lose their desire for food so that weight loss is very common. In fact, many older patients with hyperthyroidism are evaluated for depression or cancer before the correct diagnosis is made.

Therefore, it is apparent that hyperthyroidism can be easily overlooked in the elderly, because the presenting features may not conform to the usual findings in younger people. Physicians must consider the possibility of hyperthyroidism in patients who complain of a great variety of symptoms, including shortness of breath, palpitations, nervousness, weakness, loss of appetite, as well as those who seem to be emotionally ill. Fortunately, those patients whose problems are caused by hyperthyroidism can usually be identified by means of simple and inexpensive blood tests.

How Is Hyperthyroidism Diagnosed?

The techniques used by physicians to diagnose hyperthyroidism in elderly patients are usually simple and similar to those employed in younger patients. Blood tests reveal high serum concentrations of thyroid hormones and a low level of TSH (thyroid stimulating hormone) from the pituitary gland. A radioactive thyroid scan can tell whether the entire thyroid is overactive or whether there are one or more hyper-functioning nodules present.

What Is the Best Treatment?

Treatment of hyperthyroidism is similar for patients of any age, though at times physicians make minor alterations because of the presence of other underlying medical problems. The treatment of choice is almost always radioactive iodine, because of the safety and simplicity of its administration. It is taken by mouth. By damaging thyroid tissue, this treatment begins to slow the thyroid gland's output of thyroid hormone after one to two months. After the thyroid hormone levels return to normal, they need to be rechecked only once or twice a year after the first six months. However, almost all patients develop hypothyroidism (an underactive thyroid) after radioiodine. It usually occurs within the first year after treatment, but it can develop at any time. This makes lifelong monitoring of thyroid function mandatory.

About 40 percent of patients treated with radioactive iodine become hypothyroid within a year of treatment. An additional 3 percent of those treated will develop hypothyroidism each successive year.

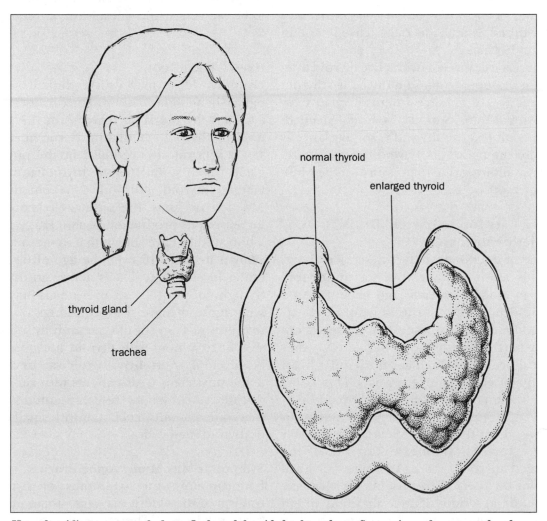

Hyperthyroidism can cause the butterfly-shaped thyroid gland to enlarge. Surgery is rarely warranted, unless the thyroid becomes so large that it interferes with breathing or swallowing.

293

Occasionally, a physician may choose to slow down an overactive thyroid by using an antithyroid drug such as propylthiouracil (PTU) or methimazole (Tapazole). These drugs block the utilization of iodine by the thyroid gland. Since iodine is necessary for the manufacture of thyroid hormone, hormone levels begin to fall in 10 days to two weeks and may become normal after just four to six weeks of such therapy. Usually, these drugs only control the thyroid as long as the patient takes them, but hyperthyroidism will again be experienced by many patients when they stop the medications. Moreover, since these drugs may cause rare side effects, including fever, hives, and a lowering of the white blood cell count, they are not used as much as radioactive iodine in older individuals.

Surgical removal of overactive thyroid nodules (or most of the gland if the entire thyroid is overactive) offers a treatment alternative for hyperthyroidism. Surgery is rarely needed, however, unless the thyroid is so very large as to cause the patient to have difficulty breathing or swallowing due to pressure on the windpipe or esophagus.

Special Uses for Antithyroid Drugs in Elderly Patients

In spite of the disadvantages described above, there is an important role for antithyroid drugs in elderly hyperthyroid patients. Antithyroid drugs are often used before radioactive iodine treatment, especially if the patient has hyperthyroidism complicated by other medical problems, such as an irregular heart rhythm or chest pain (angina). This is because radioiodine treatment is occasionally followed by temporary further increases in circulating thyroid hormone levels, presumably due to stored hormone leaking out of the damaged thyroid gland. A young individual may not be affected by this, but an older patient with a serious heart condition might experience complications from even a temporary mild increase in thyroid hormone levels.

Pre-treatment with antithyroid drugs will prevent this from happening. In addition, physicians often prescribe one of the beta adrenergic blocking drugs (for example, Inderal, Corgard, Tenormin, Lopressor), which lessen the severity of symptoms by blocking the action of circulating thyroid hormone on body tissues. Radioiodine can then be administered safely despite a possible temporary worsening of the thyroid condition.

Although hyperthyroidism is often more difficult to diagnose in an elderly patient because its presentation may be subtle or somewhat unusual, the diagnosis, once suspected, is simple to confirm. Radioiodine is considered to be the easiest and safest form of treatment.

HYPOTHYROIDISM

Hypothyroidism may also be difficult to recognize in an older patient. The earliest sign of a failing thyroid is an increase in the blood level of thyroid stimulating hormone (TSH). TSH is a hormone produced by the pituitary gland which stimulates the thyroid to manufacture thyroid hormones. When thyroid function declines, the pituitary responds by increasing its production of TSH. Large population studies have shown that as many as one woman in every 10 over the age of 65 has a blood level of TSH that is above normal. Although most of these individuals have no symptoms, all have the beginnings of hypothyroidism. They should be carefully followed so that treatment with thyroid hormone can be given if overt hypothyroidism develops. Some physicians treat patients with very mild disease, since several research studies show that some patients feel better with small doses of thyroid medication.

Symptoms May Mimic Aging Process

Unfortunately, the symptoms of hypothyroidism in the elderly are very easy to mistake for normal aging. Therefore, elderly individuals who gradually become hypothyroid may see a variety of specialists because of the various symptoms they may have, including hoarseness, dry skin, deafness, muscle cramps, numbness and weakness of the hands, unsteadiness of gait, anemia, and constipation. It is easy to see why such vague and nonspecific symptoms can often be attributed to the aging process.

Associated Disorders Suggest Need for Thyroid Screening

Physicians are aware that although hypothyroidism is very common in elderly patients, it is extremely difficult to recognize by physical examination alone. There are clues which can lead physicians to test for hypothyroidism in certain individuals within an elderly population. These include premature graying of the hair, protrusion of the eyeballs (known as exophthalmos), juvenile (type 1) diabetes which requires treatment with insulin, rheumatoid arthritis, pernicious anemia (caused by lack of vitamin B_{12}) harmless white skin spots known as vitiligo, and patchy hair loss known as alopecia areata.

The presence of these and certain other medical problems in either the patient or a close relative increases the likelihood that the particular individual will develop thyroid failure. By taking a careful family history, physicians can identify the people with the greatest risk for thyroid failure and perform thyroid testing, even in the absence of physical evidence of hypothyroidism.

How is Hypothyroidism Diagnosed?

Fortunately, the laboratory tests required for the diagnosis of hypothyroidism are simple, inexpensive, and the same as those used in younger patients. A single blood sample is obtained and the concentrations of the thyroid hormone, thyroxine (T4), and the pituitary thyroid stimulating hormone (TSH) are measured. People with obvious evidence of thyroid failure usually show both a decrease in T4 and an increase in TSH. Some patients who are just beginning to experience thyroid failure may only show an increase in TSH. Many patients also have elevated levels of antibodies directed against the thyroid (called antithyroid antibodies).

Who Needs Treatment?

Patients with obvious thyroid failure require treatment. It is not clear, however, whether individuals with only an increased TSH and still-normal thyroid hormone levels need treatment. One long-term follow-up study showed that about 20 percent of elderly patients with a high TSH progressed to true hypothyroidism each year. This suggests that patients who feel well and have only a high TSH should be retested every year to be sure that they are not becoming hypothyroid. The chances of hypothyroidism developing are highest in individuals who have a high TSH and antithyroid antibodies in their blood.

Thyroid replacement is often started when a further reduction in thyroid function is highly likely, such as in those who were treated with radioactive iodine, or when the LDL cholesterol is elevated.

On the other hand, some patients who have only mild TSH elevations actually feel better when they take enough thyroid hormone each day to normalize the TSH level. Studies have shown that thyroid hormone may improve symptoms of fatigue, constipation, and poor energy in some people with only an elevated TSH level. This has led many physicians to recommend a trial of thyroid hormone in every patient with an increased blood level of TSH.

Start with Low Doses of Thyroid Hormone

Treatment of hypothyroidism should be instituted with extreme care in elderly patients. Most of them have had this condition for months or even years without obvious symptoms, and most do not feel particularly sick. Furthermore, their requirements for thyroid hormone are usually not very great. The hypothyroid condition slows the chemical reactions within the body so that thyroid hormone is used up more slowly than normal. Therefore, most physicians recommend starting treatment with as little as 25 micrograms of thyroxine (T4) per day, increasing the dose of medication by 25 micrograms each month until the blood level of TSH falls into the normal range. In patients with heart disease, even lower initial doses and a more gradual increase in medication may be necessary. Long-term follow-up of all patients is essential. Thyroid function may continue to decline, and, therefore, yearly blood tests for T4 and TSH are necessary.

Physicians now know that taking too much thyroid hormone replacement can increase bone loss and worsen osteoporosis. To avoid this, TSH levels must be monitored closely to make sure that they don't drop too low.

Choice of Thyroid Hormone Preparation

The choice of the thyroid hormone preparation is important. Thyroxine is the drug of choice, since it is identical to the hormone produced by the thyroid gland; it is easily monitored by readily available blood tests. Since the potency of generic thyroxine products may vary considerably, your physician may specify a brand name of thyroxine to treat your hypothyroidism.

Thyroid hormone products, such as desiccated thyroid and thyroglobulin, contain both thyroxine as well as a second, more rapidly acting, thyroid hormone known as triiodothyronine (T3). It is unnecessary and probably unwise to use these combination tablets for two reasons. First, the body normally makes T3 from T4 in a very gradual fashion as it is needed by the body. Second, the blood T3 level can become abnormally high after taking medication that contains T3. The abnormally high T3 can, in turn, cause a rapid pulse and increase the workload of the heart, which could be dangerous for any elderly patient with underlying heart disease.

THYROID NODULES AND THYROID CANCER

As with younger patients, thyroid nodules (lumps) are very common among older people, while thyroid cancers are not. If an older person is found to have a nodule within the thyroid gland, every effort should be made to determine the nature of the nodule without having to subject the individual to a thyroid operation. Many nodules may be left alone if thyroid blood levels are normal, and if a thyroid scan picture shows that the nodule is functioning normally. If a nodule shows no evidence of function on a thyroid scan, a sample of the nodule can be obtained by a simple procedure called a fine needle aspiration (FNA) biopsy. Subsequent microscopic examination of the cells obtained will exclude cancer in the majority of individuals, and surgery can be avoided. Only those few individuals who are found to have thyroid cancer in the biopsy material, or those whose samples show highly suspicious cells, need to have their nodules removed surgically. Fortunately, surgery is neither difficult nor a health risk for most older patients, and recovery following surgery tends to be rapid and complete.

SUMMARY

It is apparent that thyroid disorders have no age limits. In fact, some thyroid disorders are more common in the elderly. When they occur in older individuals, they may be difficult to diagnose, require special attention to gradual and careful treatment, and require lifelong follow-up. By educating patients and those that care for them, we can recognize thyroid problems earlier and treat them with greater safety.

The Thyroid Foundation of America

The Eyes

The eye is an incredibly complex organ—particularly considering its compact size of about one inch in diameter. Like a camera, the eye has a single lens that focuses on objects in the world around us and projects an image of those objects—upside down and in miniature—onto the retina, the light-sensitive region at the back of the eyeball that processes the incoming image. But the eye is far more advanced than any camera.

The movement of the eye is controlled by six muscles attached to the eye's tough outer membrane, which is known as the sclera. (The sclera is the part you see as the "white" of your eye.) These muscles work to move both eyes simultaneously, keeping them centered on the same field of view, to provide a stereoscopic, three-dimensional image.

A layer of clear tissue called the cornea covers the lens, the pupil, and the iris (the pigmented disc that gives the eye its color). The cornea protects these delicate structures, and its rounded shape helps to bend light rays through to the eye's lens. In fact, the cornea provides about two-thirds of the eye's total focusing ability. Behind the cornea is a fluid-filled space known as the anterior chamber. The fluid, called the aqueous humor, constantly flows through the anterior chamber and other parts of the inner eye, carrying nutrients and washing away wastes. If the flow of the aqueous humor becomes blocked for any reason, pressure may build up and damage the fragile structures of the inner eye. If high eye pressure leads to damage inside the eye, the patient is said to have glaucoma.

Directly behind the anterior chamber is the iris. (People with brown eyes, incidentally, have the same pigments in the iris as people with blue or green eyes; they just have more of them. Albinos have none; their eyes appear pink from the blood vessels underlying the transparent tissue.) The pupil is the opening at the center of the iris that allows light to enter the eye. Muscles controlling the iris cause the pupil to change size to adjust to the amount of incoming light, much like the aperture of a camera.

Behind the iris and pupil is the lens, enclosed in a capsule and held in place by a network of fibers. The lens is pliant and changes shape in order to focus on an image clearly.

As we age, the lens of the eye loses its elasticity. Consequently, by around age 40, we begin to find that it is harder to focus on nearby objects. This gradual farsightedness is known as presbyopia, meaning "old eye," and it affects everyone eventually.

For many people, age may also bring about cataracts, which occur when the normally crystal-clear lens gradually becomes opaque.

Behind the lens is the largest portion of the eye—a large round chamber filled with a gelatinous clear fluid called the vitreous humor. Tiny bits of unattached cellular material may drift around in the vitreous humor, resulting in "floaters," the phenomenon whereby you see little spots or strings moving across your field of vision. Floaters are generally just a harmless occasional nuisance, but tend to occur more frequently as we age, especially among nearsighted people.

At the back of the eyeball lies the retina, the complex ten-layered structure that processes the light images projected through the cornea and lens. The retina has two distinct types of photosensitive cells—rods and cones—which transform light signals into electrical nerve impulses to be sent to the brain. Rods, which outnumber cones 20 to 1, perceive the world in black and white. The cones perceive color. They require more light than the rods to function properly, which explains why colors appear as shades of gray in faint light, even if shapes seem perfectly distinguishable.

At the center of the retina is the macula, which provides the most acute vision. If this portion of the retina begins to deteriorate (macular degeneration), central sight and the ability to read or do any kind of work requiring keen vision is greatly jeopardized.

Connected to the retina at the rear of the eyeball is the optic nerve. It conducts electro-chemical nerve impulses from the eye to the visual cortex in the rear of the brain, where these signals are then interpreted and transformed into meaningful pictures, shapes, symbols, and cues.

People over 50 should have their eyes examined at least every two years by an ophthalmologist (a medical eye doctor). Many important eye diseases, such as glaucoma, cataract, and macular degeneration, increase in prevalence in older adults. As presbyopia initially progresses, you may need new glasses fairly often. But for most people, around the age of 65, the eye's lens has lost most of its elasticity; thus, vision stabilizes and the need for new glasses tapers off sharply.   *The Editors*

CATARACTS

A cataract is a clouding of the normally clear lens of the eye. It can be compared to a window that is frosted or fogged with steam. There are many misconceptions about cataracts. A cataract is not a film over the eye; caused by overusing the eyes; a cancer; spread from one eye to the other; or a cause of irreversible blindness. Common symptoms of cataract include:

- A painless blurring of vision
- Glare, or light sensitivity
- Frequent eyeglass prescription changes
- Double vision in one eye
- Needing brighter light to read
- Poor night vision
- Fading or yellowing of colors

The amount and pattern of cloudiness within the lens can vary. If the cloudiness is not near the center of the lens, you may not be aware that a cataract is present.

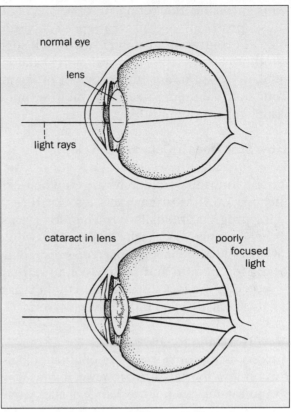

A normal, clear lens allows light to pass through unobstructed. When a cataract forms, light diffuses in the clouded lens, resulting in blurred vision.

What Causes Cataract?

The most common type of cataract is related to aging. Other causes of cataract include:

- Family history
- Medical problems, such as diabetes
- Injury to the eye
- Medications, such as steroids
- Long-term, unprotected exposure to sunlight
- Previous eye surgery

How Is a Cataract Detected?

A thorough eye examination by your ophthalmologist (medical eye doctor) can detect the presence and extent of a cataract, as well as any other conditions that may be causing blurred vision or discomfort.

There may be other reasons for visual loss in addition to the cataract, particularly problems involving the retina or optic nerve. If these problems are present, perfect vision may not return after cataract removal. If such conditions are severe, removal of the cataract may not result in any improvement in vision. Your ophthalmologist can tell you how much visual improvement is likely.

How Fast Does a Cataract Develop?

How quickly the cataract develops varies among individuals and may vary even between the two eyes. Most cataracts associated with aging progress gradually over a period of years. Other cataracts, especially in younger people and people with diabetes, may progress rapidly over a few months and cause vision to worsen. It is not possible to predict exactly how fast cataracts will develop in any given person.

How Is a Cataract Treated?

Surgery is the only way your ophthalmologist can remove the cataract. However, if symptoms from a cataract are mild, a change of glasses may be all that is needed for you to function more comfortably. There are no medications, dietary supplements, exercises, or optical devices that have been shown to prevent or cure cataracts.

Protection from excessive sunlight may help prevent or slow the progression of cataracts. Sunglasses that screen out ultraviolet (UV) light rays or regular eyeglasses with a clear, anti-UV coating offer this protection.

When Should Surgery Be Done?

Cataract surgery should be considered when cataracts cause enough loss of vision to interfere with daily activities. It is not true that cataracts need to be "ripe" before they can be removed. Cataract surgery can be performed when your visual needs require it. You must decide if you can see to do your job and drive safely, if you can perform daily tasks, such as cooking, shopping, or taking medications without difficulty. Based on your symptoms, you and your ophthalmologist should decide together when surgery is appropriate.

What Can I Expect from Cataract Surgery?

Over 1.4 million people have cataract surgery each year in the United States, 95 percent without complications. During cataract surgery, which is usually performed under local anesthesia as an outpatient procedure, the cloudy lens is removed from the eye. In most cases, the focusing power of the natural lens is restored by replacing it with a permanent intraocular lens implant.

Bifocal lens implants are arriving on the market and are expected to be widely available in a few years.

Your ophthalmologist performs this delicate surgery using a microscope, miniature instruments, and other modern technology.

Although it is a common misconception, lasers are not used to remove cataracts. In approximately one-fifth of people having cataract surgery, the natural capsule that supports the intraocular lens will become cloudy. Laser surgery (called YAG) is used to open this cloudy capsule, restoring the clear vision.

After cataract surgery, you may return almost immediately to all but the most strenuous activities. You will have to take eyedrops as your ophthalmologist directs. Several postoperative visits are needed to check on the progress of the eye as it heals.

Cataract surgery is a highly successful procedure. Improved vision is the result in over 90 percent of cases, unless there is a problem with the cornea, retina, or optic nerve. It is important to understand that complications can occur during or after the surgery, some severe enough to limit vision. As with any surgery, a good result cannot be guaranteed.

Conclusion

Cataracts are a common cause of poor vision, particularly for the elderly, but they are treatable. Your ophthalmologist can tell you if a cataract or some other problem is the cause of vision loss or discomfort and help you decide if cataract surgery is appropriate for you.

The American Academy of Ophthalmology

GLAUCOMA

Glaucoma is a leading cause of blindness in the United States, especially for older people. But loss of sight from glaucoma is preventable if you get treatment early enough. Glaucoma is a disease of the optic nerve. The optic nerve carries the images we see to the brain. Many people know that glaucoma has something to do with pressure inside the eye. The higher the pressure inside the eye, the greater the chance of damage to the optic nerve.

The optic nerve is like an electric cable containing a huge number of wires. Glaucoma can damage nerve fibers, causing blind spots to develop. Often people don't notice these blind areas until much optic nerve damage has already occurred. If the entire nerve is destroyed, blindness results. Early detection and treatment by your ophthalmologist are the keys to preventing optic nerve damage and blindness from glaucoma.

What Causes Glaucoma?

Clear liquid, called the aqueous humor, flows in and out of the eye. This liquid is not part of the tears on the outer surface of the eye. You can think of the flow of aqueous fluid as a sink with the faucet turned on all the time. If the drainpipe gets clogged, water collects in the sink and pressure builds up. If the drainage area of the eye—called the drainage angle—is blocked, the fluid pressure within the inner eye may increase, which can damage the optic nerve.

What Are the Different Types of Glaucoma?

Chronic open-angle glaucoma. This is the most common glaucoma. It occurs as a result of aging. The drainpipe, or drainage angle of the eye, becomes less efficient with time, and pressure within the eye gradually increases.

If this increased pressure results in optic nerve damage, it is known as chronic open-angle glaucoma. Over 90 percent of adult glaucoma patients have this type of glaucoma.

Chronic open-angle glaucoma can damage vision so gradually and painlessly that you are not aware of trouble until the optic nerve is already badly damaged.

Angle-closure glaucoma. Sometimes the drainage angle of the eye may become completely blocked. It is as though a sheet of paper floating near a drain suddenly drops over the opening and blocks the flow out of the sink. The iris may act like the sheet of paper closing off the drainage angle. When eye pressure builds up rapidly, it is called acute angle-closure glaucoma. The symptoms include:

- Blurred vision
- Severe eye pain
- Headache
- Rainbow haloes around lights
- Nausea and vomiting

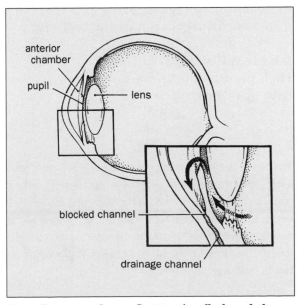

Normally, aqueous humor flows continually through the structures of the inner eye. In glaucoma, this flow is blocked, so that pressure builds up within the eye.

If you have any of these symptoms, call your ophthalmologist immediately. Unless an ophthalmologist treats acute angle-closure glaucoma quickly, blindness can result.

A more gradual and painless closing of the angle is called chronic angle-closure glaucoma. It occurs more frequently in people of African and Asian ancestry.

How Is Glaucoma Detected?

Regular eye examinations by your ophthalmologist are the best way to detect glaucoma. Your ophthalmologist can detect and treat glaucoma. During a complete and painless examination, your ophthalmologist will:

- Measure your intraocular pressure (tonometry)
- Inspect the drainage angle of your eye (gonioscopy)
- Evaluate any optic nerve damage (ophthalmoscopy)
- Test the visual field of each eye (perimetry)

Some of these tests may not be necessary for every person. You may need to repeat these tests on a regular basis, to determine if glaucoma damage is increasing over time.

Who Is at Risk for Glaucoma?

High pressure alone does not mean that you have glaucoma.

The trend is to rely less and less on intraocular pressure (IOP) to make a diagnosis, depending instead upon examination of the optic disc and visual field tests. IOP is a key risk factor for glaucoma, but not all people with high IOP have the disorder, and some with low IOP do. In fact, 15 to 20 percent of glaucoma patients have normal IOP readings.

Your ophthalmologist puts together many kinds of information to determine your risk for developing the disease, including:

- Age
- Nearsightedness
- African ancestry
- A family history of glaucoma
- Past injuries to the eyes
- A history of severe anemia or shock

Your ophthalmologist will weigh all of these factors before deciding whether you need glaucoma treatment, or whether you should be monitored closely as a glaucoma suspect. This means your risk of developing glaucoma is higher than normal, and you need to have regular examinations to detect the early signs of damage to the optic nerve.

How Is Glaucoma Treated?

As a rule, damage caused by glaucoma cannot be reversed. Eye drops, pills, and laser and surgical operations are used to prevent or slow further damage from occurring.

With any type of glaucoma, periodic examinations are very important to prevent vision loss. Because glaucoma can worsen without your being aware of it, your treatment may need to be changed over time.

MEDICINES

Glaucoma is usually controlled with eye drops taken several times a day, sometimes in combination with pills. These medications decrease eye pressure, either by slowing the production of aqueous fluid within the eye or by improving the flow leaving the drainage angle.

For these medications to work, you must take them regularly and continuously. It is also important to tell all of your doctors about the eye medications you are using.

Glaucoma medications can have side effects. You should notify your ophthalmologist immediately if you think you may be experiencing side effects. Some eye drops may cause:

- A stinging sensation
- Red eyes
- Blurred vision

LOSS OF VISION CAN BE PREVENTED

Regular medical eye exams may help prevent unnecessary vision loss. You should have an examination:

Every 3 to 5 years
• If you are age 39 and over

Every 1 to 2 years
• If a family member has glaucoma
• If you are of African ancestry
• If you have had a serious eye injury in the past
• If you are taking steroid medications

• Headaches
• Changes in pulse, heartbeat or breathing

Pills sometimes cause:
• Tingling of fingers and toes
• Drowsiness
• Loss of appetite
• Bowel irregularities
• Kidney stones
• Anemia or easy bleeding

LASER SURGERY

Laser surgery treatments may be effective for different types of glaucoma. The laser is usually used in one of two ways.

In open-angle glaucoma, the drain itself is treated. The laser is used to enlarge the drain (trabeculoplasty) to help control eye pressure.

In angle-closure glaucoma, the laser creates a hole in the iris (iridotomy) to improve the flow of aqueous fluid to the drain.

OPERATIVE SURGERY

When operative surgery is needed to control glaucoma, your ophthalmologist uses miniature instruments to create a new drainage channel for the aqueous fluid to leave the eye. The new channel helps to lower the pressure.

Though serious complications of modern glaucoma surgery are rare, they can occur, as with any surgery. Surgery is recommended only if your ophthalmologist feels that it is safer to operate than to allow optic nerve damage to continue.

What Is Your Part in Treatment?

Treatment for glaucoma requires a team made up of both you and your doctor. Your ophthalmologist can prescribe treatment for glaucoma, but only you can make sure you take your eye drops or pills.

Never stop taking or change your medications without first consulting your ophthalmologist. Frequent eye examinations and tests are critical to monitor your eyes for any changes. Remember, it is your vision, and you must do your part to maintain it.

The American Academy of Ophthalmology

MACULAR DEGENERATION

Macular degeneration is damage or breakdown of the macula of the eye. The macula is a small area at the back of the eye that allows us to see fine details clearly. Macular degeneration makes close work—like threading a needle or reading—difficult or impossible.

When the macula doesn't function cor-

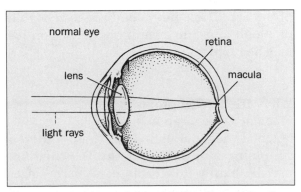

The macula is the part of the retina that distinguishes fine detail. An abnormal growth of blood vessels and scarring causes macular degeneration.

303

rectly, we experience blurriness or darkness in the center of our vision. Although macular degeneration reduces vision in the central part of the retina, it does not affect the eye's side, or peripheral, vision. For example, you could see a clock but not be able to tell what time it is. Macular degeneration alone does not result in total blindness. Most people continue to have some useful vision and are able to take care of themselves.

What Causes Macular Degeneration?

Many older people develop macular degeneration as part of the body's natural aging process. The two common types of age-related macular degeneration are "dry" and "wet."

The newest names for age-related macular degeneration emphasize the main culprits: abnormal new blood vessels. "Dry" macular degeneration is termed non-neovascular; "wet" is termed neovascular.

"Dry" macular degeneration. Most people have this form of macular degeneration. It is caused by aging and thinning of the tissues of the macula. Vision loss is usually gradual.

"Wet" macular degeneration. This type accounts for about 10 percent of all cases. It results when abnormal blood vessels form at the back of the eye. These new blood vessels leak fluid or blood and blur central vision. Vision loss may be rapid and severe.

What Are the Symptoms of Macular Degeneration?

Macular degeneration can cause different symptoms in different people. The condition may be hardly noticeable in its early stages. Sometimes only one eye loses vision while the other eye continues to see well for many years.

But when both eyes are affected, reading and close work can become difficult. Following are some common ways vision loss is detected:

- Words on a page look blurred
- A dark or empty area appears in the center of vision

How Is Macular Degeneration Diagnosed?

Many people do not realize that they have a macular problem until blurred vision becomes obvious. Your ophthalmologist can detect earlier stages of macular degeneration during a medical eye examination that includes the following:

- Viewing the macula with an ophthalmoscope
- A simple vision test in which you look at a grid resembling graph paper
- A color vision test
- Sometimes a special photograph, called an angiogram, is taken to find abnormal blood vessels under the retina. Fluorescent dye is injected into your arm, and your eye is photographed as the dye passes through the blood vessels in the back of the eye

How Is Macular Degeneration Treated?

Despite ongoing medical research, there is no cure yet for "dry" macular degeneration. Some doctors believe that nutritional supplements may slow macular degeneration, but this has not yet been proven. Treatment of this condition focuses on helping a person find ways to cope with visual impairment.

In its early stages "wet" macular degeneration can be treated with laser surgery, a brief and usually painless outpatient procedure. Laser surgery seals the leaking blood vessels that damage the macula. Although a small, permanently dark "blind spot" is left at the point of laser contact, the procedure can preserve more sight overall.

A new treatment for "wet" age-related macular degeneration (AMD), called photodynamic therapy, will likely come on the market in the near future. Researchers are also testing whether a new surgical procedure can remove from under the retina the abnormal blood vessel that causes "wet" AMD and whether mild laser treatments for those with severe cases of "dry" AMD will reduce their chance of developing the other form of the disease.

Despite advanced medical treatment, people with macular degeneration still experience some vision loss. Your ophthalmologist can prescribe optical devices or refer you to a low-vision specialist or center. Because side vision is usually not affected, a person's remaining sight can be very useful. A wide range of support services, rehabilitation programs, and devices are available to help people with macular degeneration maintain a satisfying lifestyle.

Because side vision is usually not affected, a person's remaining sight can be very useful. Often, people can continue with many of their favorite activities using low-vision optical devices such as magnifying devices, closed-circuit television, large-print reading materials, and talking or computerized devices.

The American Academy of Ophthalmology

REFRACTIVE ERRORS

For our eyes to be able to see, light rays must be refracted, or bent, so they can focus on the retina, the nerve layer that lines the back of the eye. The cornea and the lens refract light rays. The retina receives the picture formed by these light rays and sends the image to the brain through the optic nerve.

A refractive error means that the shape of your eye doesn't refract the light properly, so that the image you see is blurred. Though refractive errors are called eye disorders, they are not diseases.

What Are the Different Types of Refractive Errors?

Myopia (nearsightedness). A myopic eye is longer than normal, so that the light rays focus in front of the retina. Close objects look clear but distant objects appear blurred.

Myopia is inherited and is often discovered in children when they are eight to 12 years old. During the teenage years, when the body grows rapidly, myopia gets worse. Between the ages of 20 and 40, there is usually little change.

If the myopia is mild, it is called low myopia. Severe myopia is known as high myopia. If you have high myopia, you have a higher risk of detached retina. It is important to have regular eye examinations by an ophthalmologist to watch for any changes in the retina. If the retina does detach, a surgical operation is the only way to repair it.

Hyperopia (farsightedness). A hyperopic eye is shorter than normal. Light from close objects, such as the page of a book, cannot focus clearly on the retina.

Like nearsightedness, farsightedness is usually inherited. Babies and young children tend to be slightly hyperopic. As the eye grows and becomes longer, hyperopia lessens.

Astigmatism (distorted vision). The cornea is the clear front window of the eye. A normal cornea is round and smooth, like a basketball. When you have astigmatism, the cornea curves more in one direction than in the other, like a football.

Astigmatism distorts or blurs vision for both near and far objects. It's almost like looking into a funhouse mirror in which you appear too tall, too wide, or too thin. You can have astigmatism in combination with myopia or hyperopia.

THE BEST SUNGLASSES

A few years ago, a team of researchers from Johns Hopkins conducted a study involving over 800 fishermen from the Chesapeake Bay area, and found that the incidence of cataracts in this group was three times greater than the average. The likely culprit: the invisible but damaging ultraviolet (UV) radiation in the sun's rays. Further research, including a large-scale international study, has since confirmed these findings. Also, upon reanalyzing the data, the team discovered some evidence that the wavelengths of visible sunlight that we see as blue light may hasten macular degeneration (the deterioration of the central portion of the retina), the fastest growing cause of legal blindness among older Americans.

Fortunately, sunglasses provide simple and effective protection from these hazards, with no risk of side effects. Unfortunately, some marketers have hoped to parlay such research into profit, and are offering sunglasses that provide UV and blue-light protection at prices often approaching or even exceeding $100 a pair. But experts say protecting your eyes need not cost you an arm and a leg.

Dr. Sheila West, a professor of ophthalmology at Johns Hopkins and a specialist in light toxicity and the epidemiology of macular degeneration, as well as a co-author of the Chesapeake Bay study, points out that though the research does suggest a correlation between blue light and retinal damage, it would be premature to base any edicts on these findings. "For one thing, the study turned up only eight cases of macular degeneration. How can you make any precise claims from that? Our research is only very preliminary, and mainly indicates the need for further research." And even if the research did indicate that everyone should wear UV and blue-light-blocking sunglasses, a high price tag alone in no way ensures the best protection. In fact, when Dr. West and her team tested dozens of pairs of glasses for overall effectiveness against UV and blue light, the very best turned out to be a pair that one of the researchers had received free in a promotion at a Baltimore Orioles game. Put simply: "Wearing sunglasses is prudent and can do no harm," says Dr. West. "But spending one or two hundred dollars is throwing your money away." You should be able to find a perfectly adequate pair for under $20. If the price tag is not a reliable criterion for choosing the best sunglasses, then what factors should you consider?

Adequate UV Protection/The ANSI Label
Many makers (even of very inexpensive brands) voluntarily label their glasses in accord with American National Standard Institute (ANSI) guidelines for UV protection, which fall into three categories: cosmetic, general purpose, and special purpose.

• *Cosmetic glasses* block at least 70 percent of UVB radiation (the particular wavelengths associated with cataracts); 20 percent of UVA rays (the longer wavelengths of UV, also possibly harmful to the eyes, though probably less so than UVB); and 60 percent of

---

Presbyopia (aging eyes). When you are young, the lens in your eye is soft and flexible. The lens of the eye changes its shape easily, allowing you to focus on objects both close and far away.

After age 40, the lens becomes more rigid. Because the lens can't change shape as easily as it once did, it is more difficult to read at close range.

This perfectly normal condition is called presbyopia. You can also have presbyopia in combination with myopia, hyperopia or astigmatism.

How Are Refractive Errors Corrected?

Eyeglasses or contact lenses are the most common methods of correcting refractive errors. They work by refocusing light rays on the retina, compensating for the shape of your eye. Refractive surgery is also an option to correct or improve vision. These surgical procedures are used to permanently adjust your eye's focus by reshaping the cornea, or front surface of your eye.

There is no scientific evidence that eye exercises, vitamins, or pills can prevent or cure refractive errors.

light from the visible portion of the spectrum. These usually lightly tinted lenses are recommended for everyday, around-town wear, when constant harsh light isn't a problem.

• *General-purpose glasses* have medium to dark lenses that block at least 95 percent of UVB rays, 60 percent of UVA, and 60 to 90 percent of visible light. These are good for most outdoor activities, such as driving or playing tennis. Most sunglasses, whether they say so or not, fall into this category (even many pairs costing under $5).

• *Special-purpose sunglasses* must block 99 percent of UVB, 60 percent of UVA, and 97 percent of visible light. They tend to be very dark, and are advised for extremely bright conditions, such as you might find on ski slopes or tropical beaches.

Color

Gray and green lenses distort colors least. You can get greater protection from blue light with reddish, orange, or amber lenses. Glasses that promise 100 percent blockage of blue light are fine, but may be quite expensive, and some people who try them complain of headaches.

Darkness

One common misconception about sunglasses is that darker lenses necessarily mean greater protection. Even clear lenses can provide total UV protection if specially pretreated, while some dark ones might offer significantly less. Again, check for ANSI labels.

The most important thing is that you see well out of your glasses; they should be neither too dark nor too light. Gradient lenses are good for driving because they have less tint at the bottom, enabling you to see the dashboard better.

Size and Fit

The frames should be large enough to keep light out from around all sides. Glasses that slip down your nose even half an inch allow about 20 percent of unfiltered sunlight to reach your eyes. Wraparound styles, popular among skiers, are a good safeguard against this. Make sure the frames don't interfere with your peripheral vision.

Gimmicks

Don't let them fool you. Some companies claim that their glasses improve the clarity of your vision (only prescription lenses can do that); some sell their glasses with vitamin supplement packets that are supposed to restore or protect your vision. Such ploys are grossly misleading.

You might, however, want to consult an ophthalmologist if your job or hobby finds you outside for hours at a stretch, or if you are fair-skinned and have blue or green eyes, or are elderly—especially if you've had cataract surgery or are taking a drug (such as tetracycline) that may increase your sensitivity to ultraviolet light. If you fall into one of these high-risk groups, consider buying special-purpose sunglasses.

The Editors

Eyeglasses. Glasses are an easy method to correct refractive errors. They can also help protect your eyes from harmful light rays, such as ultraviolet (UV) light rays. A special coating that screens out UV light is available when you order your glasses.

Bifocals are glasses that are used to correct presbyopia. They have a correction for reading on the bottom half of the lens and another for seeing distance on the top. Trifocals are lenses with three different lens corrections in one set of eyeglasses. If you don't need correction for seeing distance, you can buy over-the-counter reading glasses to correct presbyopia.

No exercise or medication can reverse presbyopia. You will probably need to change your prescription from time to time between the ages of 40 and 60, because your lens will continue to lose flexibility.

Contact lenses. There are now a wide variety of contact lenses available. The type that is best for you depends on your refractive error and your lifestyle. If you want to wear contact lenses, discuss the various options with your ophthalmologist.

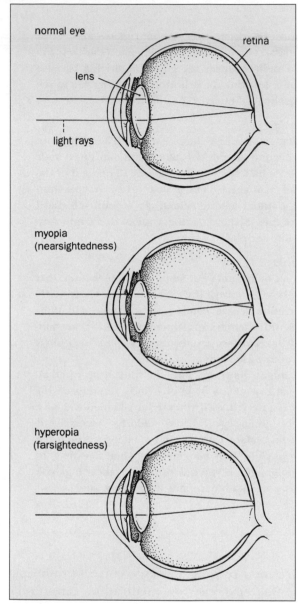

In a normal eye, light focuses precisely on the retina. In nearsightedness, light focuses short of the retina; in farsightedness, beyond the retina.

You may have heard of a process called orthokeratology to treat myopia. Orthokeratology uses a series of hard contact lenses to gradually flatten the cornea and reduce the refractive error. Improvement of sight from orthokeratology is temporary.

After the use of the lenses is discontinued, the cornea reverts to its original shape and myopia returns.

Refractive Surgery

Photorefractive keratectomy (PRK). In this procedure the excimer laser is used to reduce myopia, astigmatism, and hyperopia. Using an invisible, high-energy light, the laser precisely sculpts the cornea. No blades are used.

Laser in-situ keratomileusis (LASIK). LASIK is a combined microsurgical and excimer laser procedure to correct myopia and astigmatism. In LASIK, a highly specialized instrument (microkeratome) is used to make a thin flap in the cornea. This flap is folded back, and excimer laser is then applied to the cornea under the flap to correct myopia and astigmatism. The flap is then replaced and allowed to heal back into position. There are no stitches used in this procedure.

Radial keratotomy (RK). Radial keratotomy is a surgical operation to improve myopia by changing the curve of the cornea over the pupil. The surgeon makes several deep incisions (keratotomies) in the cornea in a radial, or spokelike, pattern. The incisions flatten out the cornea and shorten the distance light rays must travel to the retina.

Experts in the field of ophthalmological research believe that as excimer laser technology becomes widespread, the popularity of conventional RK will decrease significantly.

Astigmatic keratotomy (AK). In this microsurgical procedure the surgeon makes deep incisions in the cornea (usually one or two) in a curvilinear pattern. The incisions flatten the areas of the cornea that are too steeply curved.

Refractive surgery is elective surgery, so it is very important to make an informed decision. Complications and side effects of these procedures include temporary discomfort, blurry and fluctuating vision, glare and haloes, the need for reading glasses, poor night vision, difficulty fitting contact lenses, corneal scarring, and permanent vision loss.

The American Academy of Ophthalmology

THE CAROTID ARTERY AND THE EYE

The two carotid arteries are the main arteries in the neck which supply blood to the eyes and the brain. One carotid artery supplies the right side, and the other serves the left. Because the eye and the brain share the same source of blood supply, blockages or conditions of the carotid artery can affect either or both organs.

What Happens When the Carotid Artery Is Blocked?

When the large or small branches of the carotid artery are blocked, the brain is deprived of blood and a stroke may result. Depending on the part of the brain involved and the size of the area deprived of its blood supply, the effects of a stroke may be slight or devastating. Severe effects can include paralysis of one side of the body and loss of speech. If the part of the brain having to do with vision is involved, a stroke can lead to loss of side vision.

When the ophthalmic artery (the first main branch of the internal carotid artery) or its branch (the central retinal artery) is blocked, a sudden, near-total loss of vision usually occurs. The mechanism of damage is the same in the brain and the eye. Cells die if they are deprived of blood for too long.

Is This Damage Permanent?

Not everyone who suffers a blocked blood supply to the eye or the brain has permanent damage. A temporary blockage of blood supply to the brain, called a transient ischemic attack (TIA), may result in muscle weakness on one side of the face or numbness of an arm or leg which only lasts about an hour.

A temporary blockage of blood supply to the eye, called amaurosis fugax or fleeting blindness, can cause a temporary loss of vision in one eye. This sometimes looks as though a curtain is descending over all or part of your vision in that eye and may last for seconds or for several hours.

Both amaurosis fugax and transient ischemic attacks are possible warnings of a serious problem involving the brain's blood supply. They should be reported to an ophthalmologist, who may recommend further tests.

Are There Other Signs of Carotid Artery Disease?

As part of a routine eye exam, the ophthalmologist may dilate the pupil to examine the retina at the back of the eye. During this procedure, conditions which may indicate an increased risk of stroke are sometimes discovered.

For instance, when the carotid artery becomes gradually blocked with fat and calcium deposits, the first signs can appear in the eye, providing critical clues to a life-threatening reduction of circulation to the brain.

If a plaque is found during a routine eye exam, further evaluation may be indicated. Other plaques from the carotid artery may break off, block the brain's blood supply, and cause a stroke.

What Further Tests or Treatments May Be Needed?

Ultrasound may be helpful to measure the flow of blood through the arteries. When a more accurate view of the arteries is required, a special x-ray test called an angiogram or angiography may be ordered. Angiography involves injecting an iodine-containing dye into the artery and taking pictures of the blood flowing into the brain. If an abnormality is found, surgery may be recommended to correct the blockage. The most common operation is an endarterectomy, in which the blockage on the inner wall of the artery is removed.

Routine, comprehensive medical eye examinations can help ensure healthy vision and can provide important information concerning carotid artery disease. If problems are detected, your ophthalmologist will work with your other medical doctors to coordinate your complete medical care.

The American Academy of Ophthalmology

FLOATERS AND FLASHES

What Are Floaters?

You may sometimes see small specks or clouds moving in your field of vision. They are called floaters. You can often see them when looking at a plain background, like a blank wall or blue sky.

Floaters are actually tiny clumps of gel or cells inside the vitreous, the clear jellylike

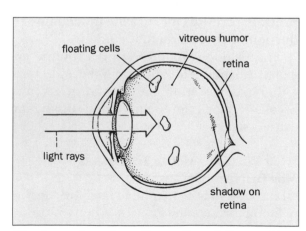

Tiny clumps of protein, or "floaters," may drift around in the vitreous humor, and often create little shadows on the retina.

fluid that fills the inside of your eye. While these objects look as though they are in front of your eye, they are actually floating inside. What you see are the shadows they cast on the retina, the nerve layer at the back of the eye that senses light and allows you to see. Floaters can have different shapes: little dots, circles, lines, clouds, or cobwebs.

What Causes Floaters?

When people reach middle age, the vitreous gel may start to thicken or shrink, forming clumps or strands inside the eye. The vitreous gel pulls away from the back wall of the eye, causing a posterior vitreous detachment. Posterior vitreous detachment, a common cause of floaters, is more common for people who:

- Are nearsighted
- Have undergone cataract operations
- Have had YAG laser surgery of the eye (to clear clouding after cataract surgery)
- Have had inflammation inside the eye

The appearance of floaters may be alarming, especially if they develop suddenly. You should see an ophthalmologist right away if you suddenly develop new floaters, especially if you are over 45 years of age.

Are Floaters Ever Serious?

The retina can tear if the shrinking vitreous gel pulls away from the wall of the eye. This sometimes causes a small amount of bleeding in the eye that may appear as new floaters. A torn retina is always a serious problem, because it can lead to a retinal detachment. You should see your ophthalmologist as soon as possible if:

- Even one new floater appears suddenly
- You see sudden flashes of light

If you notice other symptoms, like the loss of side vision, you should return to your ophthalmologist.

What Can Be Done About Floaters?

Because you need to know if your retina is torn, call your ophthalmologist if a new floater appears suddenly. Floaters can get in the way of clear vision, which may be quite annoying, especially if you are trying to read. You can try moving your eyes, looking up and then down to move the floaters out of the way.

Though some floaters may remain in your vision, many of them will fade over time and become less bothersome. Even if you have had some floaters for years, you should have an eye examination immediately if you notice new ones.

What Causes Flashing Lights?

When the vitreous gel rubs or pulls on the retina, you may see things that look like flashing lights or lightning streaks. You may have experienced this same sensation if you have ever been hit in the eye and seen stars.

The flashes of light can appear off and on for several weeks or months. As we grow older, it is more common to experience flashes. If you notice the sudden appearance of light flashes, you should visit your ophthalmologist immediately to see if the retina has been torn.

Migraine

Some people experience flashes of light that appear as jagged lines or heat waves in both eyes, often lasting 10 to 20 minutes. These types of flashes are usually caused by a spasm of blood vessels in the brain, which is called migraine.

If a headache follows the flashes, it is called a migraine headache. However, jagged lines or heat waves can occur without a headache. In this case, the light flashes are called ophthalmic migraine, or migraine without headache.

How Are Your Eyes Examined?

When an ophthalmologist examines your eyes, your pupils will be dilated with eye drops. During this painless examination, your ophthalmologist will carefully observe your retina and vitreous. Because your eyes have been dilated, you may need to make arrangements for someone to drive you home afterwards.

Floaters and flashes of light become more common as we grow older. Though not all floaters and flashes are serious, you should always have a medical eye examination by an ophthalmologist to make sure there has been no damage to your retina.

The American Academy of Ophthalmology

The Heart and Blood Vessels

OVERVIEW

The circulatory system is the network of elastic tubes through which blood flows as it carries oxygen and nutrients to all parts of the body. It includes the heart, lungs, arteries, arterioles (small arteries), and capillaries (minute blood vessels). It also includes venules (small veins) and veins, the blood vessels through which blood flows as it returns to the heart and lungs.

The circulating blood brings oxygen and nutrients to all the tissues and organs of the body, including the heart. It also picks up waste products from the body's cells. These waste products are removed as they're filtered through the kidneys, liver, and lungs.

The normal heart is a strong, muscular pump a little larger than a fist. It pumps blood continuously through the circulatory system. Each day the average heart beats (or expands and contracts) 100,000 times and pumps about 2,000 gallons of blood. In a 70-year lifetime, an average human heart beats more than 2.5 billion times.

The heart has four chambers. The upper two are the atria; the lower two, the ventricles. Blood is pumped through them, aided by four valves that open and close to allow blood to flow in only one direction when the heart contracts (beats).

The four heart valves are: 1) the tricuspid valve, located between the right atrium and right ventricle; 2) the pulmonary (pulmonic) valve, between the right ventricle and the pulmonary artery; 3) the mitral valve, between the left atrium and left ventricle; and 4) the aortic valve, between the left ventricle and the aorta. Each valve has a set of flaps (also called leaflets or cusps). The mitral valve has two flaps; the others have three. Under normal conditions, the valves permit blood to flow in only one direction. Blood flow occurs only when there's a difference in pressure across the valves that causes them to open.

The heart pumps blood to the lungs and to all the body's tissues by a sequence of highly organized contractions of its four chambers. The heart works as follows:

The right atrium receives blood from the

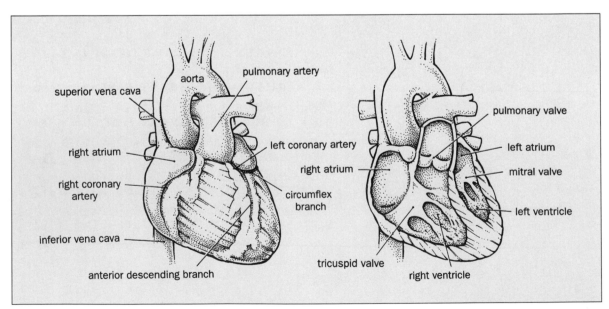

The heart (here in exterior and cutaway views) actually consists of two separate pumps. The right ventricle delivers blood to the lungs to be oxygenated; the left ventricle pumps this blood out to the body.

AORTIC STENOSIS

Aortic stenosis is a narrowing of the aortic valve opening, which causes the left ventricle of the heart to work harder to overcome the resistance of the narrowed passageway. This added workload can cause irreversible damage to the left ventricle and lead to left ventricular failure.

Aortic stenosis can be present without symptoms, and so it may be first detected as a heart murmur on a routine physical examination. However, when the stenosis is severe, then the narrowing of the valve opening causes the amount of blood pumped from the heart to be inadequate to meet the needs of the body. It may then result in such symptoms as fatigue, fainting, shortness of breath, and angina. Sudden cardiac death may occur.

More common in men than women, aortic stenosis can be caused by rheumatic fever or a congenital defect. Among older people, however, it is most often caused by deposits of calcium on a previously normal aortic valve, a phenomenon associated with the aging process. If there are significant symptoms, surgery may be required. With recent techniques of valve replacement surgery, the outlook is generally good if stenosis is relieved before extensive damage is done to the left ventricle.

The Editors

veins. This blood carries little oxygen and lots of carbon dioxide, because it's returning from the body's tissues, where much of the oxygen was removed and the carbon dioxide added. Venous blood is darker in color than arterial blood because of the difference in dissolved gases.

While the heart is relaxed, venous blood flows through the open tricuspid valve to fill the right ventricle. An electrical signal starts the heartbeat by causing the atria to contract. This contraction "tops off" the filling of the ventricle. Shortly after the atrium contracts, the right ventricle contracts. As this occurs, the tricuspid valve closes, and the partially deoxygenated blood is pumped through the pulmonary valve into the pulmonary artery and on to the lungs. In the lungs the blood gives up its carbon dioxide and gets oxygen before returning to the left atrium. This newly oxygenated blood is bright red.

At the same time the right atrium contracts, the left atrium contracts, topping off the flow of oxygenated blood through the mitral valve and into the left ventricle. Then a split second later the left ventricle contracts, pumping the blood through the aortic valve, into the aorta and on to the body's tissues.

For the heart to function properly, the four chambers must beat in an organized manner. This is governed by the electrical impulse. A chamber of the heart contracts when an electrical impulse or signal moves across it. Such a signal starts in a small bundle of highly specialized cells located in the right atrium—the sinoatrial node (SA node). A discharge from this natural pacemaker causes the heart to beat. This pacemaker generates electrical impulses at a given rate, but emotional reactions and hormonal factors can affect its rate of discharge. This allows the heart rate to respond to varying demands.

The electrical impulses generated by the SA node move throughout the right and left atrium, causing the muscle cells to contract. Shortly after both atria have contracted, the electrical signal travels down specialized fibers throughout the ventricles. The path of the signal causes the ventricles to contract together in a wringing motion, squeezing blood from them. The route of this electrical impulse is specific and produces the coordinated sequential contraction of the heart's four chambers that's necessary for the heart to work properly.

ATHEROSCLEROSIS

"Arteriosclerosis" is a general term for the thickening and hardening of arteries. Some hardening of arteries normally occurs when people grow older.

Atherosclerosis, a type of arteriosclerosis, comes from the Greek word "athero" (meaning gruel or paste) and "sclerosis" (hardness). It's characterized by deposits of fatty substances, cholesterol, cellular waste products, calcium, and fibrin (a clotting material in the blood) in the inner lining of an artery. The resulting buildup is called plaque.

Plaque may partially or totally block the blood's flow through an artery. Two things that can happen where plaque occurs are: 1) bleeding (hemorrhage) into the plaque, or 2) formation of a blood clot (thrombus) on the plaque's surface. If either of these occurs and blocks the entire artery, a heart attack or stroke may result.

Atherosclerosis affects large and medium-sized arteries. The type of artery and where the plaque develops varies with the individual.

Atherosclerosis is a slow, progressive disease that some evidence shows starts in childhood. In some people this disease progresses rapidly in their third decade; in others it doesn't become threatening until they're in their fifties or sixties.

ABDOMINAL ANEURYSM

An aneurysm—an egg-shaped ballooning out of a weakened wall of an artery—can occur in any artery in the body. It is most common, however, in the lower aorta, the main blood vessel that carries blood from the heart into the arteries of the legs. Although aneurysms can be caused by disease or injury or a congenital defect in the arterial wall, abdominal aneurysms are most often the result of atherosclerosis, and they occur most commonly among men over the age of 60. They frequently develop without symptoms, although in their advanced stage they may cause lower back pain. More often, they are found on routine examination.

Aneurysms usually grow slowly, at the rate of one-eighth to one-fourth inch a year. Although aneurysms of any size may burst—and so cause rapid hemorrhaging and death—the larger the aneurysm, the more likely it is to rupture. If your physician discovers an aneurysm, he or she may well decide simply to monitor its progress if you are not suffering any pain, and the aneurysm is not too large. But if the aneurysm is causing pain, is larger than 6 cm, or is rapidly increasing in size, surgery may be necessary. During surgery, the damaged artery is replaced by a synthetic vessel. The risk of elective surgery for such aneurysms is small, though less than half of those survive emergency surgery if they are operated on after the aneurysm ruptures.

The Editors

HOW ATHEROSCLEROSIS STARTS

The development of atherosclerosis is a complex process. Precisely how atherosclerosis begins or what causes it isn't known, but several theories have been proposed.

Many scientists believe atherosclerosis begins because the inner, protective lining of the artery (endothelium) becomes injured and can no longer do its job. When this happens, over time, fats, cholesterol, and other substances in the blood may pass through the damaged lining and become deposited in the artery wall. These and other substances linked with high blood cholesterol (possibly oxidized forms of cholesterol-carrying fats, called oxidized lipoproteins) may cause the cells of the artery wall to make certain substances. These result in more buildup of cells (white cells from the blood and cells normally found in the artery wall) in the endothelium where the atherosclerotic lesions form. These cells accumulate and many of them divide.

At the same time, fat keeps building up in and around these cells. They also form sub-

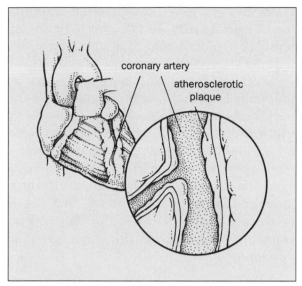

Coronary arteries narrow and harden as atherosclerotic plaque builds up inside them. Ultimately, blockage of these arteries may cause a heart attack.

stances called connective tissue. The endothelium becomes much thicker due to this buildup of cells and the surrounding material. If it's thickened enough, the deposit can reduce the amount of blood flowing through the artery. This decreases the oxygen supplied to the heart (leading to heart attack), brain (leading to stroke), or the arms and legs (leading to gangrene).

Three of the possible causes of damage to the arterial walls are: 1) elevated levels of cholesterol and triglycerides in the blood, 2) high blood pressure, and 3) cigarette smoke. Cigarette smoke particularly aggravates and speeds up the development of atherosclerosis in the coronary arteries, the aorta, and arteries of the legs.

Cholesterol is a soft, fatlike substance found in the body's cells. It's used to form cell membranes, certain hormones, and other necessary substances.

People get cholesterol in two ways. The body—primarily the liver—produces varying amounts, usually about 1,000 mg a day. An additional 400 to 500 mg or more can come directly from foods. Foods from animals—

especially egg yolks, meat, fish, poultry, and whole-milk dairy products—contain it; foods from plants don't. Typically the body makes all the cholesterol it needs, so people don't have to consume it to maintain their health.

Besides its presence in human tissues, cholesterol is also found in the bloodstream. The blood transports it to and from various parts of the body. Hypercholesterolemia is the term for high levels of cholesterol in the blood.

How Cholesterol Is Carried in the Blood

Cholesterol and other fats can't dissolve in blood and must be transported by special carriers called lipoproteins, which are created by the liver. Lipoproteins transport cholesterol and triglycerides, which are found in foods and made by the body.

The process starts when cholesterol and fats in food go to the intestine to be digested and absorbed. Chylomicrons (fatty particles containing mainly triglycerides, but also cholesterol, phospholipids, and protein) are produced in the intestinal wall. When the chylomicrons enter the bloodstream, they contact binding sites on capillaries. Many of their triglycerides break down and are released into the blood. The remainder of the chylomicron (the chylomicron remnant), now richer in cholesterol, continues in circulation until it reaches the liver and is absorbed.

The liver then produces very low density lipoprotein (VLDL), the largest type of lipoprotein. VLDL carries triglycerides made in the liver from fatty acids, carbohydrates, alcohol, and some cholesterol. VLDL is released into the bloodstream and, like chylomicrons, is transported to tissue capillaries, where the triglycerides are broken down and either used for energy or stored by muscle or fat cells.

After VLDL releases its triglycerides, what remains is a VLDL remnant called intermediate density lipoprotein (IDL). Some IDL is removed from circulation by the liver; the rest is transformed into low density lipoprotein (LDL).

LDL is the major cholesterol carrier in the blood, carrying about 60 to 80 percent of the body's cholesterol. Some of this cholesterol circulating in the bloodstream is used by tissues to build cells, some is returned to the liver. If too much LDL cholesterol circulates in the blood, cholesterol may also be deposited in artery walls and cause plaques and atherosclerosis. The tendency for high levels of LDL to produce arterial deposits is why LDL is often called "bad" cholesterol and why lower levels of LDL reflect a reduced risk of heart disease.

Another type of lipoprotein is high density lipoprotein (HDL). HDL is a flat, disklike particle produced primarily in the liver and intestines and released into the bloodstream. As VLDL and chylomicron particles release their triglycerides into the body's cells, fragments containing proteins, fats, and cholesterol break away. It's thought that HDL picks up the cholesterol and brings it back to the liver for reprocessing or excretion. Some researchers believe HDL may also remove excess cholesterol from fat-sated cells, possibly even those in artery walls. Because HDL clears cholesterol out of the system and high levels of it are associated with a decreased risk of heart disease, HDL is often called "good" cholesterol.

The levels of HDL and LDL in the blood are measured to evaluate the risk of atherosclerosis.

HDL and Triglyceride Levels

As a rule, women have higher HDL levels than men. The female sex hormone estrogen tends to raise HDL, which may help to explain why premenopausal women are usually protected from developing heart disease. Estrogen production is highest during the childbearing years.

Triglyceride levels normally range from about 50 to 250 mg/dl, depending on age and sex. As people tend to get older or fatter or both, their triglyceride and cholesterol levels tend to rise. Women also tend to have higher triglyceride levels. An elevated blood triglyc-

eride level and lower HDL are often accompanied by an increase in LDL and total cholesterol. (For more about total cholesterol, see page 336.)

Several clinical studies have shown that an unusually large number of people with coronary heart disease also have high levels of triglycerides in the blood (hypertriglyceridemia). However, some people with this problem seem remarkably free from atherosclerosis. Thus elevated triglycerides, which are often measured along with HDL and LDL, may not directly cause atherosclerosis. But they may accompany other abnormalities that speed its development.

RECENT PROGRESS IN RESEARCH

Research aimed at finding ways to prevent or reverse atherosclerosis is now under way. One of the most promising areas of research is in finding ways to control elevated levels of cholesterol and other fats in the blood.

Three advances have been especially dramatic. One is the discovery of cell-surface receptors for LDL by 1985 Nobel laureates Drs. Joseph Goldstein and Michael Brown. These receptors bind LDL circulating through the bloodstream, allowing the LDL and its cholesterol to enter cells. Research has shown that when the amount of cholesterol within cells builds up, the number of these receptors on cell surfaces is reduced and blood levels of LDL increase. This can lead to more cholesterol being available for deposit in artery walls.

Another recent research finding has resulted from the Coronary Primary Prevention Trial (CPPT). It showed that lowering a high level of blood cholesterol reduces deaths from heart attack.

A final important advance in recent years has been the development of a new class of cholesterol-lowering drugs. These compounds either block the synthesis of cholesterol by the body's cells, or force its elimination by preventing its absorption from the intestine.

The landmark 4S study, published in November 1994, showed that lowering LDL cholesterol levels substantially by drug treatment greatly improved the outlook for both men and women who had angina or a previous heart attack. Over an average period of five and a half years, compared with a placebo-treated group, those treated with a cholesterol-lowering drug had a 30 percent or greater reduction in heart attacks, deaths from coronary artery disease, and need for angioplasty or bypass surgery. In addition, for the first time, this study showed a decrease (30 percent) in overall mortality as the result of lowering LDL cholesterol levels in patients with coronary artery disease. There was no increase in deaths from cancer or other causes in the treated group, putting to rest the concern raised in some publications that lowering cholesterol levels may lead to other health problems. The west of Scotland and the AFCAPS/TEXCAPS studies proved that lowering blood cholesterol levels with statin medications also reduces cardiovascular risk in people without established heart disease.

Of course, many fundamental questions remain. Medical scientists are continuing to search for answers by studying life at its most basic level—the cell.

Even though much more work needs to be done, scientists have found some answers. For instance, they've found a definite relationship between the amount of cholesterol in the bloodstream and coronary artery disease (blockage of the arteries supplying blood to the heart muscle itself). A large body of scientific evidence shows that a diet high in saturated fats and cholesterol can raise blood cholesterol levels and contribute to atherosclerosis.

The problem of high blood cholesterol isn't limited to adults. Millions of children also have elevated levels, and thus may be at increased risk of atherosclerosis and coronary heart disease later in life.

That's why the American Heart Association recommends that healthy adults and children age two and over eat a diet that's low in saturated fats and cholesterol. Eating a proper diet helps reduce the risk of high blood cholesterol and thus the risk of heart attack.

The American Heart Association

HIGH BLOOD PRESSURE

Blood pressure is the result of two forces— one created by the heart as it pumps blood into the arteries, the other created by the arterial blood vessels as they exert resistance to the blood flow from the heart.

When the heart pumps, it causes the blood to flow through the large arteries into the smaller arteries, the arterioles. The walls of the arterioles can contract or expand (dilate), altering the resistance to blood flow and, thus, the amount of blood flow and the blood pressure. Contraction of the arterioles increases the resistance to blood flow and therefore reduces blood flow through those arterioles while increasing blood pressure. Expansion (dilation) of the arterioles has the opposite effect on resistance, blood flow, and blood pressure. Hence, regulation of the size (inner diameter) of the arterioles plays an important role in regulating blood flow and determining blood pressure. If the arterioles remain constricted, they can create a condition of hypertension or high blood pressure.

HOW BLOOD PRESSURE IS MEASURED
Blood pressure is measured by a quick, painless test using a medical instrument called a sphygmomanometer. A rubber cuff is wrapped around a person's upper arm and inflated. When the cuff is inflated, it compresses a large artery in the arm, momentarily stopping the flow of blood.

319

Next, air in the cuff is released, and the person measuring the blood pressure listens with a stethoscope. When the blood starts to pulse through the artery, it makes a sound; sounds continue to be heard until pressure in the artery exceeds the pressure in the cuff.

While the person listens and watches the sphygmomanometer gauge, he or she records two measurements. The systolic pressure is the pressure of the blood flow when the heart beats (the pressure just after the first sound is heard). The diastolic pressure is the pressure between heartbeats (the pressure just after the last sound is heard). Blood pressure is measured in millimeters of mercury, which is abbreviated mm Hg.

A typical blood pressure reading for an adult might be 127/78 mm Hg, although readings vary depending on age and other factors. The first, larger number is the systolic pressure; the second is the diastolic pressure. The important point is that the harder it is for blood to flow, the higher the numbers will be.

WHAT IS HIGH BLOOD PRESSURE?

Medical scientists have determined a norm for blood pressure after studying the blood pressure of many people over many years. These studies showed that there is no ideal blood pressure reading. Instead, acceptable (normal) blood pressure falls within a range rather than a certain pair of numbers. For most adults, a blood pressure reading that's less than 140/90 mm Hg indicates there's no cause for worry. However, in adults, high blood pressure (called hypertension) exists when systolic pressure is equal to or greater than 140 mm Hg and/or diastolic pressure is equal to or greater than 90 mm Hg for extended periods of time.

For many years, no effort was made to lower blood pressure in people with isolated systolic hypertension (ISH)—that is, a systolic pressure greater than 140 mm Hg in association with a diastolic pressure less than 90 mm Hg, which is especially common in older individuals. Treatment of ISH is now strongly recommended because a number of studies of patients with ISH show that significant benefits resulted from lowering systolic blood pressure.

Why High Blood Pressure Is Bad

High blood pressure means that the heart is working harder than normal, putting the heart and the arteries under a greater strain. This may contribute to heart attacks, strokes, kidney failure, and atherosclerosis. If high blood pressure isn't treated, the heart may have to work progressively harder to pump enough blood and oxygen to the body's organs and tissues to meet their needs.

When the heart is forced to work harder than normal for an extended time, it tends to enlarge. A slightly enlarged heart may function well, but one that's significantly enlarged has a hard time meeting the demands put on it.

Arteries and arterioles also suffer the effects of high blood pressure. Over time they become scarred, hardened, and less elastic. This may occur as people age, but high blood pressure accelerates this process, probably because hypertension speeds atherosclerosis.

Arterial damage is bad because hardened or narrowed arteries may be unable to supply the amount of blood the body's organs need. And if the body's organs don't get enough oxygen and nutrients, they can't function properly. There's also the risk that a blood clot may lodge in an artery narrowed by atherosclerosis, depriving part of the body of its normal blood supply. The heart, brain, and kidneys are especially prone to damage by high blood pressure.

Why Mortality from High Blood Pressure Seems So Low

Mortality figures for high blood pressure are deceptive. Many people die from heart attacks and strokes caused by high blood pressure. But these deaths aren't listed as deaths from hypertension; instead, they're listed as deaths from heart attack and stroke.

The result is that high blood pressure may not seem as dangerous as it really is. Because of the disguised mortality figures and, more important, because it's possible to have high blood pressure for years without knowing it, this disease is called the "silent killer."

CAUSES OF HIGH BLOOD PRESSURE

In 90 to 95 percent of high blood pressure cases, the cause is unknown. (This type of high blood pressure is called essential hypertension.) Fortunately, even though scientists don't fully understand the causes of high blood pressure, they've developed both non-drug and drug treatments that are effective over the long term in treating this disease. They also have identified some factors that contribute to the elevation of the blood pressure (arteriosclerosis or hardening of the arteries, thickening or hypertrophy of the artery wall, and excess contraction of arterioles).

In the remaining cases, high blood pressure is a symptom of a recognizable problem such as a kidney abnormality, tumor of the adrenal gland, or congenital defect of the aorta. When the root cause is corrected, blood pressure usually returns to normal. This type of high blood pressure is called secondary hypertension.

WHAT CAN BE DONE

Many medications (known as antihypertensives) are available to lower high blood pressure. Some, called diuretics, rid the body of excess fluids and salt (sodium). Others, called beta-blockers, reduce the heart rate and the heart's output of blood.

Another class of antihypertensives is called sympathetic nerve inhibitors. Sympathetic nerves go from the brain to all parts of the body, including the arterioles. They can cause the arteries to constrict or narrow, thereby raising blood pressure. This class of drugs reduces blood pressure by inhibiting these nerves from constricting blood vessels.

Yet another group of drugs is the vasodilators. These can cause the muscle in the walls of the blood vessels (especially the arterioles) to relax, allowing the arteriole to dilate (widen).

Two other classes of drugs used to treat high blood pressure are the angiotensin-converting enzyme (ACE) inhibitors and the calcium antagonists (calcium channel blockers). The ACE inhibitors interfere with the body's production of angiotensin, a chemical that causes the arterioles to constrict. The calcium antagonists can reduce the heart rate and relax blood vessels.

In most cases these drugs lower blood pressure, but quite often people respond very differently to these medications. Thus most patients must go through a trial period to find out which medications are most effective while causing the fewest side effects.

The most important points for people with high blood pressure to remember are to: 1) follow their doctor's instructions; and 2) stay on their medication. In addition, dietary and lifestyle changes may help control high blood pressure. Some people with mild hypertension can lower their blood pressure by reducing sodium in their diet. Excessive alcohol intake (more than one ounce daily) raises blood pressure in some people and should be restricted. Blood pressure also returns to normal in many obese people when they lose weight. Increasing physical activity can reduce blood pressure in some people, too. Before drugs are prescribed, these methods to control blood pressure are often recommended for people with only mildly elevated blood pressure.

FACTORS CONTRIBUTING TO
HIGH BLOOD PRESSURE

Because medical science doesn't understand the causes of most cases of high blood pressure, it's hard to say how to prevent it. Still, several factors may contribute to it. Being overweight or using excessive salt are two avoidable factors.

Age is one risk factor that can't be changed. Generally speaking, the older people get, the more likely they are to develop high blood pressure

Heredity is another factor. People whose parents have high blood pressure are more likely to develop it than those whose parents don't. African Americans are also more likely to have high blood pressure than whites.

The incidence of high blood pressure isn't directly related to a person's sex. However, doctors usually keep a close watch on a woman's blood pressure during pregnancy or when she's taking oral contraceptives. Some women who've never had high blood pressure develop it during pregnancy. Similarly, a woman taking oral contraceptives is more likely to develop high blood pressure if she's overweight, has had high blood pressure during pregnancy, has a family history of high blood pressure, or has mild kidney disease.

The American Heart Association

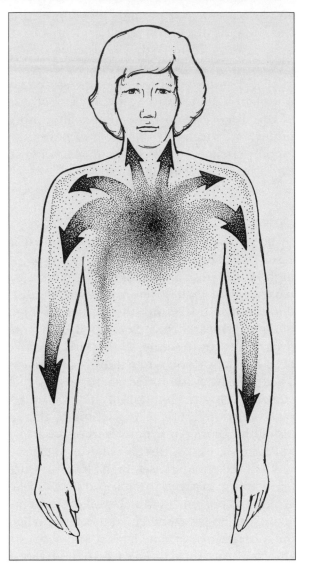

The pain of angina (radiating outward from the heart) typically comes on with exertion, and unlike the pain of a heart attack, subsides shortly with rest.

HEART ATTACK AND ANGINA

WHAT IS A HEART ATTACK?

Heart attacks result from heart disease—blood vessel disease in the heart. Coronary heart disease (CHD), sometimes referred to as coronary artery disease (CAD), and ischemic heart disease are more specific names for heart disease.

A heart attack, or myocardial infarction, occurs when the blood supply to part of the heart muscle itself (the myocardium) is severely reduced or stopped. This occurs when one of the coronary arteries (the arteries that supply blood to the heart muscle) is blocked by an obstruction, such as a blood clot that has formed on plaque due to atherosclerosis. Such an event is sometimes called a coronary thrombosis or coronary occlusion. A myocardial infarction is the damaging or death of an area of the heart muscle resulting from a reduced blood supply to that area.

If the blood supply is cut off drastically or for a long time, muscle cells suffer irreversible injury and die. Disability or death can result, depending on how much heart muscle is damaged.

Sometimes a coronary artery temporarily contracts or goes into spasm. When this happens the artery narrows and blood flow to part of the heart muscle decreases or even stops. What causes a spasm is unclear, but it can occur in normal blood vessels as well as vessels partially blocked by atherosclerosis. If a spasm is severe, a heart attack may result.

WHAT IS ANGINA?

Chest pain called angina pectoris is another result of coronary artery disease. Angina is a symptom of a condition called myocardial ischemia, which occurs when the heart muscle (myocardium) doesn't get as much blood (hence as much oxygen) as it needs for a given level of work. Lack of blood supply is called ischemia.

Angina pectoris can occur when blood circulation to the heart is enough for normal needs but not enough when the heart's needs increase, such as during physical exertion, emotional excitement, or extreme temperatures. Running to catch a bus, for example, could trigger an attack of angina while walking to a bus stop might not. Some people, such as those with a coronary artery spasm, may have angina when they're resting (variant angina pectoris). Angina can be a warning sign that someone is at risk of heart attack.

WHAT IS VARIANT ANGINA PECTORIS?

Variant angina pectoris is also called Prinzmetal's angina. It differs from typical angina in that it occurs almost exclusively when a person is at rest, and it doesn't follow a period of physical exertion or emotional stress. Attacks can be very painful and usually occur between midnight and 8 a.m. It's associated with acute myocardial infarction (heart attack), severe cardiac arrhythmias (including ventricular

tachycardia and fibrillation), and sudden cardiac death.

Variant angina is due to coronary artery spasm. About two-thirds of people with it have severe coronary atherosclerosis in at least one major vessel. The spasm usually occurs very close to the obstruction.

Many people with Prinzmetal's angina go through an acute, active phase. Anginal and cardiac events may occur frequently for six months or more. During this time, nonfatal heart attack occurs in up to 20 percent of patients; death occurs in up to 10 percent. People who develop serious heart rhythm disturbances (arrhythmias) at this time are at greater risk of sudden death.

Most people who survive an infarction or this initial three- to six-month period stabilize, and symptoms and cardiac events tend to diminish over time. Long-term survival is excellent, ranging from 89 to 97 percent at five years. Patients without significant obstructive CAD have an excellent long-term outlook.

WHAT IS SILENT ISCHEMIA?

Some people have ischemia, which means not enough blood flows to a part of the body's tissue. This occurs when the arteries bringing blood to the heart are narrowed by spasm or disease. As many as three to four million Americans may have ischemic episodes without knowing it. These people have silent ischemia. They may have a heart attack with no prior warning. In addition, people with angina also may have undiagnosed episodes of silent ischemia. Various tests, such as an exercise test or a 24-hour portable monitor of the electrocardiogram (Holter monitor), are used to diagnose silent ischemia.

WHAT IS COLLATERAL CIRCULATION?

Collateral circulation involves small arteries that connect two larger coronary arteries or different segments of the same artery. They provide an alternate route for blood flow to the heart muscle. Everyone has collateral vessels, at least in microscopic form. These vessels aren't open under normal conditions but grow and enlarge in some people with coronary heart disease. When a collateral vessel enlarges, it lets blood flow from an open artery to an adjacent artery or further downstream on the same artery. Myocardial ischemia stimulates the growth of collateral vessels, so they can form a kind of detour around a blockage and provide alternate routes of blood flow.

Research has shown that while everyone has collateral vessels, they don't open and become available in all people. People who have open collateral vessels can benefit, because collateral vessels help protect heart muscle from tissue death if the normal blood supply is cut off.

HOW ANGINA IS TREATED

Angina pectoris can be treated with drugs that affect 1) the supply of blood to the heart muscle or 2) the heart's demand for oxygen. Some drugs, called coronary vasodilators, cause blood vessels to relax. When this happens the opening inside the vessels (the lumen) gets bigger. Then blood flow improves, allowing more oxygen and nutrients to reach the heart muscle. Nitroglycerin is the drug most often used. It relaxes the veins (reducing the amount of blood returning to the heart and thus lessening the work of pumping) and the coronary arteries (increasing the blood supply to the heart).

Alternatively, the heart's demand for oxygen also can be modified. For example, a drug can be prescribed to reduce blood pressure and thus reduce the heart's workload and need for oxygen. Drugs that slow the heart rate achieve a similar effect.

Invasive techniques that improve the blood supply to the heart also may be used. One technique is percutaneous transluminal coronary angioplasty (PTCA), also known as angioplasty

---

HEART ATTACK—SIGNALS AND ACTION

Know the warning signals of a heart attack:
• Uncomfortable pressure, fullness, squeezing, or pain in the center of the chest that lasts more than a few minutes, or goes away and comes back.
• Pain that spreads to the shoulders, neck, or arms.
• Chest discomfort with light-headedness, fainting, sweating, nausea, or shortness of breath.

Not all these warning signs occur in every heart attack. But if some start to occur, don't wait. Get help immediately. Delay can be deadly!

Know what to do in an emergency:
• Find out which area hospitals have 24-hour emergency cardiac care.
• Know in advance which hospital or medical facility is nearest your home and office, and tell your family and friends to call this facility in an emergency.
• Keep a list of emergency rescue service numbers next to the telephone and in your pocket, wallet, or purse.

• If you have chest discomfort that lasts more than a few minutes, call the emergency rescue service.
• If you can get to a hospital faster by going yourself and not waiting for an ambulance, have someone drive you there.

Be a heart saver:
• If you're with someone experiencing the signs of a heart attack—and the warning signs last more than a few minutes—act immediately.
• Expect a "denial." It's normal for someone with chest discomfort to deny the possibility of something as serious as a heart attack. But don't take no for an answer. Insist on taking prompt action.
• Call the emergency service, or
• Get to the nearest hospital emergency room that offers 24-hour emergency cardiac care.
• Give CPR (mouth-to-mouth breathing and chest compression) if it's necessary and you're properly trained.

NEW CARDIAC IMAGING TESTS

Radionuclide Imaging. This includes such tests as perfusion imaging, MUGA (Multi-Gated Acquisition) scan, or acute infarct scintigraphy. These tests involve injecting substances called radionuclides into the bloodstream. Computer-generated pictures can then find them in the heart. These tests show how well the heart muscle is supplied with blood and how well the heart's chambers are functioning or identify a part of the heart damaged by heart attack.

Magnetic Resonance Imaging (MRI). This test uses powerful magnets to look inside the body. Computer-generated pictures can image the heart muscle, identify damage from a heart attack, diagnose certain congenital heart defects, and evaluate disease of larger blood vessels such as the aorta.

Contrast Echo and Doppler Echo. Echocardiography uses sound waves to evaluate the size, shape, and motion of the heart. The sound waves bounce back from the various structures of the heart, and a computer translates those waves into a two-dimensional image of a beating heart. With contrast echo, a radio-opaque substance is injected into the bloodstream, so that the velocity and direction of blood flow and the borders of the heart muscle can be precisely determined.

Digital Cardiac Angiography, Digital Subtraction Angiography (DCA or DSA). This test uses a modified form of imaging that records pictures of the heart and its blood vessels by computer.

The Editors

or balloon angioplasty. Another procedure is coronary artery bypass graft surgery.

Before performing either of these procedures, a doctor must find the blocked part of the coronary arteries. This is done using coronary arteriography, which is done during a procedure called cardiac catheterization. In this procedure, a doctor guides a thin plastic tube (a catheter) through an artery in the arm or leg and into the coronary arteries. Then the doctor injects a liquid dye visible in x-rays through the catheter. High-speed x-ray movies record the course of the liquid as it flows through the arteries. Doctors can identify obstructions in the arteries by tracing the liquid's flow.

Some new diagnostic tools are available to evaluate how well the heart works. These tests may be done before or after a heart attack.

PTCA is a procedure designed to dilate (widen or expand) narrowed coronary arteries. In it, a doctor inserts a catheter into an artery in an arm or leg and guides it to an obstructed coronary artery. Then a second catheter with a balloon tip is passed inside the first, and the balloon tip is inflated at the arterial blockage. This compresses the plaque, enlarging the inner diameter of the blood vessel so blood can flow more easily. Then the balloon is deflated and the catheters are withdrawn.

In about 25 percent of the people who've had PTCA, the dilated part of the coronary artery renarrows. This usually occurs within the first six months. Then a doctor must decide whether to repeat the operation or if open heart surgery is a better choice.

In coronary artery bypass graft surgery, surgeons take a blood vessel from another part of the body (usually the leg or from inside the chest wall) and construct a detour around the blocked part of a coronary artery. One end of the vessel is attached above the blockage; the other, to the coronary artery just beyond the blocked area. This restores blood supply to the heart muscle.

People with angina should also modify their controllable risk factors. This means they must not smoke, and should control their blood pressure and make sure their diet doesn't contribute to atherosclerosis or obesity.

SYMPTOMS OF A HEART ATTACK

Sometimes the first indications of a heart attack come as warning signals. These warning signals are outlined on the facing page.

The actual diagnosis of a heart attack must be made by a physician who has studied the results of several tests. Besides reviewing a patient's complete medical history and giving a physical examination, a doctor will use an electrocardiogram (ECG) to discover any abnormalities caused by damage to the heart. Sometimes a blood test is used to detect abnormal levels of certain enzymes in the bloodstream.

HOW A HEART ATTACK IS TREATED

When a heart attack occurs, it's critical to recognize the signals and respond immediately. Delaying may increase the damage to the heart and reduce the chance of survival. Anyone experiencing the warning signals of a heart attack should be taken immediately to the nearest hospital with 24-hour emergency cardiac care. People who become unconscious before reaching the emergency room may receive emergency cardiopulmonary resuscitation (CPR).

Most communities have an emergency cardiac care system that can quickly respond. This prompt care for heart attack victims dramatically reduces damage to the heart. In fact, 88 percent of heart attack survivors under age 65 can return to work within three months. Prompt care for heart attack victims isn't the only reason so many people recover so quickly, but it's an important one.

The importance of time cannot be overemphasized. When a coronary artery gets blocked, the heart muscle doesn't die instantaneously—damage increases the longer an artery remains blocked. If a victim gets to an emergency room fast enough, a form of reperfusion therapy (called thrombolysis) sometimes can be performed. It involves injecting a thrombolytic (clot-dissolving) agent, such as streptokinase, urokinase, or tPA (tissue plasminogen activator), to dissolve a clot in a coronary artery and restore some blood flow. These drugs must be used within a few (usually one to three) hours of a heart attack for best

IMPROVING THE CHANCES OF SURVIVING A HEART ATTACK

Research in recent years has established three major factors that can reduce the death rate from myocardial infarction:

• **Early treatment.** The sooner you get to the emergency room after a heart attack, the better. Reperfusion therapy (clearing the blockage in a coronary artery with clot-dissolving thrombolytic drugs)—especially when initiated within the first hour or two of a heart attack—consistently saves lives. Also, heart attack victims have a better chance of survival if taken to hospitals equipped with the facilities to perform direct angioplasty (opening blocked blood vessels with a balloon during a heart attack), should this procedure be warranted.

• **Aspirin.** Research has concluded that almost anyone experiencing a heart attack should immediately begin taking a daily dose of 160 to 325 milligrams of aspirin, and will be asked in the emergency room to chew the first dose. This has been shown to reduce mortality rates as well as the incidence of future heart attacks and strokes.

• **Beta-blockers.** These medications, such as metoprolol (Lopressor) and atenolol (Tenormin) help reduce the magnitude of the heart attack and the workload of the heart, and so reduce death rates. (A similar class of drugs, known as ACE inhibitors, has also been shown to improve ultimate chances of survival when administered in the days and weeks following a heart attack.)

The Editors

effect. The sooner a drug is used, the more effective it's likely to be.

According to the largest heart attack study to date—the GUSTO trial (Global Utilization of Streptokinase and tPA for Occluded Coronary Arteries)—tPA is now considered the best agent for early treatment; it produces the lowest mortality rate (6.3 percent) of all clot-dissolving drugs when administered within six hours after a heart attack. Mortality is reduced even further when the drug is administered within less than two hours. Emergency angioplasty, using a balloon to open blocked arteries during a heart attack, is an alternative to clot-dissolving medications in hospitals equipped with emergency angioplasty facilities.

In the weeks following a heart attack, either PTCA or coronary artery bypass surgery may be performed to improve the blood supply to the heart muscle. Once part of the heart muscle dies, its function can't be restored. Function may be restored to areas with decreased blood flow, however.

REDUCING THE CHANCE OF A HEART ATTACK
Many scientific studies show that certain characteristics increase the risk of coronary heart disease. These are called risk factors. The four major modifiable risk factors are cigarette/tobacco smoke, high blood cholesterol, hypertension, and physical inactivity. Other contributing risk factors are diabetes mellitus and obesity. (See page 335 for more information.)

The American Heart Association strongly urges people to control their modifiable risk factors. Also, people with angina should take episodes of chest pain seriously and see their doctor before their atherosclerosis leads to a heart attack.

The American Heart Association

ARRHYTHMIAS AND SUDDEN CARDIAC DEATH

WHAT ARE ARRHYTHMIAS?
Normal cardiac rhythm results from electrical impulses that start in the sinoatrial (SA or sinus) node. They spread in a timely way through the atria to the atrioventricular (AV) node. From there, each impulse travels over the many specialized fibers of the His-Purkinje system, distributing the electrical ignition signal to the ventricular muscle cells.

The transmission of impulses is delayed a fraction within the AV node. This allows time for the atrial contraction that helps fill the ventricles with blood.

Most people experience an occasional change in the regular beating of their heart and feel a fluttering in the chest, or a speeding up of their heartbeat, or a bout of dizziness or breathlessness. And for most people with such symptoms, these arrhythmias are harmless. In some people, however, especially if such episodes persist or become worse, the arrhythmias may be associated with heart disease. Only a physician will be able to distinguish with certainty between those arrhythmias that are serious and those that are not, so you should report any changes in the regular beating of your heart to your doctor.

The term "arrhythmia" refers to any change from this normal sequence of beginning and conducting impulses. Some arrhythmias are so brief (for example, a temporary pause or premature beat) that the overall heart rate isn't greatly affected. However, if arrhythmias last for some time, they may cause the heart rate to be too slow or too fast.

The term "bradycardia" is used to describe a rate of less than 60 beats per minute. "Tachycardia" usually refers to a heart rate of more than 100 beats per minute.

How Arrhythmias Occur
Cells in the heart's conduction system, from the sinus node down to the outer branches of the His-Purkinje system, can fire automatically and begin electrical activity. Normally, the sinus node contains the heart's most rapidly firing cells. (This allows that area to be a natural pacemaker.) Subsidiary pacemakers elsewhere in the heart provide a back-up rhythm

MONITORING YOUR HEARTBEAT

Electrocardiogram. A person's heartbeat is regulated by the heart's own natural pacemaker: a wave of electricity that passes through your heart from the sinoatrial node (a small cluster of specialized cells in the right atrium of the heart) down to the ventricles. And, because the body's tissues are good conductors of electricity, these electrical impulses can be detected by placing electrical sensors at various points on your skin.

The impulses are picked up by an electrocardiograph, which produces a printed record—an electrocardiogram (ECG). The electrical pattern of the ECG can sometimes reveal abnormalities of heart rhythm, damage to heart muscle from a previous heart attack, an insufficient blood flow to the heart muscle (possibly because of atherosclerosis), an inflammation of the membrane around the heart (pericarditis), or of the heart muscle itself (myocarditis). And all of this information about the inner workings of the heart can be obtained with an easy, painless, noninvasive test.

An ECG is commonly taken in a physician's office with the patient lying down (a resting ECG); but if your physician wants to see how your heart responds when it is subjected to added work, he is likely to recommend a stress test.

Stress Test. An exercise ECG, or stress test, is most often performed while you walk on a treadmill. As you walk for 10 or 15 minutes, your physician will gradually increase the speed and incline of the treadmill to see how your heart responds to the increasing demands placed on it. Although designed to place a strenuous demand on your cardiovascular system in order to reveal any coronary heart disease, the test itself is safe when it is performed under the supervision of a physician. If you are unable to exercise, your doctor may recommend a pharmacologic stress test. Instead of exercising, a drug is injected into your vein and pictures of the heart are obtained.

Walking ECG, or Holter Monitor. If your physician wants to evaluate your heart rhythm's response to the ordinary stresses of your daily life—rather than the artificial stress of the treadmill—he may ask you to wear a Holter monitor for 24 hours. A Holter monitor is a miniature electrocardiograph; its recording device, which is the size of an instant camera, attaches to your belt; and its tiny electrodes remain in place on your chest through a 24-hour cycle to record your ECG as you work, eat, sleep, and play. *The Editors*

---

when the sinus node doesn't work properly or when the transmission of impulses is blocked somewhere in the conduction system.

Under certain conditions, the automatic firing rate of secondary pacemaker tissue may become too fast. If such an abnormal "focus" fires faster than the sinus node, it may take over control of the heart rhythm and produce tachycardia.

Arrhythmias also may develop because of abnormalities in how impulses are conducted. Delays in the spreading of impulses can occur anywhere in the conduction system. When the transmission of impulses is intermittently or completely blocked (heart block), bradycardia may result. In such cases, subsidiary pacemaker cells (located beyond the conduction block) may maintain cardiac rhythm.

In another type of abnormal conduction, impulses get caught in a merry-go-round-like sequence. This process, called reentry, is a common cause of tachycardias. Regardless of what causes them, tachycardias may be subclassified by where they arise. Thus, ventricular tachycardias originate in the heart's lower chambers. Supraventricular tachycardias arise higher in the heart—either in the upper chambers (atria) or the middle region (AV node or the beginning portion of the His-Purkinje system).

SYMPTOMS OF ARRHYTHMIAS

Arrhythmias can produce a broad range of symptoms, from barely perceptible to cardiovascular collapse and death. When they're very brief, arrhythmias are most likely to be almost without symptoms. For example, a single premature beat may be perceived as a palpitation or skipped beat. Premature beats that are frequent or occur in rapid succession during a nonsustained or sustained tachycardia may cause a greater awareness of heart palpitations or a fluttering sensation in the chest or neck.

When arrhythmias last long enough to affect how well the heart works, more serious symptoms may develop. At slower rates, the heart may not be able to pump enough blood to the body. This can cause fatigue, light-headedness, loss of consciousness, or even death. Death occurs if the heart rate is zero or so slow that the heart and brain stop working.

Tachycardias can reduce the heart's ability to pump by interfering with the ventricular chambers' ability to properly fill with blood. They do this by reducing the time for such filling or by interfering with the booster effect normally provided by timely contraction of the atria (or both).

Loss of this atrial "kick" during tachycardia may be caused by a change from the usual sequence of atrial and ventricular activity. It also can be caused by rapid chaotic electrical activity in the upper chambers (for example, atrial fibrillation). The reduced pumping efficiency that can develop during tachycardia may be made worse by underlying heart muscle abnormalities or atherosclerotic blocks in the coronary arteries. It's not surprising, then, that tachycardias can produce shortness of breath, chest pain, light-headedness, or loss of consciousness.

When the heart's ability to work is greatly reduced for a prolonged time, cardiac arrest and death are likely. This may result from ventricular tachycardia and ventricular fibrillation (an extremely rapid, chaotic rhythm during which the heart quivers). If the heart can continue to pump normally, though, some ventricular tachycardias (even those that last for minutes or hours) may be well tol-

erated without a loss of consciousness or cardiac arrest. Tachycardia may be nonsustained (lasting only seconds) or sustained (lasting for minutes or hours).

Tachycardias sometimes can cause serious injury to other organ systems. For example, the brain, kidneys, lungs, or liver may be damaged during prolonged cardiac arrest. Also, blood clots can form in the upper heart chambers as a result of atrial fibrillation. They may break free and cause a stroke or damage other organs.

WHO IS PRONE TO ARRHYTHMIAS?

Although there's great variation in their severity, arrhythmias occur throughout the population. On an everyday level, the heart rate speeds up (sinus tachycardia) during physical activity, stress, or excitement, and slows down (sinus bradycardia) during sleep. Even beyond these daily changes, probably everyone at one time or another develops premature atrial or ventricular beats. In fact, during a 24-hour period about one-fifth of healthy adults are likely to have frequent or multiple types of ventricular premature beats. (This even includes short episodes of ventricular tachycardia in a small percentage of monitored people.)

The prevalence of atrial and ventricular arrhythmias tends to increase with age, even when there's no overt sign of heart disease. Certain congenital conditions may make a person prone to arrhythmias. For example, an incompletely developed conduction system can cause chronic heart block and bradycardia. On the other hand, people born with extra conduction pathways, either near the AV node or bridging the atria and ventricles, are prone to reentrant supraventricular tachycardias.

Still, acquired heart disease is the most important factor predisposing a person to arrhythmias. The main causes are atherosclerosis, hypertension, and inflammatory or degenerative conditions. The scarring or abnormal tissue deposits found with these diseases can cause bradycardias; they do this by interfering with the work of the sinus node or overall AV conduction. Likewise, they can cause tachycardias (originating in either the atria or ventricles) by causing cells to fire abnormally or by creating islands of electrically inert tissue. (Impulses circulate in a reentrant fashion around these areas.)

A variety of other factors may predispose a person to develop arrhythmias. Prominent among them is the part of the autonomic nervous system that's involved in cardiovascular regulation. One element of this control system slows the sinus rate and depresses AV nodal conduction. (These effects may prevail during sleep or in athletically well-trained people.) The opposing element of the autonomic nervous system tends to speed up the firing rate of the sinus node and other pacemaker tissue in the heart. Further, it may also make it easier for reentrant tachycardias to occur.

Many chemical agents may provoke arrhythmias, sometimes with serious consequences. Known factors include high or low blood and tissue concentrations of a variety of minerals, such as potassium, magnesium, and calcium. These play a vital role in starting and conducting normal impulses in the heart. Addictive substances, especially alcohol, cigarettes, and recreational drugs, can provoke arrhythmias, as can various cardiac medications. Even drugs used to treat an arrhythmia may provoke another arrhythmia.

DIAGNOSING ARRHYTHMIAS

An electrocardiogram is the standard clinical tool for diagnosing arrhythmias. Such a recording shows the relative timing of atrial and ventricular electrical events. It can be used to measure how long it takes for impulses to be transmitted through the atria, AV conduction system, and ventricles.

An arrhythmia is considered documented if it can be recorded on an electrocardiogram. Often, though, the electrocardiogram of a person who complains of symptoms that suggest arrhythmia doesn't show anything (because of the fleeting nature of arrhythmias).

Suspected arrhythmias sometimes may be documented by using a small, portable electrocardiogram recorder, called a Holter monitor. This can record 24 hours of continuous electrocardiographic signals.

For suspected arrhythmias that occur less than daily, a patient can wear an event monitor. It provides for a continuously updated memory loop and can allow the heart to be monitored by telephone.

These electrocardiographic techniques are passive; they require an arrhythmia to spontaneously occur. Other options that provoke arrhythmias and make their diagnosis (and thus their proper treatment) easier also are used. For example, treadmill testing may be considered for people whose suspected arrhythmias are clearly exercise related. In patients prone to passing out, tilt table studies may reproduce the faint when it's due to abnormal nervous system reflexes that cause the heart rate to slow down and the blood pressure to drop.

Electrophysiologic testing has become extremely valuable for provoking known, but infrequently occurring, arrhythmias and for unmasking suspected arrhythmias. This procedure is performed using local anesthesia. It involves placing temporary electrode catheters through peripheral veins (and sometimes through arteries) into the heart using fluoroscopic guidance. Then these catheters are positioned in the atria, ventricles, or both, and at strategic locations along the conduction system. Their purpose is to record cardiac electrical signals and map the spread of electrical impulses during each beat.

This technique shows where the heart block is (AV node vs. His-Purkinje system). It also shows the origin of tachycardia (supraventricular vs. ventricular) far better than is usually possible using an electrocardiogram. The ability to electrically stimulate the heart at programmed rates and induce precisely timed premature beats lets a doctor assess electrical properties of the heart's conduction system. Most significantly, it also triggers latent tachycardia or bradycardia. Induced tachycardias can usually be stopped by rapid pacing via the electrode catheters. Sometimes an externally applied shock may be required if the patient loses consciousness during the tachycardia.

Being able to turn on and turn off tachycardias during electrophysiologic studies allows antiarrhythmic drugs to be quickly tested for effectiveness. This can be done during a single study using intravenous therapy or during short follow-up studies with oral medication. Electrophysiologic testing has been performed safely worldwide; complications only rarely occur.

When Should Arrhythmias Be Treated?

Once an arrhythmia has been documented, it's important to try to find out where it starts in the heart. It's also necessary to find out whether it's abnormal or merely reflects the heart's normal physiologic processes. The arrhythmia must be abnormal and clinically significant before it justifies an antiarrhythmic intervention. In other words, it must either cause symptoms or put a person at risk for more serious arrhythmias or complications of arrhythmias in the future.

In some patients whose symptoms suggest arrhythmias, tachycardias or bradycardias may be found during diagnostic (particularly electrophysiologic) tests. In such cases, a doctor must judge whether the arrhythmia is a likely enough explanation for the patient's original symptoms to justify therapy. The risks and benefits of the intervention also must be taken into account.

How Are Bradycardias Treated?

Potentially life-threatening bradycardias may be treated acutely with medication. Such medication increases the automatic firing rate of cardiac pacemaker tissue and improves the transmission of impulses through the conduction system.

Another way to maintain the cardiac rhythm is to insert a temporary pacemaker.

ARTIFICIAL PACEMAKERS

If your heart's own natural electrical pacemaker fails to work properly—if your heart beats too quickly or slowly, or erratically—your physician may recommend an artificial pacemaker. An artificial pacemaker is a small, battery-powered, implanted device that produces electrical impulses that travel from your heart's atria down through the ventricles. Some of the pacemakers have two wires, or "leads"; one goes to the heart's right upper chamber, or right atrium, and one to the right lower chamber, or right ventricle. This allows the upper and lower chambers to retain their normal pattern of sequential contraction and relaxation and helps the ventricles to fill properly. Some pacemakers even cause the heart rate to increase, as it naturally would, in response to exercise or stress.

As with any such device, an artificial pacemaker needs some care. A minor surgical procedure is required to replace batteries when they wear down; but most people with pacemakers can take part in all the normal activities for a person of their age.   *The Editors*

This involves using a thin, flexible electrode wire. One end is positioned inside the heart; the other is connected to an external temporary pulse generator that can electrically stimulate the heart via the wire. If symptomatic bradycardia persists or is likely to recur, despite eliminating reversible causes, then implanting a permanent pacemaker is appropriate. This device consists of a pulse generator, which can be as small as a silver dollar. The pulse generator is hooked up to one or two pacemaker leads that are permanently affixed to a ventricular or atrial site, or to both.

Permanent pacemakers deliver electrical stimuli to the heart when the heart's spontaneous rate falls below a set value. Physiologic sensors are incorporated into many of these devices to make the pacemaker's rate vary according to the body's needs.

The pacemaker generator is implanted under the skin below the collarbone. It may work for up to eight to 12 years before it needs to be replaced.

How Are Tachycardias Treated?

Symptomatic tachycardias and premature beats may be treated with a variety of antiarrhythmic drugs. These may be given intravenously on an acute basis, or orally for long-term treatment. These drugs act by suppressing the abnormal firing of pacemaker tissue or by depressing the transmission of impulses in tissues that either conduct too rapidly or that participate in reentry. In patients with atrial fibrillation, a blood thinner (anticoagulant) is often added to reduce the risk of blood clots and stroke.

When tachycardias or premature beats occur often, the effectiveness of antiarrhythmic drug therapy may be gauged by electrocardiographic monitoring in a hospital, by using a 24-hour Holter monitor, or by serial drug evaluation with electrophysiologic testing.

The relative simplicity of antiarrhythmic drug therapy must be balanced against two disadvantages. One is that the drugs must be taken daily for an indefinite period. The second is the risk of side effects. While side effects are inherent in all medication, those associated with antiarrhythmic drugs can be most difficult to manage. These side effects include proarrhythmia, which is more frequent occurrence of preexisting arrhythmias or the appearance of new arrhythmias as bad as or worse than those being treated.

A host of nondrug therapies are being used to treat patients with symptomatic tachycardias. Ablative techniques refer to therapeutic methods that physically destroy the cardiac tissue that causes or contributes to a tachycardia. Until recently, such therapy was feasible only through surgery (often involving an open heart procedure). In such a surgical approach, the culprit cardiac tissue is removed or destroyed by local heating or cooling.

Newer advances now permit therapeutic ablations to be done using a transcatheter approach. In this technique, an electrode catheter inserted through a vein or artery during electrophysiologic studies is used to perform targeted electrocautery in the heart. A patient may be cured of tachycardia through ablative therapy, so that antiarrhythmic medication is no longer needed. Transcatheter ablation has become the treatment of choice for many supraventricular tachycardias.

Other types of electrical therapy are also available for treating tachycardias. On an acute basis, many pathological tachycardias can be stopped by an electric shock delivered to the heart or by rapid "overdrive" pacing with an electrode catheter. Implantable devices can provide automatic electrical therapy on a chronic basis for patients with recurrent tachycardias.

The greatest advance in this area is the implantable cardioverter defibrillator. It's used in patients at risk for recurrent sustained ventricular tachycardia or fibrillation.

The device is connected to leads positioned either inside the heart or on its surface. These leads are used to deliver electrical shocks, sense the cardiac rhythm, and sometimes pace the heart, as appropriate. These various leads are tunnelled to a pulse generator. Such generators are typically a little larger than a wallet and contain the electronics that automatically monitor and treat heart rhythms recognized as abnormal. Newer devices are smaller and have simpler lead systems that make implanting them much easier.

When the implantable cardioverter defibrillator detects ventricular tachycardia or fibrillation, it shocks the heart to restore the normal rhythm. New devices also provide overdrive pacing to electrically convert sustained ventricular tachycardia, backup pacing in the event of bradycardia, and a host of other sophisticated functions (such as storage of detected arrhythmia events and capability to perform noninvasive electrophysiologic testing).

Implantable cardioverter defibrillators have already been very useful in preventing sudden death in patients with known sustained ventricular tachycardia or fibrillation. Studies are now being done to find out whether these devices have a role in preventing cardiac arrest in high-risk patients who haven't yet had, but are at risk for, life-threatening ventricular arrhythmias.

WHAT IS SUDDEN CARDIAC DEATH (SCD)?

It's the sudden, abrupt loss of heart function (i.e., cardiac arrest) in a person who may or may not have diagnosed heart disease, but in whom the time and mode of death occur unexpectedly. The unexpected nature of the event is the key point in the definition.

How Common Is the Sudden Cardiac Death Syndrome?

About half of all deaths from heart disease are sudden and unexpected, regardless of the underlying disease. Thus 50 percent of all deaths due to atherosclerosis of the coronary arteries are sudden, as are 50 percent of deaths due to degeneration of the heart muscle or to cardiac enlargement in patients with high blood pressure. Sudden death is a major health problem: About 250,000 sudden cardiac deaths occur each year among U.S. adults. Controlling SCD might significantly reduce death from heart diseases.

What Is the Impact of Sudden Cardiac Death?

The shock of sudden cardiac death lies in its unexpectedness. Although the direct medical costs are much less than for lingering illnesses, its economic and social impacts are huge. Sudden cardiac death occurs at an average age of about 60 years, claims many people during their most productive years, and devastates unprepared families.

What Causes Sudden Cardiac Death?

SCD is the result of an unresuscitated cardiac arrest, which may be caused by almost all known heart diseases. Most cardiac arrests are due to rapid and/or chaotic activity of the heart (ventricular tachycardia or fibrillation); some are due to extreme slowing of the heart. These events are called life-threatening arrhythmias and are responsible for sudden death.

The term "massive heart attack," commonly used in the media to describe sudden death, only infrequently is responsible. "Heart attack" more properly refers to death of heart muscle tissue due to the loss of blood supply. Though a heart attack may cause cardiac arrest and sudden cardiac death, the terms aren't synonymous.

Can the Cardiac Arrest That Causes Sudden Cardiac Death Be Reversed?

Cardiac arrest is reversible in most victims if it's treated within a few minutes. This first became clear in the early 1960s with the development of coronary care units and electrical devices that shocked the heart to turn an abnormally rapid rhythm into a normal one. Before then, heart attack victims had a 30 percent chance of dying if they got to the hospital alive; 50 percent of these deaths were a consequence of cardiac arrest.

In-hospital survival after cardiac arrest in heart attack patients improved dramatically when the external defibrillator and bedside monitoring were developed. Later, it also became clear that cardiac arrest could be reversed outside a hospital by appropriately staffed emergency rescue teams trained to perform CPR and to defibrillate. Thus, the problem isn't the ability to reverse cardiac arrest, but reaching the victim in time to do so. The American Heart Association supports the concept of the need for a chain of survival to rescue the person who suffers cardiac arrest in the community.

Who's at Risk for Sudden Cardiac Death?

Underlying heart disease is nearly always found in victims of sudden cardiac death. Typically in adults, this takes the form of atherosclerotic heart disease. Two or more major coronary arteries are narrowed in 90 percent of cases; scarring from a prior heart attack is found in two-thirds of victims. It's not surprising, then, that predisposing factors for sudden cardiac death are similar to risk factors for atherosclerotic heart disease and include cigarette/tobacco smoke and high blood pressure.

A heart that's scarred or enlarged from any cause is prone to develop life-threatening ventricular arrhythmias. The first six months after a heart attack is a particularly high-risk period for sudden cardiac death in patients who have atherosclerotic heart disease. A thickened heart muscle from any cause (typically high blood pressure or valvular heart disease)—especially when there's congestive heart failure, too—is an important predisposing factor for sudden cardiac death.

Under certain conditions, various heart medications can set the stage for arrhythmias that cause sudden cardiac death. In particular, so-called antiarrhythmic drugs, even at normally prescribed doses, sometimes may produce lethal ventricular arrhythmias (proarrhythmic effect).

Regardless of whether there's organic heart disease, significant changes in blood levels of potassium and magnesium (from using diuretics, for example) also can cause life-threatening arrhythmias and cardiac arrest.

When sudden cardiac death occurs in young adults, atherosclerotic heart disease usually isn't the cause. More often these young victims have a thickened heart muscle (hypertrophic cardiomyopathy) without accompanying high blood pressure.

Certain electrical abnormalities within the heart may be responsible for sudden cardiac death in the young. These include a short circuit between the upper and lower chambers (Wolff-Parkinson-White syndrome). This sometimes can allow dangerously rapid rates to develop in the lower chamber when there's a rapid rhythm disturbance in the upper chamber and a congenitally prolonged electrical recovery after each heartbeat (long-QT syndrome). These may set the stage for fatal ventricular arrhythmias.

Less often, inborn abnormalities of the blood vessels, particularly the coronary arteries and aorta, may be present in young sudden death victims.

Adrenaline released during intense physical or athletic activity often acts as a trigger for sudden cardiac death when these predisposing conditions are present.

In young people without organic heart disease, recreational drug abuse is an important cause of sudden cardiac death.

How Can Survivors of Unexpected Cardiac Arrest Be Protected from Fatal Recurrences?

Survivors of unexpected cardiac arrest (aborted sudden cardiac death) due to ventricular tachycardia or fibrillation are at risk for recurrent arrest. This is especially true if they have underlying heart disease. Patients with atherosclerotic heart disease are at risk of recurrent cardiac arrests when the first, aborted sudden death episode occurs in the absence of a new heart attack, because this implies a persistent underlying tendency toward electrical instability.

To find the treatment program most likely to prevent recurrent cardiac arrest in a patient, it's critical to identify any predisposing anatomic or electrophysiologic abnormalities. This often requires cardiac catheterization (to show the heart and coronary blood vessels) and electrophysiologic testing. It's also necessary to determine the possible contribution of reversible causes; if they're identified and removed or corrected, the risk of recurrent cardiac arrest can be markedly reduced or eliminated. Such factors may include excessive doses of various cardiac drugs, the presence of antiarrhythmic agents, and abnormal blood levels of various minerals, especially potassium.

The treatment program used to prevent fatal recurrences in survivors of cardiac arrest due to ventricular tachycardia or fibrillation must be chosen based upon several factors that depend on the individual. These include the underlying cardiac condition, how well the heart can pump, and the demonstration of ventricular tachycardia or fibrillation during electrophysiologic testing.

For example, cardiac arrest survivors with the Wolff-Parkinson-White syndrome (who otherwise have normal hearts) may be satisfactorily treated simply with a catheter ablation procedure that destroys the short circuit between the upper and lower heart chambers. At the other extreme, a heart transplant may be recommended for patients who've had a cardiac arrest as a result of very severe structural heart disease.

In cardiac arrest survivors with atherosclerotic heart disease but without a new heart attack, attention must be paid to both the degree of narrowing in the coronary arteries and the presence of ventricular tachycardia and fibrillation that can occur during electrophysiologic testing. Therapy limited to reversing or blunting the effects of reduced blood supply to the heart (through bypass surgery, angioplasty, or medication) is likely to protect only a minority of these aborted sudden death patients from recurrent cardiac arrest. The reason is that such treatments alone don't stabilize the electrical abnormalities in scarred heart muscle that can lead to recurrent cardiac arrest.

A number of therapies exist for controlling potentially life-threatening ventricular tachyarrhythmias that result from diseased or scarred heart muscle. Antiarrhythmic medication may protect against subsequent sudden death in certain subsets of cardiac arrest survivors (for example, in persons whose hearts pump well who are given a drug that suppresses ventricular tachycardia induced during electrophysiologic testing). However, antiarrhythmic medication is limited by the need for lifelong dosing and the potential for intolerable or lethal side effects. As a result, there's been increasing reliance on the use of implantable cardioverter defibrillators. They can automatically detect ventricular tachycardia or fibrillation when it occurs and, within seconds, deliver a lifesaving electrical shock to restore the normal rhythm.

Rapid heart rhythms account for the great majority of sudden cardiac deaths. Still, very slow rhythms due to conduction system failure are sometimes responsible for cardiac arrest. Persons resuscitated from this uncommon type of cardiac arrest are treated with a permanent pacemaker after acute reversible causes, such as drug toxicity, have been ruled out.

What Are the Hopes for the Future?

If the past is any indication, there's great hope for the future. The dramatic progress during the past 30 years, focused largely on very high-risk groups (such as cardiac arrest survivors), has shown what can be achieved. At the same time, recent advances in treating heart attack victims appear to be reducing the significant risk of sudden death during the first year after a heart attack.

In the future, ways to identify potential victims need to be developed. People whose risk may not be very high account for the vast majority of sudden death victims in absolute numbers—perhaps 80 percent of the deaths per year. Once these people are identified, it will be possible to devise broader strategies to prevent sudden cardiac arrest.

RISK FACTORS FOR HEART DISEASE

Extensive clinical and statistical studies have identified several factors that increase the risk of heart attack and stroke. These risk factors can be grouped into two classifications: 1) major risk factors and 2) contributing risk factors.

Major risk factors are those that medical research has shown to be definitely associated with a significant increase in the risk of cardiovascular disease. The major risk factors for heart attack that cannot be changed are hered-ity (inherited traits), male sex, and increasing age. The major risk factors that result from modifiable lifestyle habits are cigarette/tobac-co smoke, high blood cholesterol, high blood pressure, and physical inactivity.

Contributing risk factors are those associated with in-creased risk of cardiovascular disease. For heart at-tack, these include diabetes and obesity. Stress may also be a factor. The more risk factors a person has, the greater the chance of developing heart disease.

Major Risk Factors That Can't Be Changed

Heredity. A tendency toward heart disease or atherosclerosis seems to be hereditary. That means children of parents with cardiovascular disease are more likely to develop it them-selves. Race is a consideration, too. African Americans have moderate high blood pressure twice as often as whites and severe hyperten-sion three times as often. Consequently, their risk of heart disease is greater.

Being Male. Men have a greater risk of heart at-tack than women earlier in life. After meno-pause, women's death rate from heart disease increases.

Increasing Age. About four out of five people who die of heart attack are age 65 or older. At older ages, women who have heart attacks are twice as likely as men to die from them within a few weeks.

Major Risk Factors That Can Be Changed

Cigarette/Tobacco Smoke. Smokers' risk of heart attack is more than twice that of non-smokers. In fact, cigarette smoking is the biggest risk factor for sudden cardiac death: smokers have two to four times the risk of nonsmokers. Smokers who have a heart attack are more likely to die and die suddenly (with-in an hour) than nonsmokers.

Evidence also indicates that chronic expo-sure to environmental tobacco smoke (second-hand smoke, passive smoking) increases the risk of heart disease. The risk of death due to heart disease is increased by about 30 percent among those exposed to environmental tobac-co smoke at home and could be much higher in those exposed in the workplace, where high-er levels of environmental tobacco smoke may be present.

Smoking is also the biggest risk factor for peripheral vascular disease (narrowing of blood vessels carrying blood to leg and arm muscles). In fact, this condition is almost ex-clusively confined to smokers. Smokers with peripheral vascular disease are also more likely to develop gangrene and require leg amputation. Benefits from corrective surg-ery are also reduced when patients continue to smoke.

When people stop smoking, regardless of how long or how much they've smoked, their risk of heart disease rapidly declines. Three years after quitting, the risk of death from heart disease and stroke for people who smoked a pack a day or less is almost the same as for people who never smoked.

It's important to stop smoking before the signs of heart disease appear. If you smoke, QUIT NOW. And if you don't smoke, don't start.

High Blood Cholesterol. The risk of coronary heart disease rises as blood cholesterol levels increase. When other risk factors (such as high blood pressure and cigarette/tobacco smoke) are present, this risk increases even more. A person's cholesterol level is also af-fected by age, sex, heredity, and diet.

Based on large population studies, blood cholesterol levels below 200 mg/dl (milli-grams per deciliter) in middle-aged adults seem to indicate a relatively low risk of coro-nary heart disease. A level of 240 mg/dl and over approximately doubles the risk. Blood cholesterol values from 200 to 239 mg/dl in-dicate moderate and increasing risk.

Blood cholesterol levels should be measured at least once every five years in healthy adults 20 years of age and over. HDL should be measured at the same time. People with cholesterol levels of 200 mg/dl or greater, or HDL cholesterol less than 35 mg/dl on initial testing, should have fasting lipoprotein analysis that provides measures of total cholesterol, HDL cholesterol, triglycerides, and an estimate of LDL cholesterol. If the result is from 200 to 239 mg/dl and the person has coronary heart disease or a family history of premature CHD, measuring lipoproteins is warranted.

Desirable levels of LDL are under 130 mg/dl; "borderline high" ranges from 130 to 159; 160 or more is considered "high." If you have any manifestations of heart disease or have had a heart attack, LDL levels should be kept below 100 mg/dl.

A certain amount of cholesterol in the body is necessary to build cell membranes, etc. However, the liver produces enough cholesterol to meet these needs. That's why diet is important. A diet high in saturated fat and cholesterol tends to raise blood cholesterol; a diet low in saturated fat and cholesterol usually means lower levels of blood cholesterol.

On the whole, Americans should reduce the amount of fat and cholesterol in their diet. By watching their diet, people with low levels of blood cholesterol will help minimize the tendency for cholesterol levels to rise with age. People with higher levels of blood cholesterol will benefit even more. First, controlling their diet will help reduce their blood cholesterol levels. Second, if drugs are still needed to reduce blood cholesterol, the diet will improve their effectiveness.

High Blood Pressure. High blood pressure usually has no specific symptoms and no early warning signs. It's truly a "silent killer." But a simple, quick, painless test can detect it. (See page 319.)

High blood pressure increases the heart's workload, causing the heart to enlarge and weaken over time. It also increases the risk of stroke, heart attack, kidney failure, and congestive heart failure. When high blood pressure exists with obesity, smoking, high blood cholesterol levels, or diabetes, the risk of heart attack or stroke increases several times.

As a rule, blood pressure tends to increase with age. Men have a greater risk of high blood pressure than women until age 55, when their respective risks become about equal. At age 75 and older, women are more likely to develop high blood pressure than men.

People who have high blood pressure should work with their doctor to control it. Eating a proper diet, losing weight, exercising regularly, restricting salt (sodium) intake, and following a program of medication may all be prescribed to lower blood pressure and keep it within healthy limits.

Physical Inactivity. Physical inactivity or lack of exercise is a risk factor for coronary heart disease. Regular aerobic exercise plays a significant role in preventing heart and blood vessel disease.

For some years the American Heart Association has recommended 30 to 60 minutes of aerobic exercise three to four times per week to promote cardiovascular fitness. Such activities could include aerobics, jogging, running, swimming, and sports such as tennis, racquetball, soccer, and basketball.

Even modest levels of low-intensity physical activity are beneficial if done regularly and long term. Such activities include walking for pleasure, gardening, housework, and dancing.

Physical inactivity can lead to several changes that are risk factors for heart disease. When lack of exercise is combined with overeating, excess weight and increased blood cholesterol levels can result—and these unquestionably contribute to the risk of heart disease. Middle-aged or older people who are inactive should seek medical advice before they start or significantly increase their physical activity.

Other Contributing Factors

Diabetes. Diabetes is the inability of the body to produce or respond to insulin properly. Insulin is needed for the body to metabolize or use glucose (sugar). Diabetes appears most often in middle age and among overweight people. In a mild form, it can go undetected for many years. Besides increasing the risks of kidney disease, blindness, and nerve and blood vessel damage, diabetes also seriously increases the risk of developing cardiovascular disease. In fact, more than 80 percent of people with diabetes die of some form of heart or blood vessel disease. Part of the reason for this is that diabetes affects cholesterol and triglyceride levels.

When diabetes is detected, a doctor may prescribe changes in eating habits, weight control, exercise programs, and drugs, if necessary, to keep it in check. Despite the different measures that may be taken to control glucose levels, as a contributing risk factor for heart disease, diabetes cannot be changed.

Obesity. People who are overweight or obese are more likely to develop heart disease and stroke even if they have no other risk factors. Excess weight is unhealthy because it increases the strain on the heart. It's linked with coronary heart disease mainly because it influences blood pressure and blood cholesterol and can lead to diabetes.

Recent evidence indicates that how fat is distributed on the body may affect the risk of coronary heart disease. A waist-to-hip ratio greater than 1.0 for men indicates a significantly increased risk. For women, the ratio is 0.8. This means that a man's waist measurement should not exceed his hip measurement, and a woman's waist measurement should not be more than 80 percent of her hip measurement.

Individual Response to Stress. It's almost impossible to define and measure someone's level of emotional stress. There's no way to measure the psychological impact of different experiences. All people feel stress, but they feel it in different amounts and react in different ways. Life would be dull without stress, but excessive amounts of stress over a long time may create health problems in some people.

Some scientists have noted a relationship between coronary heart disease risk and a person's life stress, behavior habits, and socioeconomic status. These factors may affect established risk factors. For example, people under stress may start smoking or smoke more than they otherwise would. The contributing risk factors just discussed may not be as significant as cigarette/tobacco smoke, high blood cholesterol, or high blood pressure in their impact on heart disease. Still, they're important and shouldn't be ignored.

The American Heart Association

STROKE

Stroke is a form of cardiovascular disease that affects the arteries of the central nervous system. A stroke (or "brain attack") occurs when a blood vessel bringing oxygen and nutrients to the brain bursts or is clogged by a blood clot or some other particle. Because of this rupture or blockage, part of the brain doesn't get the flow of blood it needs. Deprived of oxygen, nerve cells in the affected area of the brain can't function and die within minutes. And when nerve cells can't function, the part of the body controlled by these cells can't function either. The devastating effects of stroke are often permanent because dead brain cells aren't replaced.

TYPES OF STROKE

There are four main types of stroke: two caused by clots (ischemic strokes), and two by hemorrhage. Cerebral thrombosis and cerebral embolism are by far the most common, accounting for about 70 to 80 percent of all strokes. They're caused by clots that plug an artery. Cerebral and subarachnoid hemorrhages are caused by ruptured blood vessels. They have a much higher fatality rate than strokes caused by clots.

Cerebral thrombosis is the most common type of stroke. It occurs when a blood clot (thrombus) forms and blocks blood flow in an artery bringing blood to part of the brain. Blood clots usually form in arteries damaged by atherosclerosis.

One identifying feature of cerebral thrombotic strokes is that they usually occur at night or first thing in the morning, when blood pressure is low. They're often preceded by a transient ischemic attack, also called a TIA or mini-stroke (see box on page 340).

Cerebral embolism occurs when a wandering clot (an embolus) or some other particle occurs in a blood vessel away from the brain, usually in the heart. The clot is carried by the bloodstream until it lodges in an artery leading to or in the brain, blocking blood flow.

The most common cause of these emboli is blood clots that form during atrial fibrillation. In atrial fibrillation the two small upper chambers of the heart, the atria, quiver instead of beating effectively. Blood isn't pumped completely out of them when the heart beats, allowing the blood to pool and clot. About 15 percent of strokes occur in people with atrial fibrillation.

Atrial fibrillation can be brought on by hyperthyroidism, pulmonary embolus, congestive heart failure, acute heart attack, other types of long-standing heart disease, or without any specific cause. Its sudden onset may initially cause palpitations or angina. The first line of treatment is drug therapy to bring the heart rhythm

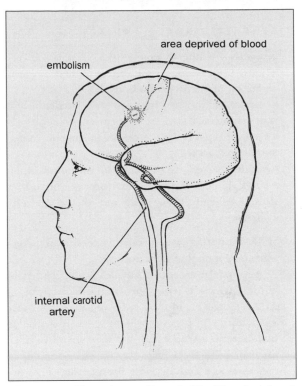

The two carotid arteries are the main bloodlines from heart to brain. In one kind of stroke, a cerebral embolism, or blood clot, blocks an artery to the brain.

back to normal. If the fibrillation is of recent onset and drugs do not bring it under control, a physician will use an electrical shock to the heart to reverse it (defibrillation). Because chronic atrial fibrillation may be associated with emboli (clots) that may cause a stroke, anticoagulants, or other drugs that will inhibit platelet aggregation, are often prescribed as a way to reduce the chance of a stroke.

Subarachnoid hemorrhage occurs when a blood vessel on the surface of the brain ruptures and bleeds into the space between the brain and the skull (but not into the brain itself). Subarachnoid hemorrhages account for about 7 percent of all strokes.

Cerebral hemorrhage is another type of stroke that occurs when a defective artery in the brain bursts, flooding the surrounding tissue

339

STROKE—SIGNALS AND ACTION

Know the Warning Signs of Stroke:
• Sudden weakness or numbness of the face, arm, or leg on one side of the body
• Sudden dimness or loss of vision, particularly in only one eye
• Loss of speech, or trouble talking or understanding speech
• Sudden, severe headaches with no known cause
• Unexplained dizziness, unsteadiness, or sudden falls, especially along with any of the previous symptoms

If you notice one or more of these signs, don't wait—see a doctor right away.

About 10 percent of strokes are preceded by "little strokes" (transient ischemic attacks or TIAs). However, of those who've had one or more TIAs, about 36 percent will later have a stroke. In fact, a person who's had one or more TIAs is 9.5 times more likely to have a stroke than someone of the same age and sex who hasn't. Thus TIAs are extremely important stroke warning signs.

TIAs are more useful for predicting if a stroke will occur than when one will happen. They can occur days, weeks, or even months before a major stroke. In about 50 percent of the cases, the stroke occurs within one year of the TIA; in about 20 percent of the cases, within one month.

TIAs occur when a blood clot temporarily clogs an artery, and part of the brain doesn't get the blood it needs. The symptoms occur rapidly and last a relatively short time. More than 75 percent of TIAs last less than five minutes. The average is about a minute, although some last several hours. By definition, TIAs can last up to—but not over—24 hours, although this is very unusual. Unlike stroke, when a TIA is over, people return to normal.

The usual TIA symptoms are very similar to those of stroke. They are: 1) temporary weakness, clumsiness or loss of feeling in an arm, leg, or the side of the face on one side of the body (or some combination thereof); 2) temporary dimness or loss of vision, particularly in one eye (also often in combination with other symptoms); 3) temporary loss of speech or difficulty in speaking or difficulty in understanding speech, particularly with a right-side weakness. Sometimes dizziness, double vision, and staggering also occur. The short duration of these symptoms and lack of permanent damage is the main distinction between TIA and stroke.

Although TIAs signal only about 10 percent of strokes, they're very strong predictors of stroke risk. Don't ignore them! Get medical attention immediately! A doctor should determine if a TIA or stroke has occurred, or if it's another medical problem with similar symptoms (seizure, fainting, migraine, or general medical or cardiac condition). Prompt medical or surgical attention to these symptoms could prevent a fatal or disabling stroke from occurring.

with blood. About 10 percent of all strokes result from cerebral hemorrhages.

Hemorrhage, or bleeding, from an artery in the brain can be caused by a head injury or a burst aneurysm. Aneurysms are blood-filled pouches that balloon out from weak spots in the artery wall. They're often caused or aggravated by high blood pressure. Aneurysms aren't always dangerous, but if one bursts in the brain, a stroke results.

When a cerebral or subarachnoid hemorrhage occurs, the loss of a constant blood supply means some brain cells can no longer function. Another problem is that accumulated blood from the burst artery may put pressure on the surrounding brain tissue and interfere with how the brain functions. Severe or mild symptoms can result, depending on the amount of pressure.

The amount of bleeding determines the severity of cerebral hemorrhages. In 50 percent of the cases, people with cerebral hemorrhages die of increased pressure on their brains. Those who live, however, tend to recover much more than those whose had strokes caused by a clot. The reason is that when a blood vessel is blocked, part of the brain dies—and the brain doesn't regenerate. But when a blood vessel in the brain bursts, pressure from the blood compresses part of the brain. If the person survives, gradually the pressure diminishes and the brain may return to its former state.

EFFECTS OF STROKE

Strokes affect different people in different ways, depending on the type of stroke and the area of the brain affected. Brain injury from a stroke can affect the senses, speech and the ability to understand speech, behavioral patterns, thought patterns, and memory. Paralysis on one side of the body is common. Stroke also can cause depression, as survivors think they're now less than whole.

Stroke often causes people to lose feeling in an arm or leg, or suffer diminished sight in one eye. The loss of feeling or visual field results in a loss of awareness, so stroke survivors may forget or ignore their weaker side, a problem called neglect. As a result, they may ignore items put on their affected side, have trouble reading, or dress only one side of their bodies and think they're completely dressed. Bumping into furniture or door jambs is also common.

A stroke can affect seeing, touching, moving, and thinking, so a person's perception of everyday objects may be changed. Stroke survivors may not be able to recognize and understand familiar objects the way they did before. When vision is affected, objects may look closer or farther away than they really are, causing spills at the table or collisions when walking.

Usually stroke doesn't cause hearing loss, although people may have problems understanding speech. They also may have trouble verbalizing what they're thinking. This is called aphasia. Aphasia affects the ability to talk, listen, read, and write. It usually occurs when a stroke weakens the right side of the body.

A related problem is that a stroke can affect muscles used in talking (those in the tongue, palate, and lips), and speech can be slowed, slurred, or distorted. Stroke survivors thus can be hard to understand. This is called dysarthria and may require the help of a speech pathologist. Chewing and swallowing food also can be a problem. One or both sides of the mouth can lack feeling, increasing the risk of choking.

Finally, a stroke can affect the ability to think clearly. Planning and carrying out even simple activities may be hard. Stroke survivors may not know how to start a task, confuse the sequence of logical steps in tasks, or forget how to do tasks they've done many times before.

RISK FACTORS FOR STROKE

When stroke occurs, there can be severe losses in mental and bodily functions—if not death. That is why preventing stroke is so important. The best way to prevent a stroke from occurring is to reduce the risk factors for stroke.

Some factors that increase the risk of stroke are hereditary. Others are a function of natural processes. Still others result from a person's lifestyle. Factors resulting from heredity or natural processes can't be changed, but environmental factors can be modified with a doctor's help.

Risk Factors That Can Be Treated

Five partly controllable risk factors are: 1) high blood pressure, 2) heart disease, 3) cigarette smoking, 4) transient ischemic attacks, and 5) high red blood cell count.

High Blood Pressure. Hypertension is the most important risk factor for stroke. In fact, stroke risk varies directly with blood pressure. What makes high blood pressure even more significant is that it afflicts about one in every four American adults. And women don't tolerate high blood pressure any better than men. The effect of hypertension doesn't ease as a person gets older either. That's why everyone should have their blood pressure checked regularly. Controlling high blood pressure reduces the risk of stroke significantly; often blood pressure can be controlled simply by eating a healthier diet and maintaining proper weight. Drugs to control blood pressure are also available. Many people think the reason the death rate from stroke has declined over the past decade is due to better control of high blood pressure.

Heart Disease. A diseased heart increases the risk of stroke. Independent of blood pressure, people with heart problems have more than twice the risk of stroke than people with normally functioning hearts. The four major controllable risk factors for heart attacks are cigarette/tobacco smoke, high blood cholesterol, high blood pressure, and physical inactivity. Controlling these factors reduces the risk of heart disease and thus the risk of stroke.

Cigarette Smoking. In recent years, studies have shown cigarette smoking to be an important risk factor for stroke. Inhaling cigarette smoke produces a number of effects damaging to the cardiovascular system. Nicotine in tobacco smoke increases a person's blood pressure. Carbon monoxide also gets in the blood, reducing the amount of oxygen the blood can supply to the body. Cigarette smoke also causes the platelets in the blood to become sticky and cluster, shortens platelet survival, decreases clotting time, and increases blood thickness.

Transient Ischemic Attacks (TIAs). Only about 10 percent of strokes are preceded by TIAs. Nevertheless, TIAs are extremely important; they're strong predictors of stroke. TIAs are usually treated with drugs that inhibit clots from forming.

A TIA is a medical emergency. Even though symptoms (which may include weakness or numbness on one side of the body, double or impaired vision, speech difficulty, light-headedness, and confusion) generally disappear on their own, prompt medical attention is nonetheless essential to prevent future strokes or other serious complications.

High Red Blood Cell Count. A marked, or even moderate increase in the red blood cell count is a risk factor for stroke. The reason is that increased red blood cells thicken the blood and make clots more likely. This problem is treatable by removing blood or administering blood thinners.

Risk Factors That Can't Be Changed

Seven risk factors for stroke can't be changed. These are: 1) increasing age, 2) being male, 3) race, 4) diabetes mellitus, 5) prior stroke, 6) heredity, and 7) asymptomatic carotid bruit.

Increasing Age. Incidence of stroke is strongly related to age. Older people have a much greater stroke risk than younger people. The risk of stroke in people aged 65 to 74 is about 1 percent a year. If they've had a TIA, it increases to 5 to 8 percent a year.

Being Male. The incidence of stroke is about 19 percent higher for men than it is for women. For men under age 65, the difference is even greater.

Race. African Americans have more than 60 percent greater risk of death and disability from stroke than whites. This may be because African Americans have a greater incidence of high blood pressure. Asian-Pacific Islanders and Hispanics also have a higher risk.

Diabetes Mellitus. Although diabetes is treatable, the fact that a person has it still makes it much more likely that he or she will suffer a stroke. This is even more true for women than for men. Many times people with diabetes also have hypertension, increasing their risk of stroke even more.

Prior Stroke. The risk of stroke for someone who's already had one is many times that of someone who has not.

Another significant risk factor for stroke is atrial fibrillation—when the upper chambers of the heart (the atria) irregularly flutter and quiver instead of pumping in a steady rhythm. This promotes the formation of blood clots that may eventually lodge in an artery supplying blood to the brain.

Heredity. Stroke risk is greater for people who have a family history of stroke.

Asymptomatic Carotid Bruit. A bruit is an abnormal sound heard when a stethoscope is placed over an artery (in this case, the carotid artery, which is in the neck). Carotid bruit clearly indicates increased stroke risk. However, a bruit mainly indicates atherosclerosis; it doesn't necessarily mean the carotid artery will become clogged and a stroke will result.

On the other hand, in cases where diagnostic tests reveal that carotid arteries are occluded by atherosclerotic plaque beyond a certain point, a stroke-preventing procedure known as carotid endarterectomy may be required to remove plaque from the arteries.

Other Risk Factors
Other, less-documented risk factors include: 1) geographic area, 2) season and climate, 3) socioeconomic factors, 4) excessive alcohol intake, and 5) certain kinds of drug abuse.

Geographic Area. Strokes are more common in the southeastern United States. The so-called "Stroke Belt" states are Alabama, Arkansas, Georgia, Indiana, Kentucky, Louisiana, Mississippi, North Carolina, South Carolina, Tennessee, and Virginia.

Season and Climate. Stroke deaths occur more often during periods of extreme temperatures.

Excessive Alcohol Intake. More than one drink per day raises blood pressure. Binge drinking can lead to stroke.

Certain Kinds of Drug Abuse. Intravenous drug abuse carries a high risk of stroke from cerebral embolisms. Cocaine use has been closely related to strokes, heart attacks, and a variety of other cardiovascular complications. Some of them have been fatal even in first-time cocaine users.

Secondary Risk Factors
Besides the risk factors listed, other (controllable) factors indirectly increase stroke risk. These include: 1) elevated blood cholesterol and lipids, 2) physical inactivity, and 3) obesity. These are secondary risk factors, because they affect the risk of stroke indirectly by increasing the risk of heart disease (which is a primary risk factor for stroke).

Finally, it's worth noting that some rather low-level risk factors—when combined with certain other risk factors—become extremely significant. Taking oral contraceptives and smoking cigarettes, for example, increases the risk of stroke considerably. More to the point, the 10 percent of the population in whom one-third of all strokes occur have a set of five risk factors. These are:

- high blood pressure
- elevated blood cholesterol levels
- abnormal glucose tolerance
- cigarette smoking
- left ventricular hypertrophy (the over-development of the left side of the heart)

People who have all these factors should have close medical supervision.

DIAGNOSING STROKE

When someone has shown symptoms of a TIA or stroke, one of the first steps a doctor must take is to gather data to make a diagnosis. He or she will take a careful history of the events that have occurred, as well as a general medical history for diabetes, hypertension, heart and blood vessel disease, and other neurological diseases. Measuring blood pressure in both arms, testing the pulse, checking the heart, listening for bruits over the neck and collarbone, checking the eyes, and giving a neurological exam are all standard practices.

A doctor might use many different tests in a neurological exam. For example, doctors may test patients' level of consciousness, orientation, memory, and emotional control.

Some doctors test patients by having them stand motionless with feet together, arms outstretched, and eyes closed; testing for facial paresis (paralysis) by having patients bare their gums and stick out their tongues is also sometimes done. Hearing might be tested by rubbing the thumb and forefinger together about 12 inches from the ear. Having patients read newsprint using one eye at a time is a test of vision; visual fields can be tested by having a person cover one eye and look into the doctor's opposite eye. (The doctor will then bring a thumb or small object from the side and ask the patient to signal when it becomes visible.) The perception of pain and light touch, muscular strength, and deep tendon reflexes are also commonly tested.

The tests described here are only examples of those that might be done. After these basic tests, many people will need laboratory tests showing a complete blood count, blood sugar, urea, and electrolytes. Some people may even be given an electrocardiogram.

TESTS THAT REVEAL A STROKE

Identifying stroke warning signals is one way to diagnose a stroke. But proper diagnosis doesn't stop there. Other tests may be run because the symptoms may not necessarily result from a stroke. For example, a brain tumor can produce similar symptoms. A doctor must eliminate other possibilities before making a diagnosis.

Remarkable advances in modern technology now make it possible to examine how the brain looks, functions, and gets its blood supply. These tests can outline the affected part of the brain and help define the problem created by stroke. Most of these newer tests are safe and painless and can be undergone as an outpatient. They fall into three categories:

- Tests that image the brain make pictures that look similar to ordinary x-rays
- Tests that measure the electrical activity of the brain, giving useful information about how it's functioning and pinpointing areas where it's functioning abnormally
- Blood flow tests to measure flow and detect blockages in blood vessels—useful in revealing areas of significant atherosclerosis in carotid arteries

A doctor must decide on a case-by-case basis whether such tests will be useful, and if so, which ones to use.

What Are Some Imaging Tests?

The computed tomographic scan (CT scan) may be the most well-known imaging test. In computerized tomography, the person's head is put in an apparatus resembling a beauty shop hair dryer and taped to avoid movement that might ruin the picture. CT scanning takes from 20 minutes to an hour to complete.

Magnetic resonance imaging scanning (MRI) is another imaging test. It uses a giant magnet to generate an image. MRI is similar to a CT scan but uses a different machine and takes longer.

Radionuclide angiography (nuclear brain scan) is a third imaging test. In it, radioactive compounds are injected into a vein in the arm, and a machine similar to a Geiger counter creates a map showing their uptake into different parts of the head. The pictures, rather than showing the brain's structure, show how it functions. This test can detect blocked blood vessels and areas where the brain is damaged.

What Tests Show the Brain's Electrical Activity?

Two basic tests show the electrical activity of the brain: an electroencephalogram (EEG) and an evoked response test. In an electroencephalogram, small metal disks (electrodes) are put on a person's scalp to pick up electrical impulses transmitted and received by brain cells. A machine equipped with pens transcribes this activity onto large pieces of paper.

Evoked responses measure how the brain handles different sensory stimuli. They can detect abnormal areas of the brain. A doctor evokes a visual response by flashing a light or checkerboard pattern in front of a patient. For auditory evoked responses, a doctor makes a sound in one of the patient's ears; for bodily evoked responses, one of the nerves in an arm or leg is electrically stimulated.

What Tests Show Blood Flow?

This category has the greatest variety of tests.

The Doppler ultrasound test is performed to detect blockages in the carotid artery. In it, a gel is put on the neck or eyelids, then a technologist puts a pencil-like probe into the gel and listens to blood flowing in the carotid artery.

In carotid phonoangiography, a sensitive microphone is put over the carotid artery and a technologist listens for a bruit. (A bruit is the sound created by turbulent blood flow as it passes through a partially blocked artery.)

In ocular plethysmography (OPG), anesthetizing drops are put into the eyes, and then small plastic cups similar to contact lenses are positioned on the eyes to detect pulses or measure pressure in the eyes.

The cerebral blood flow test (inhalation method) measures how much oxygen dissolved in the blood supply reaches different areas of the brain. A person is told to lie flat on a table, then a cap containing detectors is secured over the head. Then the person starts breathing through a mask containing air mixed with a small amount of radioactive xenon. This test lasts 30 minutes to an hour.

Finally, *digital subtraction angiography* (DSA) gives an image of the major blood vessels to the brain. It lets a doctor know if there are any blockages, how severe they are, and what can be done about them. In this test, dye is injected into a vein in the arm, and an x-ray machine quickly takes a series of pictures of the head and neck.

TREATMENT AND REHABILITATION
How Are Strokes Treated?

Surgery, drugs, acute hospital care, and rehabilitation are all accepted ways to treat stroke.

When a neck artery has become blocked, surgery might be used to remove the buildup of atherosclerotic plaque. This is called carotid endarterectomy.

Drugs may be used when a blood vessel has been blocked or blood clots are a problem. They can help prevent new clots from forming or prevent an existing clot from getting bigger.

Sometimes treating a stroke means treating the heart, because various forms of heart disease can contribute to the risk of stroke. For example, damaged heart valves may need to be surgically treated or treated with anticlotting drugs to reduce the chance of clots forming around them. If clots form, there's a chance they could travel to the brain and cause a stroke.

Can Stroke Survivors Be Rehabilitated?

Besides being the third leading cause of death in the United States, stroke is the major cause of serious disability. The initial 30-day case fatality for stroke is high, averaging 38 percent; however, about 50 percent of people who survive this critical period are still alive seven years later. Many of these survivors are left with mental and physical disabilities and receive expensive, time-consuming, and intensive rehabilitation to try to increase their independence.

In the Framingham Study, 31 percent of stroke survivors needed help caring for themselves; 20 percent needed help walking; and 71 percent had an impaired vocational capacity when examined an average of seven years after stroke. Sixteen percent had to be institutionalized. Elsewhere it's been estimated that one-third of the estimated two million cases of disability from stroke in the United States are wage earners aged 35 to 65 who have become unemployable because of disability.

Spontaneous recovery in the first 30 days following a stroke probably accounts for most gains in functional ability. Still, rehabilitation is important. To a large degree, successful rehabilitation depends on the extent of brain damage, the person's attitude, the rehabilitation team's skill, and the cooperation of family and friends. People with the least impairment are likely to benefit the most, but even when improvement is slight, rehabilitation may still mean the difference between staying in an institution and returning home.

The goal of rehabilitation is to reduce dependence and improve physical ability. Often old skills have been lost and new ones are needed. Maintaining and improving a person's physical condition whenever possible is also important. Rehabilitation begins early as nurses and other hospital personnel work to prevent such secondary complications as stiff joints, bedsores, and pneumonia. These can result from being confined to bed for a long time.

The role of the person's family in rehabilitation is also significant. A caring, able spouse can be one of the most important positive factors in rehabilitation. The knowledge of family members also matters a great deal. Family members need to understand what the stroke survivor has undergone and how disabilities can affect the person. The situation will be easier to handle if the family knows what to expect and how to handle problems that arise after the person leaves the hospital.

For a stroke survivor, the goal of rehabilitation is to be as independent and productive as possible, given the limitations resulting from the stroke. *The American Heart Association*

CONGENITAL HEART DEFECTS

"Congenital" means inborn or existing at birth. The terms "congenital heart defect" and "congenital heart disease" are often used interchangeably, but the word "defect" is more accurate. A congenital heart defect occurs when the heart or blood vessels near the heart don't develop normally before birth.

Congenital heart defects are present in about one percent of live births and are the most frequent congenital malformations in newborns. In most cases, scientists don't know why they occur. Sometimes a viral infection causes serious problems. German measles (also called rubella) is an example. If a mother contracts German measles during pregnancy, it can interfere with the development of the baby's heart or produce other malformations. Other viral diseases also may produce congenital defects.

Heredity sometimes plays a role in congenital heart disease. More than one child in a family may have a congenital heart defect, but this is rare. Certain conditions affecting multiple organs, such as Down syndrome, can involve the heart, too. A high number of congenital heart defects also result from mothers' drinking too much alcohol or using drugs such as cocaine during pregnancy.

Types of Defects That Can Occur

Most heart defects either: 1) obstruct blood flow in the heart or vessels near it or 2) cause blood to flow through the heart in an abnormal pattern. Defects rarely occur in which only one functional ventricle (single ventricle) is present, or both the pulmonary artery and aorta arise from the same ventricle (double outlet ventricle). A third rare defect occurs when the right or left side of the heart is incompletely formed (hypoplastic heart).

An obstruction is a narrowing that partially or completely blocks the flow of blood. Obstructions (stenoses) can occur in heart valves, arteries, or veins. The three most common forms of obstructed blood flow are pulmonary valve stenosis, aortic valve stenosis, and coarctation of the aorta.

In pulmonary stenosis the pulmonary valve (which lets blood flow from the right ventricle to the lungs) is narrowed. As a result, the right ventricle must pump harder than normal to overcome the obstruction.

In aortic stenosis the aortic valve (between the left ventricle and the aorta) is narrowed. making it hard for the heart to pump blood to the body. In coarctation of the aorta, the aorta is pinched or constricted. This obstructs blood flow to the lower part of the body and increases blood pressure above the constriction.

Some congenital heart defects allow blood to flow between the right and left chambers of the heart. This happens when a baby is born with an opening or defect between the wall (septum) that separates the right and left sides of the heart. This defect is sometimes called "a hole in the heart."

The two most common types of such openings are atrial septal defect and ventricular septal defect. In atrial septal defect, an opening exists between the two upper chambers of the heart. This allows some blood from the left atrium (blood that's already been to the lungs) to return via the hole to the right atrium instead of flowing through the left ventricle, out the aorta, and to the body. In ventricular septal defect, an opening exists between the two lower chambers of the heart. Some blood that has returned from the lungs and has been pumped into the left ventricle flows to the right ventricle through the hole instead of being pumped into the aorta.

Another defect, patent ductus arteriosus, allows blood to mix between the pulmonary artery and the aorta. Before birth, there's an open passageway (the ductus arteriosus) between these two blood vessels. Normally this closes within a few hours of birth. When this doesn't happen, however, some blood that should flow through the aorta and on to nourish the body returns to the lungs. Failure of the ductus to close is quite common in premature infants but rare in full-term babies.

Another classification of heart abnormalities is congenital cyanotic heart defects. In these defects, blood pumped to the body contains less-than-normal amounts of oxygen. This results in a condition called cyanosis, a blue discoloration of the skin. The term "blue babies" is often applied to infants with cyanosis.

Two examples of cyanotic defects are tetralogy of Fallot and transposition of the great arteries. Tetralogy of Fallot has four components. The two major ones are: 1) a large hole (ventricular septal defect) that allows blood to pass from the right ventricle to the left ventricle without going through the lungs; and 2) a narrowing (stenosis) at or just beneath the pulmonary valve. This narrowing partially blocks the flow of blood from the right side of the heart to the lungs. The other two components are: 3) the right ventricle is more muscular than normal; and 4) the aorta lies directly over the ventricular septal defect.

In transposition of the great arteries, the position of the pulmonary artery and the aorta are reversed. Some type of opening, such as an atrial septal defect or ventricular septal defect, also exists between the right and left sides of the heart. The aorta is connected to the right ventricle, so most of the blood returning to the heart from the body is pumped back out without first going to the lungs. The pulmonary artery is connected to the left ventricle so that most of the blood returning from the lungs goes back to the lungs again.

How a Heart Defect is Detected

Serious congenital heart defects are usually diagnosed at birth or during infancy. Sometimes a doctor hears an abnormal sound (a murmur) in the heart. In other babies, cyanosis is present.

Special tests are often necessary. A chest x-ray gives information about a child's lungs and the size and shape of the heart. An electrocardiogram (ECG) can show an abnormal heartbeat rhythm.

A Doppler echocardiogram is also usually used. An echocardiogram is a painless test that uses high-frequency sound waves to image the heart's internal structures. A Doppler test uses sound waves to measure blood flow. By combining these two tests, a doctor can learn about the heart's structure and function.

Sometimes an in-hospital test called a cardiac catheterization is required. Here a catheter is inserted into a blood vessel in the groin and is slowly advanced under x-ray guidance until it reaches the heart. This test can measure blood pressure and how much oxygen is in the blood of the heart chambers and vessels and provide other information as well. A special fluid visible by x-ray also can be injected into the blood vessels or heart, and an x-ray motion picture can be made. This procedure can help define the heart defect.

Because the Doppler echocardiogram provides a wealth of diagnostic information about congenital heart defects, there has been a marked decrease in the need for cardiac catheterization.

How Congenital Heart Defects Are Treated

Some heart defects can be treated with medicine and others with surgery. The goal of surgery is to repair the defect as completely as possible and make circulation as normal as possible. In some children more than one surgical procedure may be necessary.

The malformed part of the heart or blood vessel may be surgically repaired in several ways. Septal defects can be closed by sewing the defect shut or by sewing a patch (made of Teflon, Dacron, etc.) over the hole. Stenotic valves can be surgically widened. A narrowed segment of a blood vessel can be removed. A ductus arteriosus can be closed by tying it. These are just some examples of surgical techniques that can be used. In some cases, results can be obtained by treatment with special equipment in the cardiac catheterization laboratory.

Some congenital heart defects don't require surgery. Drugs may be used to prevent complications, relieve symptoms or both. Sometimes medical treatment is used for awhile and surgery performed later.

Most people with congenital heart defects are susceptible to bacterial endocarditis, an infection of the heart (see page 352). That's why they're often given antibiotic drugs during certain dental or surgical procedures.

The American Heart Association

RHEUMATIC HEART DISEASE

In rheumatic heart disease the heart valves are damaged by a disease process that begins with a strep throat (streptococcal infection). If it is not treated, the streptococcal infection can develop into acute rheumatic fever.

Rheumatic fever is an inflammatory disease that can affect many connective tissues of the body—especially those of the heart, the joints, the brain, or the skin. When rheumatic fever permanently damages the heart, the damage is called rheumatic heart disease.

People of all ages can develop acute rheumatic fever, but it usually occurs in children five to 15 years old. The resulting rheumatic heart disease can last for life.

Signs of Strep Throat

The most common symptoms of strep throat are the sudden onset of a sore throat (particularly with painful swallowing), fever, and tender, swollen glands under the jaw angle.

Laboratory tests can confirm inflammation and identify a streptococcal infection, but there's no specific lab test for rheumatic fever. Strep throat infections can be detected by throat cultures or more rapid laboratory antigen detection tests.

Throat cultures, blood antibody tests, and other blood tests are also used to find out if a recent strep infection could have triggered rheumatic fever.

What Happens in Acute Rheumatic Fever?

The first symptoms of rheumatic fever are a high fever that lasts from 10 to 14 days and arthritic pain and soreness that moves from one joint to another. In acute attacks of rheumatic fever, joints often swell and become red and hot.

A child suffering from rheumatic fever may have shortness of breath or chest pains; these symptoms indicate the heart has been affected. Other signs include tiring easily, eating poorly, or paleness. A doctor examining the child may hear an abnormal heart murmur or find that the heart is enlarged. Acute inflammation of the heart is a serious condition and requires direct and sometimes lengthy medical care.

Tests Used to Detect Heart Damage

Chest x-rays and an electrocardiogram are two common tests that determine if the heart has been affected. Echocardiography is a technique that sends sound waves into the chest to rebound from the heart's walls and valves. The recorded waves show the shape, texture, and movement of the valves, and also the size of the heart chambers and how well they're functioning. This technique doesn't hurt or pose a risk to people. These aren't the only ways doctors study heart damage. Cardiac catheterization is also used.

What Happens When a Heart Valve Is Damaged by Rheumatic Heart Disease?

A damaged heart valve either doesn't completely close (insufficiency) or doesn't completely open (stenosis). A heart valve that doesn't close properly lets blood leak back into the chamber from which it was pumped. This is called regurgitation or leakage. With the next heartbeat, regurgitated blood flows through the valve and mixes with blood that flows normally. This extra volume of blood passing through the heart puts added strain on the heart muscle. An insufficient heart valve can be diagnosed by listening to the heart and verified by echocardiography.

When a valve doesn't open enough, the heart must pump harder than normal to force blood through the narrowed opening. Usually there are no symptoms of this until the valve opening becomes very narrow. With modern diagnostic tools, however, doctors can discover valves that can't open fully many years before people complain of discomfort.

Symptoms of Rheumatic Heart Disease

The symptoms vary greatly from person to person. Often the damage to heart valves isn't immediately noticeable. Some people have no problem for years; others feel only mild discomfort for years.

Eventually damaged heart valves can cause serious, even disabling, problems. These problems depend on the severity of the damage and on which heart valve is affected.

Abnormalities of valves on the left side of the heart (the mitral and aortic valves) usually cause symptoms earlier than abnormalities on the right side. The reason is that blood pressures are higher on the left side of the heart. (The tricuspid valve is usually the only valve affected by rheumatic heart disease on the right side of the heart—the pulmonic valve is almost never affected.)

People with mitral or aortic valves that don't fully close find that their heart becomes overactive during vigorous work or play, or during emotional excitement. Increased physical or emotional activity puts an added strain on a heart that's already overworked because of the valve leakage.

As a result, the left ventricle gradually gets bigger to compensate for the added volume. Eventually this becomes counterproductive, and the heart can't pump adequately. Pressure builds in the ventricle and causes blood to back up into the lungs, resulting in shortness of breath. This can result in an inadequate blood supply to the body and fatigue. The body also may retain fluid.

The lungs of people with mitral valve stenosis are under added pressure. This puts an extra burden on the right side of the heart, since it must pump against the increased pressure. The added pressure in the lungs also results in fluid retention (pulmonary edema) and shortness of breath.

In aortic valve stenosis, the extra pressure and added size of the left ventricle means the heart muscle itself requires more blood. If the coronary arteries don't supply enough blood to the heart tissue, angina pectoris can result. Dizziness or fainting during exertion, shortness of breath, fatigue, and palpitations are other symptoms of the same problem. The most advanced condition is congestive heart failure.

Preventing Rheumatic Heart Disease

Rheumatic fever and rheumatic heart disease are prevented in two ways: primary and secondary prevention.

The goal in primary prevention is to prevent the first attack of rheumatic fever from ever occurring. Since rheumatic fever results from strep throat, it's important to diagnose and treat cases of strep throat early by noting the symptoms and taking a throat culture.

Often a doctor will wait for the result of a throat culture to be sure a strep infection is present and antibiotics are warranted. Most sore throats are caused by viral infections that aren't helped by antibiotic treatment. Strep throats are bacterial infections, so antibiotics are helpful for them.

When a strep throat is diagnosed, treatment with penicillin should follow. If a person is allergic to penicillin, other antibiotics can be used. By treating strep throat, doctors can usually prevent acute rheumatic fever from developing.

When someone has already had rheumatic fever, the goal is to prevent another attack. People who've already had an attack of rheumatic fever are much more susceptible to further attacks and the risk of heart damage. Such people are given continuous monthly or daily antibiotic treatment, perhaps for life. In addition, people who have heart damage are given short-term antibiotic treatment when dental or surgical procedures are used that increase the risk of bacterial endocarditis (see page 352).

What Can Be Done About a Bad Heart Valve?

When heart valves are damaged by rheumatic fever, they may not open or close properly. If they don't open properly, they block the forward flow of blood; if they don't close properly, blood may leak backwards.

When these problems occur, valve replacement surgery may be recommended. In such surgery the diseased valve is replaced with an artificial valve made of metal or plastic, or with a specially prepared valve taken from an animal (such as from a pig). Most people who have valve replacement surgery improve markedly.

The American Heart Association

CONGESTIVE HEART FAILURE

Congestive heart failure is a condition that occurs because the heart muscle is damaged or overworked. This damage can result from high blood pressure, a heart attack, atherosclerosis, a congenital heart defect, heart muscle disease (called cardiomyopathy), rheumatic fever, or high blood pressure in the lungs resulting from lung disease. Because it's damaged, the heart lacks the strength to keep blood circulating normally throughout the body. The failing heart keeps working but it does not work as efficiently as it should.

Next, as blood flow out of the heart slows, blood returning to the heart through the veins backs up, causing congestion in the tissues. Often swelling (edema) results, most commonly in the legs and ankles, but possibly in other parts of the body as well. Sometimes fluid collects in the lungs and interferes with breathing, causing shortness of breath, especially when a person is lying down.

Heart failure also affects the ability of the kidneys to dispose of sodium and water. The retained water increases the edema.

DIAGNOSIS AND TREATMENT

The most common signs of congestive heart failure are swollen legs or ankles or difficulty breathing. Another symptom is weight gain because of accumulating fluid.

Congestive heart failure usually requires a treatment program of rest, proper diet, modi-

CHF: SOME IMPORTANT DISTINCTIONS

Congestive heart failure (CHF) should not be confused with a heart attack, which involves sudden tissue death of the heart muscle. Although heart failure may occur suddenly in some cases, gradual loss of heart function is more common. Fatigue, shortness of breath on exertion, and increased frequency of nighttime urination develop and worsen over time. Shortness of breath is often worse when lying down—a condition known as orthopnea—as fluid from the lower limbs pools in the lungs. Elevating the head with pillows eases chest congestion, but in advanced stages, the patient may be unable to recline at all without severe breathlessness, and may need to sleep upright in a chair. CHF occurs most frequently in those over 60, and is the leading cause of hospitalization and death in that age group. In over 50 percent of cases, sudden death occurs due to a cardiac arrhythmia, or irregular heartbeat. Unfortunately, antiarrhythmic medications may not be effective in controlling arrhythmias caused by CHF. *The Editors*

fied daily activities, and drugs such as digitalis, diuretics, and vasodilators.

The various drugs used to treat congestive heart failure perform different functions. Digitalis increases the pumping action of the heart, while diuretics help the body eliminate excess salt and water. Vasodilators expand blood vessels and decrease resistance, allowing blood to flow more easily and making the heart's work easier.

The class of drugs known as ACE inhibitors has been shown to have the most profound impact on improving odds of survival for congestive heart failure (CHF) patients. More recently, another class of medications, called beta-blockers, has also been shown to improve the outcome in patients with CHF.

When a specific cause of congestive heart failure is discovered, it should be treated, or if possible, corrected. For example, in some cases congestive heart failure can be treated by treating high blood pressure or by surgically replacing abnormal heart valves.

Most cases of congestive heart failure are treatable. With proper medical supervision, people with heart failure don't have to become invalids.

Heart Transplantation

Sometimes the heart is irreversibly damaged by long-lasting heart disease. People with long-term heart failure that doesn't respond to all available treatment may be candidates for heart (cardiac) transplants. People with some forms of cardiomyopathy (acute or chronic disease of the heart muscle) may also become heart transplant candidates.

When the heart can no longer adequately function and a person is at risk of dying, a heart transplant may be indicated. Cardiac transplantation is now recognized as a proven procedure when performed on appropriately selected patients.

The American Heart Association

BACTERIAL ENDOCARDITIS

Bacterial endocarditis is a serious infection of the heart valves or the tissues lining the heart. It rarely occurs but is a real threat to people with structural abnormalities of the heart, artificial (prosthetic) heart valves, or people with rheumatic or other acquired heart valve dysfunction. Also, people who've previously had bacterial endocarditis are at risk for getting it again, even when they don't have heart disease.

Bacterial endocarditis is caused by bacteria in the bloodstream. Most bacteria in the bloodstream are destroyed by normal body defenses, but sometimes they can settle on an abnormal or artificial heart valve or on congenital deformations of the heart. When this occurs, bacterial endocarditis may result.

In people with abnormal or artificial heart valves or congenital defects, prevention (prophylaxis) is believed to reduce the risk of bacterial endocarditis. Thus it's necessary to take precautions before some dental and surgical procedures that may introduce bacteria into the bloodstream. The American Heart Association recommends antibiotic prophylaxis when people undergo dental procedures that may cause the gum or mouth to bleed; have tonsils and adenoids removed; and have surgery for certain gastrointestinal, genital, or urinary tract problems. This normally involves taking a dose of antibiotics an hour or two before the procedure and another one six hours after the first dose.

The American Heart Association

PERIPHERAL VASCULAR DISEASE

It's a wonderful case of the hair of the dog that bit you: The treatment for intermittent claudication (muscle pain in one or both legs that is brought on by walking) is, usually, more walking. Intermittent claudication is a symptom of peripheral vascular disease—a narrowing of the arteries in the arms and legs due to the buildup of atherosclerotic (fatty) plaque—and in 70 percent of patients, it is the only symptom.

In those with peripheral vascular disease, exercise brings on pain because the blood flow through the narrowed arteries is insufficient to provide the muscles with enough oxygen to meet the increased demands of exercise; the oxygen deficit causes muscle cramping. For some people this pain might begin after walking only a block, for others it might be close to a mile—but for anyone with intermittent claudication, the pain consistently begins at the same distance (occasionally it will be brought on only by walking uphill). A minute or two of rest brings relief. The pain is usually in the calf muscles, but it can also occur in the buttocks, hips, feet, or thighs, depending on where the arterial narrowing is located. Increased exercise helps, in part, by enlarging collateral vessels ("side streets" around the main blocked artery in the leg). There is some evidence that exercise might actually reduce some of the plaque buildup in the artery itself and can lead to better coordination of muscles.

Atherosclerosis is a process that affects the whole body; the same narrowing that causes intermittent claudication causes angina—heart pain that is brought on by exercise and relieved by rest. Angina is the cardinal symptom of narrowed coronary arteries, and 60 percent of those with intermittent claudication also have coronary artery disease. However, unlike angina (which can progress to an actual heart attack), intermittent claudication is not usually dangerous in and of itself. While patients often fear that their problems might lead to loss of a limb, this is highly unlikely. Excluding people with diabetes and smokers, who are at higher risk for progression of the condition, only about 10 percent ever require surgery, and only about 2 percent need amputation—and even these rates can be reduced with proper care.

Dr. Bruce Perler, a Johns Hopkins vascular surgeon, says, "Intermittent claudication is a fairly benign symptom that poses no immediate or even long-term danger. Patients should be cautious if surgery or other treatments such as laser angioplasty are recommended for symptoms that only appear with exercise. In the vast majority, lifestyle changes are the only treatment required." Smokers are counseled to quit, since tobacco causes constriction of peripheral veins and

WALKING AWAY THE PAIN

If you have muscle pain brought on by walking, see your doctor before starting an exercise program (there are other conditions that may mimic peripheral vascular disease but require different treatments). The following tips should help you increase the distance you can walk without pain:

• Spend several minutes stretching before you walk, and walk on level ground.

• When walking, note how far you can go before pain starts (the initial claudication distance). Continue from this point until pain becomes so severe that you have to stop.

• Rest for a few minutes until pain subsides, then resume walking.

• Repeat this pattern for 40 to 60 minutes.

• Try to walk at least four times a week. In inclement weather, walk in a mall or other indoor space.

• Keep track of initial claudication distances and the stopping distances. Both should increase within a few weeks.

• If you have heart disease, check with your physician about how much you should walk. Even if you don't have a history of heart disease but experience chest pain, shortness of breath, or rapid heartbeat while walking, stop and call your doctor.

arteries, and all patients are advised to begin a walking training program and, if overweight, lose weight (the walking will help with the weight loss).

One study reported in the *Journal of Vascular Surgery* documented the significant difference a walking program can make. Fifty-six patients with varying degrees of intermittent claudication were enrolled in a six-month supervised walking training program consisting of three one-hour sessions a week, walking on an indoor track. Patients were instructed to walk at speeds that caused some discomfort (but not severe pain), and to slow down or stop when the pain became severe. By the end of the training period, patients had, on average, more than doubled the distance they could walk without stopping. Some 84 percent of those who completed the program were able to walk more than 1.25 miles after three months of training; 70 percent could walk almost two miles or more, at an average speed of about 3.5 mph. Furthermore, 20 out of 22 patients who were retested a year later had maintained a good walking ability.

The Editors

VARICOSE VEINS

Our prehistoric ancestors' innovation of walking upright may have helped us create civilization, but it also put a lot of stress on our legs—particularly on their thin-walled veins. Blood is pumped under pressure out of the heart into arteries, and gravity helps it reach its destination in the lower extremities. But the return trip through the veins—against gravity—is not so easy. By the time blood has traveled through the tiniest arteries, through the capillaries, and into the tiniest veins, the force provided by the heart is exhausted. Veins must rely on the surrounding skeletal muscles to push and squeeze blood through as they flex.

Valves along the interior of veins permit blood to flow in one direction only. When we stand upright, these valves must bear the weight of a long column of blood—perhaps more than we are evolutionarily equipped to handle.

WHO IS AT RISK?
It is impossible to say just who will develop varicose veins, and when, but there seem to be several contributing factors:

Sedentary lifestyle. The large calf muscles are sometimes called the peripheral heart, as their motion serves to pump blood back up through the veins. Long periods of inactivity stifle this pumping action, and allow blood to pool in the veins and cause them to swell.

Sex. Women are four times more likely than men to have varicose veins. During pregnancy, heightened hormone levels weaken vein walls and lead to the failure of the valves. Similarly, for women already genetically predisposed to varicose veins, the hormones in birth control pills seem to promote it.

Genetics. People of Irish and German descent seem to have a predisposition to varicosities. And indeed, it's not uncommon for a daughter to develop varicose veins identical to her mother's.

Age. As veins and skin lose their elasticity, the veins become more susceptible to varicosity.

ARE THEY DANGEROUS?
Usually varicose veins pose more risk to your

TIPS FOR PREVENTING VARICOSE VEINS

- Avoid standing or sitting for long periods.
- Put your feet up above hip level periodically during the day. This facilitates blood flow out of the veins, back to the heart.
- Maintain proper weight—excess pounds are a strain.
- Avoid repeated heavy lifting, or straining at stool. These activities induce backflow of blood in the veins.
- Don't smoke. A possible correlation has been found between smoking and incidence of varicose veins.
- Don't wear tight shoes, garters, belts, or other restrictive clothing.
- Exercise. Action in the calf muscles staves off pooling of blood and improves circulation in the lower leg. Regular aerobic exercise will also help keep weight down.

vanity than your health. However, they may cause swelling in the calf, dull pain (particularly after standing for long periods), itching, and even skin ulcers due to poor circulation. Although rare, phlebitis (inflammation of the vein), often in association with a blood clot, can occur. Such clots cause local pain, but rarely, if ever, travel to the heart or lungs.

Thrombophlebitis (or, simply, phlebitis) is a condition that involves the inflammation of a vein or veins and the formation of blood clots in the veins. It may occur either in the superficial veins you can readily see near the surface of the skin or in the veins deep within the legs (or, less commonly, the arms). Superficial phlebitis does not usually lead to serious complications, although deep-vein phlebitis can lead to a pulmonary embolism (a blood clot that lodges in a pulmonary artery, cutting off blood flow through the affected portion of the lungs). Most commonly, phlebitis is caused by prolonged bed rest—after an operation,

for example—or even by prolonged sitting during an automobile or airplane trip. Superficial phlebitis can usually be treated with bed rest, elevation of the affected limb, heat, and the use of an anti-inflammatory drug. Deep-vein phlebitis is often treated with an anticoagulant drug and the use of antiembolism stockings, and hospitalization is often necessary.

TREATMENT OPTIONS

Fortunately, varicose veins can be safely remedied. Currently, there are two methods available: surgery and sclerotherapy. Sometimes a combination of both is used for optimal cosmetic results.

Surgery, the more drastic of the two, is being increasingly done on an outpatient basis. In most cases, a branch of the main saphenous vein, which runs down the inside of the thigh and calf, causes most of the backwards flow. These branches can be disconnected surgically, so that blood is forced to flow through veins with good valves. Only under exceptional cir-

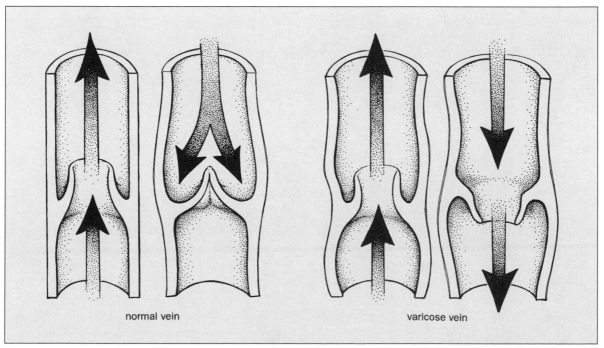

normal vein

varicose vein

In a normal vein, the valve opens to allow blood to flow in one direction, then closes securely to prevent backflow in the opposite direction. A varicose vein occurs when these valves fail.

cumstances, where the main vein itself lacks valves, is "vein stripping" (closing off the whole vein) done, because the saphenous vein is the best one to use for a graft in heart bypass procedures, should this ever become necessary.

In sclerotherapy, a chemical solution is injected into the vein to kill the cells lining it. This turns the vein into a useless but innocuous fibrous cord. After either surgery or sclerotherapy, blood reroutes itself into the healthy veins of the leg, lessening the pressure on the veins with broken valves. This, in turn, makes the varicose vein less noticeable.

The Editors

The Kidneys and Urinary Tract

OVERVIEW

Kidneys perform crucial functions that affect all parts of the body. Many other organs in our body depend upon the kidneys to function normally. The kidneys perform complex operations that keep the rest of the body in balance. But when the kidneys become damaged by disease, the other organs are adversely affected as well.

Kidney problems can range from a minor urinary tract infection to progressive kidney failure. Scientific advances over the past three decades have improved our ability to diagnose and treat those who suffer from kidney disorders.

Even when the kidneys no longer function, treatments such as dialysis and transplantation have brought hope and literally new life to hundreds of thousands of people.

Medical scientists continue to learn more about the function and structure of the kidneys and the diseases that affect them. There

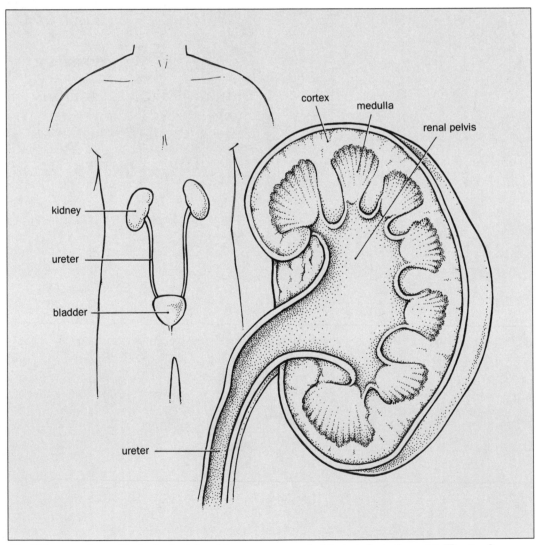

The kidneys are located in the back of the abdomen, one on each side, just above the waist. They produce urine, which flows down the ureters to the bladder, where it is stored until excretion.

is still much to learn and a need for continued support of research.

WHY THE KIDNEYS ARE SO IMPORTANT

A major function of the kidneys is to remove waste products and excess fluid from the body. These waste products and excess fluid are removed through the urine. The production of urine involves highly complex steps of excretion and reabsorption. This process is necessary to maintain a stable balance of body chemicals.

The critical regulation of the body's salt, potassium, and acid content is performed by the kidneys. The kidneys also produce hormones and vitamins that affect the function of other organs. For example, a hormone produced by the kidneys stimulates red blood cell production. In addition, other hormones produced by the kidneys help regulate blood pressure, and still others help control calcium metabolism.

Moreover, the kidneys are powerful chemical factories that perform the following functions: remove waste products from the body; balance the body's fluids; release hormones that regulate blood pressure; synthesize the vitamins that control growth; control the production of red blood cells.

LOCATION AND FUNCTION OF THE KIDNEYS

There are two kidneys, each about the size of a fist, located on either side of the spine at the lowest level of the rib cage. Each kidney contains about one million functioning units called nephrons. A nephron consists of a filtering unit of tiny blood vessels called a glomerulus attached to a tubule. When blood enters the glomerulus, it is filtered, and the remaining fluid then passes along the tubule. In the tubule, chemicals and water are either added to or removed from this filtered fluid according to the body's needs, the final product being the urine we excrete.

The kidneys perform their life-sustaining job of filtering and returning to the bloodstream about 200 quarts of fluid every 24 hours. (Approximately two quarts are eliminated from the body in the form of urine, and about 198 quarts are retained in the body.) The urine we excrete has been stored in the bladder for approximately one to eight hours.

TYPES AND CAUSES OF KIDNEY DISEASE

Kidney disease usually affects both kidneys. If the kidneys' ability to remove and regulate water and chemicals is seriously damaged by disease, waste products and excess fluid build up, causing severe swelling and symptoms of kidney failure. The kidneys may be affected by diseases such as diabetes and high blood pressure. (Diabetes is the leading cause of serious kidney disease; see also Diabetes Mellitus on page 268.) In addition, there are many different types and causes of kidney disease, and these can be characterized as hereditary, congenital, or acquired.

Hereditary Disorders

Hereditary disorders can be transmitted to both males and females and generally produce clinical symptoms from teenage years to adulthood. The most prevalent hereditary kidney condition is polycystic kidney disease. Other hereditary conditions include hereditary nephritis, primary hyperoxaluria, and cystinuria.

Congenital Disease

Congenital disease usually involves some malformation of the genitourinary tract, usually leading to some type of obstruction, which subsequently produces infection and/or destruction of kidney tissue. The destruction can eventually progress to chronic kidney failure.

Acquired Kidney Diseases

These diseases are very numerous, the general term being "nephritis" (meaning inflammation of the kidney). The most common type of nephritis is glomerulonephritis, and again this has many causes.

DIALYSIS TREATMENTS

There are many patients who have been on chronic dialysis treatment since the time it first became widely available in the late 1960s.

The total life expectancy remains unknown, but some dialysis patients may approach normal life spans. However, some patients do not tolerate dialysis well and have many complications.

Hemodialysis

In hemodialysis, an artificial kidney (hemodialyzer) is used to remove waste products from the blood and restore the body's chemical balance. In order to get the patient's blood to the artificial kidney, it is necessary to make an access to the patient's blood vessels. This requires surgery on an arm or a leg. The procedure connects an artery to a vein underneath the skin. The joining of an artery to a vein creates an enlarged vessel known as a fistula. Once healing occurs, two needles are placed, one in the artery side and one in the vein side of the fistula. Plastic tubing attached to the needles connects the patient to the artificial kidney. The patient is now ready to begin treatment.

How Does the Artificial Kidney Work?

The artificial kidney has two compartments, one for the patient's blood and one for a cleaning solution called dialysate. A thin porous membrane separates these compartments. Blood cells, protein, and other important substances in the blood remain in their compartment because they are too large to pass through the holes of the membrane. Smaller waste products in the blood, such as urea and creatinine, and excess water pass through the membrane and are washed away. Needed substances such as calcium or dextrose (sugar) can be added to the dialysate and can move from the dialysate through the membrane into the patient's blood.

How Long Does It Take and How Often Is It Necessary?

The time required for each treatment is determined

Kidney stones are very common, and when they pass, the pain can be extremely severe in your side and back. Stone formation can be an inherited disorder, secondary to a malformation and/or infection in the kidney, or can occur without any prior problem. The pain can appear suddenly, occur in waves, and disappear just as rapidly when the stone is passed.

Evaluation by your doctor can reveal a cause for the kidney stone formation in about one-third of patients who have their first stone.

When kidney stones get stuck in the kidney and ureter (and cannot pass), a new form of shock wave treatment has been used to destroy the stone. This treatment is called extracorporeal shock-wave lithotripsy.

Nephrotic syndrome refers to a large protein loss in the urine, frequently in association with low blood protein (albumin) levels, an elevated blood cholesterol, and severe retention of body fluid causing swelling (edema). This disease can be a primary disorder of the kidney or secondary to an illness affecting many parts of the body (for example, diabetes mellitus).

Long-standing high blood pressure (hypertension) can cause kidney disease itself or be a result of a kidney disorder. Uncontrolled high blood pressure can accelerate the natural course of any underlying kidney disease.

Drugs and toxins. Years of heavy use of headache compounds can slowly produce kidney failure. Certain other medications, toxins, pesticides, and "street" drugs (i.e., heroin) can also produce kidney damage.

TREATING KIDNEY DISEASE

Unfortunately, the cause of many kidney diseases is still unknown. Some of the kidney diseases noted above can be successfully treated, and others progress to advanced kidney fail-

by the patient's amount of remaining kidney function, fluid weight gain between treatments, and the buildup of harmful chemicals between treatments. On the average, each treatment lasts three to four hours and is usually necessary three times a week.

Peritoneal Dialysis
In this type of dialysis, the patient's blood is cleaned within the body. The blood stays in the blood vessels that line the patient's own abdominal (peritoneal) space. The lining of the space acts like the membrane in the artificial kidney.

A plastic tube called a catheter is surgically placed into the patient's abdomen to create an access. During the treatment, the patient's peritoneal cavity is slowly filled with dialysate through the catheter. As in hemodialysis, an exchange of waste products and chemical balancing takes place. Once a cycle (exchange) has been completed, the used dialysate is drained from the peritoneal cavity through the catheter and discarded; the process is then repeated.

The following are the types of peritoneal dialysis.

• *Continuous Ambulatory Peritoneal Dialysis (CAPD).* This is the only type of peritoneal dialysis that is done without the use of machines. Patients perform this procedure themselves, usually four or five times a day at home and at work. The patient drains a bag of dialysate into his or her peritoneal cavity by way of the catheter. The dialysate remains there for about four to five hours. After an exchange is complete, the patient drains the used dialysate back into the bag. The patient then repeats the procedure using a new bag of dialysate. While the dialysate remains inside the peritoneal cavity, the patient can go about daily activities.

• *Continuous Cycling Peritoneal Dialysis (CCPD).* This is usually done at home using a cycling machine. The process is identical to CAPD except the cycle periods are usually one and a half hours and are performed several times a night, as the patient sleeps.

ure, requiring dialysis and/or transplantation. For example, kidney infections and kidney stones can often be successfully treated. Chronic inflammation of the glomerulus (called glomerulonephritis) is the most common kidney disease, which slowly progresses to kidney failure.

TREATING ADVANCED KIDNEY FAILURE
Research is now being considered on the effect of special diets in slowing or halting progressive kidney failure, especially if the problem is approached early.

Treatments to slow the progress of kidney failure hold promise for the future. When these therapies are no longer successful, there are now several ways by which chronic, irreversible kidney failure can be treated, and often more than one type of treatment is suitable for any one person. These methods are listed below.

Dialysis
Treatment with hemodialysis (the artificial kidney) may be performed at a dialysis unit or at home. Hemodialysis treatments are usually performed in three separate sessions per week.

Peritoneal dialysis is generally done daily at home. Continuous cycling peritoneal dialysis requires the use of a machine, but continuous ambulatory peritoneal dialysis does not. A kidney specialist can explain the different approaches and suggest what type may be best.

Transplantation
Finally, there has been increasing success with kidney transplantation. In some cases, the kidney may come from a relative who donates one of his or her own kidneys to the patient. Kidney transplantation from cadaveric donors, however, is more common in the United States. Under these circumstances, individuals who have died have donated their kidneys for potential transplantation.

THE WARNING SIGNS OF KIDNEY DISEASE

Although many forms of kidney disease do not produce symptoms until late in the course of the disease, there are six warning signs of kidney diseases:

- Burning or difficulty during urination
- An increase in the frequency of urination
- Passage of bloody urine
- Puffiness around the eyes, swelling of the hands and feet
- Pain in the small of back just below the ribs
- High blood pressure

The National Kidney Foundation

URINARY TRACT INFECTIONS

An estimated 20 percent of women have at least one urinary tract infection (UTI) in their life. (Men can also develop UTIs, but such infections are far more prevalent among women, since a woman's urethra—the canal carrying urine from the bladder—is significantly shorter than that of men, facilitating the entrance of bacteria into the urinary tract.) Among adults, postmenopausal women are at greatest risk, because they are more likely to have hormonal changes that may render the urethra less able to fight infection. In older women, UTIs—usually bladder infections, also known as cystitis—are the second most common type of infection. Cystitis is sometimes associated with prolapsed bladder, in which weakened bladder walls cause the organ to protrude downward into the vagina, causing urinary difficulty. For 80 percent of first-time sufferers, this painful condition becomes a recurrent problem.

In men, UTIs are usually serious and are a sign of an underlying problem. These infections should always be evaluated and treated by a physician immediately.

About 80 percent of UTIs are caused by *Escherichia coli (E. coli)* bacteria, which usually inhabit the anal area with no ill effect. In women, the urethra is so close to the anus that *E. coli* are easily transmitted: By traveling a mere inch, they can reach the bladder. Such infections are almost always easy to treat with a three- to five-day regimen of antibiotics or sometimes with a single-dose antibiotic.

Women who have recurrent UTIs are all too familiar with the most common early symptoms, which include: a frequent and urgent need to urinate; painful urination; blood in the urine (hematuria); discomfort in the lower abdomen; and, occasionally, fever and chills. Indeed, one study revealed that 90 percent of patients (whose infections could later be documented) were able to correctly diagnose

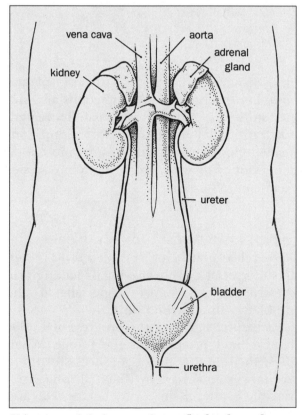

Urinary tract infections are often confined to the urethra (urethritis), but may involve the bladder (cystitis) or kidneys (pyelonephritis).

their UTIs themselves.

Early treatment is essential—not only to relieve the discomfort, but also to prevent the infection from spreading to the kidneys (a potentially dangerous complication). Some physicians might suggest a prescription for Pyridium, a bladder anesthetic that will ease the pain of cystitis before an antibiotic takes effect. (Pyridium contains an orange dye that will color your urine, as well as stain your underpants, so wearing pads is a good idea.)

SELF-TREATMENT GUIDELINES
Only women who are prone to uncomplicated UTIs, and who have had at least two episodes of recurrent cystitis (confirmed by taking a culture) in a year, should consider self-treatment. Before supplying you with antibiotics, your doctor should carry out a thorough evaluation, including: a complete urinalysis, a serum creatinine level (measure of kidney function), and a urine culture. The doctor may also ask you to keep a week's diary of your urination habits to insure that you have no voiding problems.

If your history shows uncomplicated, recurrent cystitis, your doctor may give you a prescription for a supply of antibiotics (usually enough for four infections) and, sometimes, urine dipsticks, which are used to indicate the presence of bacteria. Your doctor may also suggest you keep a record of your infections and any precipitating factors. And you should return for a follow-up appointment within three to six months. (Call your physician sooner if you use all four cycles of the antibiotics before this time.)

UTIs should not be self-managed in women who have compromised immune systems, diabetes, or a history of UTIs that develop into kidney problems or were caused by resistant organisms. Also, women who have structural abnormalities of the urinary tract, whether congenital or as a result of surgery, are not candidates for self-treatment.

PREVENTING UTIs
Women can reduce their chances of getting UTIs by taking the following steps:
• Drink at least eight glasses of water a day.
• Urinate at least once every four hours.
• Urinate after sexual intercourse.
• Use a mild soap to wash yourself and your undergarments.
• Treat yeast infections (which cause vaginal discharge, itching, odor, and pain) promptly since they, too, can cause UTIs, albeit rarely.

When You Suspect a UTI
If you and your doctor have decided you can self-manage your UTIs, follow these steps when you suspect an infection:

• Obtain a clean-catch urine specimen. Your doctor will probably give you an antiseptic wipe and directions on how to wipe yourself before collecting a specimen. After cleansing, start to urinate, stop midstream, then start again and collect the urine.
• Use a dipstick to test the specimen for bacteria.
• If the dipstick shows bacterial contamination, start on the medication.
• Call your doctor if: symptoms don't improve within 48 hours, you have a fever over 101°F, or you have symptoms despite negative dipstick results.
• Record your symptoms and their response to treatment in a diary.

The Editors

KIDNEY STONES

Kidney stones, also known as renal calculi, form when substances in the urine, such as calcium oxalate, concentrate and coalesce into hard, solid lumps in the kidney. Calcium oxalate and calcium phosphate stones account for about 80 percent of all kidney stones. The next most common type of stone is composed of uric acid. Calculi may form in the kidney if the urine becomes too concentrated, if excessive amounts of calcium are absorbed from the intestine or released from bone, or if a bacterial infection alters the pH (acidity) of the urine. The stones may pass from the kidney, through the ureter (a long, thin tube), and into the bladder, before being eliminated from the body with the urine.

Some stones are so small that they cause no symptoms and pass painlessly on their own; large stones may remain lodged in the kidney and are detected only when an abdominal x-ray is taken for another reason. Sometimes, however, a stone enters the ureter and produces intermittent but often severe pain (known as renal colic) that continues until the stone has reached the bladder; this process may take a few hours or up to several days. The pain of a single attack is usually felt only on the affected side of the body; however, stones tend to recur and may develop in the other kidney, causing pain on that side. Symptoms abate once the stone passes. Recurrence is common, and treatment is aimed at relieving symptoms, dissolving or removing existing stones, and preventing recurrence. Kidney stones are common, especially among young and middle-aged adults, and men are affected much more frequently than women.

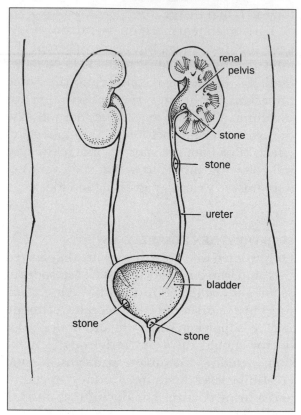

Stones can form in the kidney and may cause substantial pain when they become lodged along the urinary tract. Most kidney stones pass spontaneously.

nate except in certain positions, frequent urge to urinate but with only small amounts of urine passed, and bloody, cloudy, or darkened urine. Kidney stones may promote kidney infection, which may produce a burning sensation during urination and fever.

SYMPTOMS

The primary symptom of kidney stones is intermittent pain—sometimes excruciating—that originates in the lower back below the ribs and travels downward through the lower abdomen to the groin. The pain may be accompanied by nausea and vomiting. Men might experience genital pain as the stone passes. Urinary symptoms can include interruption of the urine stream, inability to uri-

HOW TO PREVENT KIDNEY STONES

Kidney stones are less likely to occur if you regularly drink at least eight glasses of water a day and eat a healthy, well-balanced diet. For those who have had kidney stones in the past, dietary changes may be advised to prevent recurrence. Specific changes, such as avoiding calcium or foods containing oxalic acid (found in rhubarb, spinach, leafy vegetables, and coffee), will depend on the type of kidney stone involved. Medications such as thiazide diuretics, phosphate-based compounds, allopurinol, sodium or potassium citrate, or large doses of calcium or magnesium may be prescribed to help prevent recurrence. The type of medication varies according to the exact composition of the stone. For example, an effort is made to increase urine acidity in people with calcium stones, but to decrease urine acidity in those with uric acid stones.

HOW KIDNEY STONES ARE DIAGNOSED

A urine culture may be examined for unusual cells or crystals. Imaging tests such as a CT scan, ultrasound, or x-ray may also be taken. In cases when stones recur, the doctor may ask you to collect urine over a 24-hour period in order to measure the amount of calcium and uric acid excreted. A blood test to measure calcium, uric acid, and parathyroid hormone levels should also be performed. Abdominal x-rays may be taken following injection of an iodine-based dye into the kidneys (pyelography). Any stone that is passed and captured is analyzed for its chemical content.

HOW KIDNEY STONES ARE TREATED

To encourage a small stone to pass, at least three liters of water should be consumed daily to flush the stone into the bladder. Associated bacterial infections are treated with antibiotics. In more severe cases, hospitalization may be advised, and narcotic painkillers are warranted. Antispasmodic drugs may be given to help the ureter muscles relax and thus ease the passing of the stone. Larger stones can be pulverized with a treatment called extracorporeal shock-wave lithotripsy, in which concentrated bursts of sound waves are aimed at the stones. The tiny fragments may then pass into the bladder to be excreted. For large stones, abdominal surgery is sometimes required. In some cases, stones develop due to an overactive parathyroid gland (hyperparathyroidism), which causes excess levels of calcium to be released into the blood. In such cases, removal of a portion of the parathyroid may be performed. In advanced cases that do not respond to other forms of treatment, surgery to remove the kidney may be required. Only one kidney is necessary for normal body function; if a diseased kidney is removed, the remaining one compensates for the loss. *The Editors*

VITAMIN C AND KIDNEY STONES

Vitamin C supplements have been shown to promote kidney stones in those already at risk for them. A study published in the *Journal of Urology* found that doses of 500 mg or more of vitamin C were associated with an increase in oxalate in the urine. Oxalate, a component of one type of kidney stone (called calcium stones, the most common stone in older men), forms when vitamin C is metabolized by the body. Seventy to 80 percent of all kidney stones form around crystals of calcium and oxalate or phosphate.

According to the study's authors, "patients with a history of stone disease or those who have decreased renal function should certainly be discouraged from taking more than the recommended daily allowance of vitamin C." If you do tend to form kidney stones (as 10 to 15 percent of people do), be sure to follow your doctor's advice on what foods to avoid (vitamin C is just one possible kidney stone cause), and continue to drink plenty of water and take any medication prescribed.

The Editors

GLOMERULONEPHRITIS

"Glomerulonephritis" is the term used to describe a group of diseases that damage the part of the kidney that filters blood. When the kidney is damaged, it cannot get rid of wastes and extra fluid in the body. If the illness continues, the kidneys might stop working completely. Some other terms you may hear used are "nephritis" and "nephrotic syndrome."

There are two types of glomerulonephritis—acute and chronic. The acute form develops suddenly. You may get it after an infection in your throat or on your skin. Sometimes, you may get well on your own. Other times, your kidneys may stop working unless effective treatment is started quickly. The early signs of the disease are: puffiness of your face in the morning; blood or protein in your urine (or brown urine); urinating less than usual; high blood pressure; swelling of your ankles; getting up often at night to urinate; very bubbly and foamy urine.

NEPHROTIC SYNDROME

Nephrotic syndrome (also called nephrosis) happens when you start losing large amounts of protein in your urine. As your kidneys get worse, you retain extra fluids and salt. This causes you to have swelling (edema), high blood pressure, and an increase in your blood cholesterol. Nephrotic syndrome may come from primary kidney diseases or from other illnesses such as diabetes and lupus. It may also be caused by some medicines, IV drug abuse and the AIDS virus. Sometimes, nephrotic syndrome may go away by itself or after treatment (such as prednisone). In other cases, this condition may last for many years and eventually lead to kidney failure.

ACUTE GLOMERULONEPHRITIS

Usually, you will feel ill and go to the bathroom less often. Your urine will look blood red, rusty, smoky, or coffee-colored because blood is in it. Your face, eyelids, and hands may be swollen in the morning, and your ankles may be swollen in the evening. You may be short of breath and cough because of extra fluid in your lungs.

Your blood pressure may be high. You may have one or all of these symptoms. You will need to see a doctor right away.

The acute disease may be caused by infections such as strep throat. It may also be caused by some other illnesses, including: lupus, Goodpasture's syndrome, Wegener's granulomatosis, Henoch-Schönlein purpura, and polyarteritis nodosa. Early diagnosis is important because prompt medical care may prevent severe kidney damage in some cases.

CHRONIC GLOMERULONEPHRITIS

You may go for long periods with no symptoms, but your kidneys are still being damaged. You may have protein and/or blood in your urine. As you get worse, you will begin to show symptoms such as high blood pressure and swelling of the face and legs. If your kidneys fail, you will feel:

- That you are not very hungry
- That your stomach is upset and you may throw up
- Very tired
- That it is difficult to sleep
- That your skin is dry and itchy
- Muscle cramps, especially at night

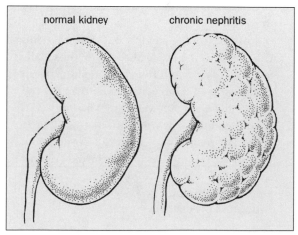

Chronic nephritis destroys kidney tissue in addition to damaging the ability of existing kidney tissue to function properly.

In a small number of cases, chronic glomerulonephritis runs in the family. This kind often shows up in young men who may also have hearing loss and vision loss. Some forms are caused by changes in the immune system. However, in many cases, the cause is not known. Sometimes, you will have one acute attack of glomerulonephritis and develop the chronic disease years later.

DIAGNOSING GLOMERULONEPHRITIS

The first clues are the signs and symptoms you will have. Finding protein and blood cells in your urine is another sign. Blood tests will help the doctor tell what type of illness you have and how much it has damaged your kidneys.

Sometimes, your doctor will need to do a kidney biopsy (take a tiny piece of your kidney with a special needle). This will help the doctor plan the best treatment for you.

CAN GLOMERULONEPHRITIS BE PREVENTED?

Not until we know more about its causes. However, good hygiene, "safe sex," and avoiding IV drugs are helpful in preventing infections that could lead to this illness.

If you have the chronic type, it is very important to control your blood pressure since this may slow down kidney damage. Your doctor may tell you to eat less protein. A dietitian who is trained to work with kidney patients (a renal dietitian) can be very helpful in planning your diet.

HOW GLOMERULONEPHRITIS IS TREATED

The acute form may go away by itself. Sometimes you may need medication or even temporary treatment with an artificial kidney machine to remove extra fluid and control high blood pressure and kidney failure. Antibiotics are not used for acute glomerulonephritis, but they are important in treating other forms of disease related to infection. If your illness is getting worse rapidly, you may be put on high doses of medicines that affect your immune system. Sometimes, your doctor may tell you to have plasmapheresis, a special blood filtering process to remove harmful proteins from your blood.

There is no specific treatment for the chronic form of the illness. Your doctor may tell you to:

- Eat less protein, salt, and potassium
- Control your blood pressure
- Take diuretics
- Take calcium supplements

HOW NEPHROTIC SYNDROME IS TREATED

Your doctor may tell you to take prednisone. This medicine helps cut down protein loss. If prednisone does not work, your doctor may suggest medicines that affect your immune system. These are especially helpful in children and patients with a form of the disease called membranous glomerulonephritis. Your doctor may also suggest a low-salt diet, diuretics, and blood pressure medications.

CONCLUSION

Many patients who have kidney failure go back to normal living after getting used to their treatment. Your National Kidney Foundation affiliate can give you information about the different kinds of treatment available for people whose kidneys have stopped working and about services and programs that are available in your area.

The National Kidney Foundation

The Lungs and Respiratory System

OVERVIEW

The respiratory system, including the lungs, brings air into the body. The oxygen in the air travels from the lungs through the bloodstream to the cells in all parts of the body. The cells use the oxygen as fuel and give off carbon dioxide as a waste gas. This waste gas is carried by the bloodstream back to the lungs to be eliminated or exhaled. The lungs accomplish this vital process—called gas exchange—using an automatic and quickly adjusting control system.

In addition to gas exchange, the lungs and respiratory system have important jobs to do related to breathing. These include:

- Bringing inhaled air to body temperature
- Moisturizing the inhaled air for necessary humidity
- Protecting the body from harmful substances by coughing, sneezing, filtering, or swallowing them, or by alerting the body through the sense of smell
- Defending the lungs with (1) cilia, microscopic hairs along the air passages; (2) phlegm (mucus or sputum)—a moving carpet of phlegm collects dirt and germs inhaled into the lungs and moves them out to be coughed up or swallowed; (3) macrophages, scavenger cells in the lungs that literally eat up dirt and germs invading the lungs

THE WARNING SIGNS OF LUNG DISEASE

The most frequent warning signs of lung disease are listed here. If you are experiencing any of these symptoms, discuss them with your doctor as soon as possible.

Chronic cough. Any cough that has lasted a month is chronic. This is an important early symptom indicating something is wrong with your breathing system, regardless of your age.

Shortness of breath. Shortness of breath that continues after a brief rest following normal exercise, or comes after little or no exertion, is not normal. Labored or difficult breathing, the feeling that it is hard to draw air into your lungs or breathe it out, is also a warning sign.

Chronic phlegm production. Phlegm, or sputum, is produced by the lungs as a defense response to infection or irritants. If your phlegm or mucus production has lasted a month, this could be an indication of an underlying problem.

Wheezing. Noisy breathing or wheezing is a sign that something unusual is blocking the airways of your lungs or making the airways too narrow.

Coughing up blood (hemoptysis). If you are coughing up blood, the blood may be coming from your lungs, upper respiratory tract, or stomach. Whatever the source of the blood, it signals the onset of a health problem.

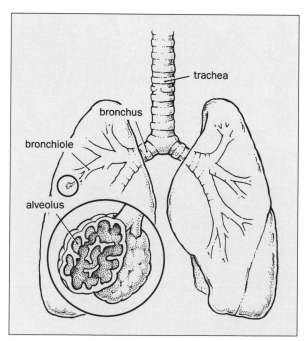

The trachea divides into two bronchi, one leading into each lung. These branch out further into the bronchioles and culminate in tiny air sacs, or alveoli.

Frequent chest colds. If you have more than two colds a year, or if one lasts more than two weeks, you may have an underlying disorder.

WHAT THE SYMPTOMS MEAN

Experts agree that your lungs are not healthy if you have any of these symptoms. You must have them checked out by your doctor. If you wait for symptoms to become severe, you have already lost valuable treatment time. Taking care of mild symptoms can actually be to your advantage.

Even if you have only one of the symptoms of lung disease—chronic cough, shortness of breath or difficult breathing, phlegm, wheezing, or frequent chest colds—you should see your doctor. Most lung conditions can be helped by treatment and can even be reversed if caught early.

DIAGNOSING LUNG DISEASE

Your doctor will usually use very simple tests to determine if you have a lung disease. He or she will take a medical history and give you a complete physical examination. Your examination may include some simple laboratory tests like a chest x-ray, blood tests, a phlegm (sputum) examination, and a pulmonary function test, which is a painless procedure that shows the doctor how well your lungs work when you breathe. Exercise testing may also be done to examine the body's response to exertion or physical activity.

Health authorities advise a tuberculosis (TB) skin test for various groups of people, including all persons who are HIV-positive, meaning that they have tested positive for the human immunodeficiency virus that causes AIDS. Because the TB test reaction may be misleading in AIDS, a chest x-ray and complete physical exam may be recommended even if the tuberculin test is negative. Based on information gathered through these quick and basic tests, your doctor will decide which lung disease, if any, exists. Then appropriate treatment can be started

COMMON LUNG HAZARDS

Any substance that is breathed in affects what happens to the lungs. Many of these substances can be hazardous and threaten the lungs' ability to work properly. Such hazards may include the following.

Cigarette smoking. The major cause of chronic obstructive pulmonary disease and lung cancer is cigarette smoking. When someone inhales cigarette smoke, irritating gases and particles cause one of the lungs' defenses—the cilia—to slow down, weakening the lungs' ability to defend themselves against infections. Cigarette smoke can cause air passages to close up and make breathing more difficult. It causes chronic inflammation or swelling in the lungs, leading to chronic bronchitis. And cigarette smoke changes the enzyme balance of the lungs, leading to destruction of lung tissue that occurs in emphysema. Macrophages—protective scavenger cells in the lungs—are also impaired.

Triggers of asthma. Asthma, the temporary narrowing of the small passages of the lungs, has many possible triggers and can be life-threatening. Infections, lung irritants, cold weather, allergies, overexertion, excitement, emotional distress, inherited factors, and workplace chemicals play a part in this disease.

Tuberculosis (TB). Tuberculosis is caused by a bacterium spread by the coughing or sneezing of a person who has active TB germs in his or her phlegm (sputum). Most people who develop TB today were infected years ago when the disease was widespread.

Years or decades later, if the natural defense systems of people's bodies begin to weaken, the barriers they built up around the germs begin to crumble, and the TB germs escape and multiply. Such waiting-to-attack infection can become real illness when a person's defenses are weakened by HIV (human immunodeficiency virus) infection or other chronic illnesses such as cancer.

Occupational hazards. Substances you breathe at work can cause lung trouble, too. Workers who are exposed to occupational hazards in the air—dusts like those from coal, silica, asbestos, or raw cotton and metal fumes or chemical vapors—can develop lung disease, including occupational asthma.

Virus, fungus, bacterium (other than TB). Hundreds of germs like these are carried in the air at all times. If they are inhaled into the lungs, the germs can cause colds, influenza, pneumonia, and other respiratory infections. When these germs lodge in your lungs, your breathing patterns can be disrupted, and you can become ill. Some of these illnesses can be prevented with vaccination.

Air pollution. Particles and gases in the air can be a source of lung irritation. Do whatever you can to reduce your exposure to air pollution. Refer to radio or television weather reports or your newspaper for air quality information. On days when the smog level is unhealthy, restrict your physical activity to early morning or evening, because smog is increased in sunlight. When pollution levels are dangerous, limit activities as necessary. People with chronic heart and lung disease should stay indoors.

PROTECTING YOUR LUNGS AND PREVENTING LUNG DISEASE

Controlling and preventing lung disease needs everyone's attention. Learn to recognize the symptoms of lung disease, such as those previously described. If you have any of these symptoms, get medical attention as soon as possible.

Everyone needs to protect the lungs by observing the following measures.

• *Don't smoke.* Quitting smoking is the best protection you can give your lungs and reduces your risk of lung disease.
• *Be honest.* Understand that chronic cough, shortness of breath, and other lung symptoms are not normal.
• *Take action.* Bring any lung disease symptom to your doctor's attention early. Then follow the doctor's advice.
• *Avoid lung hazards.* Secondhand cigarette smoke, air pollution, and lung hazards at work can cause some lung diseases.
• *Think about prevention.* Lung diseases like influenza (flu) and pneumococcal pneumonia may be prevented with vaccination. Get immunized if you are in a high risk group, which includes people over 65 or anyone with a chronic health problem such as heart disease, lung disease, and diabetes. Remember—early detection of lung disease is the key to prompt and successful treatment.

The American Lung Association

ASTHMA

Bronchial asthma is a chronic inflammatory condition in the lungs that periodically causes the bronchi (the primary airways) and their branches (the bronchioles) to constrict, leading to an episode or attack characterized by wheezing, coughing, tightness in the chest, and breathing difficulty. To feel what a severe episode is like, breathe in very deeply, hold for a second, then try to take another breath. This unpleasant sensation occurs when someone with asthma is exposed to a stimulus known as a trigger. The most common triggers include protein-based particles (allergens) from dust or mold, animal danders, pollens, or insects. Furthermore, nonallergic (irritant) factors such as strong odors, cold weather, physical exertion, and emotional stress can also induce or aggravate symptoms. Sometimes, no specific trigger is identified.

For reasons not fully understood, the bronchi of people with asthma are hypersensitive to such stimuli, so that upon exposure, the airways contract, clog up with excess mucus, and become inflamed. During an attack, the bronchial muscles go into a spasm, causing air to build up in the alveoli (tiny air sacs at the very end of the bronchioles). Eventually, the bronchioles may collapse, trapping air inside the alveoli and potentially leading to chronic breathing problems.

TREATMENT STRATEGY

New research shows that repeated episodes of asthma can cause the air passages to become permanently inflamed and constricted, which results in a gradual decline in respiratory function. It is no longer enough to focus exclusively on relieving symptoms during an acute episode by using bronchodilators (drugs that widen the airways).

Today, the goal is to prevent asthmatic episodes in the first place through careful monitoring and the use of either corticosteroids (a highly effective group of anti-inflammatory medications) or certain nonsteroidal anti-inflammatory drugs.

Effective therapy may depend upon a combination of a primary anti-inflammatory medication to suppress the underlying inflammation that characterizes asthma, in conjunction with bronchodilators to relieve acute symptoms during attacks. Choices of inhaled anti-inflammatory drugs include corticosteroids (beclomethasone, triamcinolone, flunisolide), cromolyn, and nedocromil. Short-acting bronchodilators include: albuterol, terbutaline, metaproterenol, bitolterol, and pirbuterol. In addition, theophylline preparations and salmeterol are available as long-acting bronchodilators if needed. Such multi-drug therapy can help to limit the severity and

frequency of inflammatory episodes, prevent progressive lung damage, and permit full participation in physical activities.

Successful treatment also requires careful self-monitoring of breathing capacity, much as people with diabetes must monitor their sugar levels. A peak flow meter, a device that measures how fast you can expel air from your lungs, can help you and your physician determine which medications are best for you, how much to take, and how often (see box, page 374). It can also help you identify and avoid triggers, predict attacks, detect damage to the bronchi at the earliest stages, and determine when medical attention is necessary. It's important to keep a daily diary of peak flow readings and note the timing and dose of drugs which are used.

Inhaled Corticosteroids

The most important advance in asthma therapy is the use of inhaled corticosteroid drugs, developed in England and continental Europe over the past two decades. Corticosteroids prevent inflammation and limit damage to bronchial tissue with little risk of serious side effects. They are now first-line therapy for anyone with moderate to severe asthma (more than two episodes a week). To be effective, corticosteroids must be taken daily, regardless of whether or not symptoms occur.

Steroids are administered through a device called an inhaler, which delivers a fine mist of medication directly to the bronchi. All steroid inhalers should be adapted with another device known as a spacer, which holds the vaporized medication in a chamber until you're ready to breathe in. The spacer maximizes the delivery of the drug into the lower airways and minimizes the deposition of the drug into the back of the mouth and throat, where it can't do any good. It also helps to prevent coughing during the procedure.

Inhaled corticosteroids do not have the same side effects as the anabolic steroids some athletes take illegally to enhance their performance (at the risk of causing liver damage and cardiovascular problems). Nevertheless, the use of corticosteroids requires regular checkups, as recommended by your physician. Oral yeast infections (those occurring in the mouth or throat) are the most common adverse effect. These can be minimized by using the spacer properly, and by rinsing out your mouth with water following each dose, or by taking your drugs just before meals.

For severe asthma (daily episodes and continuous discomfort), corticosteroids are sometimes taken systemically (orally or by injection). Systemic corticosteroids may cause more pronounced side effects, including increased appetite, fluid retention, weight gain, mood changes, high blood pressure, osteoporosis, muscle weakness, and easy bruising. If a prolonged course of oral corticosteroids is required, your doctor will run tests to monitor your red and white blood cells, blood sugar, potassium, skeletal strength, and vision. Meanwhile, short courses of systemic corticosteroid therapy—lasting one or two weeks—are generally recognized as safe, and at times are needed to restore the effectiveness of the inhaled medication regimen.

Bronchodilators

Bronchodilators still remain an important component of asthma treatment. They bring rapid relief by relaxing bronchial muscles when symptoms do flare up. Bronchodilators are used as soon as you realize an episode is imminent. However, the plan for using bronchodilators should always be established with your physician. Among the early signs that suggest the start of an asthma flare-up are:

- A drop in your peak flow readings
- Coughing with increased frequency
- Chest pain or tightness
- Wheezing, shortness of breath, or rapid breathing

USING A PEAK FLOW METER

A peak flow meter, which measures how fast you can blow air out of your lungs, can help you and your physician determine your peak capacity and get a sense of your asthmatic patterns. Take your readings two or three times a day, as recommended by your physician, and record them in a diary that you bring with you every time you visit the doctor. A reading around 80 percent of peak capacity may mean the beginning of an episode: You should take precautions, such as resting, taking additional medications as prescribed, and avoiding triggers. A reading between 50 to 80 percent may indicate that your overall condition is worsening: You should contact your physician to discuss the possibility of revising your treatment plan. A reading below 50 percent is in the danger zone: You should take a bronchodilator immediately and seek medical attention as soon as possible.

To use your peak flow meter properly:
- Set the scale to zero.
- Always take the reading in the same position, preferably standing up (if you are unable to stand, choose another comfortable position).
- Breathe in deeply.
- Place the meter in your mouth and close your lips around the mouthpiece.
- Don't cough or let your tongue block the mouth of the meter.
- Blow out as hard and as fast as you can.
- Check the value on the scale and write it down.
- Take two more readings.
- Record the highest of the three numbers in your peak flow diary.

- Fatigue or restlessness
- Itching eyes or sore throat
- Sneezing, stuffy head, or headache

Serious side effects are rarely associated with bronchodilators, but you may experience fleeting tremors, anxiousness, nausea, and a rapid heartbeat. Call your doctor right away if

INHALERS THAT ARE ATMOSPHERE-FRIENDLY AND EASIER TO USE

Because of a 1995 ban on fluorocarbons (gases used in aerosol spray devices, including inhalers, that destroy the atmosphere's protective ozone layer), a new generation of inhalers that deliver medication more efficiently, without Freon (a fluorocarbon), is under development. Asthma sufferers may be able to benefit from these environmentally friendly inhalers. They will use either a non-Freon propellant or a breath-activated device that delivers the drug without the need for any propellant or solvent.

you experience chest pain, a very fast or irregular heart beat, severe headache or dizziness, or vomiting. Remember that bronchodilators do not prevent inflammation or long-term damage. Furthermore, the increased use of bronchodilators may be associated with more serious complications, including cardiac arrhythmias (heartbeat irregularities).

You should not exceed a dosage of one or two puffs every three to four hours without your doctor's specific instructions. If this does not relieve your symptoms, you should notify your physician or nurse. Increased dependence on your bronchodilator can serve as an early warning sign of poor asthma control and may suggest the need to discuss increasing your primary anti-inflammatory agent with your doctor.

Additional Medications

Additional drugs are frequently prescribed to supplement corticosteroid and bronchodilator therapy. Cromolyn sodium, which has anti-inflammatory properties, can help prevent an episode when you anticipate exposure to a trigger—such as before visiting someone with a cat. It must be taken (usually in inhaled form) five to 60 minutes prior to contact with the trigger, and will last for three or four hours. The only side effect is a dry cough, which you can avoid by taking a few sips of water after inhalation.

Salmeterol is a recent addition to the choices in drug treatment. It is a long-acting bronchodilator that can help airways stay open, but should not be used to relieve the acute symptoms of an attack.

Theophylline, which is similar to the bronchodilators, may be prescribed in tablet, capsule, or liquid form when you need additional relief. Once a first-choice therapy, theophylline is now generally used only as a backup maintenance bronchodilator and is most effective when used continuously. It can be particularly useful in eliminating nighttime (nocturnal) attacks.

Theophylline can exacerbate hypertension, aggravate acid indigestion, and may interact with certain drugs, such as cimetidine (for heartburn) and erythromycin (for infection). Side effects include nausea, vomiting, and increased heart rate (tachycardia).

The Editors

CHRONIC BRONCHITIS

Bronchitis is an inflammation of the lining of the bronchial tubes. These tubes, the bronchi, connect the windpipe with the lungs. When the bronchi are inflamed and/or infected, less air is able to flow to and from the lungs, and a heavy mucus or phlegm is coughed up. This is bronchitis.

Many people suffer a brief attack of acute bronchitis with cough and mucus production when they have severe colds. Acute bronchitis is usually not associated with fever.

Chronic bronchitis is defined by the presence of a mucus-producing cough most days of the month, three months of a year for two successive years. It may precede or accompany pulmonary emphysema.

CAUSES

Cigarette smoking is by far the most common cause of chronic bronchitis. The bronchial tubes of people with chronic bronchitis may also periodically be irritated by bacterial or viral infections. Air pollution and industrial dusts are also causes of chronic bronchitis.

When the bronchial tubes have been irritated over a long period of time, excessive mucus is produced constantly, the lining of the bronchial tubes becomes thickened, an irritating cough develops, air flow may be hampered, and the lungs are endangered. The bronchial tubes then make an ideal breeding place for infections.

WHO GETS CHRONIC BRONCHITIS?

Chronic bronchitis is estimated to affect over 5 percent of the population of the United States. Cough and mucus production are more common among men than women, which is also true of cigarette smoking. Chronic bronchitis symptoms are also more common among people over 40 than younger individuals.

No matter what their occupation or lifestyle, people who smoke cigarettes are those most likely to develop chronic bronchitis. But workers with certain jobs, especially those involving high concentrations of dust and irritating fumes, are also at high risk of developing this disease. Higher rates of chronic bronchitis are found among coal miners, grain handlers, metal molders, and other workers exposed to dust. Chronic bronchitis symptoms worsen when atmospheric concentrations of sulfur dioxide and other air pollutants increase. These symptoms are intensified when individuals also smoke.

COMPLICATIONS

Chronic bronchitis is often neglected by individuals until it is in an advanced state, because people mistakenly believe that the disease is not life-threatening. By the time a patient goes to his or her doctor, the lungs may have been seriously injured. Then the patient may be in danger of developing serious respiratory problems or heart failure.

HOW CHRONIC BRONCHITIS ATTACKS

Chronic bronchitis doesn't strike suddenly. After a winter cold seems cured, an individual may continue to cough and produce large amounts of mucus for several weeks. Since people who get chronic bronchitis are often smokers, the cough is usually dismissed as only "smoker's cough." As time goes on, colds may become more damaging to the lungs. Coughing and bringing up phlegm last longer after each cold.

Without realizing it, one begins to take this coughing and mucus production as a matter of course. Soon they are present all the time—before colds, during colds, after colds, all year round. Generally, the cough is worse in the

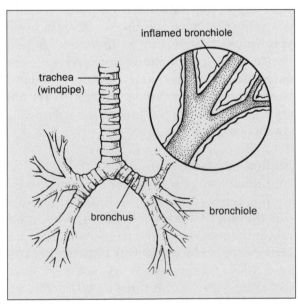

Chronic bronchitis, marked by recurrent inflammation of the lining of the bronchi or bronchioles, may narrow and obstruct the airways.

morning and in damp, cold weather. An ounce or more of yellow mucus may be brought up each day.

TREATMENT

The treatment of chronic bronchitis is primarily aimed at reducing irritation in the bronchial tubes. The discovery of antibiotics has been helpful in treating acute infection associated with chronic bronchitis. However, most people with chronic bronchitis do not need to take antibiotics continually.

Bronchodilator drugs may be prescribed to help relax and open up air passages in the lungs, if there is a tendency for these to close up. These drugs may be inhaled or taken orally.

Eliminating irritants. To effectively control chronic bronchitis, it is necessary to eliminate sources of irritation and infection in the nose, throat, mouth, sinuses, and bronchial tubes. This means an individual must avoid polluted air and dusty working conditions, and give up smoking. Your local American Lung Association office can suggest methods to help you quit smoking.

If the person with chronic bronchitis is exposed to dust and fumes at work, the doctor may suggest changing to another job or changing the work environment. All persons with chronic bronchitis must develop and follow a plan for a healthy lifestyle. Improving one's general health also increases the body's resistance to infections.

WHAT YOU SHOULD DO IF YOU HAVE CHRONIC BRONCHITIS

A good health plan for any person with chronic bronchitis should include the following rules.

- Don't smoke.
- Follow a nutritious, well-balanced diet, and maintain your ideal body weight.
- Get regular exercise daily, without tiring yourself too much.
- Ask your doctor about whether you should get vaccinated against influenza and pneumococcal pneumonia.
- Avoid exposure to colds and influenza at home or in public, and avoid respiratory irritants such as secondhand smoke, dust, and other air pollutants.

The American Lung Association

EMPHYSEMA

Emphysema is a condition in which there is overinflation of structures in the lungs known as alveoli or air sacs. This overinflation results from a breakdown of the walls of the alveoli, which causes a decrease in respiratory function (the way the lungs work) and often, breathlessness. Early symptoms include shortness of breath and cough.

HOW SERIOUS IS EMPHYSEMA?

Emphysema ranks ninth among chronic conditions that contribute to a person's lack of activity. Over 42 percent of individuals with emphysema report that their daily activities have been limited in some way by the disease.

Many of the people with emphysema are older men, but the condition is increasing among women. Males with emphysema outnumber females by 64 percent.

It is estimated that 70,000 to 100,000 Americans living today were born with a deficiency of a protein known as alpha 1-antitrypsin (AAT), which can lead to an inherited form of emphysema.

CAUSES

It is known from scientific research that the normal lung has a remarkable balance between two classes of chemicals with opposing action. The lung also has a system of elastic fibers. The fibers allow the lungs to expand and contract. When the chemical balance is altered, the lungs lose the ability to protect themselves against the destruction of these elastic fibers. This is what happens in emphysema.

There are a number of reasons this chemical imbalance occurs. Smoking is responsible for about 80 percent of chronic lung disease, including emphysema. Exposure to air pollution is one suspected cause. Irritating fumes and dusts on the job also are thought to be a factor.

A small number of people with emphysema have a rare inherited form of the disease called alpha 1-antitrypsin (AAT) deficiency-related emphysema, or early onset emphysema. This form of disease is caused by an inherited lack of the protective protein called AAT.

HOW EMPHYSEMA DEVELOPS

Emphysema begins with the destruction of air sacs in the lungs, where oxygen from the air is exchanged for carbon dioxide in the blood. The walls of the air sacs are thin and fragile. Damage to the air sacs is irreversible and results in permanent holes in the tissues of the lungs. As air sacs are destroyed, the lungs are able to transfer less and less oxygen

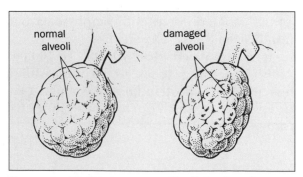

Damage to alveoli is permanent. Alveoli that have burst may fuse with one another, resulting in fewer, larger—and exceedingly less efficient—air sacs.

to the bloodstream, causing shortness of breath. The lungs lose their elasticity and the patient experiences great difficulty exhaling.

Emphysema does not develop suddenly—it comes on very gradually. Years of exposure to the irritation of cigarette smoke usually precede the development of emphysema.

A person may initially visit the doctor because he or she has begun to feel short of breath during activity or exercise. As the disease progresses, a brief walk can be enough to bring on difficulty in breathing. Some people may have had chronic bronchitis before developing emphysema.

TREATMENT

Doctors can help persons with emphysema live more comfortably with their disease. The goal of treatment is to provide relief of symptoms and prevent progression of the disease with a minimum of side effects. The doctor's advice and treatment may include:

Quitting smoking. The single most important factor for maintaining healthy lungs.

Bronchodilator drugs (prescription drugs that relax and open up air passages in the lungs) may be prescribed to treat emphysema if there is a tendency toward airway constriction or tightening. These drugs may be inhaled as aerosol sprays or taken orally.

Antibiotics, if you have a bacterial infection, such as pneumococcal pneumonia.

Exercise, including breathing exercises to strengthen the muscles used in breathing as part of a pulmonary rehabilitation program to condition the rest of the body.

Treatment with alpha 1-proteinase inhibitor (A1PI). This applies only if a person has AAT deficiency-related emphysema. A1PI is not recommended for those who develop emphysema as a result of cigarette smoking or other environmental factors.

Lung transplantation. Recent reports have been encouraging. Experience at this point in time is limited.

PREVENTION

Continuing research is being done to find answers to many questions about emphysema, especially about the best ways to prevent the disease.

Researchers know that quitting smoking can prevent the occurrence and decrease the progression of emphysema. Other environmental controls can also help prevent the disease from occurring.

If an individual has emphysema, the doctor will work hard to prevent the disease from getting worse by keeping the patient healthy and clear of any infection. The patient can participate in this prevention effort by following these general health guidelines.

See your doctor at the first sign of symptoms. Emphysema is a serious disease. It damages your lungs, and it can damage your heart.

Don't smoke. A majority of those who get emphysema are smokers. Continued smoking makes emphysema worse, especially for those who have AAT deficiency, the inherited form of emphysema.

Maintain overall good health habits, which include proper nutrition, adequate sleep, and regular exercise to build up your stamina and resistance to infections.

Reduce your exposure to air pollution, which may aggravate symptoms of emphysema. Refer to radio or television weather reports or your local newspaper for information about air quality. On days when the air quality is unhealthy, restrict your activity to early morning or evening. When pollution levels are dangerous, remain indoors and stay as comfortable as possible.

Consult your doctor at the start of any cold or respiratory infection because infection can make your emphysema symptoms worse. Ask about getting vaccinated against influenza and pneumococcal pneumonia.

The American Lung Association

PNEUMONIA

Pneumonia is a serious infection or inflammation of your lungs. The air sacs in the lungs fill with pus and other liquid. Oxygen has trouble reaching your blood. If there is too little oxygen in your blood, your body cells can't work properly—and may die. Lobar pneumonia affects a section (lobe) of a lung. Bronchial pneumonia (or bronchopneumonia) affects patches of both lungs.

Until 1936, pneumonia was the number-one cause of death in the United States. Then antibiotics brought it under control. Now this deadly enemy is making a comeback, in part because some bacteria can resist antibiotics. Pneumonia and influenza combined have ranked as the sixth leading cause of death since 1979.

CAUSES

Pneumonia is not a single disease. It can have over 30 different causes.

There are four main causes of pneumonia: bacteria, viruses, mycoplasmas, and others, such as pneumocystis.

BACTERIAL PNEUMONIA

Bacterial pneumonia can attack anyone from infants through the very old. Alcoholics, the debilitated, postoperative patients, people with respiratory diseases or viral infections, and people who have weakened immune systems are at greater risk.

How It Strikes

Pneumonia bacteria are present in some healthy throats. When body defenses are weakened in some way—by illness, old age, malnutrition, general debility, or impaired immunity—the bacteria can multiply and cause serious damage. Usually when a person's resistance is lowered, bacteria work their way into the lungs and inflame the air sacs. The tissue of part of a lobe of the lung, an entire lobe, or even most of the lung's five lobes become completely filled with liquid matter. (This is called consolidation.) The infection quickly spreads through the bloodstream, and the whole body is invaded.

The pneumococcus is the most common cause of bacterial pneumonia. It is the only form of pneumonia for which a vaccine is available.

Symptoms

The onset of bacterial pneumonia can vary from gradual to sudden. In the most severe cases, the patient may experience shaking chills, chattering teeth, severe chest pain, and a cough that produces rust-colored or greenish sputum. Body temperature often rises as high as 105°F. The patient sweats profusely, and breathing and pulse rate increase rapidly. Lips and nailbeds may have a bluish color due to lack of oxygen in the blood. A patient's mental state may be confused or delirious.

VIRAL PNEUMONIA

Half of all pneumonias are believed to be caused by viruses. More and more viruses are being identified as the cause of respiratory infection, and though most attack the upper respiratory tract, some produce pneumonia.

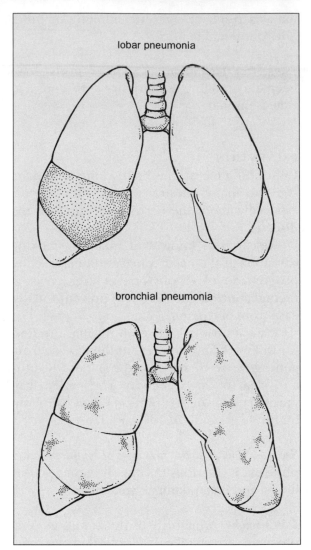

Lobar pneumonia affects a section (or lobe) of a single lung; bronchial pneumonia affects patches throughout both lungs.

Most of these pneumonias are not serious and last a short time. Influenza virus may be severe and occasionally fatal. The virus invades the lungs and multiplies, but there are almost no physical signs of lung tissue becoming filled with fluid. Many of its victims have pre-existing heart or lung disease or are pregnant.

Symptoms

The initial symptoms of viral pneumonia are the same as influenza symptoms: fever, a dry cough, headache, muscle pain, and weakness. Within 12 to 36 hours, there is increasing breathlessness; the cough becomes worse and produces a small amount of mucus. There is a high fever and there may be blueness of lips. In extreme cases, the patient has a desperate need for air and experiences extreme breathlessness.

Other viral pneumonias are complicated by an invasion of bacteria—with all the typical symptoms of bacterial pneumonia.

MYCOPLASMA PNEUMONIA
Because of its somewhat different symptoms and physical signs, and because the course of the illness differed from classic pneumococcal pneumonia, mycoplasma pneumonia was once believed to be caused by one or more undiscovered viruses and was called primary atypical pneumonia.

Identified during World War II, mycoplasmas are the smallest free-living agents of disease in man, unclassified as to whether bacteria or viruses, but having characteristics of both. They generally cause a mild and widespread pneumonia. They affect all age groups, occurring most frequently in older children and young adults. The death rate is low, even in untreated cases.

Symptoms
The most prominent symptom of mycoplasma pneumonia is a cough that tends to come in violent attacks, but produces only sparse whitish mucus. Chills and fever are early symptoms, and some patients experience nausea or vomiting. The patient's heartbeat is often slow, and in some extreme cases, he or she may suffer from breathlessness and have a bluish cast to his lips and nailbeds.

OTHER KINDS OF PNEUMONIA
Pneumocystis carinii pneumonia (PCP) is caused by an organism long thought of as a parasite but now believed to be a fungus. PCP is the first sign of illness in many persons with AIDS, and perhaps 80 percent (four out of five) will develop it sooner or later. It can be successfully treated in many cases. It may recur a few months later, but treatment can help to prevent or delay its recurrence.

Other less common pneumonias may be quite serious and are occurring more often. Various special pneumonias are caused by the inhalation of food, liquid, gases, or dust, and by fungi. Foreign bodies or a bronchial obstruction such as a tumor may promote the occurrence of pneumonia, although they are not causes of pneumonia.

Rickettsia (also considered something between viruses and bacteria) cause Rocky Mountain spotted fever, Q fever, typhus, and psittacosis—diseases that may have mild or severe effects on the lungs. Tuberculosis pneumonia is a very serious lung infection and extremely dangerous unless treated early.

TREATMENT
If you develop pneumonia, your chances of a fast recovery are greatest under certain conditions: if you're young, if your pneumonia was caught early, if your defenses against disease are working well, if the infection hasn't spread, and if you're not suffering from other illnesses.

Antibiotics. In the young and healthy, early treatment with antibiotics can cure bacterial and mycoplasma pneumonia, and a certain percentage of rickettsia cases. There is no effective treatment yet for viral pneumonia, which usually heals on its own.

The drug or drugs used are determined by the germ causing the pneumonia and the judgment of the doctor. After a patient's temperature returns to normal, medication must be continued according to doctor's instructions— otherwise the pneumonia may recur. Relapses can be far more serious than the first attack.

Supportive treatment. Besides antibiotics, patients are given supportive treatment: proper diet, and oxygen to increase oxygen in the blood when needed. In some patients, medication to ease chest pain and to provide relief from violent cough may be necessary.

RECOVERING FROM PNEUMONIA

The vigorous young person may lead a normal life within a week of recovery from pneumonia. For the middle-aged, however, weeks may elapse before they regain their accustomed strength, vigor, and feeling of well-being. A person recovering from mycoplasma pneumonia may be weak for an extended period of time. In general, a person should not be discouraged from returning to work or carrying out usual activities, but must be warned to expect some difficulties. Adequate rest is important to maintain progress toward full recovery and to avoid relapse.

PREVENTION

Because pneumonia is a common complication of influenza (flu), getting a flu shot every fall is good pneumonia prevention.

A vaccine is also available to help fight pneumococcal pneumonia—one type of bacterial pneumonia. Your doctor can help you decide if you—or a member of your family—needs the vaccine against pneumococcal pneumonia. It is usually given only to people at high risk of getting the disease and its life-threatening complications. Ask your doctor if you should be vaccinated. The greatest risk of pneumococcal pneumonia usually is among people who:

- Have chronic illnesses such as lung disease, heart disease, kidney disorders, sickle cell anemia, or diabetes
- Are recovering from severe illness
- Are in nursing homes or other chronic care facilities
- Are age 65 or older

The vaccine is generally given only once. Ask your doctor about revaccination recommendations.

Because pneumonia often follows ordinary respiratory infections, the most important preventive measure is for a person to be alert to any symptoms of respiratory trouble that linger more than a few days. Good health habits—proper diet and hygiene, plentiful rest, regular exercise, etc.—increase resistance to all respiratory illnesses. Such habits also help promote fast recovery when illness does occur.

IF YOU HAVE SYMPTOMS OF PNEUMONIA

Even though pneumonia can be satisfactorily treated, it can be an extremely serious illness. If you think you have symptoms of pneumonia, you should:

- Call your doctor immediately. Even with the many effective antibiotics, early diagnosis and treatment are important.
- Follow your doctor's advice. In serious cases, your doctor may advise a hospital stay. Or recovery at home may be possible.
- Continue to take the medicine your doctor prescribes until told you may stop. This will help prevent recurrence of pneumonia and relapse.

The American Lung Association

INFLUENZA

Influenza is a contagious disease caused by a virus. A virus is a germ that is very small. Influenza viruses infect many parts of the body, including the lungs.

When someone who has the flu sneezes, coughs, or even talks, the flu virus is expelled into the air and may be inhaled by anyone close by. Flu may be transmitted by direct hand contact.

WHAT HAPPENS WHEN YOU GET THE FLU?

When flu strikes the lungs, the lining of the respiratory tract is damaged. The tissues become swollen and inflamed. Fortunately, the damage is rarely permanent. The tissues usually heal within two weeks.

Influenza is often called a respiratory disease, but it affects the whole body. The victim usually becomes acutely ill with fever, chills, weakness, loss of appetite, and aching of the head, back, arms, and legs. The flu sufferer may also have a sore throat and a dry cough, nausea, and burning eyes.

The fever mounts quickly—temperature may rise to 104°F—but after two or three days, it usually subsides. The patient is often left exhausted for days afterwards.

IS FLU CONSIDERED SERIOUS?

For those who are healthy, influenza is typically a moderately severe illness. Most people are back on their feet within a week. For people who are not healthy or well to begin with, influenza can be very severe and even fatal. The symptoms described above have a greater impact on these persons. In addition, complications can occur.

Most of these complications are bacterial infections, because the body can be so weakened by influenza that its defenses against bacteria are low. Bacterial pneumonia is the most common complication. But the sinuses and inner ears may become inflamed and painful as well.

WHO GETS THE FLU?

Anyone can get the flu—especially when it is widespread in the community. In a flu epidemic year, from 20 to 50 percent of those not immunized may contract influenza.

People who are not healthy or well to begin with are particularly susceptible to the complications that can follow. These people are known as high risk. For anyone at high risk, influenza is a very serious illness. You may be at high risk if you have any of the following conditions:

- Chronic lung disease such as asthma, emphysema, chronic bronchitis, bronchiectasis, tuberculosis, or cystic fibrosis
- Heart disease
- Chronic kidney disease
- Diabetes or other chronic metabolic disorder
- Severe anemia
- Depressed immunity resulting from diseases or treatments

Additional high-risk features include the following:

- Residing in a nursing home or other chronic care facility
- Being over 65 years of age

A physician, nurse, or other provider of care to high-risk persons should be immunized to protect high-risk patients.

HOW ARE FLU AND COMPLICATIONS PREVENTED?

Influenza can be prevented when a person receives the current influenza vaccine. This vaccine is made each year so that the vaccine can contain influenza viruses that are expected to cause illness that year.

The viruses in the vaccine are killed or inactivated so that someone vaccinated cannot get influenza from the vaccine. Instead the person vaccinated develops protection in his or her body in the form of substances called antibodies.

The amount of antibodies in the body is greatest one or two months after vaccination and then gradually declines. For that reason and because the influenza viruses usually change each year, a high-risk person should be vaccinated each fall with the new vaccine. November is the best time to get your flu shot. Such a yearly vaccination has been found to be about 75 percent effective in preventing flu. It also may very well reduce the severity of flu and be lifesaving in vaccinated persons.

A drug called amantadine also can be used to help prevent flu. It is discussed later in the section on treatment.

WHAT ABOUT REACTIONS TO THE VACCINE?

Most people have little or no reaction to the influenza vaccine.

One in four might have a swollen, red, tender area where the vaccination was given.

A much smaller number might also develop a slight fever within 24 hours. They may have chills or a headache, or feel a little sick. People who already have a respiratory disease may find their symptoms worsened. Usually none of these reactions lasts for more than a couple of days.

In addition, adverse reactions to the vaccine, perhaps allergic in nature, have been observed in some people. These could be due to an egg protein allergy, since the egg in which the virus is grown cannot be completely extracted. These people should be vaccinated only if their own physician believes it necessary and if the vaccine is given under close observation by a physician.

WHO SHOULD BE VACCINATED?

People at high risk should be vaccinated yearly against flu. In addition, those who provide care to high-risk patients should be vaccinated.

If you are not in a high-risk group, ask your doctor if you need the vaccine.

CAN YOU HAVE A RECURRENCE OF THE FLU?

A person can have influenza more than once because the virus that causes influenza may belong to one of three different flu virus families, A, B, or C. Influenza A and influenza B are the major families.

Within each flu virus family are many viral strains, like so many brothers and sisters. Both A and B have strains that cause illnesses of varying severity. But the influenza A family has more virulent strains than the B family.

If you have the flu, your body responds by developing antibodies. The following year, a new family member or a member of another family may appear. Your antibodies are less effective or ineffective against this unfamiliar strain. If you are exposed to it, you may come down with flu again.

HOW ARE FLU AND COMPLICATIONS TREATED?

For uncomplicated flu, your doctor will probably tell you to stay in bed at home as long as the sickness is severe—and perhaps for about two days after the fever is gone.

The drug called amantadine is useful for treating someone who develops influenza A, particularly if it is given as soon as possible after the onset of flu. Amantadine also can be used as a preventive, but for prevention it must be taken daily as long as flu cases continue to occur in a community. Your doctor would have to decide whether to use amantadine either for prevention or treatment. If it is used for treating an early case of flu, it may shorten this illness and reduce the severity. Amantadine works only against influenza A viruses and should be used only if influenza A is suspected.

Amantadine sometimes causes side effects such as difficulty in sleeping, tremulousness, or depression; these are usually mild and often go away even when the medicine is continued.

The treatment of nonbacterial complications varies with the illness. If you should develop a bacterial complication, however, your doctor can give you an antibiotic.

WHY IS FLU MORE PREVALENT IN SOME YEARS THAN IN OTHERS?

Every 10 years or so, a flu virus strain appears that is dramatically different from the other members of its family. When this major change occurs, a worldwide epidemic—called a pandemic—almost inevitably follows. Few people have antibodies that are effective against the new virus. One such virus caused the 1918 flu epidemic that swept the world and left in its wake more than 20 million dead. Fear of a similar outbreak in the fall of 1976 inspired a mass vaccination effort. Fortunately, no epidemic developed.

The American Lung Association

CHAPTER 12

The Muscles and Bones

In the course of our lives, our muscles and bones change significantly. The newborn has 350 bones—nearly 150 more than the typical adult. As we grow up, certain bones (most notably those in the skull and lower spinal column) fuse together. So by about age 25, the normal complement of bones is 206—although an extra vertebra or pair of ribs is not uncommon.

Throughout our young life, the bones build and strengthen. Young people typically enjoy a relatively calcium-rich diet, and this large surplus of calcium is stored almost exclusively in the bones. As this occurs, the bones become more dense and solid, a process known as ossification. By about age 35, ossification is complete, and the bones are as hard—and as strong—as they will ever be.

In the ensuing years, people begin to ingest less calcium than they need. The bones are mined for their stores of calcium, resulting in a net loss of this important mineral. Over the decades, bones consequently become weaker: more porous, brittle, and subject to fractures.

Between the bones are joints. Ligaments are the tough fibrous cords that hold one bone to another; tendons attach muscle to bone. Cushioning the site where two bones meet is a rubbery layer of cartilage—a natural shock absorber. A fibrous joint capsule, lined by a synovial membrane, surrounds the joint. Within this capsule is the synovial fluid, a slippery lubricant that enables the surfaces of the joint to move against one another practically friction-free. Outside of the joint capsule are bursae, synovial sacks that secrete a lubricant to facilitate the movement of muscles across bones or over other muscles.

After years of strenuous use, the joints naturally begin to break down. Especially vulnerable are the joints that bear the most weight—the hips and knees. Other common sites for joint problems are the hands, feet, and lower back. By age 60, most people have at least some signs of joint problems.

The skeletal muscles—that is, the ones surrounding the bones and joints—are affected by age as well. Overall muscle mass decreases as a matter of course; this is only compounded by the fact that we tend to be less active when we're older, which further encourages muscles to atrophy. Moreover, the resilient fibers of the skeletal muscles are gradually replaced in later years by connective tissue (a process called fibrosis). The usurping connective tissue is certainly strong, but it lacks the elasticity and the power to contract that muscle tissues have.

Changes in the muscles, joints, and bones are inevitable, but whether they cause aggravating symptoms or impinge upon activities once taken for granted is another issue. Some people remain hearty and active into their nineties. Others are not as fortunate. It's only when mobility is lost or movement becomes painful that we start to feel truly old.

A number of therapies—ranging from massage to exercises to medication to surgery—can minimize, halt, or sometimes reverse the effects of aging on the musculoskeletal system. There are a variety of specialists to consult, depending on the disorder. An orthopedic surgeon specializes in problems affecting the body parts involved with movement: ligaments, tendons, muscles, and, especially, the bones. A rheumatologist specializes in arthritis and other problems particular to the joints. A physiatrist is a medical doctor whose practice concentrates on physical medicine and rehabilitation. Physical therapists are not M.D.s, but are licensed practitioners who design individual exercise regimens and other therapies to restore mobility and reduce pain.   *The Editors*

OSTEOPOROSIS

Osteoporosis is a disease characterized by a gradual loss of bone mass due to depletion of the minerals essential to bone formation

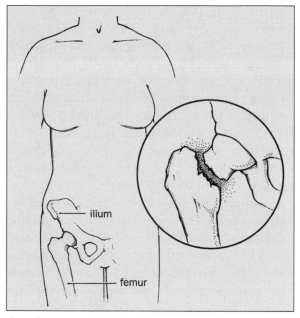

Bone fractures are a common consequence of osteoporosis. Adequate lifelong calcium intake is the best way to ensure strong bones later in life.

(phosphorous and especially calcium). Affected bones become porous and brittle and susceptible to fractures. Indeed, osteoporosis is responsible for more than one-and-a-half-million bone fractures annually—most commonly occurring in the wrists, hips, and vertebrae of the spinal column. Furthermore, each year, thousands of deaths can be attributed directly or indirectly to osteoporosis (usually due to complications following surgery for a hip fracture). The disorder is very common among people over the age of 70, and affects women four times more often than men, primarily due to hormonal changes that occur with menopause.

What Causes Bone Loss?
Up until the age of 35 or so, we continue to build bone mass. After this age, bone density is kept stable by a cyclical process called remodeling, in which new bone is built to replace old, brittle bone and repair microscopic fractures. Three types of cells are involved in this process: osteocytes, osteoblasts, and os-

teoclasts. Hormonal messages stimulate the osteocytes, which initiate the remodeling cycle by readying the bone surface to be remodeled. This activates the osteoclasts, which chew up old bone, leaving it pitted—only to be filled with new bone produced by osteoblasts. This ongoing cycle repeats itself every 90 days or so. However, hormonal and other changes that occur with age can interfere with the remodeling process, resulting in a cumulative loss of bone mass.

The skeleton is made of two types of bone: cortical (found mostly in the long bones of the arms and legs), and trabecular (found mostly in the spine and at ends of the long bones). Over time, women lose 35 percent of their cortical tissue, and 50 percent of their trabecular tissue. Men lose somewhat less—25 and 35 percent, respectively.

Sex hormones play an important role in the preservation of bone strength. A reduction in these substances may lead to an additional 15 percent decrease in cortical bone, and a 25 percent decrease in trabecular bone, regardless of gender.

Other factors that can lead to bone loss are excessive alcohol consumption, using tobacco products, taking certain prescription drugs, and prolonged use of over-the-counter antacids that contain aluminum.

Prevention
The best method of managing osteoporosis is preventing it in the first place. You can maintain bone mass by eating a balanced diet that includes foods that are rich in calcium. Men and women both should consume 1,500 milligrams of dietary calcium a day. Low-fat milk products are the best source. If you don't get enough calcium in your diet, you should discuss supplements with your doctor.

You also need a small amount of vitamin D to use calcium correctly. But most people manufacture an adequate supply when they're exposed to a minimal amount of sunlight. Vitamin D is also present in fortified foods (such as low-fat milk and cereal) and in daily multivitamin and mineral supplements.

Many experts encourage regular, moderate, weight-bearing exercise (such as walking or jogging) as another means of maintaining bone strength. Very inactive people (such as those confined to bed because of illness) lose bone 25 times faster than normal.

If you appear to be at high risk for osteoporosis, your doctor may suggest having your bone density measured to predict your risk of fracture. The most accurate method is dual-energy x-ray absorptiometry, a non-invasive imaging technique. If absorptiometry tests indicate evidence of osteoporosis, more aggressive steps can then be taken to prevent further bone loss.

Osteoporosis and Women

Women who get enough calcium (1,000 milligrams a day before menopause, and 1,500 mg daily after menopause), exercise regularly, and especially those who are on hormone-replacement therapy (HRT) following menopause are at a greatly reduced risk for developing osteoporosis. But nearly 24 million women—mostly those over 50—already have the disease. Fortunately, prevention is no longer the only hope. Research into treatment is finally paying off, providing patients with new ways to manage osteoporosis.

After menopause, when estrogen levels decline, the finely tuned cycle of bone remodeling may run amok, until loss of bone outpaces the manufacture of new bone.

Bones develop pits and tiny holes and become more fragile. In those with osteoporosis, this fragility may be so great that a minor bump causes a fracture. Drugs to treat osteoporosis are aimed at adjusting the remodeling cycle. They may either prevent bone from being reabsorbed (by interfering with osteoclasts), or build new bone (by enhancing osteoblasts).

Until recently, the only drugs that were proven effective were the antiresorptives, which work by decreasing the rate at which bone remodels. However, bone-building drugs are in the works. The first, fluoride, turned out to be a disappointment. While fluoride treatment does stimulate bone rebuilding, studies found that the new bone was weaker than usual, actually increasing the risk of fractures. However, the drug alendronate seems able to restore some of the lost bone.

Four treatments are now widely used for osteoporosis: estrogen therapy, raloxifene, calcitonin, and alendronate. Choosing a therapy is an individual matter requiring discussion with your physician. However, women with osteoporosis should be able to reduce fracture risk with one, or a combination, of these treatments.

Estrogen. Estrogen therapy—usually prescribed in combination with the sex hormone progesterone and known as hormone replacement therapy (HRT)—is probably the most common treatment for osteoporosis, although its primary benefit is to prevent the condition from developing in the first place. Estrogen bonds to bone and seems to inhibit the osteocyte response that initiates bone remodeling. When estrogen production declines at menopause, bone loss accelerates rapidly. HRT can offset this loss and actually mildly increase bone mass. Women who begin estrogen therapy at menopause have half the fractures of women who don't. But HRT can also help women who already have osteoporosis. The treatment will help avert further fractures and may increase bone mass somewhat. Studies show that even 70-year-old women who start on HRT may experience some of these benefits.

HRT is usually taken for five years or more. It may be taken as a once-a-day pill or as a skin patch that only needs to be replaced twice a week. (The progesterone component of HRT is taken either as a separate pill or in combination form.) HRT slightly increases the risk of breast cancer, and women who have had the disease or are at particularly high risk for it should probably not start HRT. (Unopposed estrogen—estrogen without progesterone—also increases the risk of endometrial cancer.) HRT may also exacerbate liver and gallbladder disease. Less significant side effects may include nausea, cramping, bloating, and weight gain. Estrogen use also causes menstrual bleeding to resume, at least temporarily.

Raloxifene. Raloxifene is a synthetic agent that mimics the effect of estrogen on bone, but opposes its action on breast and uterine tissue, thus reducing the risk of certain side effects of estrogen in these organs. It is taken once a day for the prevention of postmenopausal osteoporosis. However, direct comparisons of its effectiveness with that of other drugs are not yet available.

Calcitonin. Calcitonin, another hormone (but not a sex hormone), helps to regulate the body's use of calcium. High doses of it interfere with bone resorption by decreasing the activity of bone-chewing osteoclasts. Calcitonin treatment slows bone loss in the spine and hip, and even adds some bone mass. Whether or not this correlates with a reduction in fractures is still unknown. The drug is also a mild painkiller, so it serves a dual function in those with fractures.

In 10 to 20 percent of those treated, calcitonin causes nausea, appetite loss, and flushing. The drug is also expensive. It may be given by injection or as a nasal spray. The spray is used once daily; the injected form is usually administered once a day or every other day for two years.

Alendronate. Alendronate is the only member of a group of medications called bisphosphonates that has been approved for treatment of postmenopausal osteoporosis. Another similar medication, etidronate, has also been widely used. The bisphosphonates interfere with osteoclasts, so that bone is less pitted; when the osteoblasts then go to work, they actually add to bone rather than just replace it. Studies of alendronate have found that not only does it slow or reverse bone loss, but it also reduces fractures.

Alendronate is taken once daily. Because of a significant risk of esophageal irritation, it must be taken first thing in the morning, followed by a 30-minute period of sitting or standing upright before eating or drinking anything else.

As with the other agents, alendronate is taken in combination with vitamin D and calcium supplements.

Osteoporosis and Men
Men's bones are, on average, 20 percent more dense than those of women. This is because men are genetically programmed to have heavier skeletons than women, and their testosterone (the principal male sex hormone) levels help maintain skeletal integrity until late in life. As a result, men's bones generally stay stronger than most women's, and their risk of osteoporosis is lower.

Nonetheless, 20 percent of all cases of osteoporosis, at least one-fourth of all broken hips, and about one-seventh of all vertebral fractures occur in men. By age 70, most men have lost about one-third of the density at the top of the thigh bone (femur), which forms the hip joint at the acetabulum (a cup-shaped depression in the pelvis).

So, by age 80, one in six men has broken a hip. In addition, although men lose only about 1 percent of spinal bone mass a decade after age 40 (women lose up to 10 percent in the decade after menopause), they can still develop painful spinal fractures as they age.

Knowing if your bones are weakening is difficult, especially if you're a man. There are no obvious signals (such as the end of menstruation) to show that osteoporosis may be imminent. Low testosterone levels may go undetected, as they may have little effect on libido.

The process of mineral depletion in the bones usually takes longer in men than in women. Testosterone generally doesn't begin to decline significantly until after age 65. Even then, the reduction is slow, and concentrations of the hormone frequently remain near normal. But even though testosterone-induced bone loss occurs at a relatively slow rate, the decline can still lead to fractures.

Which Men Are at Greatest Risk?

Many men with osteoporosis have risk factors that require extra precautions. For example, about 40 percent of those with weak spines have illnesses, or take medications that interfere with calcium use when taken heavily for prolonged periods. Drugs in this group include systemic corticosteroids, the anticonvulsant phenytoin (Dilantin), the diuretic furosemide (Lasix), and over-the-counter antacids that contain aluminum (such as Amphojel, Gelusil, and Maalox).

In addition, illnesses such as prostate cancer (which may involve medication that interferes with testosterone production) and arthritis (which often involves bone erosion and corticosteroid therapy), as well as testicular surgery, and having had mumps as an adult (both of which can interfere with testosterone levels) have similar effects.

Men in these situations should be followed closely by their physicians. In addition to bone density scanning (dual-energy x-ray absorptiometry), urine and blood tests may also be ordered to measure testosterone levels and other indicators of risk factors.

If results show you're at risk, or if you're taking a drug that accelerates calcium loss, you and your physician should discuss drug therapy, generally with testosterone, bisphosphonates (such as alendronate), or dietary calcium supplements.

The Editors

OSTEOARTHRITIS

Osteoarthritis, also known as degenerative joint disease, is the most common form of arthritis. By age 40, about 90 percent of all people have x-ray evidence of osteoarthritis in the weight-bearing joints—such as the hips and knees—although symptoms generally do not begin to appear until later in life. At any given time, as many as 20 million adult Americans suffer from symptoms of osteoarthritis.

While osteoarthritis has little or no impact on the longevity of its sufferers (unlike some of the other forms of arthritis), severe involvement of the hips, knees, and spinal column may greatly limit activity and diminish overall quality of life for some patients.

CAUSES

The gradual breakdown of cartilage that comes with age is the leading cause of osteoarthritis. This damage is due to several factors, including genetics, stress on the joint (for example, caused by obesity), and an inability of the cartilage to repair itself to any degree. Metabolic changes in chondrocytes (cartilage-producing cells) and production of an enzyme (peptidase) are also thought to play roles in the breakdown of cartilage.

This type of cartilage breakdown is called primary osteoarthritis. The first alteration is roughening of articular cartilage, followed by pitting, ulceration, and progressive loss of cartilage surface. Accompanying these changes is overgrowth of the bones, forming spurs and lipping at the edge of the joint (osteophytes). Primary osteoarthritis most commonly involves joints of the fingers, hips, knees, and spine, and at the base of the thumb and the big toe. It can be present in just one of these joints or in all of them. The wrists, elbows, shoulders, and ankles are rarely involved.

Secondary osteoarthritis, on the other hand, can affect any joint. It follows trauma or chronic joint injury due to some other type of arthritis (rheumatoid arthritis, for example), or may result from overuse of a particular joint. Because trauma or overuse hastens the degeneration of cartilage, symptoms of secondary osteoarthritis become apparent at a much younger age than symptoms of primary osteoarthritis.

In the arthritic joint, the protective cartilage and synovial lining gradually erode, so that bone surfaces rub directly against each other and disintegrate.

SYMPTOMS

People rarely have symptoms of primary osteoarthritis before their forties or fifties. At first, symptoms are usually mild; morning stiffness is often the only indicator. As the disease advances, there may be mild pain when moving the affected joint. The pain is made worse by greater activity and is relieved by rest. In many people, symptoms progress no further; in others, the pain and stiffness grow gradually worse, until they limit daily activities, such as walking, going up stairs, and typing.

Enlargement of the finger joints is common in the later stages of some cases of osteoarthritis. Knobby overgrowths of the joints nearest the fingertips, called Heberden's nodes, occur most often in women, and tend to run in families. Typically, these overgrowths affect only one finger at first, but may eventually involve all of the fingers to a greater or lesser degree. Heberden's nodes may be painful and can limit flexibility. Enlargement of the middle joints of the fingers is referred to as Bouchard's nodes. A crackling may be heard or felt when an affected joint is moved.

DIAGNOSIS

When a patient complains of joint pain and stiffness, the doctor will obtain a complete medical history and conduct a thorough physical examination. These diagnostic procedures are important for two reasons: first, to identify the type of arthritis and second, to eliminate the possibility that the symptoms are caused by a more general disorder. The doctor will ask questions such as:

• Which joints are involved?
• What triggers pain?
• When is pain the worst?

393

- Does anything provide relief?
- Have the joints been red and swollen?
- Do you have morning stiffness?

The physical exam includes inspection of all of the joints of the hands, arms, legs, feet, and spine to determine how many joints are affected and whether the arthritis involves joints symmetrically on both sides of the body. In most cases, the diagnosis of osteoarthritis is apparent from the patient history and physical examination. X-ray findings of a narrowed joint space and thickened bone with spurs and cysts confirm the diagnosis and help to distinguish osteoarthritis from other forms of arthritis. Also, marked deformity in a joint is much less common with osteoarthritis than with rheumatoid arthritis or gout.

In unusual situations when the diagnosis is in doubt, a sample of synovial fluid may be drawn from the affected joint for laboratory analysis.

PREVENTION

The only preventive measures for osteoarthritis are weight control and, whenever possible, avoidance of repetitive activities that may produce secondary osteoarthritis. In one study, overweight women who lost an average of 11 pounds reduced the development of osteoarthritis symptoms in their knees by 50 percent. In this study, those who were the most overweight to begin with, and then subsequently lost weight, showed the greatest overall improvement. Although being overweight is thought to place greater stress on weight-bearing joints (such as the hips or knees) and therefore lead to cartilage damage, another study linked obesity to osteoarthritis in the nonweight-bearing joints in the hands. This finding suggested to researchers that excess body fat itself may have a direct and deleterious metabolic effect on joint cartilage. People who are overweight should make every attempt to lose weight and normal-weight people should strive to maintain their weight.

TREATMENT

The goals of osteoarthritis treatment are to relieve the pain associated with the disorder and to maintain as much normal function of the joints as possible. To accomplish these goals, physicians will apply a combination of treatment approaches. Pain management through careful use of medication, joint strengthening by physical and occupational therapy properly balanced with rest, weight loss to take stress off weight-bearing joints, and, in some cases, surgery are the treatments used most often.

Heat and Ice

While medications are the most effective treatment for pain, a warm bath or shower, a heat lamp, or warm compresses may relieve pain and ease stiffness by relaxing muscles. Paraffin (warm wax) baths can lessen pain and stiffness in fingers and feet. Heat treatments may also improve subsequent ability to exercise. In some people, however, application of cold packs or "blue ice" provides better relief of pain, especially when pain and inflammation follow activity. Warm compresses or ice should be applied for no longer than 20 minutes. Ice should be wrapped in a towel and removed when the area becomes numb.

Exercise

The treatment of arthritis requires both rest and exercise. The right balance between the two must be tailored to each individual and the stage of the disease. While rest is important when joints ache, appropriate exercise is equally essential to maintain joint motion, muscle strength, and fitness when symptoms have subsided. An exercise program should be started with the approval of a physician and, preferably, under the guidance of a physical therapist who can design and teach an exercise program for home use, as well as provide periodic monitoring of progress. The three forms of exercise are: range-of-motion, muscle-strengthening, and endurance or fitness.

Range-of-motion exercises. These exercises involve moving a joint as far as possible in every direction without causing pain. Their purpose is to maintain flexibility, reduce pain and stiffness, and improve joint function. In range-of-motion exercises, muscles and joints are moved to a point that is just mildly uncomfortable. These exercises help to relieve or prevent stiffness and are recommended as a warm-up before workouts.

Muscle-strengthening exercises. Stronger muscles provide greater structural support for the joints. Isometric exercises—pushing or pulling against a fixed object—can strengthen muscles without damaging joints, which remain immobile during the exercise. In one study, eight weeks of a muscle-strengthening program improved muscle tone and decreased pain significantly in people with osteoarthritis of the knee.

Endurance exercises. Aerobic activities—such as swimming, walking, running, and bicycling—improve overall body fitness. There has been some concern that such exercises could accelerate the breakdown of cartilage in weight-bearing joints, such as the knee, but studies have not shown this to be the case. Be sure to warm up properly before exercising—walk briskly to get your heart rate up and then do some gentle stretches. Wear comfortable, supportive exercise shoes to help absorb the shock of weight-bearing exercise.

Drug Treatment

Pain relief can be achieved with acetaminophen, or aspirin and other nonsteroidal anti-inflammatory drugs, or NSAIDs, some of which—ibuprofen (Motrin) and naproxen (Aleve)—are available over-the-counter. In some instances, injections of corticosteroid drugs or cartilage-like agents are used. Experimentation with a number of drugs may be necessary before osteoarthritis patients achieve optimal pain relief.

Acetaminophen. Because inflammation plays only a minor role in osteoarthritis, use of NSAIDs with the most potent anti-inflammatory effects (which carry the greatest risk of side effects) is not usually required. For most, the pain of osteoarthritis can be treated with acetaminophen, which is not an NSAID, but can provide adequate pain relief with fewer side effects. This was borne out in a study that compared acetaminophen with the NSAID naproxen for the treatment of osteoarthritis of the knees. No significant differences were found in how the two drugs affected the progress of the disease, and side effects for the two drugs were about the same. As is true for any drug, acetaminophen can cause side effects. These can include kidney disease, if taken regularly at doses exceeding the recommended amount, or if taken with large quantities of alcohol. Patients who use acetaminophen regularly should avoid heavy alcohol intake and see their doctor periodically to be monitored for side effects.

Nonsteroidal anti-inflammatory drugs (NSAIDs). If nondrug methods and/or acetaminophen fail to control osteoarthritis pain, NSAIDs are the next option. How well symptoms respond to a specific NSAID varies greatly from person to person. This means that finding the right one depends largely on trial and error; and since each drug's effects are cumulative, a week or two is necessary to evaluate its effectiveness. Moderate doses of NSAIDs are usually enough to control pain in those with osteoarthritis.

Although NSAIDs can provide effective treatment, long-term use of these drugs, even in moderate doses, can cause side effects. And certain patients—the elderly, those taking corticosteroids, and those who have a history of ulcer disease, alcoholism, or adverse effects from NSAIDs—are at higher risk of experiencing side effects. The most common of these is stomach irritation, bleeding, and ulceration caused by the drug's interference with the formation of protective mucus that normally coats the stomach. The recent introduction of a special class of NSAIDs called COX-2 inhibitors has markedly reduced though not eliminated the risk of these side effects. Celecoxib (Celebrex) is the first of this class to gain approval for osteoarthritis.

Corticosteroid injections. In uncommon situations, such as an acute flare-up of severe osteoarthritis or treatment of those who are not good candidates for joint replacement surgery (due to severe heart disease, for example), injection of corticosteroids directly into the joint may be helpful. Corticosteroids relieve pain by reducing inflammation, and the injection should provide pain relief lasting up to several months. Pain returning within a few weeks may indicate some problem other than inflammation. Because more frequent use increases the risk of damage to the cartilage, these injections should be given only two or three times a year.

Hyaluronate. Hyaluronic acid is the compound that gives synovial (joint) fluid its viscoelasticity. Hyaluronate (Synvisc, Hyalgan) is a derivative of hyaluronic acid that has recently been approved for injection into arthritic joints. It may decrease pain in patients with osteoarthritis but is expensive, and its effectiveness remains to be clearly proven.

Topical Products

Topical preparations for arthritis won't "banish" pain, as some advertisements claim, but they can provide temporary relief. These products work in two ways. When applied to the skin over an affected joint, they mask pain by stimulating a warm or cool sensation that sometimes distracts users from the underlying discomfort (and frequently causes a harmless, transitory reddening of the skin). Alternatively, they offer limited, direct pain relief by reducing the amount of specific neurotransmitters (chemicals that transmit pain impulses to the central nervous system and may encourage inflammation) found inside aching joints.

Preparations that mask pain, called counterirritants, are available over-the-counter. Their active ingredients are camphor, menthol, or turpentine oil. These preparations should be gently but thoroughly rubbed into the skin over the aching joint. A counterirritant can be applied three or four times a day, but patients who find they're using it regularly more than two or three times a week should consult their physicians to develop a more comprehensive treatment program.

The only topical preparation that has been shown to affect pain directly contains capsaicin, the compound that gives hot peppers their bite. This compound reduces the amount of a neurotransmitter, substance P, which is thought to release inflammation-causing enzymes and possibly carry pain impulses to the nervous system.

Ointment containing capsaicin (Zostrix) is available over-the-counter. This ointment must be applied to affected joints three or four times a day. It usually requires about two weeks for pain to diminish (and might take up to six weeks). Unlike counterirritants, capsaicin doesn't usually cause redness, but it may induce a burning sensation that disappears after the first few applications. You must keep using the product to realize its benefit: When you stop, pain quickly returns.

Topical treatments are not dangerous and have few side effects, but some precautions are necessary. Don't get any into your eyes, nose, mouth, or any open cuts. Never tightly bandage or apply heat to a treated area. If you develop an irritation, stop using the product.

Surgery

Severely disabling arthritis can be aided by one of the following surgical procedures. Joint replacement, the most extensive type of surgery, is discussed in a separate section below.

Arthroscopy. This procedure entails the insertion of an arthroscope—a thin, lighted tube that allows the surgeon to see directly into a joint. Arthroscopy is almost always performed in the knee or hip. It may be used for diagnostic purposes to determine the type of arthritis and the degree of damage it has caused. It can also be used for such surgical procedures as repairing torn cartilage or smoothing roughened cartilage and removing loose fragments.

Osteotomy. Bone tissue in the knees or spine is cut away. The bones are then reset to allow weight to be distributed to healthier areas of the joint cartilage.

Resection. All or part of a bone is removed in a joint of the hands, wrists, elbows, toes, or ankles.

Arthrodesis. In this procedure, a surgeon fuses together two bones in a finger, wrist, ankle, or foot joint to form a single bone. While this naturally results in a loss of flexibility, it relieves pain caused by the two bones rubbing against each other in the damaged joint. The "new" fused bone is more stable and can then bear weight much better than the two separate bones.

Resurfacing. This is actually a type of joint replacement (see below) and is also known as bone relining. In this procedure, damaged cartilage and ends of bone in the hip joint are removed and capped with metal; the joint capsule is sometimes lined with plastic.

Total Joint Replacement (Arthroplasty)

Arthroplasty relieves pain and restores function by removing the entire diseased or damaged joint and replacing it with a mechanical joint. Between 80 and 90 percent of joint replacements are of the hip and knee, although joints in the elbows, shoulders, hands, and feet can also be replaced. For many patients, new technology and improved operative techniques and materials have made joint replacement the best treatment alternative. Each year approximately 150,000 joint replacements are done in the U.S., primarily (but not exclusively) for arthritis sufferers. For hip replacement—the most common type—the success rate is almost 95 percent during the first 5 to 10 years, according to the Arthritis Foundation.

Before considering surgery, patients should consult their physicians about more conservative treatments—rest, ice or heat, muscle-strengthening exercises, and pain medication. Indications for joint replacement include the following:

- Failure of arthritis to respond adequately to the various antiarthritic drugs or drug combinations and lifestyle changes within six months
- Joint pain severe enough to cause awakening at night
- Joint pain that limits walking endurance to about one block
- Evidence of substantial joint degeneration on x-rays, but only if accompanied by severe pain. (Even when x-rays show significant joint deterioration, some arthritis patients have little or no pain.)

Joint replacement options. Two types of hip and knee joint replacements are available: cemented and uncemented. Cemented joints are literally glued to the natural bone; uncemented joints are covered with a porous, bumpy material into which the natural bone eventually grows and attaches itself. Cemented joints offer the advantage of faster healing; they are strong on the day they are put in place and can bear weight right away. Yet they may have a limited lifetime, because the growth of soft tissue between the cement and the bone can cause the artificial joint to loosen. At some point this loosening may necessitate further surgery, called a revision, which entails extra risks and costs. About half of all cemented hip and knee joints have to be redone within 10 to 20 years. One way to minimize the need for revision is to postpone the initial replacement procedure as long as possible.

In contrast, an uncemented joint is not initially physically connected to the natural bone, but rather wedged tightly in the proper place. It will get even stronger over time. Theoretically, uncemented joints should last longer because the bone growth into them only increases their strength. But uncemented joints have not been used long enough to prove that this theory holds true in practice. And for some unknown reason, as many as 30 percent of those with uncemented total-hip prostheses develop hip pain.

In general, uncemented joints are probably better for patients under age 65, who are more likely to need revision of a cemented joint due to the probable length of time the implant will be in place. After 65, when natural bone gets thinner, a cemented joint may be safer. The decision on the type of joint replacement is contingent not only upon the individual patient's age, but also on his or her lifestyle and general health. For example, an uncemented prosthesis may be best for a very active 65-year-old, while a sedentary 55-year-old with osteoporosis may opt for a cemented joint.

Revisions tend to be riskier operations than the initial replacement surgery. It is basically a more complicated version of the first procedure: More bone is cut away, the surgery takes longer, and blood loss is greater. On top of this, since it takes place up to 20 years after the original surgery, the patient is older and perhaps less healthy.

Significant complications of joint replacement surgery occur in about 5 percent of cases. The most frequent are blood clots, though surgeons are careful to take extra precautions to help prevent them. A potentially more serious but less common complication is infection, which usually requires removal of the prosthesis and several weeks in the hospital. Eventually, a new prosthesis may be implanted, but the joint remains unstable until then.

Rehabilitation. Immediately after the surgery, considerable pain may result—from muscles disturbed during the operation, rather than from the joint itself. Rehabilitation begins in the hospital, usually the day after surgery, with passive motion exercises to maintain the mobility of the muscles supporting the joint. The patient won't be able to get up and walk normally right away because the new joint is still unstable, but walking with assistance should be possible within a day or two. However, a walker—and then crutches—will be needed for several weeks until the joint is stable enough to bear full weight. Full recovery usually takes about six weeks. During that time a rather strict timetable of exercise, rest, and medication is crucial to the success of the surgery.

Continuous passive motion (CPM) may be used when the knee joint is replaced. This therapy utilizes a device that slowly but continually bends and straightens the patient's leg for several hours a day, gradually increasing the range of movement. The patient can read a book, watch television, or talk with visitors; the machine, stationed at the foot of the patient's bed, does all the work. Compared with standard therapy in one study, CPM combined with standard therapy improved early recovery of joint function, decreased postoperative swelling, and ultimately cost substantially less than standard therapy alone (because it eliminated the need for expensive hands-on treatment by a physical therapist).

Research shows that the success of total joint replacement depends, to a great extent, on the motivation and participation of the patient following the operation. In fact, the decision to have joint replacement surgery should be accompanied by a commitment to this period of recuperation. Successful joint replacement, especially knee replacement, requires quite an investment of time and energy in postsurgical rehabilitation, but the rewards are great, and are not exclusively physical ones. Studies of joint replacement patients have shown improvements in psychological well-being and life-satisfaction, as well as reduced pain. *The Editors*

RHEUMATOID ARTHRITIS

Less common than osteoarthritis, rheumatoid arthritis affects some 1 to 2 percent of the population. Three times more women than men suffer from rheumatoid arthritis, which strikes multiple joints as well as other tissues and organs throughout the body. Although manifestations begin most often between ages 20 and 40, rheumatoid arthritis may start at any age.

CAUSES

The joint damage caused by rheumatoid arthritis (see the illustration on page 393) begins with inflammation of the synovial membrane. Although the source of this inflammation is unknown, the disease is considered an autoimmune disorder. Such disorders result when the body initiates an immunological response against some natural body constituent that has been mistakenly recognized as foreign. The inflammation leads to a thickened synovial membrane (which is called a pannus), due to overgrowth

of synovial cells and an accumulation of white blood cells. Release of enzymes and growth factors by these cells, along with continuing growth of the pannus, can erode the articular cartilage as well as the bones, tendons, and ligaments within the joint capsule.

As rheumatoid arthritis progresses, the production of excess fibrous tissue can further limit joint motion. Inflammation of tissues surrounding the joint also contributes to joint damage.

SYMPTOMS

Most often the onset of rheumatoid arthritis is marked by nonspecific symptoms, such as fatigue, weakness, low-grade fever, and loss of appetite and weight. Such symptoms may or may not be accompanied by mild joint stiffness or pain. Stiffness is most prominent in the morning and improves during the day; the period of stiffness lengthens when the disease is more active, and tends to recur after prolonged inactivity (this result is known as gelling). The joints that most often become inflamed (red, warm, swollen, and painful) are those of the fingers, wrists, knees, ankles, and toes—typically on both sides of the body.

This symmetrical pattern, as well as the signs of inflammation, differentiates rheumatoid arthritis from osteoarthritis. Also, unlike osteoarthritis, the joints at the tips of the fingers are generally not affected by rheumatoid arthritis. Another characteristic feature of rheumatoid arthritis is the formation of chronic collections of inflammatory cells (rheumatoid nodules) that can be found in tissues throughout the body, but especially over bony prominences such as the elbows or heels.

If the disease progresses for months or years, affected joints eventually become deformed and their range of motion becomes increasingly more limited. Rheumatoid nodules are found under the skin in about 20 percent of patients. Other manifestations may include atrophy of the skin and muscles around affected joints, carpal tunnel syndrome, and dryness of the eyes, mouth, and other mucous membranes (Sjögren's syndrome). Infrequently, patients may experience serious systemic problems, such as inflammation of the membrane covering the heart (pericarditis) or of the heart muscle itself; an enlarged spleen; inflammation of the membranes surrounding the lung (pleurisy); and inflammation of the eye's outer layers that can lead to blindness.

DIAGNOSIS

It is difficult to make a diagnosis of rheumatoid arthritis in the early stages of the disease. In fact, rheumatoid arthritis cannot be definitively diagnosed until symptoms are present for six weeks because evidence supporting the diagnosis does not appear until the first month or two. Initially, then, the diagnosis is made by ruling out all other possible causes for the symptoms. The doctor will take a medical history and conduct a physical examination similar to those used in diagnosing osteoarthritis. If rheumatoid arthritis is suspected, the diagnosis can be confirmed later with x-rays and laboratory tests. Certainly, the presence of multiple red, swollen joints that are warm to the touch is strongly suggestive of rheumatoid arthritis, particularly if the joints are involved symmetrically on both sides of the body. However, these signs are present only during active stages of the disease (which can go into remission periodically), and may not be detectable in joints that are deeply buried in the body, such as the hip.

PROGNOSIS

About 10 percent of patients diagnosed with rheumatoid arthritis experience a complete remission within one year. Another 40 to 65 percent go into remission within two years. These two groups of patients often have a low or negative level of rheumatoid factor and rel-atively mild symptoms, even when the disease is active. The prognosis is much worse for those whose disease remains active for more than two years. Not only do they have a far greater chance of significant joint deformity, but they also have a lower overall survival rate because of systemic disorders that accompany the disease. The lungs, heart, gastrointestinal tract, and eyes may all be affected by rheumatoid arthritis or its treatment.

TREATMENT

The goals in the treatment of rheumatoid arthritis are to relieve pain, reduce inflammation, maintain function, and prevent deformities. Medications are required to control pain and diminish inflammation. Other therapeutic components include an appropriate mixture of rest periods and gentle exercise, as well as physical therapy and protection of the joints (for example, using splints). A thorough understanding of the disease and a positive attitude are also tremendous assets. One change that is currently taking place in treatment approaches for rheumatoid arthritis is a movement among physicians to prescribe stronger antirheumatic drugs earlier in treatment to control symptoms more quickly in hopes of lessening damage.

Patients with rheumatoid arthritis can benefit from many of the treatments for osteoarthritis, including icing the affected joints to reduce pain and inflammation, exercise to build strength and flexibility, surgery to replace damaged joints, and developing strategies to cope with the emotional and psychological factors associated with a chronic illness. However, topical preparations don't work for those with rheumatoid arthritis, and pain management with nonsteroidal anti-inflammatory drugs (NSAIDs) is different. Additional medications are employed in the treatment of rheumatoid arthritis to control inflammation. And patients with rheumatoid arthritis must pay special attention to combating fatigue, which can be the most incapacitating feature of the disease. Proper rest and the use of splints and other assistive devices when joints are inflamed can help relieve fatigue.

Rest

Inflamed joints must be rested; they are easily damaged, and rest can decrease the inflammation. Complete bed rest may be necessary during periods of severe inflammation involving multiple joints. As severe inflammation subsides, or with more moderate degrees of inflammation, it is important to employ physical therapy to avoid flexion contracture—a loss of joint motion due to shortening of the surrounding tissues—especially in the hips and knees.

Exercise

When joints are inflamed, only passive range-of-motion exercises are appropriate (see page 395). Hydrotherapy (exercise in water) is also a good exercise option for people with rheumatoid arthritis, since the buoyancy created by the water helps alleviate weight-bearing stress on the joints. Many local arthritis organizations have been instrumental in establishing accessible and affordable water-based (as well as land-based) exercise programs for patients with arthritis. More strenuous resistance exercises can be introduced gradually as joint inflammation subsides. However, an exercise should be avoided if it worsens pain an hour later. A program of moderate aerobic exercise to help increase endurance and keep joints flexible should be performed when joints are not inflamed.

Splints and Assistive Devices

Splints are over-the-counter or custom-made supports designed to relieve pain and stabilize and protect joints during periods of inflammation, when joints (especially those in the hands and wrists) are more prone to injury. Splints should be lightweight and easy to remove, allowing for range-of-motion exercises several times daily. Prolonged or improper use can increase stiffness and progressively diminish strength and joint mobility. The most effective splints are those for the hands, wrists, or both. For the hip and knee joints, the best "splint" is lying in a face-down position on a firm bed, several times a day. For the elbow and shoulder joints, judicious use of local treatments like injections of inflammation-reducing steroids and appropriate use of physical therapy are preferable to splints, which pose the risk of rapid loss of joint mobility in these areas.

Assistive devices help with the performance of daily activities. Most familiar are canes, crutches, and walkers. Other examples of simple assistive devices are raised toilet seats and firm pillows placed under the seats of chairs to help people with hip or knee arthritis to rise from a sitting position. Additional assistive devices include faucet turners, openers for jars and doors, elbow crutches, and extended handles on combs, hairbrushes, toothbrushes, and tools. In fact, an enormous array of helpful devices is available. It is probably best to use only those that are absolutely essential to maintain independence.

Occupational therapists are experts in fabricating splints, recommending assistive devices, and instructing patients on their proper use. These practitioners can help arthritis sufferers to overcome physical limitations by suggesting specific, practical lifestyle changes, in addition to selecting the proper splints and assistive devices.

Drug Treatment: Nonsteroidal Anti-inflammatory Drugs (NSAIDs)

Unless there is some contraindication (such as an allergy), aspirin is usually the first drug used, because it is effective in reducing inflammation and is less expensive than other NSAIDs. Dosage depends on a balance between the large amounts of a drug that may be needed to control symptoms and the development of toxic side effects. Enteric-coated aspirin may reduce the risk of stomach irritation.

Other NSAIDs are warranted when aspirin is ineffective or causes serious side effects. These drugs are more expensive than aspirin, but compliance may be better because they do not have to be taken as often. Although no single one of the many available NSAIDs has proven more effective in the treatment of rheumatoid arthritis, some patients respond better to one drug than to others. As in the treatment of osteoarthritis, the goal is to prescribe the NSAID that provides the greatest benefit while producing the least risk of side effects. The recent introduction of a special class of NSAIDs called COX-2 inhibitors has significantly reduced the risk of causing gastrointestinal irritation and ulcers. Celecoxib (Celebrex) is the first of this class to gain approval for rheumatoid arthritis.

Drug Treatment: Antirheumatics

The current trend is to move patients more rapidly to other, more potent antirheumatic drugs when the basic anti-inflammatories fail to control symptoms adequately. These drugs had been called disease-modifying antirheumatic drugs (DMARDs). But only some of these agents demonstrated any evidence of this effect. They are also sometimes called SAARDs (for slow-acting antirheumatic drugs).

Antimalarials. The most commonly used antimalarial is hydroxychloroquine sulfate (Plaquenil). Only about one in four patients with rheumatoid arthritis responds to this drug, and the improvement does not start for three to six months. Its advantage is a low incidence of side effects. The most serious toxicity—visual loss due to inflammation of the retina—is rare at low doses, but regular eye exams are required with long-term treatment. Other side effects include upset stomach and skin rash.

Azathioprine. Azathioprine (Imuran) is an antimetabolite (a substance that blocks a normal metabolic process due to its chemical resemblance to an essential vitamin or other compound), most commonly employed as an immunosuppressant to prevent rejection of transplanted kidneys and hearts. Azathioprine's mechanism of action in rheumatoid arthritis is unknown; and it is used only when severe symptoms fail to respond to safer drugs, since it can cause dangerous suppression of the immune system, leading to the development of serious infections. It can take several months to work.

Corticosteroids. Corticosteroids (such as prednisone) usually produce rapid and dramatic symptomatic improvement by reducing inflammation and suppressing the immune system, but disease manifestations frequently recur once the steroids are discontinued. As a result, physicians and patients alike have been tempted to continue steroid use for long periods, despite many serious side effects, which can include stomach ulcers; weight gain with deposition of fat in the trunk of the body, especially in the upper back; diabetes; high blood pressure; thinning of the skin with ready bruising and poor wound healing; acne; weakness; muscle wasting; osteoporosis; cataracts; increased susceptibility to infections; and psychiatric disturbances.

When corticosteroids are used at high doses or for a long time, the dose must be reduced very slowly to prevent a flare-up of the arthritis and to avoid the symptoms of adrenal insufficiency (since corticosteroid administration stops the normal formation of steroids by the adrenal glands). As a result, treatment with small doses of corticosteroids is often needed for long periods.

Corticosteroid use is best reserved for the treatment of incapacitating flare-ups of joint disease, other severe manifestations of rheumatoid arthritis, or when other measures are unsuccessful or cause intolerable side effects.

Cyclophosphamide. Cyclophosphamide (Cytoxan), an anticancer drug, has proven beneficial in experimental studies with rheumatoid arthritis patients who have not responded adequately to any other therapeutic measures. It is essential for people taking this drug to drink a lot of fluids to maintain good urine flow, since serious inflammation of the bladder (hemorrhagic cystitis) is one of the side effects. (Because many rheumatoid arthritis patients are young women, it should be pointed out that Cytoxan can cause fetal damage if administered to a pregnant woman. It can also cause ovarian failure, leading to premature menopause.)

Gold salts. Gold salt therapy (chrysotherapy), used in patients who do not respond to NSAIDs and are unable to take methotrexate (see below), is beneficial about 60 percent of the time. It appears to act by suppressing the inflammation of synovitis during active rheumatoid arthritis. It takes approximately eight weeks for the benefits of treatment to become apparent. Gold is administered either by weekly intramuscular injections or by twice-daily oral dosages, though injectable gold is more effective overall than the oral method. Side effects, which occur in about one-third of patients receiving gold injections, include dermatitis (skin rash), inflammation of the mucous membranes of the mouth (stomatitis), protein in the urine, and a drop in white blood cell levels. Diarrhea is common during oral gold treatment, but the other side effects, especially protein in the urine, occur less frequently.

Methotrexate. Methotrexate (Rheumatrex), an antimetabolite that acts as a mild immunosuppressant, was first used to treat various forms of cancer. It is now recognized that methotrexate may be the drug of choice for people whose severe rheumatoid arthritis does not respond to NSAIDs. It often leads to improvement within a month—much more quickly than with antimalarials, gold, or penicillamine (see below). The drug is taken oral-

ly once a week and is usually well tolerated. The most common side effects of methotrexate are irritation of the stomach and inflammation of the mucous membranes of the mouth (stomatitis). Rarely, the drug may produce a dangerous toxic reaction, causing lung inflammation, bone marrow suppression, and severe liver damage.

Because methotrexate may harm the liver, a biopsy—removal of a sample of the liver to check for damage—was previously recommended every two to three years for patients taking this drug. However, a number of studies have suggested that regular use of this procedure may be inappropriate. Biopsies are expensive and can cause complications of their own. The studies found that even if a biopsy was performed every five years, the risk of complications from the biopsy was equal to the chance of finding liver damage. Instead, they recommend blood tests every four to 12 weeks to monitor liver function. A biopsy is performed if blood tests indicate liver damage.

Penicillamine. Penicillamine has proven effective, particularly in studies carried out in England, among patients who are unresponsive to all other measures. But its use is limited by a large number of possible untoward reactions, which occur in about half the people taking this drug. Side effects include fever, rash, mouth ulcers, loss of taste, protein in the urine, and low levels of white blood cells and blood platelets.

Leflunomide. Leflunomide (Arava) is a recently approved antimetabolite that improves symptoms of rheumatoid arthritis and appears to slow joint erosion. It is taken once a day. Its safety and effectiveness are similar to methotrexate, though it is considerably more expensive than that drug.

Etanercept. Etanercept (Enbrel) is a newly approved agent created using recombinant DNA technology, which blocks the action of tumor necrosis factor—one of the major cytokines involved in the inflammation associated with rheumatoid arthritis. It is given by injection twice a week. Proven effective in reducing symptoms of active disease, etanercept has not been shown to slow joint erosion.

Cyclosporine A. Used primarily to prevent rejection of transplanted organs, cyclosporine A has been found useful in the management of severe rheumatoid arthritis. Because of its toxicity, cyclosporine A should be tried only when less toxic agents are ineffective.

Surgery

Patients with rheumatoid arthritis can benefit from the same surgical procedures as those with osteoarthritis (see page 397). Also, when rheumatoid arthritis involves the wrists, elbows, shoulders, hips, or knees, a synovectomy may be effective. This procedure consists of removing only the diseased synovium from the joint. Symptoms can recur, however, because the synovium often grows back within several years following the surgery.

The Editors

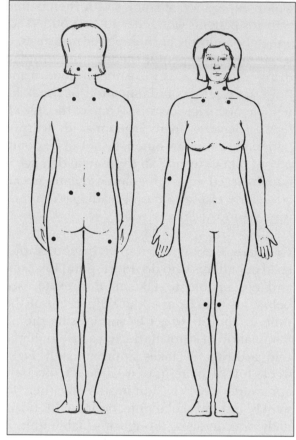

The dots indicate the locations of "tender points" common to fibromyalgia. Patients experience undue soreness when pressure is applied to these regions.

FIBROMYALGIA

About 6 million Americans suffer from fibromyalgia, a condition characterized by fatigue, stiffness, and chronic pain in the muscles, tendons (which connect muscle to bone), and ligaments (which connect bone to bone). Women are 10 times more likely to have the condition than men, and typically begin to develop symptoms between ages 20 and 60. Twenty percent of those with rheumatoid arthritis may also have fibromyalgia.

Symptoms can be debilitating; indeed, in a study of 280 women, the participants with fibromyalgia had lower quality of life scores than those with osteoarthritis, rheumatoid arthritis, insulin-dependent diabetes, and advanced lung disease. And yet—while fibromyalgia is one of the most common arthritis-related diseases (second only to osteoarthritis)—the average patient waits five years before being properly diagnosed.

The delay is largely because fibromyalgia is difficult to positively identify. Symptoms can be associated with many other medical problems, including other types of arthritis, chronic fatigue syndrome, Lyme disease, and even the flu. Furthermore, laboratory tests and diagnostic imaging studies cannot confirm the presence of fibromyalgia. Consequently, physicians must rely on conclusions drawn from the patient's medical history and a physical examination; objective clinical criteria for these procedures were not readily available until guidelines were published in 1990.

IDENTIFYING FIBROMYALGIA

Unlike most other rheumatic conditions, fibromyalgia is not progressive, nor does it damage the joints, involve detectable inflammation, or cause joint deformities. It is distinguished from other medical problems when there is tenderness in at least 11 of 18 specific locations on the body. Most patients always have some amount of general discomfort, but the severity varies according to the time of day, activity level, weather, sleep patterns, and stress. About 90 percent of patients are also fatigued, leading to decreased exercise tolerance and eventual exhaustion.

The fatigue may be due in part to the abnormal sleep patterns seen in most patients. Some studies have shown that in those with fibromyalgia, delta sleep (the deepest stage of sleep) is usually disrupted by alpha waves (a much faster type of brain wave pattern). However, a recent study demonstrated that this finding may not be unique to fibromyalgia.

All people need a certain amount of undisturbed delta sleep to feel rested. How much depends on age and other individual criteria. Interestingly, disturbing the sleep of people who don't have fibromyalgia can produce fibromyalgia-like symptoms—but only in subjects who are not physically fit, leading some researchers to speculate that physical deconditioning is an important risk factor for the condition.

Other symptoms associated with fibromyalgia are mood changes, headaches, abdominal pain, alternating constipation and diarrhea, urinary urgency, and sensitivity to temperature changes. Tingling sensations in the hands, arms, feet, legs, and face are also sometimes present.

HOW FIBROMYALGIA IS TREATED

If you have undiagnosed muscle or joint pain that has lasted for more than six months, it's important to ask your physician about seeing a rheumatologist (a specialist in joint disorders).

Once identified, fibromyalgia can be treated with medications to diminish pain and improve sleep, exercises to stretch muscles and increase cardiovascular fitness, and relaxation techniques to help release tense muscles. It's also important not to smoke, because the chemicals in tobacco smoke deprive muscles of oxygen and make them more vulnerable to insults from other health problems or injuries. You should also avoid large amounts of any substance that hinders sleep, such as alcohol (which may make you feel sleepy, but actually interferes with deep sleep) and caffeine.

Medication

Over-the-counter medications, such as aspirin, ibuprofen, and acetaminophen, may help to minimize pain and stiffness. Even though these drugs can be purchased without a prescription, you should take them only under the supervision of your doctor. Frequent, long-term use requires careful monitoring in order to reap the maximum benefit without side effects, such as stomach irritation.

Antidepressant drugs such as amitriptyline (Elavil), nortriptyline (Pamelor), and doxepin (Sinequan) may also be useful. Because they're taken in small doses before bedtime, these medications act, at least in part, as muscle relaxants and sleep aids, rather than as antidepressants.

Physiotherapy

The benefits of exercise may be great. Although at first they may cause soreness, stretching and aerobic activities will soon lead to less pain. Low-impact exercises such as walking, biking, swimming, and water aerobics are best. Start slowly in a program supervised by a physical therapist or other trained professional. (Your physician can refer you to

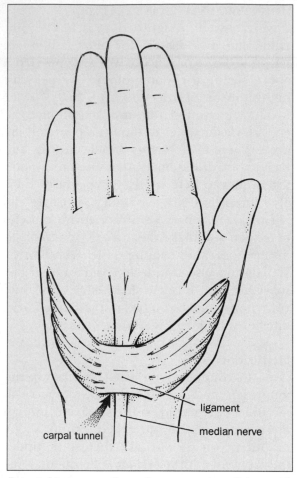

ligament

carpal tunnel — median nerve

Repeated pressure on the median nerve can result in carpal tunnel syndrome. Symptoms include numbness and pain in the hand or wrist.

a qualified practitioner.) The goal is usually 30 minutes of continuous, comfortably paced aerobic activity three to four times a week, in addition to stretching.

Your physical therapist may also incorporate heat, ice, massage, whirlpool, ultrasound, or electrical stimulation treatments into your routine. Relaxation techniques, such as biofeedback or yoga, may also be useful for soothing aching muscles.

For more information about fibromyalgia, write to the Arthritis Foundation, 1330 West Peachtree Street, Atlanta, GA 30309.

The Editors

CARPAL TUNNEL SYNDROME

Carpal tunnel syndrome (CTS) is a painful and often debilitating condition that occurs when the median nerve, which passes through a narrow tunnel of wrist (carpal) bones and soft tissues at the base of the hand, becomes compressed by surrounding tissue or excess fluid. Symptoms, including numbness and pain in the hand and wrist, may appear suddenly or gradually, and often affect both hands. The disorder occurs most often among women between the ages of 30 and 60. A study showing increased incidence of CTS among pregnant and menopausal women suggests that hormonal factors may play a role. Rheumatoid arthritis, which causes joint inflammation and deformity, is another commonly reported factor, as are diabetes mellitus and thyroid disease, among others.

Perhaps the most stressful actions implicated in CTS are wringing motions and the movements associated with playing a musical instrument, knitting, using power tools that vibrate, typing, using a computer mouse, and tightly gripping a steering wheel for long periods. Fortunately, using your hands wisely can help to prevent CTS (see box on page 407). Furthermore, if CTS does occur, early diagnosis and treatment can generally ensure relief and full recovery.

SYMPTOMS AND DIAGNOSIS
Derived from the Greek word "karpos," meaning wrist, the carpal tunnel is a passageway into the hand for the median nerve (which provides sensory and motor function to the thumb, index, and middle fingers, and the side of the ring finger toward the thumb) and nine tendons (which flex the fingers). As the fingers move, the tendons that control them ordinarily slide back and forth beside the

bones and ligaments that form the corridor. CTS develops when the membrane that lubricates the tendons (the tendon sheath) becomes inflamed and swollen, thus pressing the median nerve against the carpal bones.

Symptoms usually begin with tingling or numbness in the hand, often the dominant one, and are often first noticed at night. Pain, burning, weakness, and stiffness sometimes follow. All fingers except the pinky may be affected. You may find yourself shaking your hands and fingers frequently because they feel as if they are asleep, or you may notice yourself dropping things.

If you have any of these symptoms, rest your hands until they subside. You should also see your physician. If left untreated, CTS can lead to muscle atrophy and permanent nerve damage, and may cause pain throughout the length of the arm.

If your physician suspects CTS, you may be referred to a specialist, who will perform tests to assess the extent of your sensory and motor loss. A nerve conduction velocity test pinpoints how much the median nerve is pinched; electromyography (EMG) assesses motor control; x-rays may be taken to rule out a bone fracture or arthritis as the cause of your symptoms.

TREATMENT OPTIONS

The goal of initial treatment is to decrease the inflammation in the carpal tunnel through rest or drug therapy. The wrist may be immobilized with a lightweight, plastic splint that still permits use of the hand for most daily tasks. Your physician will probably recommend wearing the splint all day. However, some patients get relief just by wearing the splint at night.

Nonsteroidal anti-inflammatory drugs (NSAIDs), such as aspirin and ibuprofen, may also ease pain. If this approach is unhelpful, injection of a corticosteroid drug into the carpal tunnel may decrease swelling. Results

PREVENTING CTS

If you use your hands for prolonged, repetitive tasks, or if you have sprained your wrist, have arthritis, or are menopausal, you may be at increased risk of developing carpal tunnel syndrome. The following tips may help you reduce this risk:

• If your hand hurts during a repetitive activity, give it a rest. Even if hand pain hasn't occurred, take short preventive breaks from hand-intensive work every half hour or so.

• Lift objects with your whole hand and all your fingers, not just your thumb and index finger.

• Don't hold your hands in the same position or keep your wrists flexed for long periods of time.

• Don't prop your head on your hands when you sleep.

• When typing, use a light stroke and do not rest your wrists on the keyboard or desk. Your fingers should be lower than your wrists; a pad on which to rest your wrists can be useful.

• When driving, hold the steering wheel gently.

of these injections are often dramatic, but the duration of relief is limited.

If these measures fail and symptoms persist for several months, you may need to undergo surgery—especially if muscle and nerve fibers have deteriorated. In the standard practice, called open release, the thick, fibrous band of tissue (transverse ligament) that forms the floor of the carpal tunnel is severed, thus relieving pressure and creating more room in the passageway. Severing the ligament creates a slight change in wrist anatomy without noticeably impairing function. If muscles and nerves have not been damaged by inflammation, most patients can expect complete recovery.

Open release is an outpatient surgery. A regional or local anesthesia is given, and an incision of about two inches is made across the wrist. The surgeon then examines the inside of the wrist directly, cuts the ligament, and closes the incision. The procedure may take up to an hour, and patients go home the same day. Rehabilitation can take as long as seven weeks.

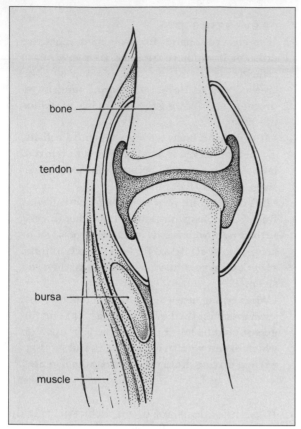

Bursitis is inflammation of the small, fluid-filled bursa inside the joint; tendinitis is inflammation of a tendon attaching a muscle to a bone.

A New Treatment Technique

A new procedure using an endoscope—a slender, flexible, lighted tube about the thickness of a pencil—has dramatically reduced recovery time for some patients. The endoscope is inserted into the wrist through an incision a little larger than the instrument. A miniaturized camera and knife are then inserted into the carpal tunnel through or alongside the endoscope. The surgeon examines and severs the ligament while controlling the knife from outside the wrist, watching the procedure on a video monitor that receives an image from the camera.

Endoscopy is an outpatient procedure that lasts about an hour, and can be performed under general or a re-gional anesthetic. Its chief advantage is that less tissue is disturbed, cutting recuperation time in half.

Endoscopy is not for everyone with CTS, however. People with arthritis or limited wrist mobility should have only the traditional open-release procedure. These conditions require maximum visibility for the surgeon.

Complications for both techniques include the possibility of an incompletely severed transverse ligament, and damage to nerve tissue and arteries. The risk of these complications is less than 1 percent with open release, but rises to between 2 and 8 percent with endoscopy. The method you select depends on how much time you have for recovery, what margin of risk you are comfortable with, and which procedure your physician favors.

The Editors

BURSITIS

The human body has approximately 150 small, fluid-filled sacs tucked into the spaces where muscles or tendons move over bones or other

PREVENTION TIPS
Here are some ways to prevent bursitis:
• **Wear protective pads and other gear when playing sports. Check with a coach, trainer, or pro to be sure that you are using proper techniques, since poor form can easily lead to soft tissue injuries.**
• **Avoid overly strenuous or repetitive physical activities, if possible.**
• **If you must work in a kneeling position, use knee pads or cushions, change positions often, and take frequent breaks.**
• **To prevent bursitis in the feet, wear high heels only when you have to; buy new running shoes when old ones wear out.**

muscles. These little sacs, called bursae (from the Greek for wine skins), produce a lubricating fluid and serve to cushion the muscles, bones, and other parts of the joints so they can move easily, without friction. But, irritation, overuse, or injury to a joint can cause inflammation of a bursa—the painful condition known as bursitis. Common causes include:

- Activities that put constant pressure on a bursa (such as kneeling or resting your elbow on a desk)
- Repetitive and vigorous joint movement (such as hammering or swinging a tennis racquet)
- A blow or other injury to a bursa
- Arthritis, gout, and certain infections
- Calcium deposits in, or degeneration of, an adjacent tendon

The shoulders, elbows, hips, knees, heels, and the base of the big toe are among the sites most commonly affected. Bursitis has acquired a number of familiar names, depending on the body part involved. These include "student's elbow" (for inflammation of the olecranon bursa in the elbow, due to habitual resting of an elbow on a desk), "pump bumps" (for the effect of high-heeled shoes on the Achilles bursa), and "housemaid's knee" (for inflammation of the bursae over the kneecap, due to excessive kneeling).

The primary symptoms are pain and swelling in or around the affected bursa, with restricted and painful movement. Bursitis in the shoulder can produce pain in the neck or arms. Fortunately, with proper treatment, the acute pain of bursitis usually subsides within a few days, and all traces of symptoms usually vanish within two weeks, although recurrence is common, and subsequent flare-ups often take longer to respond to treatment.

TREATMENT
When bursitis strikes, rest and avoid putting pressure on the affected area. Use ice packs for the first 48 hours to relieve pain, swelling, and inflammation. Then, if desired, switch to heat packs, which stimulate blood flow and ease pain. If necessary, use over-the-counter pain relievers such as aspirin or acetaminophen. Doctors generally do not recommend liniments, however, since topical treatments are usually not very effective, nor do they help to repair the underlying damage.

If pain or swelling persists for more than two weeks despite self-treatment, make an appointment with your doctor, who may provide you with a splint, brace, or sling to help you keep the joint still. In more serious cases, your doctor may administer injections of corticosteroids to reduce inflammation, or a local anesthetic (such as Xylocaine) to ease pain. To reduce swelling, excess fluid may be drawn from the bursa with a syringe, and the joint is then tightly bandaged. During the healing period, gradually resume joint movement to prevent stiffening, but avoid any activities that aggravate the condition. In severe, persistent cases of bursitis, surgery to remove the bursa may be necessary.   *The Editors*

TENDINITIS

Tendinitis (literally, inflammation of a tendon) is characterized by microscopic tears in a tendon, most often brought about gradually from a repetitive activity such as cycling, running, or hitting a tennis ball. Anytime you move a muscle too suddenly, too frequently, or with too much force, you may injure the tendon that connects it to the bone. Almost all active people eventually suffer some form of tendon injury. Even if you're sedentary, you can develop tendinitis from repetitive activities such as playing a musical instrument or slot machine for long hours, carrying a heavy briefcase every day, or sustaining a sudden physical injury, such as falling on an arm, twisting an ankle, or trying to lift an object that's too heavy for you.

Nearly every sport and activity has its vulnerable tendon or tendons. Sites most commonly affected include the rotator cuff or shoulder ("golfer's shoulder"), the elbow ("tennis elbow"), the wrist ("de Quervain's wrist"), the fingers ("trigger finger"), and the ankle ("Achilles heel"). Pain usually develops gradually with overuse. When the muscles in the affected area are used regularly despite the initial pain, the injured tendon may be slow to heal. While many cases of tendinitis last no more than two weeks and are usually alleviated by rest and proper conditioning, repeated use of the injured area may lead to chronic tendinitis, characterized by scarring of the involved tissues and limited flexibility. Those over 40 are most prone to chronic tendinitis.

TREATMENT

At the first signs of tendinitis—pain and swelling—you should stop any activity that aggravates the condition. It's usually wise at this stage to consult your doctor (who may refer you to a physical therapist), unless it's an injury you've had before and know how to treat. For the first 72 hours, rest and periodically ice the affected area to reduce inflammation. A compression bandage can help minimize swelling. After that you should start applying heat—or alternate heat and cold—to increase circulation and speed healing. Take over-the-counter anti-inflammatories, such as ibuprofen, if necessary. Start stretching to restore flexibility, and then gradually add strengthening exercises with light weights to strengthen the muscle.

If muscle or joint pain persists for more than two weeks and interferes with ordinary activities despite self-treatment, notify your doctor, who may provide you with slings or splints to immobilize the injured area for a few days. In serious cases, corticosteroids may be injected directly into the affected area to ease pain and inflammation. (However, such therapy is not recommended for Achilles tendinitis, where injections may weaken or rupture the tendon.) A more seriously torn or ruptured tendon may require surgical repair.

PREVENTION

Here are a few simple things you can do to minimize your risk of developing tendinitis:

- Don't overdo it. Suddenly increasing the number of miles you normally run or working out more strenuously or longer than usual can produce muscle fatigue leading to an injury.
- Warm up and stay flexible. Exercising with tight muscles puts extra stress on tendons. Always warm up and stretch thoroughly before exercising, and stretch again afterwards during the cooling down period.
- Exercise caution as you grow older. Starting as early as your thirties, tendons gradually lose elasticity and become more brittle.
- Develop the right technique. An improperly executed backhand is often the cause of tennis elbow, just as the wrong golf swing can lead to a rotator cuff injury. A coach, trainer, or professional can give you pointers on proper technique.
- Get the right equipment. A bike that's too small can cause tendinitis in the knee; running shoes with worn-down heels can lead to Achilles tendinitis.
- Listen to your body. If you feel pain or discomfort signaling a tendon injury, reduce the intensity of your workout or try a different activity until the tendon heals. Temporarily switch to low-impact exercise like swimming if you suspect high-impact exercise is causing a problem.
- Compensate for musculoskeletal problems. For instance, if your feet roll inward (overpronate) as you run, or your legs are different lengths, you may develop the form of tendinitis called runner's knee.

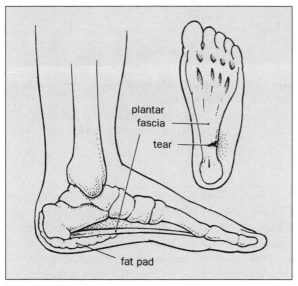

The plantar fascia runs from the heel bone to the underside of the toes. A tear can occur where this fibrous band connects to the heel, causing pain.

You may need to consult a physical therapist, podiatrist, orthopedist, or other specialist about diagnosis and treatment.

• Counter muscle imbalances. If your calf muscles are very strong but you don't strengthen the opposing muscles in the shins, you increase the chances of injuring your Achilles tendon. Strengthen the important muscle groups for your activity.

The Editors

FOOT PROBLEMS

Every day, the average person takes about 10,000 steps; in a lifetime, you may walk 115,000 miles—the equivalent of four and a half strolls around the planet. Each one of those steps exerts a force even greater than your body weight on certain bones and muscles of your feet. Running triples that force. It's no wonder that this cumulative pounding, complicated by ill-fitting shoes and the natural changes that occur with aging, can conspire to cause aching feet.

Healthy feet are crucial for an active and independent lifestyle, but four out of five adults experience foot pain—and the great majority of them are over 50. Yet, according to a poll conducted by the Gallup Organization, 62 percent of Americans think foot pain is normal—which may be why the foot problems that tend to worsen with age are too often ignored. Left untreated, foot ailments can result in altered gait and posture, which can progress to pain in the ankles, knees, hips, and lower back. However, pain in your feet is not normal, nor need it be tolerated. To counteract the effects of aging feet, it's important that you care for them properly, and seek professional care when problems occur.

HOW FEET AGE

As you get older, various changes in the feet combine to increase the likelihood of problems. The normal aging of the skin—which, for instance, causes it to become more easily dehydrated and lose its elasticity—may have more serious consequences on the feet than elsewhere, because it makes them more susceptible to bacterial and fungal infections. Calluses, which can make walking painful, tend to develop on the weight-bearing points because the soles and heels lose fat and become less padded. As the skin on the top (the dorsum) of your feet thins, it is more easily bruised by tight-fitting or tight-laced shoes. The nails, too, become thicker, brittle, and generally more difficult to care for.

The internal structure of your feet changes as well, as ligaments and tendons lose their elasticity, and muscle tone diminishes. This alters the shape of your feet so much that you may even have to switch shoe sizes. Usually, the feet become more splayed, necessitating shoes with larger forefoot space. Furthermore, foot problems can be caused or exacerbated by underlying conditions such as obesity, poor circulation, arthritis, and diabetes.

COMMON FOOT PROBLEMS AND TREATMENTS

	Foot Problem	*Self-Care/Products*
Bunion	Deformity at the big toe joint that causes the first joint to slant outward and rub against your shoe, leading to irritation, swelling, and inflammation (bursitis) of the joint.	• Wear low-heeled shoes with plenty of extra space for toes. • Do use doughnut-shaped bunion cushions or moleskin cut to size, which will take the pressure off the joint.
Calluses and Corns	A callus is a thickened pad of skin, usually on the weight-bearing portion of the sole, that results from chafing and pressure. A corn is a highly concentrated callus that occurs at a pressure point such as the top of the toe or under a toe joint. Either can become painful when they press on sensitive nerves in the surrounding skin, which may become red and inflamed.	• Soak feet daily for at least five minutes in warm water to soften skin. Use a rough towel, callus file, or pumice stone to remove the dead tissue. • Cover the area with a light pad or bandage. • Do not use medicated corn or callus pads, salicylic acid, or chemical corn removers. • Do use an unmedicated circular pad with a hole for the corn or callus, or moleskin cut to size and shape, to relieve pressure.
Hammertoe	A permanently bent, clawlike deformity in which the middle joint of a toe (usually the second digit) is bent downward. As the toe contracts and the joint extends upward, inflammation occurs on the top of the joint where it rubs against your shoes. Over time, hammertoes may impair walking.	• Wear shoes with resilient soles and enough forefoot room to protect the joints of the toes from irritation. • Do use toe caps—padded sleeves that wrap around the joint and raise the toe tips.
Heel Pain	Inflammation around a heel spur (a hook of bony overgrowth at the bottom of the heel bone), plantar fasciitis (inflammation of a band of tissue that connects the heel bone to the toes), or simply the stress of multiple impacts on hard surfaces can lead to redness, tenderness, or bruising in the heel or a burning sensation either directly under or just in front of the heel bone. Pain can occur after a long walk or without apparent reason, especially when you first arise in the morning.	• Wear low-heeled (but not flat), supportive, and well-cushioned shoes. Regular calf-stretching exercises are usually the best prevention and treatment for the pain of a heel spur and plantar fasciitis. • Do not use heel cups or cushions without consulting your podiatrist. If a precut variety is the wrong shape or size for your foot, it may do more harm than good.
Ingrown Toenail	A toenail edge that curves into the skin on the side of the toe, causing redness, swelling, and pain.	• To prevent, cut nails straight across. Wear wide, roomy shoes. To treat, soak feet until the nail is soft. If this doesn't work, see a podiatrist. • Do not use chemical "ingrown toenail relievers," which may remove healthy tissue as well.

What a Podiatrist May Do

Prescribe an orthotic—a custom-designed, molded plastic insert for your shoe that redistributes weight to take pressure off the big toe, supports the foot, and helps realign the toe. In severe cases, surgery (bunionectomy) may be needed.

Prescribe an orthotic, since the problem may be due to changes in the positions of the bones in the toes and forefoot region. Occasionally, surgery to remove a piece of bone or change the bone's position may be necessary to reduce these internal pressures.

Prescribe an orthotic (see bunion), which will not cure the problem, but can reposition the foot so that the muscles do not pull as hard on the toes. Surgery may be necessary in extreme cases.

Relieve inflammation with ibuprofen or other analgesics, or with steroid injections into the heel. May also prescribe an orthotic (see bunion). Will probably look for any underlying ailment, such as gout or arthritis, which may contribute to the problem. Surgery is rarely required.

Cut out edge of nail, possibly using a local anesthetic. If the toe is infected, your podiatrist will prescribe antibiotics.

REGULAR FOOT CARE

It is all too easy to ignore your feet until they give you pain and call for attention. But periodic care of your feet can often prevent problems from occurring at all, or at least minimize their severity.

- Wash your feet every day in warm water. Dry them by blotting with a towel, rather than rubbing.
- Dust your feet lightly with hygienic foot powder or plain talc if they perspire a lot. Sprinkle powder into your shoes as well. Don't use cornstarch powder because it feeds fungus.
- Examine your feet for red spots, sores, or any unusual skin lesions. Diabetics should perform such inspections daily.
- Trim your nails shortly after you have taken a bath or shower, when they are softer. Cut straight across with a toenail clipper.

ACTIVE FOOT CARE

The best way to take care of your feet is to use them as intended: for walking. Regular walking and other exercise will improve circulation, increase flexibility, reduce fatigue, and maintain bone and muscle strength.

Walking is crucial for maintaining the foot's overall condition. It improves strength, flexibility, and coordination in the supporting muscles of the shins and calves, and enhances circulation to the feet and legs. Try to schedule a brisk walk in your daily routine. Wear specially designed walking shoes, or ones that are flexible and provide good heel support. To fend off any injuries, warm up your muscles before walking.

Massaging your feet is a good way to relax them after an exercise session or just after a busy day. It also improves circulation to the skin and superficial tissues. You can massage your own feet, or have someone do it for you. Apply moisturizer to your hands, then gently stroke the entire foot, from the bottom of the shin to the end of the toes. Next, press on the ball of the foot and hold for 10 seconds. Press your thumbs into the heel of the foot and, moving in a circular motion, cover the sole from the heel to the ball. Now press your thumb into the spaces between the bones in the midfoot. Conclude by gently pulling on each toe and holding it for 10 seconds. (If you have diabetes, consult your doctor before doing foot massage.)

FINDING A FOOT SPECIALIST

When foot problems don't respond to home treatment, the right specialist depends in part on the nature of the problem. Orthopedists, for instance, will be able to help you with bone and joint disorders such as bunions and hammertoes. Few general physicians specialize in problems of the feet, although many are qualified to treat them.

The best all-around foot specialists are generally doctors of podiatric medicine (D.P.M.), or podiatrists. Although not M.D.s, they are medically trained, and can relate foot problems to overall health. They can prescribe medication and perform minor surgery, such as the removal of corns, calluses, and bunions. You should choose a podiatrist by asking for a referral from your primary-care physician or by contacting your local podiatry association. Most health insurance plans, including Medicare, cover certain podiatric services.

THE FOOT AND DIABETES

Foot care takes on crucial dimensions if you're a diabetic. Poor circulation to the extremities due to atherosclerosis of the large blood vessels as well as specific diabetic changes in the capillaries allow serious foot problems to develop more quickly in people with diabetes. Diabetic nerve damage can make such problems harder to detect, however, so that injuries and infections may go unnoticed for some time. Look for a persistent sensation of coldness, numbness, tingling, or burning. Other symptoms are dry and discolored skin, hair loss on your feet and legs, and muscle cramping or tightness.

Poor circulation can open the door for serious foot infections, skin ulceration, and other conditions. If you have diabetes, be especially vigilant about observing the aforementioned foot care pointers. In addition, it's very important for people with diabetes to wear comfortable shoes with plenty of support and room for their forefeet. To prevent cuts and bruises, don't go barefoot or wear sandals. Inspect your feet daily for cuts, blisters, and scratches. Consult your doctor immediately if you develop an ingrown toenail, athlete's foot, a cut or sore that doesn't heal quickly, or persistent discoloration. Be sure to tell your podiatrist that you have diabetes (see also Diabetes Mellitus, page 268.)

COMMON FOOT PROBLEMS

The problems listed in the box on pages 412–413 are among the most common foot ailments of people over 50. Most cases can be treated with self-care. But if pain persists or the problem causes changes in your gait, consult a podiatrist. If surgery is recommended, be sure to seek a second opinion. Also, check with your insurance company to make sure the surgery is covered.

The Editors

CHAPTER 13

The Skin

SKIN AND AGING

As we grow older, we see and feel certain changes in our skin, the body's largest and most visible organ. It becomes drier and more wrinkled, and spots and growths may appear. The skin tends to heal more slowly.

Some of these changes are natural, unavoidable, and harmless. Others are annoying or painful, but can be prevented or treated. Some other changes in the skin, such as skin cancers, are serious and require immediate medical attention.

Whether avoidable or not, health endangering or merely cosmetically undesirable, most unwanted aging-associated skin problems can be addressed by therapies that are now available.

Wrinkles

As skin ages, it loses its elasticity. Collagen and elastin, the tissues that keep the skin elastic, weaken. The skin becomes thinner and loses fat, so it looks less plump and smooth. While all these changes are taking place, gravity is also at work, pulling at the skin, causing it to sag.

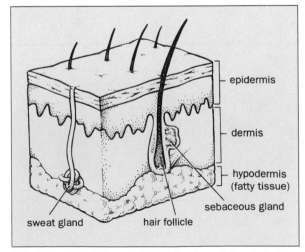

Skin has two main layers: the epidermis and dermis (with fatty tissue underneath). Cells on the surface are constantly shed and replaced by cells from below.

Can Wrinkles Be Avoided?

How wrinkled your skin becomes depends largely on how much sun you've been exposed to in your lifetime. The sun is the major cause of skin aging. Cigarette smoking can contribute to wrinkles. Wrinkles also depend on your parents—the tendency to wrinkle is inherited.

The good news is, some wrinkles can be prevented. To avoid wrinkles caused by the sun, always wear a sunscreen with an SPF (sun protection factor) of at least 15, a hat with a brim, and other protective clothing when in the sun. Don't deliberately sunbathe, and limit sun exposure between 10 a.m. and 3 p.m.

Over-the-counter "wrinkle" creams and lotions may help dry skin and make it look and feel better, but they do nothing to prevent or reverse wrinkles.

Treatments for Aging Skin

There are some promising treatments for aging skin. Retinoic acid, a cream that has been used successfully in treating acne, has been shown to improve the surface texture of the skin and reduce irregular pigmentation. Recent studies show that this cream can also reverse some of the effects of sun damage. However, it has not been approved by the FDA for that purpose. Alpha hydroxy acids are showing promise in reversing some of the effects of the sun. Creases caused by facial expressions such as squinting, frowning, or smiling can be treated by a dermatologist, using what are called dermal fillers.

Wear sunglasses when outside on bright days. Not only do sunglasses help protect against cataract formation, but they decrease the risk of wrinkle formation associated with squinting.

None of these remedies can guarantee eternally youthful skin, but they can improve the overall appearance of your skin. Severely wrinkled skin can be improved with surgery, lasers, or chemical peels. Before you undertake any self-treatment or surgery, discuss your options with your dermatologist.

Dry Skin

As we age, our skin becomes drier. This can result in flaky and itchy skin, especially in cold, dry, windy climates. Milder cases of dry skin can be treated with a moisturizer used after bathing while the skin is still damp. Bath oils, which have a limited effect, should be applied after bathing. Oils should not be added to the bath water because the tub can become dangerously slippery.

Petrolatum, an ingredient in many lotions, creams, and ointments, is an excellent moisturizer. Many moisturizers contain chemicals such as urea, alpha hydroxy acids, lactic acid, and ammonium lactate to reduce scaling and help the skin hold water. But some of these chemicals can irritate the skin. Your dermatologist can help you decide which is best for you.

Bathing less often and using milder soaps or a soap substitute, or soaking in a tub of warm water without soap, can help relieve dry skin. Hot water is more irritating to dry skin than cooler water. After bathing and patting dry, a moisturizer should be applied immediately to seal in moisture.

If dry skin continues to be a problem, consult your dermatologist. Severe flaky, itchy, and cracked skin may be a sign of a more serious problem.

The American Academy of Dermatology

SKIN LESIONS

Lesions or skin growths become more common as we age. They may range from harmless "seborrheic warts" or "age spots" to skin cancers that require immediate treatment. Most are caused by years of sun exposure.

SYMPTOMS OF MORE SERIOUS CONDITIONS

Although most of the changes we experience in our skin as we age are harmless, there are certain signs of more serious problems that shouldn't be ignored. See your dermatologist if you notice any of the following symptoms.

SYMPTOM	MAY INDICATE
• A scaly red spot • A change in color, shape, or size of a mole • Any new skin growth • Bleeding in a mole or other growth	• Skin cancer
• Excessive dryness and itching that doesn't respond to moisturizers	• Dermatitis • Psoriasis • Internal problem
• Vague or sharp local pain or headache followed by itching and formation of groups of blisters	• Shingles
• Bulging or tender veins in the leg	• Varicose veins
• A cut that fails to heal	• Skin cancer • Circulatory problem • Diabetes

Among the most common are red, scaly spots called actinic keratoses. If ignored, they may become skin cancers and will eventually have to be removed surgically. In the early stages they can be removed by applying a cream, a topical form of chemotherapy, or by freezing them with liquid nitrogen.

Squamous cell carcinoma typically develops on the rim of the ear, the face, the lips, and the back of hands. These skin cancers can increase in size and spread to internal organs.

The most common form of skin cancer, basal cell carcinoma, usually appears as a small, shiny bump on the face, neck, or chest. It's more common in older fair-skinned people with blond or red hair and blue or green

PROTECTING YOUR SKIN WITH SUNSCREENS

For people over the age of 50, the advice is the same as it is for a teenager on the beach: Wear a sunscreen. The notion that we did the crucial damage to our skin when we were sunbathing youths—and so don't need to think about sun damage anymore—is simply not true. In fact, sun damage increases with age. For one thing, older people have thinner skin, which increases vulnerability to environmental assaults. Also, they tend not to tan as readily because the skin's pigment cells, or melanocytes—the body's primary protective barrier against sunlight—disappear at a rate of 10 to 20 percent each decade.

Some recent research has suggested that people over the age of 50 should not protect themselves too thoroughly against the sun, lest they develop a vitamin D deficiency (the vitamin is synthesized when a certain compound is exposed to ultraviolet radiation).

But most people get enough sun in 15 or 20 minutes to meet their vitamin D needs. The research is applicable to people who are totally confined indoors—and the best advice for them is not to seek the sun for any presumed therapeutic benefits, but to take a vitamin D supplement.

Sunproofing

The Skin Cancer Foundation offers these tips for people of any age:

• Wear a hat, long-sleeved shirt, and long pants as much as you can outdoors. The tighter the weave, the better it will keep out the sun.

• Apply a sunscreen half an hour before you go out, so that it has time to penetrate the skin and provide optimum protection.

• Because perspiration will diminish its effectiveness, reapply a sunscreen every couple of hours.

Also be sure to reapply sunscreen after you go swimming.

• The fairer your skin, the higher the SPF (sun protection factor) you need. Use a sunscreen that indicates on the label it has an SPF of at least 15. An SPF tells you how long you may remain safely in the sun. If you normally burn after 10 minutes, for example, an SPF of 15 allows you to stay in the sun 15 times longer—150 minutes, or two and a half hours—before burning.

• Put sunscreen on with a liberal hand. Most people apply it so sparingly that they get only half the protection advertised.

• Don't forget to cover any bald spots.

• Consult your pharmacist or your physician to see if you are taking any drug that increases your skin's sensitivity to sunlight—such as certain diuretics, antihistamines, antidepressants, antibiotics, or oral hypoglycemics. You may need some extra protection.

• If one sunscreen irritates your skin, try another; there are dozens of good ones. Look for the Skin Cancer Foundation seal of recommendation on the label of any product you buy.

• Look for double protection. Research has demonstrated that ultraviolet B (UVB) rays are not the only ones that damage the skin; longer-wave ultraviolet A rays can also cause harm, leading to premature aging and possible predisposition to skin cancer.

Most sunscreens protect only against the sun's ultraviolet B rays. However, ultraviolet A rays also promote skin damage, although to a lesser degree. Some new products that protect against UVA and UVB rays are now available; consider using one of these, especially if you are very fair.

The Editors

eyes. Untreated, these skin cancers may begin to bleed and crust over. They grow slowly and rarely spread to other parts of the body. When treated early, squamous cell and basal cell skin cancers have a 95 percent cure rate.

A less common but more serious form of skin cancer is called malignant melanoma.

Men over the age of 50 are at the highest risk for melanoma, but it can affect anyone of any age. Melanoma has been associated with severe childhood sunburns. This skin cancer usually appears as a dark brown or black mole-like growth with irregular borders and irregular color. The most frequent sites for melanoma are the upper back in both men and women, the chest and abdomen in men, and the lower legs of women.

Any change in an existing mole or the emergence of a new mole could be a sign of melanoma and should be examined immediately by a dermatologist. Melanoma spreads to other organs and can be fatal.

Other Growths

Several other skin growths are common in older individuals. These include:

"Age" or "liver" spots. These flat, brown spots are called solar lentigos. Caused by the sun, they usually appear on the face, hands, back, and feet. (They have nothing to do with the liver.) These spots are generally harmless—but any large flat irregular dark area can be a form of melanoma and so requires evaluation.

Prescription and over-the-counter "fade" creams will make solar lentigos lighten in color. Laser therapies are also available that can remove them.

Seborrheic keratoses. These brown or tan raised spots or wartlike growths look as though they were stuck on the skin surface. They are not cancerous and are very common in older people. If annoying, they can be removed easily.

Cherry angiomas. These are harmless, small, bright red domes created by dilated blood vessels. They occur in more than 85 percent of middle-aged and elderly people, usually on the torso. Electrocautery or laser therapy can remove these spots.

Broken capillaries or telangiectasia. These dilated facial blood vessels are usually related to sun damage. They respond to the same treatments as angiomas.

The American Academy of Dermatology

**MOLE INSPECTION—
LEARNING YOUR ABCDs**

Mole inspection becomes simpler if you keep in mind the American Cancer Society's ABCD rule for distinguishing a normal mole or other skin blemish from an abnormal (dysplastic) one. But remember, any mole, however small, is suspect, especially if it appears in an area of previous sunburn.

Asymmetry. One half of the mole does not match the other.

Border. The edges are irregular—ragged, notched, or blurred.

Color. The color is not uniform, but may be differing shades of tan, brown, or black, sometimes with patches of white, red, or blue.

Diameter. The mole is larger than the size of a pencil eraser (about six millimeters or a quarter of an inch) or is increasing in size.

SKIN DISEASES

Some skin diseases more common in older people are shingles (herpes zoster), varicose veins, leg ulcers, and seborrheic dermatitis.

Shingles/Herpes Zoster. Shingles is an inflammation of a nerve caused by the same virus as chicken pox. Early symptoms are localized pain, headache, or fatigue. Shingles can affect people of all ages but is more common (and painful) in older adults.

The shingles virus attacks a nerve root and follows the course of that nerve, resulting in lines of blisters on the skin. The disease usually confines itself to one side of the body.

Shingles can become serious and cause complications. A dermatologist should be contacted immediately if shingles is suspected, especially if the condition appears near the eyes. Treatments are most effective if started within three day of onset. (See page 192 for more information on shingles.)

Seborrheic Dermatitis. The signs of seborrheic dermatitis are redness and flaking. It usually affects areas of the skin with a high concentration of oil glands, such as the scalp, sides of the nose, eyebrows, eyelids, behind the ears, and the middle of the chest. It occasionally affects other areas such as the navel, breasts, buttocks, and skin folds under the arms.

Seborrheic dermatitis can be successfully treated and may even go away on its own, but it tends to recur. Frequent shampooing and washing are very helpful, and your dermatologist may prescribe topical medications, including low-strength cortisone preparations and special shampoos.

Varicose Veins. These are enlarged veins that appear blue and bulging. They are common in older individuals. The veins become twisted and swollen when blood returning to the heart against gravity flows back into the veins through a faulty valve. This condition is rarely dangerous.

The symptoms of varicose veins can be eased by avoiding standing for long periods, by keeping feet elevated when sitting or lying down, and by wearing support hose or elastic bandages. More severe cases can be treated with surgery or injections. (See page 354 for more information.)

Varicose Ulcers. The same sluggish blood flow that results in varicose veins can cause varicose ulcers, also known as venous or stasis ulcers. Varicose ulcers often develop at the ankles and may be preceded by swelling and red, itchy, flaky skin before turning into a sore. These ulcers are shallow wounds that occasionally become infected.

Another cause of ulcers on the legs is insufficient blood supply. This condition is associated with medical disorders such as atherosclerosis, hypertension, and diabetes.

It is best to prevent varicose ulcers by addressing the preceding signs of swelling and irritation. Once ulcers develop, healing may take months or even years while causing discomfort and requiring daily self-care and frequent doctor visits.

Bruising (Purpura). Many seniors complain of black-and-blue marks, or bruises, particularly on the arms and legs. These are usually a result of the skin becoming thinner with age due to sun damage. Loss of fat and connective tissue weakens the support around blood vessels, making them more susceptible to injury. Bruising in areas always covered by clothing should be evaluated. Bruising sometimes is caused by medications, clotting disturbances, or internal disease.

Itching. A very common problem with aging skin is itching. Although often associated with dry skin, itching also has other causes. Elderly skin appears to be more sensitive to fabric preservatives, wool, plastics, detergents, bleaches, soaps, and other irritants. Identifying and limiting exposure to the cause is important. Prolonged itching may lead to lack of sleep and fatigue. Your dermatologist can offer some medical remedies for itching if moisturizing alone is ineffective.

The American Academy of Dermatology

Health Problems of Men

A number of physiological changes occur with age—and some of them occur only in men. More than half of the men in their sixties and as many as 90 percent in their seventies or eighties have some symptoms of prostate enlargement; 30 percent of men age 65 have had recurrent episodes of erectile dysfunction. While problems such as these may be difficult to talk about initially, help is there for the asking. Your physician can guide you in such matters—perhaps referring you to a urologist, the appropriate specialist for such problems.

The Editors

ERECTILE DYSFUNCTION

Nearly every man experiences temporary erectile dysfunction (impotence) from time to time, due to such routine difficulties as fatigue or stress or acute illness. Some men, however, are troubled and embarrassed by chronic impotence—the inability to achieve and sustain an erection for a long enough time to engage in sexual intercourse.

More than 10 million American men are chronically impotent. By the age of 55, 18 percent of men report the problem; by age 65, that figure increases to 30 percent; and by age 75, 55 percent of men report suffering from impotence.

Until just a decade ago, more than 90 percent of all cases of impotence were blamed simply on emotional causes. During the past 10 years, however, doctors have recognized that only about 15 percent of all cases have a psychological basis. And in many cases, a man's potency can be restored by a combination of medical and psychological treatment.

An erection is caused by a complex neurological mechanism: a sensory stimulus—a touch, a sight, a scent—triggers a message that travels from the brain down the spinal cord to release a chemical messenger, which causes the corpora cavernosa two rod shaped bundles of spongy muscle that run along each side of the penis—to relax and fill with blood. As they fill, the corpora cavernosa expand and press against the veins that would normally drain blood from the penis. Thus engorged, the penis enlarges and stiffens.

CAUSES
Physiological
Erectile dysfunction can result from faults in any part of this mechanism. Among the most common disrupters are medical problems such as diabetes, multiple sclerosis, Parkinson's disease, lower back problems, severe arthritis, liver or kidney disease, congestive heart failure, and extreme obesity; habits such as alcoholism, drug abuse, and, especially, smoking; injury to the spinal cord; certain surgical procedures; and the side effects of prescription medications—especially those for hypertension.

Antihypertensive drugs known to cause impotence include Aldomet, Catapres, propranolol, Ismelin, and thiazide diuretics; vasodilators and calcium channel blockers usually do not cause potency problems. In addition, antihistamines taken for allergies and decongestants taken for colds may cause temporary erectile dysfunction.

A low level of the male sex hormone testosterone also can result in impotence and decreased sexual desire.

Psychological
Impotence can have solely emotional causes, and in that case, diagnosis can be difficult. Often a conversation with a physician will turn up reasons of fatigue, tension, or depression from overwork—or stress, anger, or other psychological interferences in an intimate relationship—that result in impotence.

Few experts rely on the presence of morning erections or carry out extensive tests to document erections during sleep. In the past the presence of such erections was thought to indicate that erectile dysfunction was not due to a physical problem. It is now clear that men may have morning erections but be unable to maintain an erection that allows intercourse. This problem can be caused by physical as well as psychological factors.

WHAT CAN BE DONE

If a physiological cause is suspected, the doctor will test reflexes that could be affected by spinal cord problems. He or she will also measure blood testosterone levels and, if they are low, prescribe testosterone replacement by regular intramuscular injections or by daily applications of a testosterone skin patch.

Behavioral Changes

If there is reason to believe impotence is caused by smoking, alcohol, or drugs, the remedy is apparent. Cutting out smoking and drinking or changing medications will often cure the problem.

Some physicians have prescribed the drug yohimbine—long a constituent of folk remedies—to help men whose organic erectile difficulties are minimal. In fact, there is no evidence at all that yohimbine does any good.

Vacuum Device

Nearly all forms of impotence can be treated with a special vacuum device. An acrylic tube is placed around the penis and the air is pumped out of the tube. The resultant vacuum causes blood to flow into the penis; an erection is produced in three to five minutes. The device is then removed and a rubber band is slipped onto the base of the penis to keep the blood from flowing out and so hold the penis erect for a half hour. The sensory nerves that convey the sensation of inter-course and ejaculation are not affected by the device, although using it may initially seem cumbersome and embarrassing. But, with practice, the vacuum device is effective for virtually all forms of impotence, and those who have used it generally report very high levels of sexual satisfaction. Such a vacuum device normally costs about $450.

Injections

If these remedies do not work, your physician may suggest injections of alprostadil (Caverject) as a treatment option. Alprostadil can be self-injected directly into the base of the penis (with instructions from your physician) using a tiny syringe and needle. By dilating the blood vessels, the drug causes an erection that lasts for a half hour to 45 minutes.

Alprostadil injections can, however, cause pain and prolonged erections (priapism)—for as long as four to five hours—which can require immediate treatment to prevent permanent damage to the penis. Thus, alprostadil should only be used where medical care is quickly available. In addition, researchers are still studying the question of whether long-term use of alprostadil can cause scar tissue to form.

Alprostadil can also be inserted into the urethra. Pain is the major side effect of erections induced by urethral application.

The latest and most effective drug to stimulate an erection is sildenafil (Viagra). This drug should never be used by men who are taking nitrates for angina or who have severe coronary artery disease. A significant number of deaths have occurred among users of sildenafil who fall into either group.

Implants

Finally, ordinarily as a last resort, prosthetic devices can be surgically implanted in the penis. Some are simply rigid rods that are implanted in the corpora cavernosa as a substitute for the effect of blood flowing into these areas of spongy muscle. The rods are flexible and can be manually bent to be erect or to remain close to the body.

Other implants are more complex inflatable devices, which are implanted along with fluid reservoirs and a tiny pump that are operated manually to move the fluid from the reservoir into the device and so make the prosthesis enlarge and stiffen. Penile implants are reliable, although—as with any mechanical device—they may break down, and surgery is required to make the repair.

Vascular Surgery

Some physicians may recommend vascular surgery to enhance the blood flow through the arteries into the corpora cavernosa, although such surgery is still considered experimental. The results of this type of surgery have generally been unsatisfactory when tried in men over the age of 50.

The Editors

PROSTATE ENLARGEMENT

The prostate makes some of the milky fluid (semen) that carries sperm. The gland is the size of a walnut and is found just below the bladder, which stores urine. The prostate wraps around a tube (the urethra) that carries urine from the bladder out through the tip of the penis.

During a man's orgasm (sexual climax), muscles squeeze the prostate's fluid into the urethra. Sperm, which are made in the testicles, also go into the urethra during orgasm. The milky fluid carries the sperm through the penis during orgasm.

WHAT IS BPH?

Benign prostatic hyperplasia or BPH means that the prostate gland has grown larger than normal. BPH is not cancer and does not cause cancer. "Benign" means the cells are not cancerous. "Hyperplasia" means there are more cells than normal. BPH results from growing older and cannot be prevented. Your chances of having prostate trouble increase as you age. BPH is common in men over age 50. More than half of all men over age 60 have BPH. By age 80, about eight out of 10 men have it.

BPH does not always cause problems. Fewer than half of all men with BPH ever show any symptoms of the disease. And only some men with symptoms will need treatment.

WHAT ARE THE SYMPTOMS OF BPH?

The most common symptom of BPH is trouble urinating. Many men with BPH have no bothersome symptoms. But BPH may cause some men to have problems urinating. Common symptoms include:

- Feeling that bladder is not completely emptied after urination
- Frequent urination
- Stopping and starting on attempts to urinate
- A strong and urgent need to urinate
- Weak or hesitant urine stream
- The need to push or strain to start the urine stream
- Frequent awakening at night to urinate

What Causes Symptoms?

As the prostate grows in BPH, it squeezes the urethra (urinary tube). This narrows the tube and can cause problems with urination. Sometimes with BPH you can also have urinary infection or bleeding.

In the early stages of BPH, the bladder muscle can still force urine through the narrowed urethra by squeezing harder. But if the blockage continues, the bladder muscle gets stronger, thicker, and more sensitive. The result is a stronger need to urinate.

In some cases, you may have trouble forcing urine through the urethra. This means the bladder cannot empty completely. Some men may find that they suddenly cannot urinate (a condition called acute urinary retention). Over time, a few men might have bladder or kidney problems or both. Sometimes BPH causes infection of the urinary tract. This can cause burning or pain when you urinate. The urinary tract is the path that urine takes as it leaves the body. The tract includes the kidneys, ureters, bladder, and urethra (see illustration, next page).

HOW IS BPH DIAGNOSED?

If you have symptoms that bother you, see a doctor. He or she can find out if BPH—or another disease—is the cause. If you do have BPH, your doctor can also see if it has caused other problems. During your visit, the doctor will most likely:

- Give you a list of questions about your symptoms. Your answers are important; they will help the doctor decide if your symptoms are mild, moderate, or severe.
- Take your medical history. Your doctor will ask you about past and current medical problems.
- Examine your prostate gland by inserting a gloved, lubricated finger into your rectum.
- Do a physical exam to see if other medical problems may be causing your symptoms.
- Check your urine for blood or signs of infection (a urinalysis).
- Test your blood to see if the prostate has affected your kidneys. Your doctor may also recommend a blood test to help detect prostate cancer.

These tests are not painful or costly. They are done to help confirm that you have BPH and to find any problems it has caused. But tests used to diagnose your condition cannot predict if BPH will cause problems later if not treated now. Your doctor may also recommend other tests. They may help find if BPH has affected your bladder or kidneys and make sure your problems are not caused by cancer.

These tests may help some patients but not everyone:

- *Uroflowmetry* measures how fast your urine flows and how much you pass. This test can help find how much the urine is blocked.
- *Residual urine measurement* shows how much urine is left in your bladder after you urinate. This test can help find how much your bladder has been affected by BPH. The test can be done several ways. You and your doctor should talk about the method used.
- *Pressure-flow studies* measure the pressure in your bladder as you urinate. Some doctors feel this test is the best way to find out how much your urine is blocked. The test can help most if results of other tests are confusing or if your doctor thinks you have bladder problems. In the test, a small tube called a catheter is inserted into the penis, through the urethra, and into the bladder. The test may cause discomfort for a short time. In a few men, it may cause a urinary tract infection.
- *Prostate-specific antigen* (PSA) is a blood test that can help find prostate cancer. BPH does not cause cancer.

  But some men do have BPH and cancer at the same time. The PSA test is not always accurate. PSA test results can suggest cancer in BPH patients who do not have prostate cancer. The results can also sometimes suggest no cancer in men who do have cancer. Not all doctors agree that being tested for PSA levels lowers a patient's chance of dying from prostate cancer. Each man with BPH is different. You and your doctor may want to discuss this test.

Your doctor may also suggest other tests such as x-rays, cystoscopy, and ultrasound.

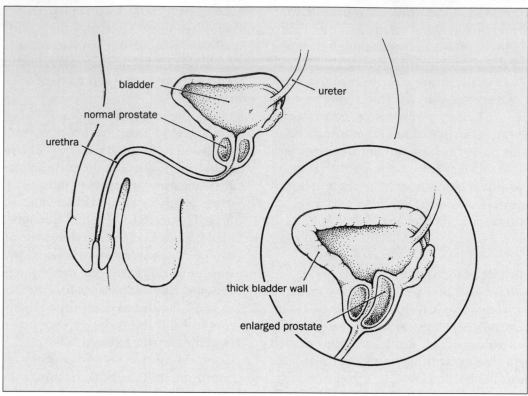

As the prostate enlarges, it may restrict urine flow, creating a frequent, urgent need to empty the bladder. Urine retention places excess demand upon the bladder wall, which can cause it to thicken.

Many men do not need these tests. They are costly and not very helpful for most men with BPH. Also, cystoscopy and x-rays can cause discomfort or problems for some men. But the tests can help patients with some BPH problems or men with other problems such as blood in the urine.

- *Cystoscopy* lets the doctor look directly at the prostate and bladder. This test helps the doctor find the best method in men who choose invasive treatments (such as surgery). In cystoscopy, a small tube is inserted into the penis, through the urethra, and into the bladder. Some men may have discomfort during and after the test. A few may get urinary infections or blood in the urine; a few may not be able to urinate for a short time after the test.

- *A urogram,* a type of x-ray, lets the doctor see blockage in the urinary tract. A dye injected into a vein makes the urine show up on the x-ray. Some men are allergic to the dye.

- *Ultrasound* lets the doctor see the prostate, kidneys, and bladder without a catheter or x-rays. A probe put on the skin sends sound waves (ultrasound) into the body. The echoes result in pictures of the prostate, kidneys, or bladder on a TV screen. This test is not harmful or painful. A special probe put in the rectum can give a better view of the prostate when the doctor wants to check for prostate cancer.

BPH needs to be treated only if the symptoms are severe enough to bother you, or your urinary tract is seriously affected. An enlarged prostate gland alone is not reason enough to get treatment. Your prostate may not get any bigger than it is now, and your symptoms may not get worse.

Ask yourself how much your symptoms really bother you:

- Do they keep you from doing the things you enjoy, such as fishing or going to sports events?
- Would you be a lot happier or do more if the symptoms went away?
- Do you want treatment now?
- Are you willing to accept some risks to try to get rid of your symptoms?
- Do you understand the risks?

TREATMENT OPTIONS

Your answers to these questions can help you choose a treatment that is right for you. Currently, the five ways of treating BPH are watchful waiting, alpha blocker drug treatment, finasteride drug treatment, balloon dilation, and surgery.

Surgery will do the best job of relieving your urinary symptoms, but it also has more risk than the other treatments. Unless you have a serious complication of BPH that makes surgery the only good choice, you can choose from a range of treatments.

Which treatment option you choose—if any—depends on how much your symptoms bother you. Your choice also depends on how much risk you are willing to take to improve your symptoms. You and your doctor will decide together.

Watchful Waiting

If you have BPH but are not bothered by your symptoms, you and your doctor may decide on a program of "watchful waiting." Watchful waiting is not an active treatment like taking medicine or having surgery. It means getting regular exams—about once a year—to see if your BPH is getting worse or causing problems.

At these exams, your doctor will ask about any problems you have. He or she may also order some simple tests to see if your BPH is causing kidney or bladder problems.

A small number of men in watchful waiting become unable to urinate at all. Some also get infections or bleed, or their bladder or kidneys are damaged. But such major problems are uncommon. Your doctor may suggest some tips to help control your symptoms. One is to drink fewer liquids before going to bed. Another is not to take over-the-counter cold and sinus medicines with decongestants, which can make a prostate condition worse.

Without treatment, BPH symptoms may get better, stay the same, or get worse. If your symptoms become a problem, talk to your doctor about treatment choices.

Alpha Blocker Drug Treatment

Alpha blocker drugs are taken by mouth, usually once or twice a day. The drugs help relax muscles in the prostate, and some men will notice that their urinary symptoms get better.

During the first three or four weeks, the doctor may see you regularly to make sure everything is okay. The doctor will check your symptoms and see if the medicine's dosage (how much you take and how often) is right for you. After that, you will visit the doctor from time to time to have your symptoms checked and prescription refilled. There is no evidence that alpha blockers reduce the rate of BPH complications or the need for future surgery.

Side effects can include headaches or feeling dizzy, light-headed, or tired. Low blood pressure is also possible. Because alpha blocker treatment for BPH is new, doctors do not know its long-term benefits and risks.

Alpha blockers include doxazosin (Cardura), prazosin (Minipress), and terazosin (Hytrin). Hytrin is the only alpha blocker now approved for BPH treatment by the Food and Drug Administration.

Finasteride Drug Treatment

Finasteride (Proscar) is taken by mouth once a day. It can cause the prostate to shrink, and some men will notice that their urinary symptoms get better. It may take six months or more before you notice the full benefit of finasteride. You still need to see your doctor on a regular basis while you take this drug. There is no evidence that finasteride reduces the rate of BPH complications or the need for future surgery.

Finasteride has proven effective mainly in men with especially large prostates.

Finasteride drug treatment is relatively new, and doctors do not know its long-term benefits and risks. Also, finasteride lowers the blood level of prostate-specific antigen. Doctors do not know if this affects the ability of the PSA test to detect prostate cancer.

Side effects of finasteride include less interest in having sex, problems getting an erection, and problems with ejaculation.

Balloon Dilation

Balloon dilation is done in the operating room in a hospital or doctor's office. After the patient gets anesthesia (medicine to reduce pain), the doctor inserts a catheter (plastic tube) into the penis. The catheter goes through the urethra and into the bladder. The catheter has a limp balloon at the end.

The doctor inflates the balloon to stretch the urethra where it has been squeezed by the prostate. In some patients, this can allow urine to flow more easily.

Balloon dilation can cause bleeding or infection. It can also make patients unable to urinate for a time. If there are no problems, you may go home the same day. Some patients have to stay overnight at the hospital.

Balloon dilation is a fairly new treatment for BPH, and doctors do not know all its long-term benefits and risks. In many patients, this treatment seems to work for only a short time.

Because relief is generally short-lived, balloon dilation is mainly reserved for patients who have troublesome symptoms but have other disorders that make them poor candidates for surgery.

Surgery

Because surgery has been used for many years to treat BPH, its benefits and risks are fairly well known. Compared with other treatments, surgery has the best chance for relief of BPH symptoms. Although surgery is also most likely to cause major problems, most men who undergo surgery have no major problems.

By itself, an enlarged prostate does not mean you need surgery. An enlarged prostate may not become larger. Also, no operation for BPH lowers the chance of getting prostate cancer in the future.

Surgery is almost always recommended for men with certain problems caused by BPH. These include:

- Not being able to urinate at all
- Urine backup into the kidneys that damages the kidneys
- Frequent urine infection
- Major bleeding through the urethra caused by BPH
- Stones in the bladder

If you do not have any of these serious problems, but you are bothered by your BPH, you may still want to consider surgery. There are three types of surgery for BPH:

- Transurethral resection of the prostate (TURP)
- Transurethral incision of the prostate (TUIP)
- Open prostatectomy

TURP. TURP is the most common surgical procedure. It is a proven way to treat BPH effectively. TURP relieves symptoms by reducing pressure on the urethra. After the patient gets anesthesia, the doctor inserts a special instrument into the urethra through the penis. No skin needs to be cut. The doctor then removes part of the inside of the prostate.

After TURP, patients usually need to wear a catheter (a tube in the penis for draining urine) for two to three days and stay in the hospital for about three days. Most patients find that their symptoms improve quickly after TURP. These men do well for many years.

TUIP. TUIP may be used when the prostate is not enlarged as much. In TUIP, tissue is not removed. Instead, an instrument is passed through the urethra to make one or two small cuts in the prostate. These cuts reduce the prostate's pressure on the urethra, making it easier to urinate. TUIP may have less risk than TURP in certain cases.

Open prostatectomy. This procedure may be used if the prostate is very large. In this procedure, an incision is made in the lower abdomen to remove part of the inside of the prostate.

Surgery for BPH improves symptoms in most patients, but some symptoms may remain. For example, the bladder might be weak because of blockage. This means there still could be problems urinating even after prostate tissue is removed.

New Treatments

New treatments for BPH appear every year. Examples are laser surgery, microwave thermal therapy, prostatic stents, and new drugs. Use of a laser is still surgery, and doctors do not yet know if its benefits and risks are higher or lower than standard surgery.

There is not yet enough information about these treatments to include them at present. If your doctor suggests a treatment not dis-

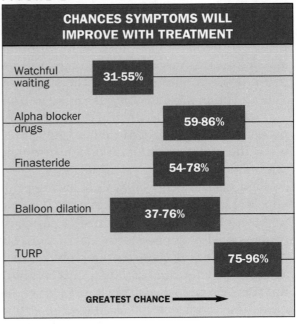

FIGURE 2

CHANCES SYMPTOMS WILL IMPROVE WITH TREATMENT

Watchful waiting — 31-55%

Alpha blocker drugs — 59-86%

Finasteride — 54-78%

Balloon dilation — 37-76%

TURP — 75-96%

GREATEST CHANCE →

cussed here, ask for the same type of information on risks and benefits given below for other treatments.

WHAT ARE THE BENEFITS AND RISKS?

Each treatment may improve your symptoms. But each treatment has different chances of success. All treatments, even watchful waiting, have some risks. Ask your doctor these questions about each treatment:

- What is my chance of getting better?
- How much better will I get?
- What are the chances that the treatment will cause problems?
- How long will the treatment work?

Both benefits and risks are given below for each treatment. This can help you and your doctor make the best choice for you.

Figure 2 shows that the chance your symptoms will improve after TURP surgery is greater than if you simply watch and wait.

But even with TURP, your chances for improvement are somewhat uncertain. This is because doctors do not know the exact chances that each patient's symptoms will improve. In general, the worse your symptoms are before treatment, the more they will improve if the treatment works. The success of TUIP and open prostatectomy is similar to TURP.

Figure 3 shows the amount of symptom improvement for each treatment. Again, TURP gives the greatest amount of improvement and watchful waiting gives the least.

Figure 4 shows the chances of having problems during or soon after treatment.

Most of the time, treatments do not cause problems. Most problems are not serious, but some are. TURP can cause serious problems such as urinary infection, bleeding that requires transfusion, or blocked urine flow. Few patients have these serious problems after surgery.

For patients taking alpha blocker drugs, the most common side effects are feeling dizzy and tired and having headaches.

With finasteride, about five out of 100 patients have some kind of sexual problem such as a lower sex drive or trouble getting an erection.

With watchful waiting, there is no active treatment and no added chance of problems right away. But over time, the BPH itself can cause symptoms to grow worse or cause other problems. Only TURP clearly reduces that risk. Doctors do not know if alpha blocker drugs, finasteride, or balloon dilation lowers the risk of future BPH problems.

Figure 5 shows the chance of dying from treatment. There are probably no added chances of dying from watchful waiting, alpha blocker drugs, and finasteride. There is now no information for balloon dilation.

The average age of men diagnosed with BPH is 67. The chances that a 67-year-old man might die from any cause are about eight out of 1,000 in a three-month period. There is a greater chance (although small) of dying up to three months after TURP—about 15 out of 1,000 patients. If you are healthy, your chance of dying after TURP is lower.

FIGURE 3

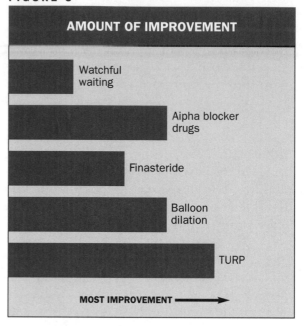

AMOUNT OF IMPROVEMENT

Watchful waiting

Aipha blocker drugs

Finasteride

Balloon dilation

TURP

MOST IMPROVEMENT ➝

FIGURE 4

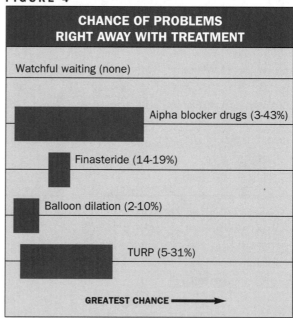

CHANCE OF PROBLEMS RIGHT AWAY WITH TREATMENT

Watchful waiting (none)

Aipha blocker drugs (3-43%)

Finasteride (14-19%)

Balloon dilation (2-10%)

TURP (5-31%)

GREATEST CHANCE ➝

Some BPH treatments can make it hard to control urine, leading to leakage (urinary incontinence). Over time, BPH itself can cause incontinence. Also, men treated with alpha blocker drugs, finasteride, or balloon dilation may have future risk of incontinence from BPH.

FIGURE 5

CHANCE OF DYING WITHIN 3 MONTHS AFTER TREATMENT	
Treatment	**Risk**
Watchful waiting	No known added risk
Alpha blocker drugs	
Finasteride	
Balloon dilation	Not certain; probably less than TURP
TURP	Less than 2 out of 100 men; less than 1 out of 100 men if healthy.

FIGURE 6

UNCONTROLLABLE URINE LEAKAGE AFTER TREATMENT	
Treatment	**Risk**
Watchful waiting	None
Alpha blocker drugs	
Finasteride	
Balloon dilation	None reported; possible
TURP	1 out of 100 men

Although it is rare, some men have severe, uncontrollable incontinence after treatment (Figure 6). About seven to 14 out of 1,000 men have this problem after TURP. Men in a program of watchful waiting have no immediate risk of uncontrollable incontinence.

The chance of needing surgery in the future differs for each treatment. Some men who at first choose watchful waiting or non-surgical treatment may later decide to have surgery to relieve bothersome symptoms. Also, some men who have surgery may need to have surgery again. One reason is that the prostate may grow back. Another is that a scar may form and block the urinary tract.

Within eight years after TURP, five to 15 out of every 100 men will need another operation Doctors are uncertain if treatment with alpha blocker drugs, finasteride, or balloon dilation lowers the chance that surgery will be needed in the future.

Figure 7 shows the chance of becoming impotent (not being able to get an erection) because of BPH treatment. Each year, about two out of every 100 men 67 years old will become impotent without BPH treatment.

There is probably no added risk of impotence with watchful waiting and alpha blocker drugs. Finasteride has a small added risk of impotence, but the problem should stop when the drug is stopped. The risk with balloon dilation is unknown, but probably low. With TURP, the risk of impotence ranges from three to 35 out of 100 patients. If your erections are normal before surgery, however, the risk of impotence after surgery may be no higher than with watchful waiting.

Figure 8 shows about how many days you can expect to lose from work or from what you normally do over the first year. Time at the doctor's office and in the hospital is included.

One other problem—retrograde ejaculation—can result. It is common with surgery and rare with alpha blocker drug treatment. Retrograde ejaculation means that during sexual climax, semen flows back into the bladder rather than out of the penis.

Men with this problem may not be able to father children. But it does not affect the ability to get an erection or have sex and does not cause other problems. You may want to talk to your doctor about retrograde ejaculation.

Between 40 and 70 out of 100 patients have this problem after surgery. About seven

FIGURE 7

CHANCE OF IMPOTENCE (Loss of Erection)	
Treatment	Risk
Watchful waiting	Probably no added risk
Alpha blocker drugs	
Finasteride	4 out of 100 men. Impotence may end when drug is stopped.
Balloon dilation	Unknown
TURP	For most, 5-10 out of 100 men; may be higher in men with sexual problems before surgery.

FIGURE 8

LOSS OF WORK AND ACTIVITY TIME, FIRST YEAR	
Treatment	Days
Watchful waiting*	1
Alpha blocker drugs*	3.5
Finasteride*	2
Balloon dilation	4
TURP	7-21

*Mainly from visits to doctor's office.

out of 100 patients have the problem while taking alpha blocker drugs. Retrograde ejaculation does not occur with watchful waiting or finasteride. Some men who take finasteride notice that they make less semen.

WHAT IS THE NEXT STEP?

Before choosing a treatment, ask yourself these two important questions:

- If my BPH is not likely to cause me serious harm, do I want any treatment other than watchful waiting?
- If I do want treatment, which is best for me based on the benefits and risks of each?

No matter what you decide, talk it over with your doctor. Together, you and your doctor can choose the treatment best for you.

U.S. Department of Health and Human Services

Health Problems of Women

Our entire body changes as we age—but for women, the most obvious and profound changes occur with the onset of menopause. Beyond this, certain other issues are of special concern to women over age 50. Questions about breast lumps, urinary incontinence, or vaginitis may be difficult to raise initially, but your family doctor, internist, or gynecologist can be a terrific resource in such matters. *The Editors*

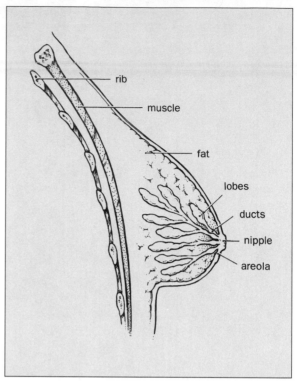

Regular breast self-exams can help a woman distinguish abnormal lumps from the lumps caused by ribs, muscles, lobes, and fat deposits in the breast.

BENIGN BREAST CONDITIONS

Over her lifetime, a woman can encounter a broad variety of breast conditions. These include normal changes that occur during the menstrual cycle as well as several types of benign lumps. What they have in common is that they are not cancer. Even for breast lumps that require a biopsy, some 80 percent prove to be benign.

Each breast has several sections, called lobes, each with many smaller lobules. The lobules end in dozens of tiny bulbs that can produce milk. Lobes, lobules, and bulbs are all linked by thin tubes called ducts. These ducts lead to the nipple, which is centered in a dark area of skin called the areola. The spaces between the lobules and ducts are filled with fat. There are no muscles in the breast, but muscles lie under each breast and cover the ribs. These normal features can sometimes make the breasts feel lumpy.

From the time a girl begins to menstruate, her breasts undergo regular changes each month. Eventually, about half of all women will experience symptoms such as lumps, pain, or nipple discharge. Generally these disappear with menopause.

Some studies show that the chances of developing benign breast changes are higher for a woman who has never had children or has a family history of breast cancer. Benign breast conditions are less common among women who take birth control pills. Because they generally involve the glandular tissues of the breast, benign breast conditions are more of a problem for women of childbearing age, who have more glandular breasts.

TYPES OF BENIGN BREAST CHANGES
Common benign breast changes fall into several categories. These include generalized breast changes, solitary lumps, nipple discharge, and infection and/or inflammation.

Generalized Breast Changes
Generalized breast lumpiness is known by several names, including fibrocystic disease

changes and benign breast disease. Such lumpiness, which is sometimes described as "ropy" or "granular," can often be felt in the area around the nipple and areola and in the upper-outer part of the breast. Such lumpiness may become more obvious as a woman approaches middle age and the milk-producing glandular tissue of her breasts increasingly gives way to soft, fatty tissue. Unless she is taking replacement hormones, this type of lumpiness generally disappears for good after menopause.

The menstrual cycle also brings cyclic breast changes. Many women experience swelling, tenderness, and pain before and sometimes during their periods.

At the same time, one or more lumps or a feeling of increased lumpiness may develop because of extra fluid collecting in the breast tissue. These lumps normally go away by the end of the period.

During pregnancy, the milk-producing glands become swollen and the breasts may feel lumpier than usual. Although very uncommon, breast cancer has been diagnosed during pregnancy. If you have any questions about how your breasts feel or look, talk to your doctor.

Solitary Lumps

Benign breast conditions also include several types of distinct, solitary lumps. Such lumps, which can appear at any time, may be large or small, soft or rubbery, fluid-filled or solid.

Cysts are fluid-filled sacs. They occur most often in women ages 35 to 50, and they often enlarge and become tender and painful just before the menstrual period. They are usually found in both breasts. Some cysts are so small they cannot be felt; rarely, cysts may be several inches across. Cysts are usually treated by observation or by needle aspiration. They show up clearly on ultrasound.

Fibroadenomas are solid and round benign tumors that are made up of both structural (fibro) and glandular (adenoma) tissues. Usually, these lumps are painless and found by the woman herself. They feel rubbery and can easily be moved around. Fibroadenomas are the most common type of tumors in women in their late teens and early twenties, and they occur twice as often in African American women as in other American women.

Fibroadenomas have a typically benign appearance on mammography (smooth, round masses with a clearly defined edge), and they can sometimes be diagnosed with needle biopsy. Although fibroadenomas do not become malignant, they can enlarge with pregnancy and breastfeeding.

Fat necrosis is the name given to painless, round, and firm lumps formed by damaged and disintegrating fatty tissues. This condition typically occurs in obese women with very large breasts. It often develops in response to a bruise or blow to the breast, even though the woman may not remember the specific injury. Sometimes the skin around the lumps looks red or bruised. Fat necrosis can easily be mistaken for cancer, so such lumps are removed in a surgical biopsy.

Sclerosing adenosis is a benign condition involving the excessive growth of tissues in the breast's lobules. It frequently causes breast pain. Usually the changes are microscopic, but adenosis can produce lumps, and it can show up on a mammogram, often as calcifications. Short of biopsy, adenosis can be difficult to distinguish from cancer. The usual approach is surgical biopsy, which furnishes both diagnosis and treatment.

Nipple Discharge

Nipple discharge accompanies some benign breast conditions. Since the breast is a gland, secretions from the nipple of a mature woman are not unusual, nor even necessarily a sign of disease. Small amounts of discharge commonly occur in women taking birth control pills or certain other medications, including sedatives and tranquilizers. If the discharge is being caused by a disease, the disease is more likely to be benign than cancerous.

Nipple discharges vary in color and texture. A milky discharge can be traced to many causes, including thyroid malfunction and oral contraceptives or other drugs. Women with generalized breast lumpiness may have a sticky discharge that is brown or green.

Benign sticky discharges are treated chiefly by keeping the nipple clean. A discharge caused by infection may require antibiotics.

One of the most common sources of a bloody or sticky discharge is an intraductal papilloma, a small, wartlike growth that projects into breast ducts near the nipple.

Single intraductal papillomas usually affect women nearing menopause. The diseased duct can be removed surgically without damaging the appearance of the breast. Multiple intraductal papillomas, in contrast, are more common in younger women. They often occur in both breasts and are more likely to be associated with a lump than with nipple discharge.

Infection and/or Inflammation

Infection or inflammation, including mastitis and mammary duct ectasia, are characteristic of some benign breast conditions.

Mastitis (also called "postpartum mastitis") is an infection most often seen in women who are breastfeeding. A duct may become blocked, allowing milk to pool, causing inflammation, and setting the stage for infection by bacteria. The breast appears red and feels warm, tender, and lumpy. In its earlier stages, mastitis can be cured by antibiotics. If a pus-containing abscess forms, it will need to be drained or surgically removed.

A word of caution: If you find a lump or other change in your breast, do not try to diagnose it yourself. There is no substitute for a doctor's evaluation.

INFLUENCE ON BREAST CANCER RISK

Most benign breast changes do not increase a woman's risk for getting cancer. Recent studies show that only certain very specific types of microscopic changes put a woman at higher risk. These changes feature excessive cell growth, or hyperplasia.

About 70 percent of the women who have a biopsy showing a benign condition have no evidence of hyperplasia. These women are at no increased risk for breast cancer.

About 25 percent of benign breast biopsies show signs of hyperplasia, including conditions such as intraductal papilloma and sclerosing adenosis. Hyperplasia slightly increases the risk of developing breast cancer.

The remaining 5 percent of benign breast biopsies reveal both excessive cell growth (hyperplasia) and cells that are abnormal (atypical). A diagnosis of atypical hyperplasia moderately increases breast cancer risk.

IF YOU FIND A LUMP

If you discover a lump in one breast, check the other breast. If both breasts feel the same, the lumpiness is probably normal. You should, however, mention it to your doctor at your next visit.

But if the lump is something new or unusual and does not go away after your next menstrual period, it is time to call your doctor. The same is true if you discover a discharge from the nipple or skin changes such as dimpling or puckering.

You should not let fear delay you. It is natural to be concerned if you find a lump in your breast. But remember that four-fifths of all breast lumps are not cancer. The sooner any problem is diagnosed, the sooner you can have it treated.

CLINICAL EVALUATION

No matter how your breast lump was discovered, the doctor will want to begin with your medical history. He or she will then carefully examine your breasts and will probably schedule you for a diagnostic mammogram, to obtain as much information as possible about the changes in your breast—either those that can be felt or those discovered on a screening mammogram. The doctor will want to compare the diagnostic mammograms with any previous mammograms. Your doctor may ask you to have an ultrasound.

Aspirating a Cyst

When a cyst is suspected, some doctors proceed directly with aspiration. This procedure, which uses a very thin needle and a syringe, takes only a few minutes and can be done in the doctor's office.

Holding the lump steady, the doctor inserts the needle and attempts to draw out any fluid. If the lump is indeed a cyst, removing the fluid will cause the cyst to collapse and the lump to disappear. If the cyst reappears at a later date, it can simply be drained again.

If the lump turns out to be solid, it may be possible to use the needle to withdraw a clump of cells, which can then be sent to a laboratory for further testing. (Cysts are so rarely associated with cancer that the fluid removed is not usually tested unless it is bloody.)

Biopsy

Biopsy is the only certain way to learn whether a breast lump or suspicious area seen on a mammogram is cancer. Tissue is removed and examined under a microscope by a pathologist. A pathologist is a doctor who specializes in identifying tissue changes that are characteristic of disease, including cancer.

Tissue samples for biopsy can be obtained by either surgery or needle. The doctor's choice of biopsy technique depends on such things as the nature and location of the lump, as well as the woman's general health.

Excisional biopsy. An excisional biopsy removes the entire lump or suspicious area. In effect, it is similar to a lumpectomy, surgery to remove the lump and some surrounding tissue. The surgeon makes an incision along the contour of the breast and removes the lump along with a small margin of normal tissue. Because no skin is removed, the biopsy scar is usually small. The procedure typically takes less than an hour, and the woman usually goes home the same day.

If no cancer is detected anywhere in the excised tissue, the lump may be considered benign.

Needle biopsies. Needle biopsies can be performed with either a very fine needle or a cutting needle large enough to remove a small nugget of tissue.

- *Fine needle aspiration* uses a very thin needle and syringe to remove either fluid from a cyst or clusters of cells from a solid mass.
- *Core needle biopsy* uses a somewhat larger needle with a special cutting edge. The needle is inserted, under local anesthesia, through a small incision in the skin and a small core of tissue is removed. This technique may not work well for very hard or very small lumps. It may cause some bruising, but rarely leaves an external scar. The procedure is over in a matter of minutes.

Core needle biopsy directed by mammogram or ultrasound guidance is a very accurate way to diagnose a breast abnormality.

Localization biopsy. This procedure uses mammography to locate and a needle to biopsy breast abnormalities that can be seen on a mammogram but not felt. It can be used with surgical biopsy, fine needle aspiration, or core needle biopsy.

437

Surgical biopsy. A radiologist locates the abnormality on a mammogram and inserts a fine needle or wire so that the tip rests in the suspicious area. The surgeon locates and cuts out the targeted area.

Stereotactic localization biopsy. Stereotactic localization biopsy is a newer approach that relies on a three-dimensional x-ray to guide the needle biopsy of a mass that cannot be felt.

TISSUE STUDIES

The cells or tissue removed through needle or surgical biopsy are promptly sent (along with the x-ray of the specimen, if one was made) to the pathology lab. A more thorough assessment takes several days, while the pathologist processes "permanent sections" of tissue that can be examined in greater detail.

The pathologist looks for abnormal cell shapes and unusual growth patterns. In many cases the diagnosis will be clear-cut. When in doubt, pathologists readily consult their colleagues. If there is any question about the results of your biopsy, you will want to make sure your biopsy slides have been reviewed by more than one pathologist.

DECIDING TO BIOPSY

Not every lump or mammographic change merits a biopsy. Nearly all mammographic masses that look smooth and clearly outlined, for instance, are benign. Your doctor needs to thoughtfully weigh the findings from your physical exam and mammogram along with your background and your medical history when making a recommendation about a biopsy.

In general, doctors feel it is wise to biopsy any distinct and persistent lump.

Although benign lumps rarely, if ever, turn into cancer, cancerous lumps can develop near benign lumps and can be hidden on a mammogram. Even if you have had a benign lump removed in the past, you cannot be sure any new lump is also benign.

In some cases, the doctor may suggest watching the suspicious area for a month or two. Because many lumps are caused by normal hormonal changes, this waiting period may provide additional information.

Similarly, if the changes on your mammogram show all the signs of benign disease, your doctor may advise waiting several months and then taking another mammogram. This would be followed by more diagnostic mammograms over the next 3 years. If you choose this option, however, you must be strongly committed to regularly scheduled follow-ups.

If you feel uncomfortable about waiting, express your concerns to your doctor. You may also want to get a second opinion, perhaps from a breast specialist or surgeon. Many cities have breast clinics where you can get a second opinion.

BIOPSY: ONE STEP OR TWO?

Not too many years ago, all women undergoing surgery for breast symptoms had a one-step procedure: If the surgical biopsy showed cancer, the surgeon performed a mastectomy immediately. The woman went into surgery not knowing if she had cancer or if her breast would be removed.

Today a woman facing biopsy has a broader range of options. In most cases, biopsy and diagnosis will be separated from any further treatment by an interval of several days or weeks. Such a two-step procedure does not harm the patient, and it has several benefits. It allows time for the tissue sample to be examined in detail and, if cancer is found, it gives the woman time to adjust to the diagnosis. She can review her treatment options, seek a second opinion, receive counseling, and arrange her schedule.

No single solution is right for everyone. Each woman should consult with her doctors

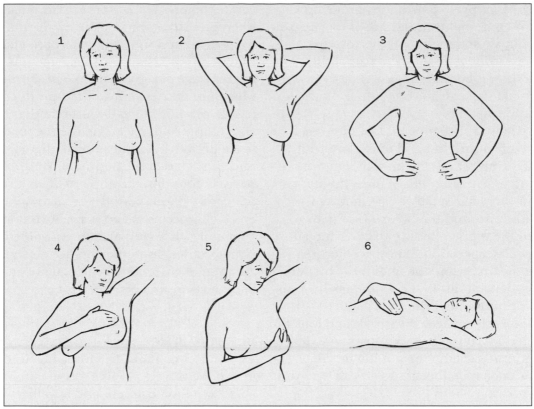

Though regular mammograms are essential in the early detection of breast cancer, many lumps are detected during monthly breast self-exams. The text below explains each of the steps as shown here.

and her family, weigh the alternatives, and decide what approach is appropriate. Being involved in the decision-making process can give a woman a sense of control over her body and her life.

BREAST SELF-EXAMINATION

Breast self-examination (BSE) should be done once a month so you become familiar with the usual appearance and feel of your breasts. Familiarity makes it easier to notice any changes in the breast from one month to another. Early discovery of a change from what is normal is the main idea behind BSE. The outlook is much better if you detect cancer in an early stage.

If you menstruate, the best time to do BSE is two or three days after your period ends, when your breasts are least likely to be tender or swollen. If you no longer menstruate, pick a day such as the first day of the month to remind yourself it is time to do BSE.

Here is one way to perform BSE (as illustrated above):

(1) Stand before a mirror. Inspect both breasts for anything unusual such as any discharge from the nipples or puckering, dimpling, or scaling of the skin.

The next two steps are designed to emphasize any change in the shape or contour of your breasts. As you do them, you should be able to feel your chest muscles tighten.

(2) Watching closely in the mirror, clasp your hands behind your head and press your hands forward.

(3) Next, press your hands firmly on your hips and bow slightly toward the mirror as you pull your shoulders and elbows forward.

Some women do the next part of the exam in the shower because fingers glide over soapy skin, making it easy to concentrate on the texture underneath.

(4) Raise your left arm. Use three or four fingers of your right hand to explore your left breast firmly, carefully, and thoroughly. Beginning at the outer edge, press the flat part of your fingers in small circles, moving the circles slowly around the breast. Gradually work toward the nipple. Be sure to cover the entire breast. Pay special attention to the area between the breast and the underarm, including the underarm itself. Feel for any unusual lump or mass under the skin.

(5) Gently squeeze the nipple and look for a discharge. (If you have any discharge during the month—whether or not it is during BSE—see your doctor.) Repeat steps 4 and 5 on your right breast.

(6) Steps 4 and 5 should be repeated lying down. Lie flat on your back with your left arm over your head and a pillow or folded towel under your left shoulder. This position flattens the breast and makes it easier to examine. Use the same circular motion described earlier. Repeat the exam on your right breast.

The National Cancer Institute

MENOPAUSE

More than one-third of the women in the United States, about 36 million, have been through menopause. With a life expectancy of about 81 years, a 50-year-old woman can expect to live more than one-third of her life after menopause. Scientific research is just beginning to address some of the unanswered questions about these years and about the poorly understood biology of menopause.

Menopause is the point in a woman's life when menstruation stops permanently, signifying the end of her ability to have children. Known as the "change of life," menopause is the last stage of a gradual biological process in which the ovaries reduce their production of female sex hormones—a process that begins about three to five years before the final menstrual period. This transitional phase is called the climacteric, or perimenopause. Menopause is considered complete when a woman has been without periods for one year. On average, this occurs at about age 50. But like the beginning of menstruation in adolescence, timing varies from person to person. Cigarette smokers tend to reach menopause earlier than nonsmokers.

HOW IT HAPPENS

The ovaries contain structures called follicles that hold the egg cells. You are born with about 2 million egg cells and by puberty there are about 300,000 left. Only about 400 to 500 ever mature fully to be released during the menstrual cycle.

The rest degenerate over the years. During the reproductive years, the pituitary gland in the brain generates hormones that cause a new egg to be released from its follicle each month. The follicle also increases production of the sex hormones estrogen and progesterone, which thicken the lining of the uterus. This enriched lining is prepared to receive and nourish a fertilized egg following conception. If fertilization does not occur, estrogen and progesterone levels drop, the lining of the uterus breaks down, and menstruation occurs.

For unknown reasons, the ovaries begin to decline in hormone production during the mid-thirties. In the late forties, the process accelerates and hormones fluctuate more, causing irregular menstrual cycles and unpredictable episodes of heavy bleeding. By the early to mid-fifties, periods finally end altogether. However, estrogen production does not completely stop. The ovaries decrease their output significantly, but still may produce a small amount. Also, another form of estrogen is produced in fat tissue with help from the adrenal glands (near the kidney). Although this form of estrogen is weaker than that produced by the ovaries, it increases with age and with the amount of fat tissue.

Progesterone, the other female hormone, works during the second half of the menstrual cycle to create a lining in the uterus as a viable home for an egg, and to shed the lining if the egg is not fertilized. If you skip a period, your body may not be making enough progesterone to break down the uterine lining. However, your estrogen levels may remain high even though you are not menstruating.

At menopause, hormone levels don't always decline uniformly. They alternately rise and fall again. Changing ovarian hormone levels affect the other glands in the body, which together make up the endocrine system. The endocrine system controls growth, metabolism, and reproduction. This system must constantly readjust itself to work effectively. Ovarian hormones also affect all other tissues, including the breasts, vagina, bones, blood vessels, gastrointestinal tract, urinary tract, and skin.

SURGICAL MENOPAUSE

Premenopausal women who have both their ovaries removed surgically experience an abrupt menopause. They may be hit harder by menopausal symptoms than are those who experience it naturally. Their hot flashes may be more severe, more frequent, and last longer. They may have a greater risk of heart disease and osteoporosis, and may be more likely to become depressed. The reasons for this are unknown. When only one ovary is removed, menopause usually occurs naturally. When the uterus is removed (hysterectomy) and the ovaries remain, menstrual periods stop but other menopausal symptoms (if any) usually occur at the same age that they would naturally. However, some women who have a hysterectomy may experience menopausal symptoms at a younger age.

WHAT TO EXPECT

Menopause is an individualized experience. Some women notice little difference in their bodies or moods, while others find the change extremely bothersome and disruptive. Estrogen and progesterone affect virtually all tissues in the body, but everyone is influenced by them differently.

Hot Flashes

Hot flashes, or flushes, are the most common symptom of menopause, affecting more than 60 percent of menopausal women in the U.S. A hot flash is a sudden sensation of intense heat in the upper part or all of the body. The face and neck may become flushed, with red blotches appearing on the chest, back, and arms. This is often followed by profuse sweating and then cold shivering as body temperature readjusts. A hot flash can last a few moments or 30 minutes or longer.

Hot flashes occur sporadically and often start several years before other signs of menopause. They gradually decline in frequency and intensity as you age. Eighty percent of all women with hot flashes have them for two years or less, while a small percentage have them for more than five years. Hot flashes can happen at any time. They can be as mild as a light blush, or severe enough to wake you from a deep sleep. Some women even develop insomnia. Others have found that caffeine, alcohol, hot drinks, spicy foods, and stressful or frightening events can sometimes trigger a hot flash. However, avoiding these triggers will not necessarily prevent all episodes.

The flashes appear to be a direct result of decreasing estrogen levels. In response to falling estrogen levels, your glands release higher amounts of other hormones that affect the brain's thermostat, causing body temperatures to fluctuate. Hormone therapy relieves the discomfort of hot flashes in most cases.

Some women claim that vitamin E offers minor relief, although there has never been a study to confirm it. Aside from hormone therapy, which is not for everyone, here are some suggestions for coping with hot flashes:

- Dress in layers so you can remove them at the first sign of a flash.
- Drink a glass of cold water or juice at the onset of a flash.
- At night keep a thermos of ice water or an ice pack by your bed.
- Use cotton sheets, lingerie, and clothing to let your skin "breathe."

Vaginal and Urinary Tract Changes

With advancing age, the walls of the vagina become thinner, dryer, less elastic, and more vulnerable to infection. These changes can make sexual intercourse uncomfortable or painful. Most women find it helpful to lubricate the vagina. Water-soluble lubricants are preferable, as they help reduce the chance of infection. Try to avoid petroleum jelly; many women are allergic, and it damages condoms. See your gynecologist if problems persist.

Tissues in the urinary tract also change with age, sometimes leaving women more susceptible to involuntary loss of urine (incontinence), particularly if certain chronic illnesses or urinary infections are also present. Exercise, coughing, laughing, lifting heavy objects, or similar movements that put pressure on the bladder may cause small amounts of urine to leak. Lack of regular physical exercise may contribute to this condition. It's important to know, however, that incontinence is not a normal part of aging, to be masked by using adult diapers. Rather, it is usually a treatable condition that warrants medical evaluation. Recent research has shown that bladder training is a simple and effective treatment for most cases of incontinence and is less expensive and safer than medication or surgery.

Within four or five years after the final menstrual period, there is an increased chance of vaginal and urinary tract infections. If symptoms such as painful or overly frequent urination occur, consult your doctor. Infections are easily treated with antibiotics, but often tend to recur. To help prevent these infections, urinate before and after intercourse, be sure your bladder is not full for long periods, drink plenty of fluids, and keep your genital area clean. Douching is not thought to be effective in preventing infection.

MANAGING MENOPAUSE

Menopause is a natural part of aging and does not necessarily require treatment. But if you experience great discomfort at this time, consult your physician.

Hormone Replacement Therapy (HRT)

To combat the symptoms associated with falling estrogen levels, doctors have turned to hormone replacement therapy (HRT). HRT is the administration of the female hormones estrogen and progesterone. Estrogen replacement therapy (ERT) refers to administration of estrogen alone. The hormones are usually given in pill form, though sometimes skin patches and vaginal creams (just estrogen) are used. ERT is thought to help prevent the devastating effects of heart disease and osteoporosis, conditions that are often difficult and expensive to treat once they appear. The cardiovascular effects of progesterone, however, are still unknown.

Hormone treatment for menopause is still quite controversial. Its long-term safety and efficacy remain matters of great concern. There is not enough existing data for physicians to suggest that HRT is the right choice for all women. Several large studies are currently attempting to resolve the questions, though it will take several more years to reach any definitive answers.

Estrogen and the Bones

HRT and ERT are successful methods of combatting osteoporosis. As previously discussed, estrogen halts bone loss but cannot necessarily rebuild bone. Long-term estrogen use (10 or more years) may be required to prevent postmenopausal bone loss. Why estrogen helps protect the skeleton is still unclear. We do know that estrogen helps bones absorb the calcium they need to stay strong. It also helps conserve the calcium stored in the bones by encouraging other cells to use dietary calcium more efficiently. For instance, muscles require calcium to contract. If there is not enough calcium circulating in the blood for muscles to use, calcium is "borrowed" from the bone. Calcium is also needed for blood clotting, sending nerve impulses, and secreting various hormones. Prolonged borrowing from bone calcium for these processes speeds bone loss. That's why it's important to consume adequate amounts of calcium in your diet. (See Osteoporosis on page 388 for more information.)

Estrogen and the Heart

The majority of past clinical studies have shown that women who use estrogen substantially reduce their risk of developing and dying from heart disease. One or two studies demonstrate conflicting evidence, but they are far outnumbered by the positive reports. Results from a 1991 study showed that after 15 years of estrogen replacement, risk of death by cardiovascular disease (CVD) was reduced by almost 50 percent and overall deaths were reduced by 40 percent. Some researchers credit this reduction to oral estrogen's ability to maintain HDL and LDL cholesterol at their healthier, premenopausal levels, through its interaction with proteins in the liver. Others believe it is estrogen's direct ef-

fect on the blood vessels themselves (through receptors on the vessel walls) that creates this benefit. In the latter case, both oral estrogen and the skin patch would be effective. Studies are under way to determine which mechanism contributes most to a healthy heart.

Drawbacks of HRT: The Cancer Risk

A major issue surrounding HRT and ERT is the influence of estrogen on breast cancer. Researchers believe that the longer your lifetime exposure to naturally occurring estrogen, the greater your risk of breast cancer. It has not been proven, however, that estrogen administered at menopause has the same effect. There is disagreement on the many trials conducted to date because of wide variations in the populations studied and the doses, timing, and types of estrogen used.

Most studies, however, have not demonstrated an increase in breast cancer mortality associated with long-term ERT (10 to 15 years of use).

A recent analysis of previous studies suggests that low-dose estrogen taken on a short-term basis (10 years or less) does not pose increased risk of breast cancer. Long-term use (more than 10 years) at a high dose may significantly increase the risk. By how much is still a matter of heated debate.

At the very most, researchers think long-term use could possibly increase the risk of getting breast cancer by 30 percent. This means that incidence would rise from 10 women per 10,000 each year to 13 women per 10,000 each year. To reach any consensus, however, more women need to be monitored for an extended period of time. The fear of cancer is one of the most common reasons that women are unwilling to use HRT. Interestingly, actual death rates for breast cancer have not risen at all. This may be because estrogen users have more frequent medical visits and obtain more preventive care, including yearly mammograms.

While no one can determine who will eventually develop breast cancer, there are certain risk factors you should be aware of when considering HRT. A family history of breast cancer (sister or mother) is probably the most important risk factor of all. You may also be at an increased risk if you menstruated before age 12; delayed motherhood until later in life; or have a late menopause (after age 50). Also, the older you are, the higher the risk. Most doctors believe that if you are not in a high-risk category for breast or endometrial cancer, the benefits of HRT far outweigh the risks. However, for some women, the side effects of therapy make it impossible to use. This is a personal decision to be made by each woman with help from her doctor.

Other Risks

Physicians usually caution women not to use HRT if they are already at high risk for developing blood clots. Obesity, severe varicose veins, smoking, and a history of blood clots put you in this category. A history of gall bladder disease could also be cause to avoid HRT, as women taking estrogen may have a greater chance of developing gallstones.

Pros and Cons of HRT

While more research is under way, here is what scientists can say so far about the advantages and disadvantages of HRT (estrogen and progesterone) and ERT (estrogen):

- HRT and ERT relieve hot flashes.
- HRT and ERT reduce the risk of heart disease.
- HRT and ERT may improve mood and psychological well-being. ERT increases the risk of cancer of the uterus (endometrial cancer).
- HRT can have unpleasant side effects, such as bloating or irritability.
- HRT and ERT may increase risk of breast cancer; long-term use may pose the greatest risk.
- In women with blood clots, HRT and ERT may be dangerous.

MENOPAUSE AND MENTAL HEALTH

A popular myth pictures the menopausal woman shifting from raging, angry moods into depressive, doleful slumps with no apparent reason or warning. However, a study by psychologists at the University of Pittsburgh suggests that menopause does not cause unpredictable mood swings, depression, or even stress in most women.

In fact, it may even improve mental health for some. This gives further support to the idea that menopause is not necessarily a negative experience. The Pittsburgh study looked at three different groups of women: menstruating, menopausal with no treatment, and menopausal on hormone therapy. The study showed that the menopausal women suffered no more anxiety, depression, anger, nervousness, or feelings of stress than the group of menstruating women in the same age range. In addition, although more hot flashes were reported by the menopausal women not taking hormones, surprisingly they had better overall mental health than the other two groups. The women taking hormones worried more about their bodies and were somewhat more depressed.

However, this could be caused by the hormones themselves. It's also possible that women who voluntarily take hormones tend to be more conscious of their bodies in the first place. The researchers caution that their study includes only healthy women, so results may apply only to them. Other studies show that women already taking hormones who are experiencing mood or behavioral problems sometimes respond well to a change in dosage or type of estrogen.

Studies indicate that women of childbearing age, particularly those with young children at home, tend to report more emotional problems than women of other ages.

The Pittsburgh findings are supported by a New England Research Institute study which found that menopausal women were no more depressed than the general population: About 10 percent are occasionally depressed and 5 percent are persistently depressed. The exception is women who undergo surgical menopause: Their depression rate is reportedly double that of women who've had natural menopause.

Studies also have indicated that many cases of depression relate more to life stresses or "mid-life crises" than to menopause. Such stresses include an alteration in family roles, as when your children are grown and move out of the house, no longer "needing" mom; a changing social support network, which may happen after a divorce if you no longer socialize with friends you met through your husband; interpersonal losses, as when a parent, spouse, or other close relative dies; and your own aging and the beginning of physical illness. People have very different responses to stress and crisis. Your best friend's response may be negative, leaving her open to emotional distress and depression, while yours is positive, resulting in achievement of your goals. For many women, this stage of life can actually be a period of enormous freedom.

MENOPAUSE AND SEXUALITY

For some women, but by no means all, menopause brings a decrease in sexual activity. Reduced hormone levels cause subtle changes in the genital tissues and are thought to be linked also to a decline in sexual interest. Lower estrogen levels decrease the blood supply to the vagina and the nerves and glands surrounding it. This makes delicate tissues thinner, drier, and less able to produce secretions to comfortably lubricate before and during intercourse. Avoiding sex is not necessary. Estrogen creams and oral estrogen can restore secretions and tissue elasticity. Water-soluble lubricants can also help.

While changes in hormone production are cited as the major reason for changes in sexual behavior, many other interpersonal, psychological, and cultural factors can come into play. For instance, a Swedish study found that many women use menopause as an excuse to stop sex completely after years of disinterest. Many physicians, however, question whether declining interest is the cause or the result of less frequent intercourse.

Some women actually feel liberated after menopause and report an increased interest in sex. They say they feel relieved that pregnancy is no longer a worry.

For women in perimenopause, birth control is a confusing issue. Doctors advise all women who have menstruated, even if irregularly, within the past year to continue using birth control. Unfortunately, contraceptive options are limited. Hormone-based oral and implantable contraceptives are risky in older women who smoke. Only a few brands of IUD are on the market. The other options are barrier methods—diaphragms, condoms, and sponges—or methods requiring surgery, such as tubal ligation.

LOOKING AHEAD

Good nutrition and regular physical exercise are thought to improve overall health. Some doctors feel these factors can also affect menopause. Although these areas have not been well studied in women, anecdotal evidence is strongly in favor of eating well and exercising to help lower the risks for CVD and osteoporosis.

Clearly, no one has all the answers about menopause. Medical research is beginning to give us more accurate information, but myths and negative attitudes remain deep-seated. Women are challenging stereotypes, gaining support from other women, learning about what takes place in their bodies, and taking more responsibility for their health.

The National Institute on Aging

URINARY INCONTINENCE

It's hard to imagine 5 million people keeping a secret. But experts estimate that's just how many older Americans suffer in secret—and, more often than not, needlessly—from urinary incontinence, or the involuntary loss of urine. And this shroud of secrecy is perpetuated by the manufacturers of adult diapers, who imply—erroneously—in their advertisements that urinary incontinence is a result of normal aging, and that diapers are the best recourse for the incontinent adult. In fact, incontinence is almost always treatable. As such, it requires an evaluation by a doctor and specific treatment, not a diaper. (Recently in New York State, two of the biggest manufacturers of adult diapers agreed to alter their advertising after the state's Attorney General demanded that the ads clearly state that incontinence should be treated by a doctor.)

A recent consensus conference of the National Institutes of Health concluded that there may be up to 10 million adult Americans, most of them older, who are incontinent. One study of a county in Michigan found that 38 percent of women and 19 percent of men over 60 suffered from incontinence. And these figures exclude nursing home residents. At least half of the 1.5 million Americans in nursing homes cannot control urination. In fact, incontinence is the second most common reason stated for admission to a nursing home—which, in part, explains why the national bill for the condition tops $10.3 billion each year. And, if left untreated, incontinence can lead to urinary tract infections, rashes, and other skin disorders. On a social level, embarrassment about odor and fear of being far from a restroom can make the incontinent person avoid outings, friends, and social activities.

Although incontinence is more prevalent among the older population, the condition is not, as myth would have it, an inevitable consequence of aging. Rather it is a symptom of some underlying disorder—and treatment for the conditions that cause incontinence can be highly successful.

A combination of techniques ranging from behavior modification to medication, and sometimes surgery, can cure or at least greatly improve the condition in 90 percent of sufferers. The first step to treatment, then, is acknowledging the problem and telling your physician about it.

CAUSES AND PROBLEMS

Control of urination, something continent people take for granted, is actually a complex synchronized process involving the kidneys, the ureters (the tubes connecting the kidneys to the bladder), the bladder itself, the urethra (the tube through which urine passes from the bladder to outside the body), and the muscles of the pelvic floor and abdominal wall.

The process of urination is coordinated by the central nervous system. Urine is produced by the kidneys, then passes into the bladder, where it is stored. When the bladder, which is like a continually inflating and deflating balloon, reaches a certain degree of fullness, it signals nerves in the spinal cord. These nerves activate the voiding reflex, which causes the muscles of the bladder to contract and squeeze the urine into the urethra. However, the brain, in the toilet-training process of childhood, has learned to identify and control this reflex by tightening the muscles of the pelvic floor—a sling of muscles that support the bladder, urethra, and other pelvic organs—until the toilet is reached.

Disruption of nearly any part of this system can lead to incontinence. Underlying causes range from neurological problems that affect central nervous system control to anatomical abnormalities or an infection of the genital or urinary systems. Incontinence can begin suddenly (transient incontinence) or develop into a chronic condition (persistent incontinence).

Transient Incontinence

This is less common than the persistent type, and any sudden onset of incontinence should prompt a call to your physician. Most often, the problem is reversible. Common causes are infections of the genitourinary system, such as cystitis, urethritis, and vaginitis; various medications, especially diuretics, sleeping pills, tranquilizers, and antidepressants; any illness that limits movement or causes confusion, such as a high fever; depression; and fecal impaction (a mass of stool in the rectum) that presses on the bladder.

Persistent Incontinence

This condition can be the outcome of untreated transient incontinence or can gradually develop on its own. There are four patterns of persistent incontinence, although at least one-third of older patients have a combination of patterns simultaneously.

Urge incontinence is caused by difficulties suppressing the sense of bladder fullness and the subsequent urge to void. Usually, the bladder contracts involuntarily, causing such an uncontrollable need to release urine that the sufferer is unable to heed the voiding reflex in time to get to a toilet. People with urge incontinence are likely to have large-volume accidents. Central nervous system disturbances such as stroke or dementia, or a bladder problem such as a tumor, can cause urge incontinence, although sometimes no underlying cause is found.

Stress incontinence is associated with problems of the urethra and the muscles of the pelvic floor. The kind of abdominal muscle contraction that occurs with sneezing, lifting, or coughing increases pressure on the bladder. In stress incontinence, the muscles surrounding the urethra are not able to resist the sudden increase in bladder pressure, so there is uncontrolled leakage of urine—usually a few drops, but occasionally a large amount. Stress incontinence is largely a women's problem, attributed to the strain of childbirth on the muscles of the pelvic floor, and the thinning of the pelvic floor muscles and other tissues in the vaginal area that can occur after estrogen levels drop following menopause.

Eighty-five percent of incontinence sufferers have stress or urge incontinence, or a combination pattern known as mixed incontinence. The two less common types of incontinence are functional and overflow.

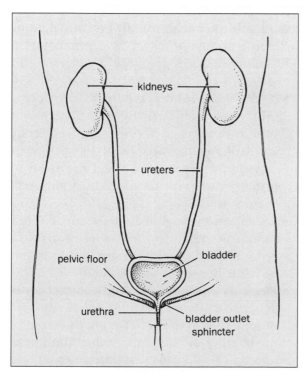

Urine flows from the kidneys, through the ureters, to the bladder. Muscles surrounding the urethra normally stem the flow of urine until urination is initiated.

THREE STEPS IN THE TREATMENT OF THE COMMON TYPES OF INCONTINENCE

Typo	Behavioral Therapy	Drug Therapy	Surgery
Stress	• Muscle strengthening exercises • Biofeedback	• Alpha adrenergic agonists (drugs that increase sphincter strength): pseudoephedrine, ephedrine, phenylpropanolamine (Propagest) • Estrogens (female hormones that increase sphincter and pelvic muscle strength)	• Vaginal sling operation (creation of a "hammock" under the urethra in order to support it) • Surgical tightening of the pelvic muscles and elevation of the bladder • Implantation of an artificial urinary sphincter
Urge	• Bladder training • Muscle strengthening exercises • Biofeedback	• Anticholinergics and combination anticholinergics/antispasmodics (drugs that reduce bladder contractions): propantheline (Pro-Banthine), imipramine (Norfranil, Tofranil), oxybutynin (Ditropan) • Estrogens	

Overflow incontinence occurs when the bladder cannot empty completely, usually due to a partial obstruction of the urethra or a drug that relaxes the bladder muscle. Even after urinating, the bladder remains full; if it becomes too full, urine leaks out through the urethra. The problem can also be caused by a dysfunction in the nerves controlling the bladder muscle or in the muscle itself, due to diabetes, injury, nervous system disorders, or drugs.

Functional incontinence develops when a person becomes unable to use the bathroom. This can be caused by a degenerative condition or illness that restricts movement, or unwillingness to use the toilet, as might occur with a psychiatric illness.

DIAGNOSTIC PROCEDURES

The most important step to the diagnosis and subsequent treatment of incontinence is to ask for help. Once you have informed your doctor of your problem, determining the un-derlying causes often requires only a simple examination that can usually be done by your internist, family physician, or gynecologist. The components of diagnosis are:

- *A detailed medical history.* Your doctor should ask very specific questions about your symptoms, including how frequently you urinate, the approximate volume of urine, how urgently you feel the need to urinate. Also, you should report all medications used.
- *Laboratory tests.* A urinalysis and culture should be performed, to check for infection or other possible diseases that might be contributing to the problem.
- *Physical examination.* Your doctor will probably do a manual rectal, genital, and abdominal exam to check for enlargement of the bladder or to identify other abnormalities that could cause incontinence.
- *Special tests.* Your doctor may perform a test to determine if the bladder is truly empty following urination. This procedure is

usually done by catheterization of the bladder immediately after voiding. In a provoked full-bladder stress test, you will be asked to cough, bend over, or walk after the bladder has been filled to capacity through a catheter, to see if leakage occurs.

Most often, your medical history coupled with these procedures will be enough to determine what treatment you need. If not, or if the initial treatment plan doesn't relieve your symptoms, your physician should refer you to a specialist, usually a urologist.

TREATMENT OPTIONS

There are three types of treatment for urinary incontinence: behavior modification, medication, and surgery.

Generally, behavioral techniques are tried first, because they are the safest and, for many people, highly effective. Two methods are commonly used: bladder training, and exercises of the pelvic muscles (such as Kegel exercises) and bladder sphincter. Such treatments demand a commitment of time and practice. For example, Kegel exercises may need to be done for two to three months before they strengthen muscles enough to correct incontinence. Both Kegel exercises and bladder training can be done at home. Biofeedback uses sophisticated equipment that gives visual and auditory feedback to help patients identify and use their bladder-control muscles more effectively. It can thus be used to enhance bladder training and pelvic muscle exercises, and has led to complete control of incontinence in up to 25 percent of patients and significant improvement in another 30 to 50 percent.

Also, there are a number of medications that may improve bladder control by relaxing the bladder, or by tightening the sphincter muscles and muscles of the pelvic floor. However, as with all medications, these drugs can have undesirable side effects, especially in those with other medical conditions.

Finally, surgery may be very effective for some cases of incontinence—especially pure stress incontinence in women.

The box opposite outlines treatment options for the two primary types of incontinence.

Several newer treatments are currently in the testing phase. For stress incontinence, the injection of collagen into the urethra is being tested as an alternative to surgery in several clinical trials around the country. The substance creates a tissuelike mass that strengthens the urethra and allows it to close fully. Also for stress incontinence, weighted vaginal cones designed to increase the effectiveness of muscle strengthening exercises are being evaluated. For urge incontinence, a new antispasmodic medication called Micturin, which needs to be taken only once a day, is in clinical trials.

Some of these new treatments are quite promising. However, until more long-term results on these devices and procedures are in, advertisements for a quick (and costly) fix for incontinence should be ignored as much as ads for adult diapers. "None of these newer treatments should yet be used, except in clinical trials," states Dr. John Burton, director of Geriatric Medicine and Gerontology at Johns Hopkins. "Furthermore, the therapies currently in use are highly effective."

How to Treat Incontinence at Home

Two of the most effective methods of treating incontinence cost no money and can be done at home. Muscle strengthening exercises, such as Kegel exercises, increase the strength of the pelvic floor, which supports the base of the bladder and the bladder outlet sphincter. These exercises help with both stress and urge incontinence. To locate the proper muscles, when you are urinating, tighten up and try to stop the flow. Another technique is to tighten your anal sphincter—because of its proximity to the bladder sphincter, this helps identify muscles necessary for maintaining continence. Once you have located the correct muscles, you should practice the exercise regularly. Try to do between 15 and 20 squeezes three times a day; work up to holding each for 10 seconds. Practice during different activities, such as walking, sitting, or lying down.

Bladder training is effective for urge, stress, and mixed incontinence. Follow these steps:

- Schedule toileting every two hours, whether you have to go or not.
- Every other day, extend the interval between toileting by 30 minutes, aiming for four-hour intervals.
- If you have an urge to urinate in between your scheduled visits to the bathroom, stay still, relax, and use the muscle strengthening exercises described above. After the urge has passed, move slowly to a bathroom.
- Maintain the schedule whether you have accidents or not.
- Maintain the schedule when you are out of your home but avoid drinking excess fluids before or while you are away from home.

The Editors

VAGINITIS

Vaginitis causes redness, swelling, and irritation of the outer genital area and discharge from the vagina. Although some types of vaginal discharge are normal, others are signs of infection or problems.

Vaginitis is a common problem that affects up to one-third of women at some point in their lives. Most often it is caused by an infection, but other factors that cause changes in the normal vagina can also result in the symptoms of vaginitis.

Vaginitis is rarely a serious threat to a woman's health. It can be annoying and uncomfortable, though. It usually does not go away without treatment. For treatment to work, the cause of the vaginitis should be found so that the treatment used matches the disease.

Some types of vaginitis are hard to get rid of. There are many types of drugs that can be used for treatment, though. With time, a treatment that works can usually be found. Long-term treatment may be needed in some cases, and sometimes changes in a woman's personal habits are required.

THE VAGINA

The vagina leads from a woman's uterus to the outside of the body. The area around the outside entrance to the vagina is called the vulva. Some conditions that affect the vulva also affect the vagina.

A healthy vagina has a balance of many microorganisms (such as yeast and bacteria). They work together to create an acidic environment. This maintains a natural barrier against infection and keeps organisms that may be harmful in check.

The vagina has a normal discharge (a small amount of fluid that passes out of the vagina). A normal discharge helps to keep the vagina healthy. It is clear or cloudy and whitish. It does not have a strong odor or cause itching or burning. How much and what kind of discharge a woman normally has may vary. It may change during the menstrual cycle, and it usually increases during pregnancy. An abnormal discharge is one that causes itching and burning or has an unpleasant odor. This is one of the most common signs of vaginitis. It should prompt you to see your doctor.

CAUSES OF VAGINITIS

Vaginitis can result from anything that causes a change in the normal environment of the vagina:

- Antibiotics
- Changes in the body's normal hormone

levels (such as those that occur with pregnancy, breastfeeding, or menopause)
- Douches
- Spermicides
- Sexual intercourse
- Sexually transmitted diseases (STDs)

A change in the normal balance can allow either yeast or bacteria to increase and result in vaginitis. Vaginitis can result from irritation, from growth of organisms in the vagina, or from infection.

TREATMENT

Treatment works best when matched to the cause of vaginitis. Your doctor will need to know what symptoms you have had. A sample of the discharge may be taken to be studied under a microscope. A sample may also be used for a culture. In this test, the organisms in the sample are allowed to multiply so that they are easier to identify. There are other tests your doctor may suggest, too. To ensure the accuracy of these tests, do not douche or use any vaginal medications or spermicide for one to two days before you visit the doctor.

Treatment may depend not only on the cause of the vaginitis but also on your personal circumstances. For instance, the creams and gels used to treat vaginitis may cause side effects of itching and burning. Some women are allergic to these medications. Another treatment may be tried if this is the case. Also, some medications may not be used during the early part of pregnancy because of possible effects on the fetus.

If you are found to have vaginitis, there are things you can do to lessen your chances of getting it again (see What You Can Do, page 452).

TYPES OF VAGINITIS
Yeast Infection

Yeast infection is also known as candidiasis.

This is one of the most common types of vaginal infection.

Cause. Yeast infection is caused by a fungus called Candida. It is found in small numbers in the normal vagina. However, when the balance of the vagina is changed, the yeast may overgrow and cause infection.

Many women who take antibiotics will get yeast infections. The antibiotics kill normal vaginal bacteria, and the yeast then has a chance to overgrow. A woman is more likely to get yeast infections if she is pregnant or has diabetes. Overgrowth of yeast can also occur if the body's immune system, which protects the body from disease, isn't working well. For example, in women infected with HIV (human immunodeficiency virus), yeast infections may be severe. They may not go away, despite treatment, or may recur often. In many cases, the cause of a yeast infection is not known.

Symptoms. The most common symptoms of a yeast infection are itching and burning of the vagina and vulva. The burning may be worse with urination or sex. The vulva may be red and swollen. The vaginal discharge is usually white and has no odor. It may look like cottage cheese. Some women with yeast infections notice an increase or change in discharge. Others do not notice a discharge at all. Some women may have no symptoms.

Treatment. Yeast infections are usually treated by placing medication into the vagina. Some doctors may prescribe a single dose you take by mouth. In most cases, treatment of male sex partners is not necessary. You can now buy an over-the-counter treatment for yeast infection but be sure to see your doctor if:

- This is the first time you've had a vaginal infection.
- Symptoms do not go away after treatment.
- The vaginal discharge is yellow or green or has a bad odor.

451

WHAT YOU CAN DO

There are a number of things you can do in your daily life to try to keep from getting vaginitis. Especially if you are prone to repeat bouts, keep in mind these points:
• Do not use feminine hygiene sprays or scented, deodorant tampons. You should not try to cover up a bad odor. It could be a sign of infection that should prompt you to see your doctor.
• Do not douche. It is better to let the vagina cleanse itself.
• Thoroughly clean diaphragms, cervical caps, and spermicide applicators after each use.
• Use condoms during sex.
• Check with your doctor about preventing yeast infections if you are prescribed antibiotics for another type of infection.

Follow your doctor's instructions to the letter, even if the discharge or other symptoms go away before the medication is finished. Even though the symptoms disappear, the infection could still be present. Stopping the treatment may cause it to come back. If symptoms recur after the treatment is finished, see your doctor again—a different treatment may be needed.

• There is a chance that you have a sexually transmitted disease.

Sometimes a woman thinks she has a yeast infection when she actually has another problem. The medication may mask another cause for vaginitis. If there is another cause, it may be harder to find if a woman is taking medication for a yeast infection.

Bacterial Vaginosis

Causes. The bacteria that cause bacterial vaginosis occur naturally in the vagina. Bacterial vaginosis is caused by overgrowth of several of these bacteria. It is not clear whether it can be passed through sex.

Symptoms. The main symptom is increased discharge with a strong fishy odor. The odor is stronger during your menstrual period or after sex. The discharge is thin and dark or dull gray. Itching is not common, but may be present if there is a lot of discharge. Some women may have no symptoms.

Treatment. Two antibiotics are used to treat bacterial vaginosis. One is a drug called metronidazole. It can be taken by mouth or applied to the vagina as a gel. The other drug is called clindamycin. It can also be taken by mouth or applied to the vagina as a cream.

When metronidazole is taken by mouth, it can cause side effects in some patients. These include nausea, vomiting, and darkening of urine. Do not drink alcohol when taking metronidazole. The combination can cause severe nausea and vomiting.

Usually there is no need to treat a woman's sex partner. But if the woman has repeated infections, treatment of the partner may be helpful. Some doctors may suggest that the couple not have sex or that they use a condom during treatment.

Bacterial vaginosis often comes back. It may require long-term or repeated treatment. In most cases, treatment eventually works in time. Sometimes when bacterial vaginosis keeps coming back it may mean that you have an STD. Your doctor may test you for other infections.

Trichomonas Vaginitis (Trichomoniasis)

Causes. Trichomonas is a parasite that is spread through sex. Women who have trichomonas vaginitis are at higher risk for infection with other STDs.

Symptoms. Signs of trichomoniasis may include a yellow-gray or green vaginal discharge. The discharge may have a fishy odor. There may be burning, irritation, redness, and swelling of the vulva and vagina. Sometimes there is pain during urination.

Treatment. Trichomoniasis is usually treated with a single dose of metronidazole by mouth. Do not drink alcohol for 24 hours when taking this drug because it causes nausea and vomiting. Sexual partners must be treated at the same time for the treatment to work.

Atrophic Vaginitis

This type of vaginitis is linked with not having enough estrogen. It can occur during breastfeeding and after menopause. Symptoms include vaginal dryness and burning. Atrophic vaginitis is treated with estrogen, either taken by mouth or applied as a vaginal cream. If for some reason a woman cannot take estrogen, she may find a water-soluble lubricant helpful.

Sexually Transmitted Diseases

Symptoms of vaginitis, such as itching, burning, and irritation, can be caused by infection with viruses and bacteria that are spread through sexual contact. A woman with this type of infection can pass it to her sexual partner. Although men have symptoms of these types of infections less often than women do, men can still spread the infection to their sexual partners. Using condoms during sex can help prevent the spread of these infections.

Human papillomavirus (HPV) and genital herpes are viruses. Infection with HPV or herpes is marked by sores, blisters, or growths on the outer genitals.

Infections caused by bacteria are gonorrhea, chlamydia, and syphilis. Symptoms of gonorrhea and chlamydia can include vaginal discharge, itching, burning, and irritation. Symptoms of syphilis can include a sore or a rash.

See your doctor right away if you notice any type of growth or sore in the genital area or if you have any of these symptoms.

OTHER CAUSES

Vaginitis is not always caused by an infection. Vaginal burning, itching, and irritation can also result from other causes. An allergic reaction to chemicals or perfumes, such as those in soaps, bubble baths, or deodorant tampons or pads, can result in these symptoms. In other cases, a reaction to the chemicals in douches, sprays, or spermicides may be the cause. Some women are allergic to the latex used to make some condoms.

Douching can upset the natural balance of the vagina. It can also help to spread organisms higher in the genital tract (up through the cervix and into the uterus and fallopian tubes). For this reason, most doctors advise against routine douching. The vagina cleanses itself naturally by producing a normal discharge.

Another cause of vaginitis is irritation of the vaginal walls. This can result from a tampon, vaginal sponge, diaphragm, or cervical cap that has been left in too long.

CONCLUSION

Vaginitis is common in women of all ages. It can occur whether or not you are sexually active. At the first sign of any abnormal discharge or other symptoms of vaginitis, see your doctor. Yeast infection is the only type of vaginitis with an over-the-counter treatment.

At the first sign of any abnormal discharge or symptoms of vaginitis, contact your doctor so that the problem can be properly diagnosed and treated. Although vaginitis can be annoying and uncomfortable, it can almost always be successfully treated once the cause has been found.

The American College of Obstetricians and Gynecologists

453

Mental Health

The period of late adulthood generally brings with it quite a number of major life changes, including shifts in work status, social situation, and health. By age 65, for example, less than 20 percent of men, and even fewer women, are still in the work force. Not having to go to a job every morning after 40-some years of working is a relief for many—but, for some, it's hard to get used to. Learning to live on a fixed income during retirement can be stressful, too. Also in later years, some decline in physical health often sets in: Four out of five people over 65 have at least one chronic illness such as arthritis or heart disease. Furthermore, one out of every four persons over 65 lives alone. Feelings of loneliness are bound to occur after a spouse dies or when grown children move away.

Any of these major transitions can understandably affect our sense of emotional well-being. Depression, insomnia, or feelings of anxiety may develop. Fortunately, in the past several decades, more and more people have felt comfortable about seeking professional help in such circumstances. In many cases, emotional or psychiatric distress can be treated by your family physician. Appropriate therapy can significantly relieve such problems. Sometimes referral to a specialist is best.

The Editors

DEPRESSION

Everyone feels "blue" at certain times during his or her life. In fact, transitory feelings of sadness or discouragement are perfectly normal, especially during particularly difficult times. But a person who cannot "snap out of it" or get over these feelings within two weeks may be suffering from the illness called depression.

Depression is one of the most common and treatable of all mental illnesses. In any six-month period, 17 million Americans suffer from this disease. One in four women and one in 10 men can expect to develop it during their lifetime. Eighty to 90 percent of those who suffer from depression can be effectively treated, and nearly all people who receive treatment derive some benefit.

Unfortunately, many fail to recognize the illness and get the treatment that would alleviate their suffering. They or their loved ones fail to notice a pattern and instead may attribute the physical symptoms to the flu, the sleeping and eating problems to stress, and the emotional problems to lack of sleep or improper eating. But if people looked at all of these symptoms together and noticed that they occur over long periods of time, they might recognize them as signs of depression.

WHAT IS DEPRESSION?

The term "depression" can be confusing because it's often used to describe normal emotional reactions. At the same time, the illness may be hard to recognize because its symptoms may be so easily attributed to other causes. People tend to deny the existence of depression by saying things like, "She has a right to be depressed! Look at what she's gone through." This attitude fails to recognize that people can go through tremendous hardships and stress without developing depression, and that those who do fall victim can and should seek treatment.

Nearly everyone suffering from depression has pervasive feelings of sadness. In addition, depressed people may feel helpless, hopeless, and irritable. For many victims of depression, these mental and physical feelings seem to follow them night and day, appear to have no end, and are not alleviated by happy events or good news. Some people are so disabled by feelings of despair that they cannot even build up the energy to call a doctor. If someone else calls for them, they may refuse to go because they are so hopeless that they think there's no point to it.

RECOGNIZING SYMPTOMS OF DEPRESSION

You should seek professional help if you or someone you know has had four or more of the following symptoms continually for more than two weeks:
• Noticeable change of appetite, with either significant weight loss not attributable to dieting, or weight gain
• Noticeable change in sleeping patterns, such as fitful sleep, inability to sleep, early morning awakening, or sleeping too much
• Loss of interest and pleasure in activities formerly enjoyed
• Loss of energy, fatigue
• Feelings of worthlessness
• Persistent feelings of hopelessness
• Feelings of inappropriate guilt

• Inability to concentrate or think, or inordinate difficulty making decisions
• Recurring thoughts of death or suicide, wishing to die, or attempting suicide
• Melancholia (defined as overwhelming feelings of sadness and grief), accompanied by waking at least two hours earlier than normal in the morning, feeling more depressed in the morning, and moving significantly more slowly
• Disturbed thinking, a symptom developed by some severely depressed persons (For example, severely depressed people sometimes have beliefs not based in reality about physical disease, sinfulness, or poverty.)
• Physical symptoms, such as stomachaches or headaches

Family, friends, and co-workers offer advice, help, and comfort. But over time, they become frustrated with victims of depression because their efforts are to no avail. The person won't follow advice, refuses help, and denies the comfort. But persistence can pay off.

Many doctors think depression is the illness that underlies the majority of suicides in our country. Suicide is the eighth leading cause of death in America; it is the third leading cause of death among people aged 15 to 24. Every day 15 people aged 15 to 24 kill themselves. One of the best strategies for preventing suicide is the early recognition and treatment of the depression that so often leads to self-destruction.

Depression can appear at any age. Current research suggests that treatable depression is very prevalent among children and adolescents, especially among offspring of adults with depression. Depression can also strike late in life, and its symptoms—including memory impairment, slowed speech, and slowed movement—may be mistaken for those of senility or stroke.

Scientists think that more than half of the people who have had one episode of major depression will have another at some point in their lives. Some victims have episodes separated by several years and others suffer several episodes of the disorder over a short period. Between episodes, they can function normally. However, 20 to 35 percent of the victims suffer chronic depression that prevents them from maintaining a normal routine.

Sadness at the loss of a loved one or over a divorce is normal, but these losses can also be the trigger for a depressive episode. In fact, most major environmental changes can trigger depression. Job promotions, moves to new areas, changes in living space—all can bring on depressive illness.

TYPES OF DEPRESSION
Depression strikes in several forms. When a psychiatrist makes a diagnosis of a patient's depressive illness, he or she may use a number of terms—such as bipolar, clinical, endogenous, major, melancholic, or unipolar—to describe it. These labels confuse many people who don't understand that they can overlap.

People with depressive illness may also receive more than one diagnosis since the illness is often linked with other problems, such as alcoholism or other substance abuses, eating disorders, or anxiety disorders.

Clinical Depression

When you hear the term "clinical depression," it merely means the depression is severe enough to require treatment. When a person is badly depressed during a single severe period, he or she can be said to have had an episode of clinical depression. More severe symptoms mark the period as an episode of major depression. Many mental health experts say the key to judging this gradation lies in the amount of change a person undergoes in his or her normal patterns along with a loss of interest and a lack of pleasure in them. An almost-daily tennis player, for instance, who began to break her court dates frequently, or a regular bridge player who lost interest in weekly games, might be edging into an episode of major depression. The more severe the depression, the more it is likely to affect its sufferer's life.

Dysthymia

While many people have single or infrequent episodes of severe depression, some suffer with recurrent or long-lasting depression. For these people, who almost always seem to have symptoms of a mild form of the illness, the diagnosis is dysthymia. A major depressive episode can hit the dysthymic person, too, causing double depression, a condition that demands careful treatment and close follow-up.

Bipolar Depression

In bipolar depression, the lows alternate with terrible highs in an often bewildering oscillation. Scientists now believe this up-and-down mood roller coaster is the product of an imbalance in the brain chemistry which can be treated successfully about 80 percent of the time with balance-restoring medications.

THEORIES ABOUT CAUSES

Medical research has contributed much to our understanding of depression. However, scientists do not know the exact mechanism that triggers depressive illness. Probably no single cause gives rise to the illness, and researchers continue to piece the puzzle together.

Genetic Factors

Scientists now believe genetic factors play a role in some depressions. Researchers are hopeful, for instance, that they are closing in on genetic markers for susceptibility to manic-depressive disorder.

Recent genetic research also supports earlier studies reporting family links in depression. For example, if one identical twin suffers from depression or manic-depressive disorder, the other twin has a 70 percent chance of also having the illness. Other studies that looked at the rate of depression among adopted children supported this finding. Depressive illnesses among adoptive family members had little effect on a child's risk of depression; however, the disorder was three times more common among adopted children whose biological relatives suffered depression.

Chemical Imbalances

Additional research data indicate that people suffering from depression have imbalances of neurotransmitters, natural substances that allow brain cells to communicate with one another. Two transmitters implicated in depression are serotonin and norepinephrine. Scientists think a deficiency in serotonin may cause the sleep problems, irritability, and anxiety associated with depression. Likewise, a decreased amount of norepinephrine, which regulates alertness and arousal, may contribute to the fatigue and depressed mood of the illness.

Other Factors

Other body chemicals also may be altered in depressed people. Among them is cortisol, a hormone that the body produces in response to stress, anger, or fear. In normal people the level of cortisol in the bloodstream peaks in the morning, then decreases as the day progresses. In depressed people, however, cortisol peaks earlier in the morning and does not level off or decrease in the afternoon or evening.

Researchers don't know if these imbalances cause the disease or if the illness gives rise to the imbalances. They do know that cortisol levels will increase in anyone who must live with long-term stress.

Other factors may also cause depression. For example, medications are known to cause some kinds of depression. About 30 years ago, physicians realized that some people taking reserpine, a medication for high blood pressure, developed symptoms of depression.

TREATMENTS

Depression is one of the most treatable mental illnesses. Between 80 and 90 percent of all depressed people respond to treatment, and nearly all depressed people who receive treatment see at least some relief from their symptoms. Along with the great strides made in understanding the causes of depression, scientists are closer to understanding how treatment of the illness works.

Before any treatment program begins, however, a complete evaluation is essential. Depression is a complex illness, and many factors in a depressed person's life may feed into their condition. For example, a number of prevalent illnesses (such as hypothyroidism or hypertension) and commonly used medications can bring on depression. An evaluation will reveal the presence of these conditions or medicines to the psychiatrist. The evaluation will also include a medical/psychiatric history that will outline the patient's physical and emotional background, and a mental status examination, to uncover changes in the patient's mood, thoughts, patterns of speech, and memory that are manifestations of de-

pression. The psychiatrist may also perform or order a physical exam for the patient to rule out undiagnosed medical problems that might lead to depressive illness.

Medication Therapy

Since the 1950s, physicians have learned much more about the effects of medication on depression. The effectiveness of a drug depends on a person's general health, weight, metabolism, and other characteristics unique to that patient. Medication must be used at an adequate dosage level and for a long enough time. Sometimes a psychiatrist will prescribe several medications, or will try a combination of medications to determine what works best. Generally, antidepressant drugs become fully effective within three to six weeks after a person begins taking them.

Physicians generally prescribe one of four major types of medication used to treat depression: heterocyclics, serotonin reuptake blockers, MAO inhibitors, and lithium.

Heterocyclics and serotonin reuptake blockers. The oldest of the heterocyclics, the tricyclics, and the serotonin reuptake blockers are most often prescribed for people whose depressions are characterized by fatigue; feelings of hopelessness, helplessness, and excessive guilt; inability to feel pleasure; and loss of appetite with resulting weight loss.

MAO inhibitors may be prescribed for people whose depressions are characterized by increased appetite; excessive sleepiness; and anxiety, phobic, and obsessive-compulsive symptoms in addition to the depression. These medications may also be prescribed for people whose depression has not been reached by other drugs.

Lithium is used for people who have manic-depressive (bipolar) illness. It is also prescribed for people suffering from recurrent depression without mania.

459

Newer antidepressants have recently become available, and more are being developed. The newer drugs can help patients who either do not respond to the more traditionally prescribed medications or have trouble with those medications' side effects.

Like medications for any other illness, antidepressants can have side effects. With tricyclic antidepressants, for instance, these may include dry mouth, blurred vision, drowsiness, lowered blood pressure, and constipation, and tend to lessen as the body adjusts to the medication.

Psychotherapies

Psychotherapy involves the verbal interaction between a trained professional and a patient with emotional or behavioral problems. The therapist applies techniques based on established psychological principles to help the patient gain insights about him or herself and thus change his or her maladaptive thoughts, feelings, and behavior. There are several forms of this "talk treatment" that have proven useful in helping the depressed person.

In the spring of 1986, scientists announced results of research into the effectiveness of short-term psychotherapy in treating depression. Their findings indicated that for some categories of patients and under certain circumstances, some types of cognitive/behavioral therapy and interpersonal therapy were as effective as medications for depressed patients. Medications relieved the symptoms more quickly, but patients who received psychotherapy instead of medicine had as much relief from symptoms after 16 weeks.

The data from this study will help scientists better identify the depressed patients who will do best with psychotherapy alone and which patients may benefit from medications. In general, psychiatrists agree that severely depressed patients do best with a combination of medication and psychotherapy.

Interpersonal psychotherapy. This therapy is based on the theory that disturbed social and personal relationships can cause or precipitate depression. The illness, in turn, may make these relationships more problematic. The therapist helps the patient understand his or her illness and how depression and interpersonal conflicts are related.

Cognitive/behavioral therapy. This treatment approach is based on the theory that people's emotions are controlled by their views and opinions of the world. Depression results when patients constantly berate themselves, expect to fail, make inaccurate assessments of what others think of them, feel hopeless, and have a negative attitude toward the world and the future. The therapist uses various techniques of talk therapy and behavioral prescriptions to alleviate the negative thought patterns and beliefs.

Psychoanalysis. This therapy is based on the concept that depression is the result of past conflicts which patients have pushed into their unconscious. The therapist meets three to five times a week with the patient to identify and resolve the patient's past conflicts that have given rise to depression in later years.

Psychodynamic psychotherapy. Based on the principles of psychoanalysis, this therapy is less intense and often is provided once or twice a week over a shorter span of time. It is based on the premise that human behavior is determined by one's past experience, genetic endowment, and current reality. It recognizes the significant effects that emotions and unconscious motivation can have on human behavior.

Electroconvulsive therapy (ECT). Scientists believe ECT works by affecting the same transmitter chemicals in the brain that are affected by medications. As more effective medications have been developed, the use of ECT for the treatment of depression has decreased.

However, ECT is very effective for treating patients who cannot take medications due to heart conditions, old age, severe malnourishment, or for patients who do not respond to antidepressant medication. It can be a lifesaving treatment technique that is considered when other therapies have failed or when a person is very likely to commit suicide.

Before ECT is administered, patients receive anesthesia and a muscle relaxant to protect them from physical harm and pain. Electrodes are placed on the head and a small amount of electricity is applied. This procedure is repeated two or three times a week until the patient improves or it becomes evident that further treatment will be ineffective.

Side effects of ECT are largely transitory. Some people may experience mild problems with memory of events that occurred within several months of the therapy.

Recent research has also found that a subtype of depression called seasonal affective disorder (SAD) exists. Research suggests that SAD arises from some people's sensitivity to seasonal changes in the amount of available daylight. A therapeutic session spent bathed in light from a special full-spectrum light source, called a "light box," has been shown to be an effective treatment.

In summary, medication or psychotherapy, or a combination of the two treatment methods, usually relieves symptoms of depression in weeks. Even the most severe forms of depression can respond to treatment rapidly.

The American Psychiatric Association

ANXIETY DISORDERS

Anxiety is as much a part of life as eating and sleeping. Under the right circumstances, anxiety is beneficial. It heightens alertness and readies the body for action. Faced with an unfamiliar challenge, a person is often spurred by anxiety to prepare for the upcoming event. For example, many people practice speeches and study for tests as a result of mild anxiety. Likewise, anxiety or fear and the urge to flee are a protection from danger.

Fears are not normal, however, when they become overwhelming and interfere with daily living. They are symptoms of an anxiety disorder, the most common and most successfully treated form of mental illness.

As a group, anxiety disorders afflict nearly 9 percent of Americans during any six-month period. Symptoms can be so severe that patients are almost totally disabled—too terrified to leave their homes, to enter the elevator that takes them to their offices, to attend parties, or to shop for food.

"Anxiety" is a word so commonly used that many people don't understand what it means in mental health care. Complicating matters is the fact that "anxiety" and "fear" are often used to describe the same thing. When the word "anxiety" is used to discuss a group of mental illnesses, it refers to an unpleasant and overriding mental tension that has no apparent identifiable cause. Fear, on the other hand, causes mental tension due to a specific, external reason, such as when your car skids out of control on ice.

THE DISORDERS

Anxiety disorders comprise a group of illnesses: generalized anxiety disorder, phobias, panic disorders, post-traumatic stress disorder, and obsessive-compulsive disorders. When people suffering from anxiety disorders talk about their condition, they often include these descriptions: unrealistic or excessive worry; unrealistic fears concerning objects or situations; exaggerated startle reactions; flashbacks of past trauma; sleep disturbances; ritualistic behaviors as a way of dealing with anxieties; shakiness; trembling; muscle aches; sweating; cold/clammy hands; dizziness; jitteriness; tension; fatigue; racing or pounding heart; dry mouth; numbness/tingling of hands, feet, or other body part; upset stomach; diarrhea; lump in throat; and high pulse and/or breathing rate.

In addition, people suffering from anxiety disorders are often apprehensive and worry that something bad may happen to themselves or loved ones. They often feel impatient, irritable, and easily distracted.

Generalized Anxiety Disorder

People with generalized anxiety disorder suffer with unrealistic or excessive anxiety and worry about life circumstances. For example, they may feel panicky about financial matters even though they have a good bank balance and have paid their debts. Or they may be preoccupied constantly about the welfare of a child who's safe at school. People with generalized anxiety disorder may have stretches of time when they're not consumed by these worries, but they are anxious most of the time. Patients with this disorder often feel "shaky," reporting that they feel "keyed up" or "on edge" and that they sometimes "go blank" because of the tension that they feel. They often suffer also with mild depression.

Phobias

This type of anxiety disorder afflicts over 12 percent of all Americans during their lifetimes. People who suffer from this illness feel terror, dread, or panic when confronted with the feared object, situation, or activity.

Many have such an overwhelming desire to avoid the source of fear that it interferes with their jobs, family life, and social relationships. They may lose their jobs because they can't go to business lunches for fear of eating in front of others. They may quit a job in a high-rise office to work on the ground floor because they fear elevators. They may become so fearful of leaving their homes that they live like hermits with their window shades down for added protection.

The following are common phobias:

Social phobia is the fear of situations in which a person can be watched by others, such as public speaking, or in which the behaviors that arise from the person's feelings might prove embarrassing, such as eating in public. It begins in late childhood or early adolescence.

Simple phobia is the fear of specific objects or situations that cause terror. The condition can begin at any age. Examples are fear of snakes, fear of flying, or fear of closed spaces.

Agoraphobia is the fear of being alone or in a public place that has no escape hatch (such as a public bus). This is the most disabling phobia because victims can become housebound. The illness can begin any time from late childhood through early adulthood and, left untreated, worsens with time.

Panic Disorders

Panic disorders afflict 1.5 million Americans during any six-month period. Victims suddenly suffer intense, overwhelming terror for no apparent reason. The fear is accompanied by at least four of the following symptoms: sweating; heart palpitations; hot or cold flashes; trembling; feelings of unreality; choking or smothering sensations; shortness of breath; chest discomfort; faintness; unsteadiness; tingling; fear of losing control, dying, or going crazy.

Often, people suffering a panic attack for the first time rush to the hospital, convinced they are having a heart attack.

Sufferers can't predict when the attacks will occur. Certain situations, however, such as driving a car, can become associated with them if the first attack occurred in those situations. Untreated, panic sufferers can despair and become suicidal.

Obsessive-Compulsive Disorders

Obsessive-compulsive disorders (OCD) afflict 2.4 million Americans. People with OCD suffer with obsessions, which are repeated, intrusive, unwanted thoughts that cause distress and extreme anxiety. They may also suffer with compulsions, which psychiatrists define as rituals—such as hand-washing—that the person with the disorder goes through in an attempt to reduce the anxiety. People who suffer from obsessive disorders do not automatically have compulsive behaviors. However, most people with compulsions also have obsessions.

Victims of obsessions are plagued with involuntary, persistent thoughts or impulses that are distasteful to them. Examples are thoughts of violence or of becoming infected by shaking hands with others. These thoughts can be fleeting and momentary or they can be a lasting rumination.

The most common obsessions focus on a fear of hurting others or violating socially acceptable behavior standards such as swearing or making sexual advances. They also can focus on religious or philosophical issues, which the patient never resolves.

People with compulsions go through senseless, repeated, and involuntary ritualistic behaviors which they believe will prevent or produce a future event. However, the rituals themselves have nothing to do with that event. For example, a person may constantly wash his or her hands or touch a particular object. Often, people with this disorder also suffer from a complementary obsession such as worries over infection.

Examples of compulsive rituals include:

- *Cleaning,* which affects women more often than men. If victims come in contact with any dirt, they may spend hours washing and cleaning even to the point that their hands bleed.
- *Repeating a behavior,* such as repeatedly saying a loved one's name several times whenever that person comes up in conversation.
- *Checking,* which tends to affect men more than women. For example, victims check and recheck that doors are locked or electric switches, gas ovens, and water taps are turned off. Other patients will retrace a route they have driven to check that they did not hit a pedestrian or cause an accident without knowing it.

Obsessive-compulsive disorders often begin during the teens or early adulthood. Generally they are chronic and cause moderate to severe disability in their victims.

Post-Traumatic Stress Disorder (PTSD)

Often associated with war veterans, post-traumatic stress disorder can occur in anyone who has experienced a severe and unusual physical or mental trauma. People who have witnessed a midair collision or survived a life-threatening crime may develop this illness. The severity of the disorder increases if the trauma was unanticipated. For that reason, not all war veterans develop PTSD, despite prolonged and brutal combat. Soldiers expect a certain amount of violence. Rape victims, however, are unsuspecting of the attack on their lives.

People who suffer from PTSD re-experience the event that traumatized them in the following ways:

- Nightmares, night terrors, or flashbacks of the event. In rare cases, the person falls into a temporary dislocation from reality in which he or she relives the trauma. This can last for seconds or days.
- Psychic numbing, or emotional anesthesia. Victims have decreased interest in or involvement with people or activities they once enjoyed.
- Excessive alertness and highly sharpened startle reaction. A car backfiring may cause people once subjected to gunfire to instinctively drop to the ground.
- General anxiety, depression, inability to sleep, poor memory, difficulty concentrating or completing tasks, survivor's guilt.

463

THEORIES ABOUT CAUSES

Probably no single situation or condition causes anxiety disorders. Rather, physical and environmental triggers may combine to create a particular anxiety illness.

Psychoanalytic theory suggests that anxiety stems from unconscious conflicts that arose from discomfort during infancy or childhood. For example, a person may carry the unconscious conflict of sexual feelings toward the parent of the opposite sex. Or the person may have developed problems from experiencing an illness, fright, or other emotionally laden event as a child. By this theory, anxiety can be resolved by identifying and resolving the unconscious conflict. The symptoms that symbolize the conflict would then disappear.

Learning theory says that anxiety is a learned behavior that can be unlearned. People who feel uncomfortable in a given situation or near a certain object will begin to avoid it. However, such avoidance can limit a patient's ability to live a normal life.

More recently, research has indicated that biochemical imbalances are culprits. Many scientists say all thoughts and feelings result from complex electrochemical interactions in the central nervous system. Moreover, some studies indicate that infusions of certain biochemicals can cause a panic attack in some people. According to this theory, treatment of anxiety should correct these biochemical imbalances. Although medications first come to mind with this theory, remember that studies have found biochemical changes can occur as a result of emotional, psychological, or behavioral changes.

No doubt each of these theories is true to some extent. A person may develop or inherit a biological susceptibility to anxiety disorders. Events in childhood may lead to certain fears that, over time, develop into a full-blown anxiety disorder.

TREATMENTS

Generally, anxiety disorders are treated by a combination approach. Phobias and obsessive-compulsive disorders often are treated by behavior therapy. This involves exposing the patient to the feared object or situation under controlled circumstances, until the fear is cured or significantly reduced. Successfully treated with this method, many phobia patients have long-term recovery.

Medications are effective treatments, sometimes used alone and often in combination with behavior therapy or other psychotherapy techniques. In addition to behavior modification techniques and medication, talking issues out in psychotherapy can be crucial.

There is good reason for optimism about treatment of even the most severe anxiety disorders. Research indicates that 65 percent of the phobic and obsessive-compulsive patients who can cooperate with the therapist and conscientiously follow instructions will recover with behavior therapy. Studies have shown that while they are taking the medications, 70 percent of the patients who suffer from panic attacks improve. Medication is effective for about half of those suffering from obsessive-compulsive disorder.

The American Psychiatric Association

MANIC-DEPRESSIVE (BIPOLAR) DISORDER

Manic-depressive illness, known in medical terms as bipolar disorder, is the most distinct and dramatic of the depressive or affective disorders. Unlike major depression, which can occur at any age, manic-depressive illness generally strikes before the age of 35. Nearly one in 100 people will suffer from the disorder at some time in their lives.

People with bipolar disorder differ from

those with other depressive disorders in that their moods swing from depression to mania, generally with periods of normal mood between the two extremes. The length of this cycle, from towering elation to near despair, varies from person to person.

SYMPTOMS
Manic Phase
When patients first suffer a manic phase, they develop elation, euphoria, or extreme irritability that increases in a matter of days to a serious impairment. Symptoms of the manic phase include the following:

- A mood that seems excessively good, euphoric, expansive, or irritable. The patient feels on top of the world, and nothing—bad news, horrifying event, or tragedy—will change his happiness. However, this euphoria can quickly change into irritability or anger. In either case, the mood is way out of bounds, given the situation and the individual's personality.
- Expressions of unwarranted optimism and lack of judgment. Self-confidence reaches the point of grandiose delusions in which the person thinks he has a special connection with God, celebrities, or political leaders. Or he may think that nothing—not even the laws of gravity—can stop him from accomplishing any task. As a result, he may think he can step off a building or out of a moving car without being hurt.
- Hyperactivity and excessive plans or participation in numerous activities that have a good chance for painful results. Patients become so enthusiastic about activities or involvements that they fail to recognize they haven't enough time in the day for all of them. For example, a person with bipolar disorder may book several meetings, parties, deadlines, and other activities in a single day, thinking he or she can make all of them on time. Added to the expansive

mood, mania also can result in reckless driving, spending sprees, foolish business investments, or sexual behavior unusual for the person.
- Flight of ideas. The person's thoughts race uncontrollably like a car without brakes careening down a mountain. When the person talks, his or her words come out in a nonstop rush of ideas that abruptly change from topic to topic. In its severe form, the loud, rapid speech becomes hard to interpret because the patient's thought processes become so totally disorganized and incoherent.
- Decreased need for sleep, allowing the patient to go with little or no sleep for days without feeling tired.
- Distractibility in which the patient's attention is easily diverted to inconsequential or unimportant details.
- Sudden irritability, rage, or paranoia when the person's grandiose plans are thwarted or his excessive social overtures are refused.

Untreated, the manic phase can last as long as three months. As it abates, the patient may have a period of normal mood and behavior. But eventually the depressive phase of the illness will set in. In some, depression occurs immediately or within the next few months. But with other patients there is a long interval before the next manic or depressive episode.

Depressive Phase
The depressive phase has the same symptoms as major or unipolar depression:

- Feelings of worthlessness, hopelessness, helplessness, total indifference and/or inappropriate guilt; prolonged sadness or unexplained crying spells; jumpiness or irritability, withdrawal from formerly enjoyable activities, social contacts, work, or sex.
- Inability to concentrate or remember details.
- Thoughts of death or suicide attempts.

465

- Loss of appetite or noticeable increase in appetite; persistent fatigue and lethargy, insomnia or noticeable increase in the amount of sleep needed.
- Aches and pains, constipation, or other physical ailments that cannot be otherwise explained.

THEORIES ABOUT CAUSES
Genetic Factors

Recent studies of the roots of bipolar disorder have centered on genetic research. Scientists believe these studies will eventually help them identify the genetic culprits that cause manic-depressive illness in its various forms among different populations. This research will also help psychiatrists to understand the biochemical reactions that are controlled by these genes and that contribute to the disorder.

Close relatives of people suffering from bipolar disorder are 10 to 20 times more likely to develop either depression or manic-depressive illness than the general population. In fact, between 80 and 90 percent of people suffering from manic-depressive illness have relatives who suffer from some form of depression.

If one parent suffers from manic-depressive illness, a child has a 12 to 15 percent risk of suffering from a depressive disorder; if both parents suffer from manic-depressive illness, the children have a 25 percent chance each of developing a depressive disorder or manic-depressive illness.

Environmental Factors

Other studies hint that environmental factors may contribute to the illness. Psychoanalytic studies suggest that such environmental factors as difficult family relationships may aggravate manic-depressive illness.

Chemical Imbalances

Still other studies suggest that imbalances in the biochemistry controlling a person's mood could contribute to manic-depressive illness. For example, people suffering from either manic-depressive illness or major depression often respond to certain hormones or steroids in a way that indicates they have irregularities in their hormone production and release. Some research points to the possibility that bipolar patients' neurotransmitters—chemicals by which brain cells communicate—become imbalanced during various phases of the disease. Finally, some people suffering from depressive illnesses have sleep patterns in which the dream phase begins earlier in the night than normal.

These studies indicate that manic-depressive illness and major depression may be caused by biochemical imbalances. Such research also helps develop scientific theories about how medications work and offers hope that psychiatrists some day will use laboratory tests to identify unipolar or bipolar illnesses.

DIAGNOSIS

Anyone who suspects he or she or a loved one suffers from manic-depressive illness should receive a complete medical evaluation to rule out any other mental or physical disorders. Many other medical disorders can mimic manic-depressive illnesses. For example, a person with symptoms of manic depression could be reacting to substances such as amphetamines or steroids or could suffer from thyroid, liver, or kidney problems or other illnesses, such as multiple sclerosis. A comprehensive medical and psychiatric evaluation by a qualified psychiatrist or other physician is vital to an accurate diagnosis. With this diagnosis a psychiatrist can then work with the patient to design the right treatment plan.

TREATMENT

Though manic-depressive illness can become disabling, it is also among the most treatable of the psychiatric illnesses. Proper medication is essential to this treatment, and psychotherapy may also be helpful.

Medication

The most common medication, lithium carbonate, successfully reduces the number and intensity of manic episodes for 70 percent of those who take the medication. Twenty percent of those who use lithium become completely free of symptoms. Those who respond best to lithium are patients who have a family history of depressive illness and who have periods of relatively normal mood between their manic and depressive phases. In recent years psychiatrists have been successful with several other medications—such as carbamazepine and valproate—in treating those for whom lithium is not effective.

Very effective in treating the manic phase, lithium also appears to prevent repeated episodes of depression. Lithium works by bringing various neurotransmitters in the brain into balance. Scientists think the medication may affect the impact neurotransmitters have on the brain cells, thus altering moods.

Like all medications, lithium can have side effects and must be carefully monitored by a psychiatrist. The physician should measure the level of lithium in the patient's blood and determine how well the patient's kidneys and thyroid gland are working. Among the side effects are weight gain, excessive thirst and urination, stomach and intestinal irritation, hand tremors, and muscular weakness. If a patient overdoses on medication, it may cause confusion, delirium, seizures, and coma and may result, rarely, in death.

However, when properly monitored, lithium, sometimes used with other medications, has returned thousands of people to happy, functioning lives that would not be possible without medication.

Psychotherapy

Like all serious illnesses, manic-depressive disorders disrupt a person's self-esteem and relationships with others, especially with spouses and family. Without treatment, people with the illness may risk consequences such as financial and occupational disintegration, or even suicide. Because of these consequences of their illness, people under treatment for manic-depressive illness also benefit from psychotherapy.

The patient and the psychiatrist work out the problems created by the disorder and reestablish the relationships and healthy self-image that are shaken by the illness. In many cases, a patient needs the psychiatrist's support to ensure that he complies with his treatment.

Family members of manic-depressive patients also may benefit from professional care. This illness can cause serious disruptions of the family's life, as the stresses of living with a person suffering from manic depression are intense. Not only may family members learn coping strategies from the psychiatrist, but they can also learn to be an active part of the treatment team.

The American Psychiatric Association

SLEEP DISORDERS

Like changes in hair color, vision, and other signs of aging, the "graying" of sleep usually develops gradually. Aging makes sleep more fragile even in extremely healthy older people.

Earlier in life, most of us fell asleep fast and could sleep through a thunderstorm. As we grow older, we may find it harder to settle down. Most of us awaken more often and take longer to fall back to sleep. The honk of a car horn or bark of a neighbor's dog down the street may be enough to rouse us. During the day, we doze off more easily, when watching TV, for example, or reading the newspaper.

Persistent trouble falling asleep at night is not, however, normal or inevitable at any age. Nor is frequently falling asleep in the daytime.

Normal age-related changes frequently mask recognition of sleep disorders that become more common with advancing years. Medical or psychiatric illnesses, particularly those involving pain or depression, go hand-in-hand with sleep disorders. Sleep specialists often cannot tell which comes first.

More than half of all people aged 65 and older experience disturbed sleep, according to a panel of experts convened by the National Institutes of Health in 1990 to develop consensus on the treatment of sleep disorders of older people. Insomnia is the most common problem.

The overuse of both prescription drugs and over-the-counter medications to aid sleep in older people worries physicians and other health professionals. While people over age 65 constitute about 13 percent of the American population, they consume more than 30 percent of prescription drugs and 40 percent of all sleeping pills. Yet recent studies show that some commonly used drugs may not work well in older people or may even make their sleep problems worse.

Such concerns fuel further research into how sleep changes as we grow older and how to improve both sleep and daytime alertness in the later years. Sleep experts say there are many steps you can take to improve your sleep and to maintain healthy, restful sleep as you grow older. New understanding also benefits those who need professional help.

WHAT HAPPENS TO SLEEP AS WE GET OLDER?

It's a myth that we need less sleep as we grow older. But it's a fact that most of us sleep less at a single stretch than we did when we were younger. Our bodies become less adept at sustaining sleep.

On the other hand, it's easier to nap during the daytime. Fortunately, we also often have more time to nap than we did in earlier years. Recent research suggests our bodies were designed for at least one afternoon nap a day. Only late in life, freed from constraints of a nine-to-five workplace and societal attitudes that frown on napping, can we let ourselves do what comes naturally.

As we grow older, we get less of the deeper stages of sleep and more of the lighter ones. We also awaken more often. But all throughout adulthood, well into old age, we spend about the same amount of time in dreaming sleep.

Sleep laboratory studies show that the number of awakenings colors our perception of the quality of our sleep. People in their sixties and older awaken for a few seconds an astounding 150 times a night. By contrast, young adults awaken briefly about five times. Even though transient awakenings usually go unremembered in the morning, they may create the subjective impression of fitful nights. Moreover, most people over age 65 awaken more fully at least once a night for a trip to the bathroom.

WHAT PROBLEMS ARE MOST COMMON?

Some people focus on trouble with sleep, and others on trouble with mood or performance during the day.

Trouble Falling Asleep

Trouble falling asleep sometimes stems from simple, easily correctable causes, such as consuming caffeine or a heavy meal, or exercising too late in the day. It may be the aftermath of hospitalization, recovery after surgery, or travel. It may flare up during times of worry or smolder under persistent stress.

In the quiet of the bedroom, some people find their minds race and worries overwhelm them. The solution here: Set aside another time as "worry" time, when you can write down both problems and possible solutions. At bedtime, focus on sleep-inducing situations. Imagine, for example, basking in the sun on a beach after lunch.

The hours we keep program our bodies for

sleeping and waking at the same time the following day. If you still work, particularly if you frequently change your hours of work and sleep, you probably have noticed that it takes longer to adapt to schedule changes. The older we become, the harder it is for the body to adapt to irregular hours. If you travel frequently across time zones, you may find jet lag lasts longer than it used to.

If you lead a sedentary lifestyle, particularly if you have restricted mobility, you may doze more during the day than you suspect. People with insomnia prove less active during the day than those who are better sleepers. A 1988 Gallup survey found that active retirees had fewer sleep problems than those who were less active. Try to confine sleep to nighttime or nap time.

Sleep Apnea

Some people who feel lethargic during the day don't suspect that anything is wrong with their sleep. Or they may find sleep unsatisfactory without being able to pinpoint the nature of the problem. Disturbed breathing, known as sleep apnea, may trigger both day and night complaints. It disrupts sleep in varying degrees in an estimated one out of every four people aged 60 and over.

In some cases, disturbed breathing is obvious to bed partners or others. The sleeper snores raucously. The snoring reflects partial blockage of the airway during sleep. Snoring increases with age and usually is more of a nuisance to others than a medical problem.

A particular type of snoring, however, demands a visit to the doctor. Such snoring follows a crescendo pattern, with each breath becoming louder. It ends with a loud gasp before the pattern then repeats. Or it may involve loud snorts with gasping.

With each gasp, the person awakens, although usually too briefly to remember doing so in the morning. Some people with this problem, obstructive sleep apnea, awaken hundreds of times a night. As a result, they feel excessively drowsy during the daytime. Indeed, some sleep specialists think sleep apnea may contribute to difficulty thinking and concentrating during waking hours that is often blamed on dementia.

Weight loss and sleeping on one's side may be helpful. Severe obstructive sleep apnea may require surgery or use of mechanical devices that keep the airway open.

People with central sleep apnea may or may not snore excessively. When respiratory muscles fail to work properly, sleepers may sigh frequently or appear to breathe shallowly. In the morning, they may remember the frequent awakenings and complain of light and fragmented sleep. When this problem is severe, medication or use of oxygen may prove helpful.

Interrupted Sleep

Not only is the sleep process less robust as we get older, but we also are more likely to develop chronic medical illnesses that interfere with sleep. Asthma and other lung diseases, heart disease, and arthritis are notorious offenders. Pain, fever, itching, and coughing often contribute to insomnia. Many drugs that are necessary to treat these problems also disrupt sleep.

Talk with your doctor; sometimes adjusting the timing or amount of medication brings about substantial improvement. Paying attention to sleep habits and using relaxation techniques may help, too. Some people benefit from having sleeping pills on hand for occasional use when they feel desperate.

Early Awakening

Waking too early may represent a rebound from use of alcohol at bedtime or even from certain types of sleeping pills.

It also is a hallmark symptom of depression. Some people sink into depression gradually. Feeling blue eventually becomes a chronic way of living. Others focus on poor sleep, telling themselves and others, "Life

469

would be much better if only I could get a decent night's sleep."

They also may not be eating regularly or may have lost their usual interest and pleasure in activities of daily life. Loss of a loved one commonly triggers insomnia and depression. Surveys show that more than three-quarters of the bereaved report trouble sleeping a month after the death of a spouse. One year later, half still report persistent sleep problems.

Often a concerned family member or friend may have to take the initiative in making an appointment with the doctor. Fortunately, most cases of depression respond well to a variety of drugs, along with counseling. Sleep improves as mood brightens.

Advanced Sleep Phase Syndrome (ASPS)
The tendency to be "early to bed and early to rise" increases as we grow older. Most of us adapt successfully. But some of us find that our bodies say, "It's bedtime," earlier than we desire, often well before 9 p.m.

Known as the advanced sleep phase syndrome or ASPS, this problem can wreak havoc with social life. Additionally, it's hard to find oneself awake for hours when most other people are still asleep.

Most people with ASPS try numerous strategies to help them stay up late. Even if they succeed in pushing bedtime later, however, they may not be able to sleep any later because their body clocks still awaken them in the early morning hours.

One solution is chronotherapy, literally, time therapy. For ASPS, this involves following a schedule of prescribed bedtimes that move backwards around the clock in, for example, three-hour intervals every two days, until reaching the desired bedtime. Regular hours from then on help maintain the new bedtime and wake time. With chronotherapy, a 65-year-old man moved his bedtime from 7 p.m. to 11 p.m. He then slept later in the morning, too.

A newer treatment, still under investigation, involves exposure in the evening to artificial lights several times brighter than ordinary room lights. Recent studies show such lights may shift both bedtime and arising time to later, more desirable, hours.

Periodic Limb Movements
Perhaps half of all people aged 65 and over experience twitching in the legs, and sometimes arms, during the night. These muscle jerks may occur infrequently or as often as once or twice each minute for an hour or two at a time. This disorder, known as periodic limb movement disorder or PLMD, seldom awakens the sleeper fully, but it understandably prevents sound sleep.

When it is mild, a person may be unaware of any impact on sleep or daytime functioning. When it is moderate, sleepers often complain of insomnia, reporting restless nights and waking to find bed sheets in disarray. When it is more severe, people often feel excessively sleepy during the day.

Many people with PLMD during sleep experience "restless legs" when awake, a peculiar crawling sensation in calves or thighs that occurs when they are sitting or lying down. A variety of medications can ease these problems. Such behavior challenges the traditional view of sleep as a time of rest.

Dream Disturbances
Some people literally act out their dreams. They may crash into furniture, break windows, or fall down stairs, often injuring themselves and sometimes others as well.

Ordinarily the body lies virtually paralyzed during dreaming sleep (called REM sleep for the rapid eye movements that accompany it). But this normal paralysis vanishes in people with the REM sleep behavior disorder. Most are men over age 50, a finding that suggests aging plays a contributory role. Fortunately, the drug clonazepam improves sleep in people with this problem and eliminates the dream disturbances.

GUIDELINES FOR SLEEPING WELL

The following measures will help you to sleep well and feel alert during the day.

• *Get up about the same time every day, regardless of when you go to bed.* Recent research suggests that lingering in bed a short while in the morning eases the transition between sleep and waking and improves alertness in older people.

• *Go to bed only when sleepy.* Establish relaxing presleep rituals, such as a warm bath, light bedtime snack, or watching the news on TV.

• *Keep active.* Exercise regularly and as vigorously as you can in the late afternoon. Two or three hours before bedtime, take a walk or do some simple stretching.

• *Organize your day.* Regular times for meals, taking medicines, performing chores, and other activities help keep inner clocks running smoothly. Spend time outdoors, particularly in the afternoon, when weather permits; recent studies suggest that regular exposure to bright light also helps synchronize body clocks. People with certain types of sleep and mood disorders may benefit from use of artificial lights several times brighter than ordinary room lights. A sleep specialist will tell you if this treatment is appropriate for you.

• *Avoid caffeine within six hours of bedtime.* Don't drink alcohol or smoke at bedtime.

• *Use alcohol sparingly, especially when sleepy.* Even a small dose of alcohol will have a much more potent effect when you are sleepy.

• *If you nap, try to nap at the same time each day.* Midafternoon is best for most people.

• *Use sleeping pills conservatively.* Most doctors seldom prescribe them for use every night or for longer than three weeks. Current recommendations call for taking a sleeping pill for a night or two, then skipping a night or two or longer if you sleep better. Don't take a sleeping pill after drinking alcohol.

OTHER COMPLICATIONS

Seventy percent of caregivers cite sleep disturbances, wandering, and confusion, sometimes called "sundowning," as a factor in their decision to institutionalize an elderly person. Most caregivers report their charges' problems disrupt their own sleep, too.

Two-thirds of those living in long-term care facilities suffer sleep disturbances. In a nursing home or hospital, nocturnal problems typically continue or increase, prompting widespread use of tranquilizing drugs. The drugs in turn may contribute to further confusion and an increased likelihood of falls.

Some specialists in the field believe that sleep disorders, particularly those of breathing, may contribute to a significant proportion of reversible dementias. They urge family physicians, internists, and others to rule out sleep disorders when evaluating an elderly person afflicted with nocturnal symptoms.

WHEN TO SEE THE DOCTOR

If you sleep poorly for a month or more or if you find that sleepiness during the day interferes with normal tasks, see your family doctor or internist or ask your doctor to refer you to a sleep disorders specialist. Your medical history, along with a physical exam and laboratory tests, such as those of hormone function, may help identify certain disorders. Ask your bed partner or other members of your household whether you snore loudly or kick or flail around. Let the doctor know.

When you make an appointment at a sleep center, you may be asked to log your sleep and waking patterns for a week or two before your visit. At the sleep center, expect a comprehensive physical and psychological exam.

You may be asked to spend a night or two having your sleep monitored—sometimes the only way to uncover a disorder that occurs only during sleep. Before you go to bed, technicians will position dime-sized sensors at various places on head and body to record brain waves, muscle activity, leg and arm movements, heart rhythms, breathing, and other bodily functions while you sleep. These monitoring devices cause little or no discomfort and will not hamper your movements during the night. Sleep specialists will compare the results from your night in the lab against norms for healthy people of all ages.

The specialists also may wish to study your sleep during the day by asking you to try to nap at two-hour intervals. The speed with which people fall asleep on this test, known as the multiple sleep latency test, documents the extent of daytime sleepiness.

Although evaluation at a sleep center may run $1,000 or more a night because of the many specialists involved, most medical insurance polices and Medicare cover this expense when it is medically indicated. Researchers are working to devise less costly alternatives, such as in-home sleep monitoring, now undergoing testing.

CAN SLEEPING PILLS HELP?

Although sleeping pills are used mostly by the elderly, and more often by women than men, they are tested mainly in young men. Doctors say many uncertainties remain about how sleeping pills and other drugs affect older people of both sexes. As we grow older, we metabolize and excrete drugs less efficiently than when we were younger. Because drugs stay in the body longer, their effects may last longer, too. Drowsiness—desirable at bedtime—is not welcome when you awaken to go to the bathroom during the night or when you drive a car the next day.

Ideally, a sleeping pill would help you fall asleep faster and awaken less often, with no "hangover" the next day. The most commonly prescribed sleeping pills, members of the benzodiazepine chemical family, come in both shorter- and longer-acting forms.

The shorter-acting drugs help induce and solidify sleep, but they usually wear off faster. The longer-acting drugs help maintain sleep through the night, but they sometimes cause sleepiness the next day. Your doctor will try to tailor the type of drug and the particular dose to your individual needs. Shorter-acting drugs commonly used to aid sleep include triazolam (Halcion) and temazepam (Restoril). A longer-acting drug is flurazepam (Dalmane).

A new class of medications, including zolpidem (Ambien), may be effective in inducing sleep in the elderly population, but may not necessarily promote longer or less interrupted sleep during the middle and late parts of the night.

Sleeping pills you can buy without a prescription, known as over-the-counter or OTC drugs, get their drowsiness-inducing effect from antihistamines. Like prescription sleep aids, they may cause sleepiness the next day. They require similar caution.

Warning: A complaint of insomnia sometimes signals disturbed breathing during sleep. If you have this problem, it may be a mistake to use sleeping pills. They may make interruptions in breathing occur more often and last longer. If you have more than occasional bad nights, see your doctor before using any drug for sleep.

Be wary of using multiple drugs. One 81-year-old woman entered the hospital for gallstone surgery. On learning that she had taken barbiturates nightly for years and felt "going to sleep" meant "taking a pill," her doctor switched her to a safer benzodiazepine. After she returned home, she became agitated and irritable. Another doctor prescribed a tranquilizer. Meanwhile, she continued a long-time habit, consumption of an evening vodka martini. The result: confusion, forgetfulness, and depression. Once doctors suspected that her medicines might be the culprit and stopped them, she rapidly returned to her former alert self.

The American Sleep Disorders Association

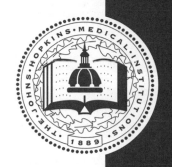

DIRECTORY
OF THE
AMERICAN MEDICAL
CARE SYSTEM

CONTENTS

Using the Directory

Your own physician will doubtless be able to refer you to the care of a specialist if you need one. But if you have just moved into a new community and your previous physician had no recommendations for you, or if a friend recommends a physician to you, you might well consult the following list of medical specialty (and subspecialty) boards. These boards can refer you to a board certified physician in your area.

You can also find out whether a physician is board certified by contacting the appropriate specialty board directly or by calling the American Board of Medical Specialties Certification Line at 800-776-2378. Descriptions of the specialties covered in this Directory are included after the list of boards.

Certification is not required for a licensed physician to practice a specialty. And certification by a medical specialty board is not a guarantee of excellence; in fact, there are many excellent physicians who are not board certified. But a board certified physician has taken and passed a written exam, thereby demonstrating a certain amount of knowledge to other specialists practicing in the same field. The boards might refer you to a "board eligible" physician. Physicians who have met a board's requirements but have not yet passed the written test are called "board eligible." Those who have passed the test are called "board certified."

Another way to find a good physician is to ask for a referral from one of the Academic Medical Center Hospitals that are members of the Association of American Medical Colleges' Council of Teaching Hospitals. Look for these hospitals under Teaching Hospitals by Disorder. The names of the Academic Medical Center Hospitals are printed in bold; those with an asterisk are privately owned.

If you do not live close to one of these hospitals, you might ask the nearest one for the name of a physician who trained there and now lives in or near your community. Also, the health information organizations listed in the back of this Directory will sometimes make referrals, so you should check with them.

MEDICAL SPECIALTY BOARDS WITH SUBSPECIALTIES

American Board of Allergy and Immunology
510 Walnut St., Suite 1701
Philadelphia, PA 19106-3699
215-592-9466

American Board of Anesthesiology
4101 Lake Boone Trail, Suite 510
Raleigh, NC 27607-7506
919-881-2570
Subspecialties include:
Pain Management

American Board of Colon and Rectal Surgery
20600 Eureka Rd., Suite 713
Taylor, MI 48180
734-282-9400

American Board of Dermatology
Henry Ford Hospital
1 Ford Pl.
Detroit, MI 48202-3450
313-874-1088

American Board of Emergency Medicine
3000 Coolidge Rd.
East Lansing, MI 48823-6319
517-332-4800

American Board of Family Practice
2228 Young Dr.
Lexington, KY 40505
606-269-5626
Subspecialties include:
Geriatric Medicine

American Board of Internal Medicine
University City Science Center
3624 Market St.
Philadelphia, PA 19104
215-446-3500
Subspecialties include:
Cardiovascular Disease, Endocrinology and Metabolism, Gastroenterology, Geriatric Medicine, Hematology, Infectious Diseases, Medical Oncology, Nephrology, Pulmonary Disease, Rheumatology

The American Board of Medical Specialties
1007 Church St., Suite 404
Evanston, IL 60201-5913
847-491-9091

**American Board of
Neurological Surgery**
Smith Tower
6550 Fannin St., Suite 2139
Houston, TX 77030-2701
713-790-6015

**American Board of
Nuclear Medicine**
900 Veteran Ave.
Los Angeles, CA 90024-1786
310-825-6787

**American Board of Obstetrics
and Gynecology**
2915 Vine St.
Dallas, TX 75204-1069
214-871-1619
Subspecialties include:
Gynecologic Oncology

American Board of Ophthalmology
111 Presidential Blvd., Suite 241
Bala Cynwyd, PA 19004
610-664-1175

**American Board of
Orthopaedic Surgery**
400 Silver Cedar Ct.
Chapel Hill, NC 27514
919-929-7103
Subspecialties include:
Hand Surgery

American Board of Otolaryngology
2211 Norfolk St., Suite 800
Houston, TX 77098
713-528-6200

American Board of Pathology
PO Box 25915
5401 W. Kennedy Blvd.
Tampa, FL 33622-5915
813-286-2444
Subspecialties include:
Blood Banking/Transfusion Medicine

**American Board of Physical
Medicine and Rehabilitation**
Nor'west Center, Suite 674
21 First St., SW
Rochester, MN 55902
507-282-1776

American Board of Plastic Surgery
7 Penn Center, Suite 400
1635 Market St.
Philadelphia, PA 19103-2204
215-587-9322
Subspecialties include:
Hand Surgery

**American Board of
Preventive Medicine**
9950 W. Lawrence Ave., Suite 106
Schiller Park, IL 60176
847-671-1750

**American Board of Psychiatry
and Neurology**
500 Lake Cook Rd., Suite 335
Deerfield, IL 60015
847-945-7900
Subspecialties include:
Geriatric Psychiatry, Clinical
Neurophysiology

American Board of Radiology
5255 E. Williams Circle
Suite 3200
Tucson, AZ 85711-7401
520-790-2900

American Board of Surgery
1617 John F. Kennedy Blvd.
Suite 860
Philadelphia, PA 19103-1847
215-568-4000
Subspecialties include:
Hand Surgery, General
Vascular Surgery

**American Board of
Thoracic Surgery**
1 Rotary Center, Suite 803
Evanston, IL 60201
847-475-1520

American Board of Urology
2216 Ivy Rd., Suite 210
Charlottesville, VA 22903
804-979-0059

DESCRIPTIONS OF THE MEDICAL SPECIALTIES

The basic training of a physician specialist includes four years of premedical education in a college or university, four years of medical school, and after receiving an M.D. or D.O. degree, at least three years of specialty training under supervision (called a "residency").

Specialists are doctors who concentrate on certain body systems, specific age groups, or on complex scientific techniques developed to diagnose or treat particular types of disorders. Specialties in medicine have developed because of the rapidly expanding body of knowledge about health and illness and the constantly evolving new treatment techniques for disease.

A subspecialist is a physician who has com-pleted training in a general medical specialty and then takes additional training in a more specific area of that specialty, called a "subspecialty." This training serves to increase the depth of knowledge of the specialist in that particular field.

Resident physicians dedicate themselves for three to seven years to full-time experience in a hospital or ambulatory care setting, caring for patients under the supervision of experienced teaching specialists. Educational conferences and research experience are also part of that training. A doctor in training to be a specialist is called a "resident," although the first year of residency used to be called an "internship."

In each state, the privilege to practice medicine is governed by state law and is not designed to recognize the knowledge and skills of a trained specialist. Specialty boards certify physicians only as having met certain published standards.

Allergy/Immunology

An allergist/immunologist is a certified internist or pediatrician expert in the evaluation, physical and laboratory diagnosis, and management of disorders potentially involving the immune system. Selected examples of such conditions include asthma, anaphylaxis, rhinitis, eczema, urticaria, and adverse reactions to drugs, foods, and insect stings, as well as immune deficiency diseases (both acquired and congenital), defects in host defense, and problems related to autoimmune disease, organ transplantation, or malignancies of the immune system.

Anesthesiology

The anesthesiologist is a physician specialist who, following medical school graduation and at least four years of postgraduate training, has the principal task of providing pain relief and maintenance, or restoration of a stable condition during and immediately following an operation or an obstetric or diagnostic procedure.

The anesthesiologist assesses the risk of the patient undergoing surgery and optimizes the patient's condition prior to, during, and after surgery.

Anesthesiologists guide the resuscitation efforts in the care of patients with cardiac or respiratory emergencies, including the provision of artificial ventilation.

Colon and Rectal Surgery

As a result of their extensive training and experience, colon and rectal surgeons develop the knowledge and skills necessary to diagnose and treat various diseases of the intestinal tract, colon, rectum, anal canal, and perianal area by medical and surgical means. They are also able to deal surgically with other organs and tissues (such as the liver, urinary, and female reproductive systems) involved with primary intestinal disease.

Dermatology

A dermatologist is a physician who has expertise in the diagnosis and treatment of pediatric and adult patients with benign and malignant disorders of the skin, mouth, external genitalia, hair, and nails, as well as a number of sexually transmitted diseases. Dermatologists have extensive training and experience in the diagnosis and treatment of skin cancers, melanomas, moles, and other tumors of the skin; contact dermatitis and other allergic and nonallergic disorders; and in the recognition of the skin manifestations of systemic (including internal malignancy) and infectious diseases.

The dermatologist also has expertise in the management of cosmetic disorders of the skin, such as hair loss and scars.

Internal Medicine

The general internist is a personal physician who provides comprehensive, long-term care in the office and the hospital, managing both common illnesses and complex problems for adolescents, adults, and the elderly. General internists are trained in the essentials of primary care internal medicine, which incorporates an understanding of disease prevention, wellness, substance abuse, mental health, and effective treatment of common problems of the eyes, ears, skin, nervous system, and reproductive organs.

Care by an internist is characterized by extensive knowledge and skill in diagnosis and treatment; by the humanistic qualities of integrity, support, sensitivity, and compassion; and by personal commitment to patients.

Well-trained internists are unique in their ability to deliver care with great professional expertise and often act as consultants to other specialists. Internists can subspecialize in the following areas:

Cardiovascular Disease. Cardiologists subspecialize in diseases of the heart, lungs, and blood vessels and manage complex cardiac conditions, such as heart attacks and life-threatening abnormal heartbeat rhythms. They often perform complicated diagnostic procedures, such as cardiac catheterization, and consult with surgeons on heart surgery.

Endocrinology and Metabolism. The endocrinologist concentrates on disorders of the internal (endocrine) glands, such as the thyroid and adrenal glands. Endocrinology also deals with disorders such as diabetes, metabolic and nutritional disorders, pituitary diseases, and menstrual and sexual problems.

Gastroenterology. The subspecialty of the digestive organs involves the stomach, bowels, liver, and gallbladder. The gastroenterologist treats conditions such as abdominal pain, ulcers, diarrhea, cancer, and jaundice. Gastroenterologists perform complex diagnostic and therapeutic procedures using lighted scopes to see internal organs.

Geriatric Medicine. The internist certified in geriatric medicine has special knowledge of the aging process and special skills in the diagnostic, therapeutic, preventive, and rehabilitative aspects of illness in the elderly. Geriatricians are trained to recognize the unusual presentations of illness and drug interactions. Some examples of common geriatric conditions are incontinence, falls, Parkinson's disease, Alzheimer's disease, and other dementias.

Hematology. Hematologists subspecialize in diseases of the blood, spleen, and lymph glands. They treat conditions such as anemia, clotting disorders, sickle cell disease, hemophilia, leukemia, and lymphoma. They perform special types of transfusions and biopsy the bone marrow for analysis.

Infectious Diseases. These subspecialists deal with infectious diseases of all types and in all organs. Conditions requiring selective use of antibiotics call for this special skill.

Medical Oncology. The medical oncologist specializes in the diagnosis and treatment of all types of cancer and other benign and malignant tumors. These subspecialists decide on and administer chemotherapy for malignancy, as well as consulting with surgeons and radiotherapists on other treatment for cancer.

Nephrology. The nephrologist is concerned with disorders of the kidneys, high blood pressure, fluid and mineral balance, dialysis of body wastes when the kidneys do not function, and consultation with surgeons about kidney transplantation.

Pulmonary Disease. Pulmonary disease is the subspecialty concerned with diseases of the lungs and airways. The pulmonologist diagnoses and treats pneumonia, cancer, pleurisy, asthma, certain occupational diseases, bronchitis, sleep disorders, emphysema, and other complex disorders of the lungs.

Rheumatology. The rheumatologist is concerned with diseases of the joints, muscles, bones, and tendons. He or she diagnoses and treats arthritis, back pain, muscle strains, common athletic injuries, and collagen diseases, which affect connective tissue.

Neurological Surgery

Neurological surgery is a discipline of medicine and specialty of surgery that deals with the diagnosis, evaluation, and treatment of disorders of the central, peripheral, and autonomic nervous systems, including their supporting structures and vascular supply.

This specialty also focuses on the evaluation and treatment of pathological processes that modify the function or activity of the nervous system, including the pituitary gland, and on the management of pain.

Neurology

The neurologist is concerned with the diagnosis and treatment of all categories of disease or impaired function of the brain, spinal cord, peripheral nerves, muscles, and autonomic nervous system, as well as the blood vessels that relate to these structures.

Obstetrics and Gynecology

Obstetrician/gynecologists are physicians who, through satisfactory completion of a defined course of graduate medical education and appropriate certification, possess special knowledge, skills, and professional capability in the medical and surgical care of the female reproductive system and associated disorders. This training distinguishes them from other physicians and enables them to serve as consultants to other physicians and as primary physicians for women.

Ophthalmology

Ophthalmologists have the knowledge and professional skills needed to provide comprehensive eye and vision care. They are the only practitioners medically trained to diagnose, monitor, and medically or surgically treat all eyelid and orbital problems affecting the eye and visual pathways and to diagnose, monitor, and treat all eye disorders. In so doing, they often prescribe vision services (glasses and contact lenses). The ophthalmologist also serves as a consultant to physicians and other professionals.

Orthopedic Surgery

Orthopedic surgery is the medical specialty that includes the preservation, investigation, and restoration of the form and function of the extremities, spine, and associated structures by medical, surgical, and physical means.

Otolaryngology

An otolaryngologist provides comprehensive medical and surgical care of patients with diseases and disorders that affect the ears, the respiratory and upper alimentary systems, and related structures—the head and neck in general.

Physical Medicine and Rehabilitation

Physical medicine and rehabilitation, also referred to as rehabilitation medicine, is the medical specialty concerned with diagnosing, evaluating, and treating patients with impairments and/or disabilities that involve musculoskeletal, neurological, cardiovascular, or other body systems.

Psychiatry

A psychiatrist is a physician who specializes in the prevention, diagnosis, and treatment of mental, addictive, and emotional disorders, such as psychoses, depression, anxiety disorders, substance abuse disorders, developmental disabilities, sexual dysfunctions, and adjustment reactions.

Radiation Oncology

Radiation oncology is the branch of radiology that deals with the therapeutic applications of radiant energy and its modifiers and with the study and management of disease, especially malignant tumors.

Surgery

A general surgeon is a specialist prepared to manage a broad spectrum of surgical conditions affecting almost any area of the body. The surgeon establishes the diagnosis and provides the preoperative, operative, and postoperative care to surgical patients and is usually responsible for the comprehensive management of the trauma victim and the critically ill.

Hand Surgery. A hand surgeon has special qualifications in the management of surgical disorders of the hand and wrist.

Vascular Surgery. The vascular surgeon brings special qualifications to the management of surgical disorders of the blood vessels, excluding those immediately adjacent to the heart, lungs, or brain.

Thoracic Surgery

Thoracic surgery encompasses the operative, perioperative, and critical care of patients with pathological conditions within the chest. Included is the surgical care of coronary artery disease; cancers of the lung, esophagus, and chest wall; abnormalities of the great vessels and heart valves; congenital abnormalities; tumors of the mediastinum (or middle chest); and diseases of the diaphragm.

Urology

A urologist is competent to manage benign and malignant medical and surgical disorders of the adrenal gland and of the genitourinary system. These subspecialists have comprehensive knowledge of, and skills in, endoscopic, percutaneous, and open surgery of congenital and acquired conditions of the reproductive and urinary systems and their contiguous structures.

Descriptions excerpted from Which Medical Specialist for You, *by the American Board of Medical Specialties*
Revised 2/95

FINDING THE RIGHT HOSPITAL

Your doctor is your best resource for finding the right hospital. He or she is familiar with many of the hospitals in your community and will know about others through colleagues. If you do not have a regular doctor, ask the physician who made your diagnosis about the hospitals that he or she knows.

Where you go for treatment depends on your illness and the kind of surroundings that make you feel comfortable. Hospitals vary enormously in size and in the level of personalized care that they can deliver. (The latter depends more on the nursing staff than anything else.) Some treatments are well carried out in the setting of your community hospital, whereas other treatments should be handled by the expertise of an Academic Medical Center Hospital.

If your illness does not require the cutting edge of technology or highly trained specialists, then you might consider a community hospital, particularly if a doctor you trust is affiliated with one. This will make it easier for friends and family to visit often and will give you the reassurance of being close to home.

Expertise and experience of staff and the latest equipment for diagnostics and treatment are the advantages of a large teaching hospital. For a physician to remain on the staff of a teaching hospital, he or she must be eminently qualified. And should the doctor need consultation on an unusual problem, it is likely that one of the leading experts in the field is already on staff. Teaching hospitals treat a wide range of disorders every day, so their personnel are familiar with disorders or conditions that a small community hospital might see only a few times a year. Teaching hospitals also have much more experience in carrying out procedures that are done infrequently in a community hospital.

The research conducted at a teaching hospital can play an important role in the outcome of a patient's treatment. The same staff that will be treating you will, through their research, also have access to the latest in diagnostics, drugs, and treatments. But do not choose a hospital just because it does research. Keep in mind that research centers are funded for the quality of their research and not necessarily for the quality of their patient care.

The lists in this Directory provide a good place to start looking for a teaching hospital. Each hospital listed participates in either a Graduate Medical Education Program accredited by the Accreditation Council for Graduate Medical Education or an Advanced Dental Educational Program accredited by the American Dental Association's Commission on Dental Education. There are two ways to look: by location or by disorder. The list of Teaching Hospitals by State and City allows you simply to look up what hospitals are in your area. Under each listing you will find the hospital's name, address, phone number, and selected specialties for which it has a medical education program. For explanations of what each medical specialty covers, see page 477.

The list of Teaching Hospitals by Disorder will give you the names of the hospitals that have teaching programs related to the disorders covered in the Handbook. To guide you, the hospitals are arranged by state, then by name. Once you have located a hospital in this listing, you can find its address and phone number in the geographic listing. Because any number of teaching specialties could qualify a hospital for inclusion under one of the disorders, check the list of teaching specialties under the hospital's listing to see if it has the specific specialty that you need.

The Teaching Hospitals by Disorder section also identifies in bold type those hospitals that are among the Academic Medical Center Hospitals in the United States. The Academic Medical Center Hospitals are designated by the Association of American Medical Colleges' Council of Teaching Hospitals. This means that the hospital must meet the following criteria: have a signed affiliation agreement with a medical school accredited by the Liaison Committee on Medical Education, be a non-Federal member of the council under either common ownership with a medical school or closely associated with one through its chiefs of service, and provide a short-stay, general hospital service.

An asterisk identifies the Academic Medical Center Hospitals that are nonprofit and privately owned, which, as a group, scored best on factors predicting good outcomes and had the lowest mortality rates per hospital stays in a study done by the *New England Journal of Medicine.*

Hospitals that are associated with treatment centers currently funded by the National Institutes of Health are marked by the symbol ▼ or † or ■ under certain disorders in the list of Teaching Hospitals by Disorder. Heart and liver transplant centers approved by Medicare are shown in italic type.

One final note: Remember that medical centers are often spread out over a wide area, so before you visit, call to get the exact location of the department you need.

FINDING A DENTAL CARE FACILITY

Chances are your dentist can provide all the care that you will ever need. But there might come a time when you want a second opinion or require a procedure unusual enough for your dentist to prefer to send you to a facility that has the extensive experience necessary for the best outcome.

Included in the list of Teaching Hospitals by State and City are those dental schools, hospitals, and organizations that run Advanced Dental Educational Programs accredited by the American Dental Association's Commission on Dental Education. These facilities have "Dentistry" listed in their teaching specialties.

In the section called Health Information and Support Organizations by Disorder, you will find a listing of a number of organizations that you can contact for more information on your particular disorder. There are also dental certification boards included in the organizations list should you wish to find out whether a dentist has been board certified.

Before calling any of the dental education programs, talk to your dentist, who will probably already know the right place for you to go for the second opinion or procedure. If he or she has more than one name to choose from or if you wish to do more checking on your own, sit down together and formulate questions that you should ask when contacting these programs for more information. They should be aimed at finding out how much experience each program has with your problem. Also, do not forget that, just as in medical surgery, there are other specialists who may be required in order to perform your procedure (such as anesthesiologists). Be sure to find out about their training too.

In general, your best bets are dental education programs that are affiliated with a den-tal or medical school. Although it is true that some good programs happen not to have such an affiliation, the programs that do can offer the widest experience in even uncommon dental disorders. The smaller programs tend to work in just a few specialties. When considering a small dental education program, check to see if its director is full-time and still actively practices dentistry. This makes it more likely that the program itself is up-to-date and professional.

Two notes on using this list: Hospitals with dental education programs have their main phone number listed, so when you call, ask for their dental education department. Also, remember that medical centers are often spread out over a wide area, so before you visit, call to get the exact location of the department you need.

FINDING A HEALTH INFORMATION ORGANIZATION

Health information organizations vary greatly in what services they can provide. The smallest can send you literature on a specific illness. The major ones can do everything from keeping you up-to-date on the latest progress in treatment, to making referrals to physicians or hospitals, to helping you locate a support group.

Because you want reliable health-related information, finding a good organization requires some careful checking. Start with your physician and ask if he or she can recommend a health information organization for you to contact.

The Health Information and Support Organizations in this Directory are listed either by the disorders covered in the Handbook or in a "general" section. If you use the "by disorder" list and have trouble deciding which organization to call, start with the ones that provided material for the corresponding chapter in the Handbook. If they cannot help you directly, they should still be able to tell you who can.

The Federal Government provides a referral service called the Office of Disease Prevention and Health Promotion National Health Information Center at PO Box 1133, Washington, DC 20013-1133; phone: 800-336-4797 or 301-565-4167. Using their database, staff members can find a health information organization to help you, or they can answer questions about what a particular health information organization does.

Another way to find a health information organization is to ask for a referral from one of the listed Academic Medical Center Hospitals. Look for these hospitals under your disorder in the list of Teaching Hospitals by Disorder. The Academic Medical Center Hospitals are in bold. Those in bold with an asterisk are nonprofit and privately owned.

FINDING A GOOD SUPPORT GROUP

Sometimes medical treatment can do only so much. You may feel the need to address the personal aspect of your illness as well. Many people in difficult situations find that meeting with other people in the same predicament can be very helpful. Self-help or support groups can provide you with a sense of community, reinforcing the knowledge that you are not alone, that there are others who understand what you are feeling.

In the Health Information and Support Organizations section of the Directory, the organizations listed under "Support Groups" in Organizations by Disorder can provide you with information on how to contact one of their local offices. If you do not find a support group geared to your specific disorder in the "by disorder" lists, look in General Organizations under "National Self-Help Clearinghouses" or "Regional Self-Help Clearinghouses." These organizations operate at the state and national levels and can tell you if there is a support group nearby that can help. Just as in searching for a hospital or health information organization, check with your physician. Find out what your doctor knows about the groups you have found and whether he or she can suggest any.

You might also try calling one of the health information organizations or Academic Medical Center Hospitals (listed in bold type in the Teaching Hospitals by Disorder section). The Office of Disease Prevention and Health Promotion National Health Information Center can also provide you with information on support groups. It can be reached at PO Box 1133, Washington, D.C. 20013-1133; phone: 800-336-4797 or 301-565-4167.

One caveat: These groups are social entities. As a whole, they have an agenda and a certain perspective on issues relating to their specialty. Keep this in mind when you contact a group. If you do not feel at ease with the people in the group, then there is no reason to stay. Remember, if you feel a certain way, there are bound to be countless others who feel exactly as you do, so the right group for you does exist.

Teaching Hospitals

To find a hospital in this section, look under the state and then city where it is located. Each listing shows the name of the hospital, its main address, its phone number, and selected medical specialties for which it has an education program.

To find a hospital that has medical education programs that correspond to one of the disorders covered in the Handbook, turn to page 539 for the list of Teaching Hospitals by Disorder.

ALABAMA

Birmingham

Baptist Medical Center-Montclair
800 Montclair Rd.
Birmingham, AL 35213
205-592-1000
Teaching Specialties:
Internal Medicine, Surgery

Baptist Medical Center-Princeton
701 Princeton Ave., SW
Birmingham, AL 35211
205-783-3000
Teaching Specialties:
Internal Medicine, Surgery

Carraway Methodist Medical Center
1600 Carraway Blvd.
Birmingham, AL 35234
205-226-6000
Teaching Specialties:
Anesthesiology, Internal Medicine, Obstetrics/Gynecology, Surgery

Cooper Green Hospital
1515 Sixth Ave. South
Birmingham, AL 35233
205-930-3225
Teaching Specialties:
Anesthesiology, Internal Medicine, Obstetrics/Gynecology, Ophthalmology, Orthopedic Surgery, Surgery, Urology

Eye Foundation Hospital
1720 University Blvd.
Birmingham, AL 35233
205-325-8100
Teaching Specialties:
Ophthalmology

University of Alabama Hospitals
619 S. 19th St.
Birmingham, AL 35233
205-934-4011
Teaching Specialties:
Anesthesiology, Dermatology, Hand Surgery, Internal Medicine, Internal Medicine-Cardiovascular Disease, Internal Medicine-Endocrinology and Metabolism, Internal Medicine-Gastroenterology, Internal Medicine-Geriatric Medicine, Internal Medicine-Hematology, Internal Medicine-Infectious Diseases, Internal Medicine-Medical Oncology, Internal Medicine-Nephrology, Internal Medicine-Rheumatology, Neurological Surgery, Neurology, Obstetrics/Gynecology, Ophthalmology, Orthopedic Surgery, Otolaryngology, Physical Medicine and Rehabilitation, Psychiatry, Radiation Oncology, Surgery, Thoracic Surgery, Urology

University of Alabama School of Dentistry
UAB Station
Birmingham, AL 35294
205-934-3000
Teaching Specialties:
Dentistry

Fairfield

Lloyd Noland Hospital and Ambulatory Center
701 Lloyd Noland Pkwy.
Fairfield, AL 35064
205-783-5121
Teaching Specialties:
Surgery

Mobile

University of South Alabama Medical Center
2451 Fillingim St.
Mobile, AL 36617
334-471-7000
Teaching Specialties:
Anesthesiology, Internal Medicine, Internal Medicine-Cardiovascular Disease, Internal Medicine-Hematology, Internal Medicine-Infectious Diseases, Internal Medicine-Medical Oncology, Neurology, Obstetrics/Gynecology, Ophthalmology, Orthopedic Surgery, Psychiatry, Surgery

Montgomery

Baptist Medical Center
2105 E. South Blvd.
Montgomery, AL 36116-2498
334-286-2970
Teaching Specialties:
Internal Medicine

Montgomery Regional Medical Center
301 S. Ripley St.
Montgomery, AL 36104
334-269-8000
Teaching Specialties:
Internal Medicine

Mt. Vernon

Searcy Hospital
PO Box 1001
Mt. Vernon, AL 36560
334-829-9411
Teaching Specialties:
Psychiatry

ARIZONA

Phoenix

Good Samaritan Regional Medical Center
1111 E. McDowell Rd.
Phoenix, AZ 85006
602-239-2000
Teaching Specialties:
Internal Medicine, Internal Medicine-Cardiovascular Disease, Obstetrics/Gynecology, Psychiatry, Surgery

Maricopa Medical Center
2601 E. Roosevelt St.
Phoenix, AZ 85008
602-267-5011
Teaching Specialties:
Anesthesiology, Internal Medicine, Neurological Surgery, Obstetrics/Gynecology, Orthopedic Surgery, Psychiatry, Surgery

St. Joseph's Hospital and Medical Center
350 W. Thomas Rd.
Phoenix, AZ 85013
602-406-3196
Teaching Specialties:
Internal Medicine, Obstetrics/Gynecology

St. Joseph's Hospital and Medical Center
Barrow Neurological Institute
350 W. Thomas Rd.

Phoenix, AZ 85013
602-285-3000
Teaching Specialties:
Neurological Surgery, Neurology

Tucson

Carondelet St. Joseph's Hospital
350 N. Wilmot Rd.
Tucson, AZ 85711
520-296-3211
Teaching Specialties:
Ophthalmology

Kino Community Hospital
2800 E. Ajo Way
Tucson, AZ 85713
520-294-4471
Teaching Specialties:
Dermatology, Internal Medicine, Internal Medicine-Endocrinology and Metabolism, Internal Medicine-Gastroenterology, Obstetrics/Gynecology, Ophthalmology, Psychiatry, Surgery

Tucson Medical Center
5301 E. Grant Rd.
Tucson, AZ 85712
520-327-5461
Teaching Specialties:
Internal Medicine, Neurology, Surgery

University Medical Center
1501 N. Campbell Ave.
Tucson, AZ 85724
520-694-0111
Teaching Specialties:
Anesthesiology, Dermatology, Internal Medicine, Internal Medicine-Cardiovascular Disease, Internal Medicine-Endocrinology and Metabolism, Internal Medicine-Gastroenterology, Internal Medicine-Hematology, Internal Medicine-Infectious Diseases, Internal Medicine-Medical Oncology, Internal Medicine-Nephrology, Internal Medicine-Rheumatology, Neurology, Obstetrics/Gynecology, Ophthalmology, Orthopedic Surgery, Psychiatry, Radiation Oncology, Surgery, Surgery-Vascular Surgery, Thoracic Surgery, Urology

ARKANSAS

Little Rock

Arkansas State Hospital
4313 W. Markham St.
Little Rock, AR 72205
501-686-9000
Teaching Specialties:
Psychiatry

Baptist Rehabilitation Institute of Arkansas
9601 Interstate 630, Exit 7

Little Rock, AR 72205
501-223-7507
Teaching Specialties:
Physical Medicine and Rehabilitation

University Hospital of Arkansas
4301 W. Markham St.
Little Rock, AR 72205
501-686-7000
Teaching Specialties:
Anesthesiology, Dermatology, Internal Medicine, Internal Medicine-Cardiovascular Disease, Internal Medicine-Endocrinology and Metabolism, Internal Medicine-Gastroenterology, Internal Medicine-Geriatric Medicine, Internal Medicine-Hematology, Internal Medicine-Infectious Diseases, Internal Medicine-Medical Oncology, Internal Medicine-Nephrology, Internal Medicine-Rheumatology, Neurological Surgery, Neurology, Obstetrics/Gynecology, Ophthalmology, Orthopedic Surgery, Otolaryngology, Physical Medicine and Rehabilitation, Psychiatry, Surgery, Surgery-Vascular Surgery, Thoracic Surgery, Urology

CALIFORNIA

Anaheim

Kaiser Foundation Hospital
441 N. Lakeview Ave.
Anaheim, CA 92807
714-978-4000
Teaching Specialties:
Internal Medicine-Geriatric Medicine, Otolaryngology

Bakersfield

Kern Medical Center
1830 Flower St.
Bakersfield, CA 93305
805-326-2000
Teaching Specialties:
Internal Medicine, Obstetrics/Gynecology, Surgery

Camarillo

Camarillo State Hospital and Development Center
PO Box 6022
1878 S. Lewis Rd.
Camarillo, CA 93011
805-484-3661
Teaching Specialties:
Psychiatry

Daly City

Seton Medical Center
1900 Sullivan Ave.
Daly City, CA 94015
415-992-4000

Teaching Specialties:
Orthopedic Surgery, Radiation Oncology

Downey

**Los Angeles County-Rancho
Los Amigos Medical Center**
7601 E. Imperial Hwy.
Downey, CA 90242
310-940-7022
Teaching Specialties:
Internal Medicine-Infectious Diseases, Orthopedic Surgery, Otolaryngology

Duarte

City of Hope National Medical Center
1500 E. Duarte Rd.
Duarte, CA 91010
818-359-8111
Teaching Specialties:
Radiation Oncology

Fairfield

Solano County Mental Health Clinic
2101 Courage Dr.
Fairfield, CA 94533
707-435-2080
Teaching Specialties:
Psychiatry

Fontana

Kaiser Foundation Hospital
9961 Sierra Ave.
Fontana, CA 92335
909-427-5000
Teaching Specialties:
Obstetrics/Gynecology, Surgery, Thoracic Surgery

Fresno

Valley Medical Center of Fresno
445 S. Cedar Ave.
Fresno, CA 93702
209-453-4000
Teaching Specialties:
Dentistry, Internal Medicine, Internal Medicine-Cardiovascular Disease, Obstetrics/Gynecology, Psychiatry, Surgery

Glendale

Glendale Adventist Medical Center
1509 Wilson Terr.
Glendale, CA 91206
818-409-8000
Teaching Specialties:
Obstetrics/Gynecology

Greenbrae

Community Mental Health Services
250 Bonair Rd.
Greenbrae, CA 94904
415-499-6835
Teaching Specialties:
Psychiatry

Hayward

Kaiser Foundation Hospital
27400 Hesperian Blvd.
Hayward, CA 94545
510-784-4000
Teaching Specialties:
Urology

Inglewood

Centinela Hospital Medical Center
555 E. Hardy St.
Inglewood, CA 90301
310-673-4660
Teaching Specialties:
Orthopedic Surgery

La Jolla

Green Hospital of Scripps Clinic
10666 N. Torrey Pines Rd.
La Jolla, CA 92037
619-455-9100
Teaching Specialties:
Allergy/Immunology, Internal Medicine, Internal Medicine-Cardiovascular Disease, Internal Medicine-Endocrinology and Metabolism, Internal Medicine-Gastroenterology, Internal Medicine-Hematology, Internal Medicine-Medical Oncology, Internal Medicine-Rheumatology

Loma Linda

Loma Linda University Medical Center
25333 Barton Rd.
Loma Linda, CA 92354
909-796-7311
Teaching Specialties:
Anesthesiology, Dermatology, Hand Surgery, Internal Medicine, Internal Medicine-Cardiovascular Disease, Internal Medicine-Gastroenterology, Internal Medicine-Nephrology, Internal Medicine-Rheumatology, Neurological Surgery, Neurology, Obstetrics/Gynecology, Ophthalmology, Orthopedic Surgery, Otolaryngology, Physical Medicine and Rehabilitation, Psychiatry, Radiation Oncology, Surgery, Surgery-Vascular Surgery, Thoracic Surgery, Urology

Loma Linda University School of Dentistry
11092 Anderson St.
Loma Linda, CA 92350

909-824-4222
Teaching Specialties:
Dentistry

Long Beach

Long Beach Memorial Medical Center
2801 Atlantic Ave.
Long Beach, CA 90806
310-933-2000
Teaching Specialties:
Internal Medicine, Internal Medicine-Cardiovascular Disease, Internal Medicine-Geriatric Medicine, Obstetrics/Gynecology, Ophthalmology, Physical Medicine and Rehabilitation, Radiation Oncology, Surgery

St. Mary Medical Center
1050 Linden Ave.
Long Beach, CA 90813
310-491-9000
Teaching Specialties:
Internal Medicine, Internal Medicine-Cardiovascular Disease, Surgery

Los Angeles

California Medical Center-Los Angeles
1401 S. Grand Ave.
Los Angeles, CA 90015
213-748-2411
Teaching Specialties:
Obstetrics/Gynecology, Radiation Oncology, Surgery

Cedars-Sinai Medical Center
PO Box 48750
8700 Beverly Blvd.
Los Angeles, CA 90048
310-855-5000
Teaching Specialties:
Dentistry, Internal Medicine, Internal Medicine-Cardiovascular Disease, Internal Medicine-Endocrinology and Metabolism, Internal Medicine-Gastroenterology, Internal Medicine-Hematology, Internal Medicine-Infectious Diseases, Internal Medicine-Medical Oncology, Internal Medicine-Nephrology, Internal Medicine-Rheumatology, Obstetrics/Gynecology, Physical Medicine and Rehabilitation, Psychiatry, Surgery

Century City Hospital
2070 Century Park East
Los Angeles, CA 90067
310-553-6211
Teaching Specialties:
Hand Surgery

Hospital of the Good Samaritan
616 S. Witmer St.
Los Angeles, CA 90017
213-977-2121

Teaching Specialties:
Thoracic Surgery

Kaiser Foundation Hospital
4867 Sunset Blvd.
Los Angeles, CA 90027
213-667-4011
Teaching Specialties:
Allergy/Immunology, Internal Medicine, Internal Medicine-Cardiovascular Disease, Internal Medicine-Gastroenterology, Internal Medicine-Hematology, Internal Medicine-Infectious Diseases, Internal Medicine-Nephrology, Neurology, Obstetrics/Gynecology, Radiation Oncology, Surgery, Urology

Kaiser Foundation Hospital-West Los Angeles
6041 Cadillac Ave.
Los Angeles, CA 90034
213-857-2201
Teaching Specialties:
Internal Medicine

Los Angeles County-King-Drew Medical Center
12021 S. Wilmington Ave.
Los Angeles, CA 90059
310-668-5201
Teaching Specialties:
Anesthesiology, Dentistry, Dermatology, Internal Medicine, Internal Medicine-Cardiovascular Disease, Internal Medicine-Gastroenterology, Internal Medicine-Infectious Diseases, Obstetrics/Gynecology, Ophthalmology, Orthopedic Surgery, Otolaryngology, Psychiatry, Surgery

Los Angeles County-University of Southern California Medical Center
1200 N. State St.
Los Angeles, CA 90033
213-226-2622
Teaching Specialties:
Allergy/Immunology, Anesthesiology, Dentistry, Dermatology, Internal Medicine, Internal Medicine-Cardiovascular Disease, Internal Medicine-Endocrinology and Metabolism, Internal Medicine-Gastroenterology, Internal Medicine-Hematology, Internal Medicine-Infectious Diseases, Internal Medicine-Medical Oncology, Internal Medicine-Nephrology, Internal Medicine-Rheumatology, Neurological Surgery, Neurology, Obstetrics/Gynecology, Ophthalmology, Orthopedic Surgery, Otolaryngology, Psychiatry, Radiation Oncology, Surgery, Thoracic Surgery, Urology

Orthopaedic Hospital
2400 S. Flower St.
Los Angeles, CA 90007
213-742-1000
Teaching Specialties:
Orthopedic Surgery

St. Vincent Medical Center
2131 W. Third St.
Los Angeles, CA 90057
213-484-7111
Teaching Specialties:
Internal Medicine-Cardiovascular Disease, Internal Medicine-Nephrology

University of California, Los Angeles Medical Center
10833 LeConte Ave.
Los Angeles, CA 90024
310-825-9111
800-825-2631 (physician referral)
Teaching Specialties:
Allergy/Immunology, Anesthesiology, Dermatology, Hand Surgery, Internal Medicine, Internal Medicine-Cardiovascular Disease, Internal Medicine-Endocrinology and Metabolism, Internal Medicine-Gastroenterology, Internal Medicine-Geriatric Medicine, Internal Medicine-Hematology, Internal Medicine-Infectious Diseases, Internal Medicine-Medical Oncology, Internal Medicine-Nephrology, Internal Medicine-Rheumatology, Neurological Surgery, Neurology, Obstetrics/Gynecology, Orthopedic Surgery, Otolaryngology, Radiation Oncology, Surgery, Surgery-Vascular Surgery, Thoracic Surgery, Urology

University of California, Los Angeles Medical Center
Jules Stein Eye Institute
100 Stein Plaza, UCLA
Los Angeles, CA 90024
310-825-5000
Teaching Specialties:
Ophthalmology

University of California, Los Angeles Neuropsychiatric Hospital
760 Westwood Plaza
Los Angeles, CA 90024
310-825-9548
Teaching Specialties:
Psychiatry

University of California, Los Angeles School of Dentistry
Center for the Health Sciences
10833 LeConte Ave.
Los Angeles, CA 90024-1668
310-825-2337
Teaching Specialties:
Dentistry

University of Southern California
The Kenneth Norris Jr. Cancer Hospital
1441 Eastlake Ave.
Los Angeles, CA 90033
323-865-3000

Teaching Specialties:
Radiation Oncology, Urology

University of Southern California School of Dentistry
925 W. 34th St.
University Park MC-0641
Los Angeles, CA 90089-0641
213-740-2800
Teaching Specialties:
Dentistry

White Memorial Medical Center
1720 Cesar Chavez Ave.
Los Angeles, CA 90033
213-268-5000
Teaching Specialties:
Internal Medicine, Obstetrics/Gynecology, Ophthalmology, Urology

Modesto

Stanislaus Medical Center
830 Scenic Dr.
Modesto, CA 95350
209-558-7171
Teaching Specialties:
Surgery

Napa

Napa State Hospital
2100 Napa-Vallejo Hwy.
Napa, CA 94558
707-253-5454
Teaching Specialties:
Psychiatry

Oakland

Highland General Hospital
1411 E. 31st St.
Oakland, CA 94602
510-437-4397
Teaching Specialties:
Dentistry, Internal Medicine, Neurology, Ophthalmology, Orthopedic Surgery, Surgery

Kaiser Foundation Hospital
280 W. MacArthur Blvd.
Oakland, CA 94611
510-596-1000
Teaching Specialties:
Internal Medicine, Obstetrics/Gynecology, Otolaryngology, Surgery

Orange

St. Joseph Hospital
1100 W. Stewart Dr.
Orange, CA 92668
714-633-9111
Teaching Specialties:
Radiation Oncology

489

University of California, Irvine Medical Center
101 The City Dr. South
Orange, CA 92868
714-456-5678
Teaching Specialties:
Allergy/Immunology, Anesthesiology, Dermatology, Internal Medicine, Internal Medicine-Cardiovascular Disease, Internal Medicine-Endocrinology and Metabolism, Internal Medicine-Gastroenterology, Internal Medicine-Geriatric Medicine, Internal Medicine-Hematology, Internal Medicine-Infectious Diseases, Internal Medicine-Medical Oncology, Internal Medicine-Nephrology, Internal Medicine-Rheumatology, Neurological Surgery, Neurology, Obstetrics/Gynecology, Ophthalmology, Orthopedic Surgery, Otolaryngology, Physical Medicine and Rehabilitation, Psychiatry, Radiation Oncology, Surgery, Urology

Pasadena

Huntington Memorial Hospital
100 W. California Blvd.
Pasadena, CA 91105
818-397-5000
Teaching Specialties:
Internal Medicine, Neurological Surgery, Surgery

Reedley

Kings View Hospital
42675 Rd. 44
Reedley, CA 93654
209-638-2505
Teaching Specialties:
Psychiatry

Riverside

Riverside General Hospital
University Medical Center
9851 Magnolia Ave.
Riverside, CA 92503
909-358-7100
Teaching Specialties:
Neurology, Obstetrics/Gynecology, Ophthalmology, Otolaryngology, Surgery

Sacramento

Kaiser Foundation Hospital
2025 Morse Ave.
Sacramento, CA 95825
916-973-5000
Teaching Specialties:
Internal Medicine, Neurological Surgery, Obstetrics/Gynecology, Orthopedic Surgery, Surgery, Urology

Sutter General Hospital
2801 L St.
Sacramento, CA 95816
916-454-2222
Teaching Specialties:
Obstetrics/Gynecology, Surgery

Sutter Memorial Hospital
515 F St.
Sacramento, CA 95819
916-454-3333
Teaching Specialties:
Obstetrics/Gynecology, Surgery

University of California, Davis Medical Center
2315 Stockton Blvd.
Sacramento, CA 95817
916-734-2011
Teaching Specialties:
Allergy/Immunology, Anesthesiology, Dermatology, Internal Medicine, Internal Medicine-Cardiovascular Disease, Internal Medicine-Endocrinology and Metabolism, Internal Medicine-Gastroenterology, Internal Medicine-Geriatric Medicine, Internal Medicine-Hematology, Internal Medicine-Infectious Diseases, Internal Medicine-Medical Oncology, Internal Medicine-Nephrology, Internal Medicine-Rheumatology, Neurological Surgery, Neurology, Obstetrics/Gynecology, Ophthalmology, Orthopedic Surgery, Otolaryngology, Physical Medicine and Rehabilitation, Psychiatry, Surgery, Urology

San Bernardino

San Bernardino County Medical Center
780 E. Gilbert St.
San Bernardino, CA 92415
909-387-8111
Teaching Specialties:
Anesthesiology, Hand Surgery, Obstetrics/Gynecology, Orthopedic Surgery, Otolaryngology, Surgery, Urology

San Diego

Kaiser Foundation Hospital
4647 Zion Ave.
San Diego, CA 92120
619-528-5000
Teaching Specialties:
Neurological Surgery, Obstetrics/Gynecology, Otolaryngology

Mercy Hospital and Medical Center
4077 Fifth Ave.
San Diego, CA 92103
619-294-8111
Teaching Specialties:
Internal Medicine, Internal Medicine-Cardiovascular Disease, Urology

Sharp Memorial Hospital
7901 Frost St.
San Diego, CA 92123
619-541-3400
Teaching Specialties:
Internal Medicine-Cardiovascular Disease, Thoracic Surgery

University of California, San Diego Medical Center
200 W. Arbor Dr.
San Diego, CA 92103
619-543-6222
Teaching Specialties:
Allergy/Immunology, Anesthesiology, Dermatology, Internal Medicine, Internal Medicine-Cardiovascular Disease, Internal Medicine-Endocrinology and Metabolism, Internal Medicine-Gastroenterology, Internal Medicine-Geriatric Medicine, Internal Medicine-Hematology, Internal Medicine-Infectious Diseases, Internal Medicine-Medical Oncology, Internal Medicine-Nephrology, Internal Medicine-Rheumatology, Neurological Surgery, Neurology, Obstetrics/Gynecology, Ophthalmology, Orthopedic Surgery, Otolaryngology, Psychiatry, Surgery, Thoracic Surgery, Urology

San Francisco

California-Pacific Medical Center
2333 Buchanan St.
San Francisco, CA 94115
415-563-4321
Teaching Specialties:
Internal Medicine, Internal Medicine-Cardiovascular Disease, Internal Medicine-Gastroenterology, Ophthalmology, Psychiatry

Kaiser Foundation Hospital
2425 Geary Blvd.
San Francisco, CA 94115
415-202-2000
Teaching Specialties:
Internal Medicine, Obstetrics/Gynecology, Orthopedic Surgery, Otolaryngology, Surgery

Langley Porter Psychiatric Hospital and Clinics
401 Parnassus Ave.
San Francisco, CA 94122
415-476-7000
Teaching Specialties:
Psychiatry

Mt. Zion Medical Center of University of California, San Francisco
1600 Divisadero St.
San Francisco, CA 94115
415-567-6600
Teaching Specialties:
Internal Medicine, Internal Medicine-Cardio-

vascular Disease, Internal Medicine-Geriatric Medicine, Internal Medicine-Infectious Diseases, Obstetrics/Gynecology, Orthopedic Surgery, Radiation Oncology

San Francisco General Hospital and Medical Center
1001 Potrero Ave.
San Francisco, CA 94110
415-206-8000
Teaching Specialties:
Anesthesiology, Dermatology, Internal Medicine, Internal Medicine-Gastroenterology, Internal Medicine-Hematology, Internal Medicine-Infectious Diseases, Internal Medicine-Medical Oncology, Internal Medicine-Nephrology, Internal Medicine-Rheumatology, Neurological Surgery, Neurology, Obstetrics/Gynecology, Ophthalmology, Orthopedic Surgery, Otolaryngology, Psychiatry, Surgery, Urology

St. Mary's Hospital and Medical Center
450 Stanyan St.
San Francisco, CA 94117
415-668-1000
Teaching Specialties:
Internal Medicine, Internal Medicine-Cardiovascular Disease, Orthopedic Surgery, Radiation Oncology

University of California, San Francisco Medical Center
505 Parnassus Ave.
San Francisco, CA 94122
415-476-1000
Teaching Specialties:
Allergy/Immunology, Anesthesiology, Dermatology, Hand Surgery, Internal Medicine, Internal Medicine-Cardiovascular Disease, Internal Medicine-Endocrinology and Metabolism, Internal Medicine-Gastroenterology, Internal Medicine-Hematology, Internal Medicine-Infectious Diseases, Internal Medicine-Medical Oncology, Internal Medicine-Nephrology, Internal Medicine-Rheumatology, Neurological Surgery, Neurology, Obstetrics/Gynecology, Ophthalmology, Orthopedic Surgery, Otolaryngology, Psychiatry, Radiation Oncology, Surgery, Surgery-Vascular Surgery, Thoracic Surgery, Urology

University of California, San Francisco School of Dentistry
Box 0430
San Francisco, CA 94143-0430
415-476-1323 (dean's office)
Teaching Specialties:
Dentistry

University of the Pacific School of Dentistry
2155 Webster St.
San Francisco, CA 94115

415-929-6400
Teaching Specialties:
Dentistry

San Jose

Santa Clara Valley Medical Center
751 S. Bascom
San Jose, CA 95128
408-299-5100
Teaching Specialties:
Anesthesiology, Dermatology, Internal Medicine, Internal Medicine-Endocrinology and Metabolism, Internal Medicine-Gastroenterology, Internal Medicine-Infectious Diseases, Internal Medicine-Rheumatology, Neurological Surgery, Neurology, Obstetrics/Gynecology, Ophthalmology, Orthopedic Surgery, Otolaryngology, Physical Medicine and Rehabilitation, Surgery, Urology

San Mateo

San Mateo County General Hospital
222 W. 39th Ave.
San Mateo, CA 94403
415-573-2222
Teaching Specialties:
Psychiatry

Santa Barbara

Sansum Medical Clinic
317 W. Pueblo St.
Santa Barbara, CA 93105
805-682-2621
Teaching Specialties:
Colon and Rectal Surgery

Santa Barbara Cottage Hospital
Pueblo at Bath Sts.
Santa Barbara, CA 93105
805-682-7111
Teaching Specialties:
Colon and Rectal Surgery, Internal Medicine, Surgery

Santa Clara

Kaiser Foundation Hospital
900 Kiely Blvd.
Santa Clara, CA 95051
408-236-6400
Teaching Specialties:
Internal Medicine, Obstetrics/Gynecology, Otolaryngology, Psychiatry, Surgery

Stanford

Stanford University Hospital
300 Pasteur Dr.
Stanford, CA 94305
650-723-4000

Teaching Specialties:
Anesthesiology, Dermatology, Internal Medicine, Internal Medicine-Cardiovascular Disease, Internal Medicine-Endocrinology and Metabolism, Internal Medicine-Gastroenterology, Internal Medicine-Geriatric Medicine, Internal Medicine-Hematology, Internal Medicine-Infectious Diseases, Internal Medicine-Medical Oncology, Internal Medicine-Nephrology, Internal Medicine-Rheumatology, Neurological Surgery, Neurology, Obstetrics/Gynecology, Ophthalmology, Orthopedic Surgery, Otolaryngology, Physical Medicine and Rehabilitation, Psychiatry, Radiation Oncology, Surgery, Surgery-Vascular Surgery, Thoracic Surgery, Urology

Stockton

San Joaquin General Hospital
PO Box 1020
Stockton, CA 95201
209-468-6000
Teaching Specialties:
Internal Medicine, Surgery

Sylmar

Olive View Medical Center
14445 Olive View Dr.
Sylmar, CA 91342
818-364-1555
Teaching Specialties:
Internal Medicine, Internal Medicine-Endocrinology and Metabolism, Internal Medicine-Hematology, Obstetrics/Gynecology, Otolaryngology, Psychiatry, Surgery, Urology

Torrance

Los Angeles County Harbor-University of California, Los Angeles Medical Center
1000 W. Carson St.
Torrance, CA 90509
310-222-2345
Teaching Specialties:
Allergy/Immunology, Anesthesiology, Dentistry, Dermatology, Internal Medicine, Internal Medicine-Cardiovascular Disease, Internal Medicine-Endocrinology and Metabolism, Internal Medicine-Gastroenterology, Internal Medicine-Hematology, Internal Medicine-Infectious Diseases, Internal Medicine-Medical Oncology, Internal Medicine-Nephrology, Internal Medicine-Rheumatology, Neurological Surgery, Neurology, Obstetrics/Gynecology, Ophthalmology, Orthopedic Surgery, Psychiatry, Surgery, Urology

Ventura

Ventura County Mental Health Center
300 N. Hillmont Ave.
Ventura, CA 93003

805-652-6737
805-652-6792 (administration)
Teaching Specialties:
Psychiatry

Walnut Creek

Kaiser Permanente Medical Center
1425 S. Main St.
Walnut Creek, CA 94595
510-295-4000
Teaching Specialties:
Urology

COLORADO

Denver

Denver Health and Hospitals
777 Bannock St.
Denver, CO 80204-4507
303-436-6000
Teaching Specialties:
Anesthesiology, Dentistry, Dermatology, Internal Medicine, Internal Medicine-Cardiovascular Disease, Internal Medicine-Endocrinology and Metabolism, Internal Medicine-Gastroenterology, Internal Medicine-Hematology, Internal Medicine-Infectious Diseases, Internal Medicine-Medical Oncology, Internal Medicine-Nephrology, Neurological Surgery, Neurology, Obstetrics/Gynecology, Ophthalmology, Orthopedic Surgery, Otolaryngology, Psychiatry, Surgery, Urology

National Jewish Center for Immunology and Respiratory Medicine
1400 Jackson St.
Denver, CO 80206
303-388-4461
Teaching Specialties:
Allergy/Immunology

Presbyterian-St. Luke's Medical Center
1719 E. 19th Ave.
Denver, CO 80218
303-839-6000
Teaching Specialties:
Internal Medicine, Obstetrics/Gynecology, Radiation Oncology

Rose Medical Center
4567 E. Ninth Ave.
Denver, CO 80220
303-320-2121
Teaching Specialties:
Internal Medicine, Obstetrics/Gynecology, Surgery

St. Joseph Hospital
1835 Franklin St.
Denver, CO 80218
303-837-7111
Teaching Specialties:
Dentistry, Internal Medicine, Obstetrics/Gynecology, Otolaryngology, Surgery

University of Colorado Health Sciences Center
University Hospital
4200 E. Ninth Ave.
Denver, CO 80220
303-270-6328
Teaching Specialties:
Allergy/Immunology, Anesthesiology, Dermatology, Internal Medicine, Internal Medicine-Cardiovascular Disease, Internal Medicine-Endocrinology and Metabolism, Internal Medicine-Gastroenterology, Internal Medicine-Geriatric Medicine, Internal Medicine-Hematology, Internal Medicine-Infectious Diseases, Internal Medicine-Medical Oncology, Internal Medicine-Nephrology, Internal Medicine-Rheumatology, Neurological Surgery, Neurology, Obstetrics/Gynecology, Ophthalmology, Orthopedic Surgery, Otolaryngology, Physical Medicine and Rehabilitation, Psychiatry, Surgery, Thoracic Surgery, Urology

University of Colorado School of Dentistry
Box C-284
4200 E. Ninth Ave.
Denver, CO 80262
303-315-7259
Teaching Specialties:
Dentistry

Englewood

Craig Hospital
3425 S. Clarkson St.
Englewood, CO 80110
303-789-8000
Teaching Specialties:
Physical Medicine and Rehabilitation

CONNECTICUT

Bridgeport

Bridgeport Hospital
267 Grant St.
Bridgeport, CT 06610
203-384-3000
Teaching Specialties:
Internal Medicine, Internal Medicine-Cardiovascular Disease, Internal Medicine-Gastroenterology, Obstetrics/Gynecology, Surgery

St. Vincent's Medical Center
2800 Main St.

Bridgeport, CT 06606
203-576-6000
Teaching Specialties:
Internal Medicine, Internal Medicine-Cardiovascular Disease

Danbury

Danbury Hospital
24 Hospital Ave.
Danbury, CT 06810
203-797-7000
Teaching Specialties:
Dentistry, Internal Medicine, Obstetrics/Gynecology, Psychiatry

Derby

Griffin Hospital
130 Division St.
Derby, CT 06418
203-735-7421
Teaching Specialties:
Internal Medicine, Internal Medicine-Gastroenterology, Surgery

Farmington

University of Connecticut Health Center
John Dempsey Hospital
263 Farmington Ave.
Farmington, CT 06030
203-679-2000
Teaching Specialties:
Anesthesiology, Internal Medicine, Internal Medicine-Cardiovascular Disease, Internal Medicine-Endocrinology and Metabolism, Internal Medicine-Gastroenterology, Internal Medicine-Geriatric Medicine, Internal Medicine-Hematology, Internal Medicine-Infectious Diseases, Internal Medicine-Medical Oncology, Internal Medicine-Nephrology, Internal Medicine-Rheumatology, Neurological Surgery, Obstetrics/Gynecology, Orthopedic Surgery, Otolaryngology, Psychiatry, Surgery, Urology

University of Connecticut School of Dental Medicine
263 Farmington Ave.
Farmington, CT 06030-3915
203-679-2808
Teaching Specialties:
Dentistry

Greenwich

Greenwich Hospital
5 Perryridge Rd.
Greenwich, CT 06830
203-863-3000
Teaching Specialties:
Internal Medicine, Psychiatry

Hartford

Hartford Hospital
80 Seymour St.
Hartford, CT 06115
203-545-5555
Teaching Specialties:
Anesthesiology, Dentistry, Internal Medicine, Internal Medicine-Cardiovascular Disease, Internal Medicine-Infectious Diseases, Neurological Surgery, Obstetrics/Gynecology, Orthopedic Surgery, Otolaryngology, Psychiatry, Surgery, Urology

Institute of Living
400 Washington St.
Hartford, CT 06106
203-545-7000
Teaching Specialties:
Psychiatry

Mt. Sinai Hospital
500 Blue Hills Ave.
Hartford, CT 06112
203-286-4600
Teaching Specialties:
Dentistry, Internal Medicine, Internal Medicine-Cardiovascular Disease, Internal Medicine-Infectious Diseases, Obstetrics/Gynecology, Physical Medicine and Rehabilitation, Psychiatry, Surgery

St. Francis Hospital and Medical Center
114 Woodland St.
Hartford, CT 06105
203-548-4000
Teaching Specialties:
Anesthesiology, Colon and Rectal Surgery, Dentistry, Internal Medicine, Obstetrics/Gynecology, Orthopedic Surgery, Otolaryngology, Psychiatry, Surgery, Urology

Middletown

Connecticut Valley Hospital
PO Box 351
Middletown, CT 06457
860-262-5000
Teaching Specialties:
Psychiatry

New Britain

New Britain General Hospital
100 Grand St.
New Britain, CT 06050
860-224-5011
Teaching Specialties:
Internal Medicine, Obstetrics/Gynecology, Otolaryngology, Surgery, Urology

New Haven

Connecticut Mental Health Center
PO Box 1842
New Haven, CT 06508
203-789-7290
Teaching Specialties:
Psychiatry

Hospital of St. Raphael
330 Orchard St., Suite 105
New Haven, CT 06511
203-789-3000
Teaching Specialties:
Dentistry, Internal Medicine, Internal Medicine-Cardiovascular Disease, Internal Medicine-Gastroenterology, Internal Medicine-Nephrology, Orthopedic Surgery, Otolaryngology, Psychiatry, Radiation Oncology, Surgery

Yale-New Haven Hospital
20 York St.
New Haven, CT 06510
203-785-4242
Teaching Specialties:
Allergy/Immunology, Anesthesiology, Dentistry, Dermatology, Internal Medicine, Internal Medicine-Cardiovascular Disease, Internal Medicine-Endocrinology and Metabolism, Internal Medicine-Gastroenterology, Internal Medicine-Geriatric Medicine, Internal Medicine-Hematology, Internal Medicine-Infectious Diseases, Internal Medicine-Medical Oncology, Internal Medicine-Nephrology, Internal Medicine-Rheumatology, Neurological Surgery, Neurology, Obstetrics/Gynecology, Ophthalmology, Orthopedic Surgery, Otolaryngology, Psychiatry, Radiation Oncology, Surgery, Thoracic Surgery, Urology

Yale Psychiatric Institute
184 Liberty St.
New Haven, CT 06519
203-785-7200
Teaching Specialties:
Psychiatry

Norwalk

Norwalk Hospital
34 Maple St.
Norwalk, CT 06856
203-852-2000
Teaching Specialties:
Internal Medicine, Internal Medicine-Cardiovascular Disease, Internal Medicine-Gastroenterology, Psychiatry

Norwich

Norwich Hospital
PO Box 508
Norwich, CT 06360
203-823-5200
Teaching Specialties:
Psychiatry

University of Connecticut Health Center
Uncas on Thames Hospital
401 W. Thames St.
Norwich, CT 06360
860-823-4675
Teaching Specialties:
Radiation Oncology

William W. Buckus Hospital
326 Washington St.
Norwich, CT 06360
203-889-8331
Teaching Specialties:
Psychiatry

Southbury

Southbury Training School
Route 172
Southbury, CT 06488-0901
203-586-2000
Teaching Specialties:
Dentistry

Stamford

Stamford Hospital
Shelburne Rd. & W. Broad St.
Stamford, CT 06904
203-325-7000
Teaching Specialties:
Internal Medicine, Obstetrics/Gynecology, Psychiatry, Surgery

Waterbury

St. Mary's Hospital
56 Franklin St.
Waterbury, CT 06706
203-574-6000
Teaching Specialties:
Dentistry, Internal Medicine, Surgery

Waterbury Hospital
64 Robbins St.
Waterbury, CT 06708
203-573-6000
Teaching Specialties:
Dentistry, Internal Medicine, Internal Medicine-Gastroenterology, Surgery, Urology

DELAWARE
New Castle

Delaware State Hospital
1901 N. Dupont Hwy.
New Castle, DE 19720
302-577-4000
Teaching Specialties:
Psychiatry

Wilmington

Alfred I. Dupont Institute
1600 Rockland Rd.
Wilmington, DE 19803
302-651-4000
Teaching Specialties:
Orthopedic Surgery, Urology

Medical Center of Delaware
501 W. 14th St.
Wilmington, DE 19801
302-733-1000
Teaching Specialties:
Dentistry, Internal Medicine, Neurology, Obstetrics/Gynecology, Psychiatry, Surgery, Thoracic Surgery

DISTRICT OF COLUMBIA
Washington

District of Columbia General Hospital
1900 Massachusetts Ave., SE
Washington, DC 20003
202-675-5000
Teaching Specialties:
Allergy/Immunology, Internal Medicine, Internal Medicine-Cardiovascular Disease, Internal Medicine-Endocrinology and Metabolism, Internal Medicine-Gastroenterology, Internal Medicine-Hematology, Internal Medicine-Medical Oncology, Internal Medicine-Nephrology, Internal Medicine-Rheumatology, Neurology, Obstetrics/Gynecology, Ophthalmology, Orthopedic Surgery, Surgery, Urology

George Washington University Hospital
901 23rd St., NW
Washington, DC 20037
202-994-1000
Teaching Specialties:
Anesthesiology, Dermatology, Internal Medicine, Internal Medicine-Cardiovascular Disease, Internal Medicine-Endocrinology and Metabolism, Internal Medicine-Gastroenterology, Internal Medicine-Geriatric Medicine, Internal Medicine-Hematology, Internal Medicine-Infectious Diseases, Internal Medicine-Medical Oncology, Internal Medicine-Nephrology, Internal Medicine-Rheumatology, Neurological Surgery, Neurology, Obstetrics/Gynecology, Ophthalmology, Orthopedic Surgery, Physical Medicine and Rehabilitation, Psychiatry, Radiation Oncology, Surgery, Thoracic Surgery, Urology

Georgetown University Hospital
3800 Reservoir Rd., NW
Washington, DC 20007
202-784-3000
Teaching Specialties:
Allergy/Immunology, Anesthesiology, Den-

tistry, Internal Medicine, Internal Medicine-Cardiovascular Disease, Internal Medicine-Endocrinology and Metabolism, Internal Medicine-Gastroenterology, Internal Medicine-Hematology, Internal Medicine-Infectious Diseases, Internal Medicine-Medical Oncology, Internal Medicine-Nephrology, Internal Medicine-Rheumatology, Neurological Surgery, Neurology, Obstetrics/Gynecology, Ophthalmology, Orthopedic Surgery, Otolaryngology, Physical Medicine and Rehabilitation, Psychiatry, Radiation Oncology, Surgery, Urology

Greater Southeast Community Hospital
1310 Southern Ave., SE
Washington, DC 20032
202-574-6000
Teaching Specialties:
Internal Medicine, Obstetrics/Gynecology, Orthopedic Surgery, Surgery

Howard University College of Dentistry
600 W St., NW
Washington, DC 20059
202-806-0100
Teaching Specialties:
Dentistry

Howard University Hospital
2041 Georgia Ave., NW
Washington, DC 20060
202-865-6100
Teaching Specialties:
Allergy/Immunology, Anesthesiology, Dermatology, Internal Medicine, Internal Medicine-Cardiovascular Disease, Internal Medicine-Endocrinology and Metabolism, Internal Medicine-Gastroenterology, Internal Medicine-Hematology, Internal Medicine-Infectious Diseases, Internal Medicine-Medical Oncology, Internal Medicine-Nephrology, Internal Medicine-Rheumatology, Neurology, Obstetrics/Gynecology, Ophthalmology, Orthopedic Surgery, Psychiatry, Radiation Oncology, Surgery, Urology

National Rehabilitation Hospital
102 Irving St., NW
Washington, DC 20010
202-877-1000
Teaching Specialties:
Physical Medicine and Rehabilitation

Providence Hospital
1150 Varnum St., NE
Washington, DC 20017
202-269-7000
Teaching Specialties:
Internal Medicine, Obstetrics/Gynecology, Orthopedic Surgery

Sibley Memorial Hospital
5255 Loughboro Rd.

Washington, DC 20016
202-537-4000
Teaching Specialties:
Orthopedic Surgery, Surgery, Urology

St. Elizabeth's Hospital
DC Commission on Mental Health Services
2700 Martin Luther King Jr. Ave., SE
Washington, DC 20032
202-373-7166
Teaching Specialties:
Dentistry, Psychiatry

Washington Hospital Center
110 Irving St., NW
Washington, DC 20010
202-877-7000
Teaching Specialties:
Dentistry, Dermatology, Internal Medicine, Internal Medicine-Cardiovascular Disease, Internal Medicine-Infectious Diseases, Internal Medicine-Medical Oncology, Internal Medicine-Rheumatology, Neurological Surgery, Neurology, Obstetrics/Gynecology, Ophthalmology, Orthopedic Surgery, Otolaryngology, Physical Medicine and Rehabilitation, Surgery, Thoracic Surgery, Urology

FLORIDA
Coral Gables

Doctors' Hospital
5000 University Dr.
Coral Gables, FL 33146
305-666-2111
Teaching Specialties:
Orthopedic Surgery

Fort Lauderdale

Cleveland Clinic Hospital
2835 N. Ocean Blvd.
Fort Lauderdale, FL 33308
954-568-1000
Teaching Specialties:
Colon and Rectal Surgery

Gainesville

Shands Hospital at the University of Florida
1600 S.W. Archer Rd.
Gainesville, FL 32610
352-395-0111
Teaching Specialties:
Anesthesiology, Hand Surgery, Internal Medicine, Internal Medicine-Cardiovascular Disease, Internal Medicine-Endocrinology and Metabolism, Internal Medicine-Gastroenterology, Internal Medicine-Geriatric Medicine, Internal Medicine-Hematology, In-

ternal Medicine-Infectious Diseases, Internal Medicine-Medical Oncology, Internal Medicine-Nephrology, Internal Medicine-Rheumatology, Neurological Surgery, Neurology, Obstetrics/Gynecology, Ophthalmology, Orthopedic Surgery, Otolaryngology, Psychiatry, Radiation Oncology, Surgery, Surgery-Vascular Surgery, Thoracic Surgery, Urology

University of Florida College of Dentistry

J. Hillis Miller Health Center
PO Box 100405
Gainesville, FL 32610-0405
352-392-2946
Teaching Specialties:
Dentistry

Jacksonville

Baptist Medical Center

800 Prudential Dr.
Jacksonville, FL 32207
904-393-2000
Teaching Specialties:
Obstetrics/Gynecology

University Medical Center

655 W. Eighth St.
Jacksonville, FL 32209
904-549-5000
Teaching Specialties:
Dentistry, Internal Medicine, Internal Medicine-Cardiovascular Disease, Internal Medicine-Endocrinology and Metabolism, Internal Medicine-Gastroenterology, Internal Medicine-Hematology, Obstetrics/Gynecology, Orthopedic Surgery, Surgery

Miami

Bascom Palmer Eye Institute-Anne Bates Leach Eye Hospital

900 N.W. 17th St.
Miami, FL 33136
305-326-6190
Teaching Specialties:
Ophthalmology

Dade County Dental Research Clinic

750 N.W. 20th St.
Miami, FL 33127
305-243-6506
Teaching Specialties:
Dentistry

Jackson Memorial Hospital

1611 N.W. 12th Ave.
Miami, FL 33136
305-585-1111
Teaching Specialties:
Anesthesiology, Dentistry, Dermatology, Hand Surgery, Internal Medicine, Internal Medicine-Cardiovascular Disease, Internal Medicine-Endocrinology and Metabolism, Internal Medicine-Gastroenterology, Internal Medicine-Geriatric Medicine, Internal Medicine-Hematology, Internal Medicine-Infectious Diseases, Internal Medicine-Medical Oncology, Internal Medicine-Nephrology, Internal Medicine-Rheumatology, Neurological Surgery, Neurology, Obstetrics/Gynecology, Ophthalmology, Orthopedic Surgery, Otolaryngology, Psychiatry, Radiation Oncology, Surgery, Thoracic Surgery, Urology

Miami Beach

Mt. Sinai Medical Center

4300 Alton Rd.
Miami Beach, FL 33140
305-674-2121
Teaching Specialties:
Anesthesiology, Dentistry, Dermatology, Internal Medicine, Internal Medicine-Cardiovascular Disease, Internal Medicine-Gastroenterology, Internal Medicine-Infectious Diseases, Neurological Surgery, Surgery, Thoracic Surgery

South Shore Hospital and Medical Center

630 Alton Rd.
Miami Beach, FL 33139
305-672-2100
Teaching Specialties:
Internal Medicine-Geriatric Medicine

Orlando

Florida Hospital Medical Center

601 E. Rollins St.
Orlando, FL 32803
407-896-6611
Teaching Specialties:
Colon and Rectal Surgery

Orlando Regional Medical Center

1414 Kuhl Ave.
Orlando, FL 32806
407-841-5111
Teaching Specialties:
Colon and Rectal Surgery, Internal Medicine, Obstetrics/Gynecology, Orthopedic Surgery, Surgery

Pensacola

Baptist Hospital

PO Box 17500
Pensacola, FL 32522
904-434-4011
Teaching Specialties:
Obstetrics/Gynecology

Sacred Heart Hospital of Pensacola

5151 N. Ninth Ave.
Pensacola, FL 32504
904-474-7000
Teaching Specialties:
Obstetrics/Gynecology

St. Petersburg

Bayfront Medical Center

701 Sixth St. South
St. Petersburg, FL 33701
813-823-1234
Teaching Specialties:
Obstetrics/Gynecology

Tampa

Tampa General Hospital

Davis Island
Tampa, FL 33601
813-251-7000
Teaching Specialties:
Anesthesiology, Dermatology, Internal Medicine, Internal Medicine-Cardiovascular Disease, Internal Medicine-Geriatric Medicine, Internal Medicine-Infectious Diseases, Internal Medicine-Nephrology, Internal Medicine-Rheumatology, Neurology, Obstetrics/Gynecology, Ophthalmology, Otolaryngology, Psychiatry, Surgery, Surgery-Vascular Surgery, Urology

University of South Florida

H. Lee Moffitt Cancer Center
12902 Magnolia Dr.
Tampa, FL 33612
813-972-4673
Teaching Specialties:
Anesthesiology, Internal Medicine-Endocrinology and Metabolism, Internal Medicine-Infectious Diseases, Internal Medicine-Medical Oncology, Urology

University of South Florida Psychiatry Center

3515 E. Fletcher Ave.
Tampa, FL 33613
813-974-8900
Teaching Specialties:
Psychiatry

Tarpon Springs

The Manors

1527 Riverside Dr.
Tarpon Springs, FL 34689
813-937-4211
Teaching Specialties:
Psychiatry

GEORGIA

Atlanta

Crawford Long Hospital of Emory University

550 Peachtree St., NE
Atlanta, GA 30308

404-686-4411
Teaching Specialties:
Internal Medicine, Neurological Surgery, Obstetrics/Gynecology, Orthopedic Surgery, Surgery, Thoracic Surgery

Emory University Hospital
1364 Clifton Rd., NE
Atlanta, GA 30322
404-727-7021
Teaching Specialties:
Allergy/Immunology, Anesthesiology, Dermatology, Internal Medicine, Internal Medicine-Cardiovascular Disease, Internal Medicine-Endocrinology and Metabolism, Internal Medicine-Gastroenterology, Internal Medicine-Hematology, Internal Medicine-Infectious Diseases, Internal Medicine-Medical Oncology, Internal Medicine-Nephrology, Internal Medicine-Rheumatology, Neurological Surgery, Neurology, Obstetrics/Gynecology, Ophthalmology, Orthopedic Surgery, Otolaryngology, Physical Medicine and Rehabilitation, Psychiatry, Surgery, Surgery-Vascular Surgery, Thoracic Surgery, Urology

Emory University School of Medicine
1440 Clifton Rd., NE
Atlanta, GA 30322
404-727-5640 (dean's office)
404-727-6652 (appointments)
Teaching Specialties:
Dentistry

Georgia Baptist Medical Center
303 Parkway Dr., NE
Atlanta, GA 30312
404-265-4000
Teaching Specialties:
Internal Medicine, Obstetrics/Gynecology, Orthopedic Surgery, Surgery

Grady Memorial Hospital
80 Butler St., SE
Atlanta, GA 30335
404-616-4252
Teaching Specialties:
Allergy/Immunology, Anesthesiology, Dermatology, Internal Medicine, Internal Medicine-Cardiovascular Disease, Internal Medicine-Endocrinology and Metabolism, Internal Medicine-Gastroenterology, Internal Medicine-Hematology, Internal Medicine-Infectious Diseases, Internal Medicine-Medical Oncology, Internal Medicine-Nephrology, Internal Medicine-Rheumatology, Neurological Surgery, Neurology, Obstetrics/Gynecology, Ophthalmology, Orthopedic Surgery, Otolaryngology, Physical Medicine and Rehabilitation, Psychiatry, Surgery, Thoracic Surgery, Urology

HCA West Paces Ferry Hospital
3200 Howell Mill Rd., NW
Atlanta, GA 30327

404-351-0351
Teaching Specialties:
Psychiatry

Piedmont Hospital
1968 Peachtree Rd., NW
Atlanta, GA 30309
404-605-5000
Teaching Specialties:
Surgery

Augusta

Medical College of Georgia
Georgia Radiation Therapy Center at Augusta
St. Sebastian Way
Augusta, GA 30912
706-721-2971
Teaching Specialties:
Radiation Oncology

Medical College of Georgia Hospital and Clinics
1120 15th St.
Augusta, GA 30912
706-721-0211
Teaching Specialties:
Allergy/Immunology, Anesthesiology, Dermatology, Internal Medicine, Internal Medicine-Cardiovascular Disease, Internal Medicine-Endocrinology and Metabolism, Internal Medicine-Gastroenterology, Internal Medicine-Hematology, Internal Medicine-Infectious Diseases, Internal Medicine-Medical Oncology, Internal Medicine-Nephrology, Internal Medicine-Rheumatology, Neurological Surgery, Neurology, Obstetrics/Gynecology, Ophthalmology, Orthopedic Surgery, Otolaryngology, Psychiatry, Radiation Oncology, Surgery, Thoracic Surgery, Urology

Medical College of Georgia School of Dentistry
1120 15th St.
Augusta, GA 30912
706-721-0211
Teaching Specialties:
Dentistry

University Hospital
1350 Walton Way
Augusta, GA 30901-2629
706-722-9011
Teaching Specialties:
Dermatology, Internal Medicine, Neurology, Obstetrics/Gynecology, Orthopedic Surgery, Surgery, Urology

Columbus

Hughston Sports Medicine Hospital
100 Frist Ct.

Columbus, GA 31909
706-576-2100
Teaching Specialties:
Orthopedic Surgery

Decatur

Georgia Regional Hospital at Atlanta
3073 Panthersville Rd.
Decatur, GA 30034
404-243-2100
Teaching Specialties:
Psychiatry

Macon

Medical Center of Central Georgia
777 Hemlock St.
Macon, GA 31201
912-633-1000
Teaching Specialties:
Internal Medicine, Obstetrics/Gynecology, Surgery

Savannah

Memorial Medical Center
4700 Waters Ave.
Savannah, GA 31404
800-350-8000
Teaching Specialties:
Internal Medicine, Obstetrics/Gynecology, Surgery

Smyrna

Brawner Psychiatric Institute
3180 Atlanta St., NW
Smyrna, GA 30080
707-436-0081
Teaching Specialties:
Psychiatry

Ridgeview Institute
3995 S. Cobb Dr.
Smyrna, GA 30080
434-434-4567
Teaching Specialties:
Psychiatry

H A W A I I
Honolulu

Kaiser Permanente Medical Center
3288 Moanalua Rd.
Honolulu, HI 96819
808-834-5333
Teaching Specialties:
Internal Medicine, Internal Medicine-Geriatric Medicine, Surgery

Kapiolani Medical Center for Women and Children
1319 Punahou St.
Honolulu, HI 96826
808-973-8511
Teaching Specialties:
Obstetrics/Gynecology, Surgery

Kuakini Medical Center
347 N. Kuakini St.
Honolulu, HI 96817
808-536-2236
Teaching Specialties:
Internal Medicine, Internal Medicine-Geriatric Medicine, Surgery

Queen's Medical Center
1301 Punchbowl St.
Honolulu, HI 96813
808-547-4798
Teaching Specialties:
Dentistry, Internal Medicine, Obstetrics/Gynecology, Orthopedic Surgery, Psychiatry, Surgery

St. Francis Medical Center
2230 Liliha St.
Honolulu, HI 96817
808-547-6011
Teaching Specialties:
Internal Medicine, Psychiatry, Surgery

Straub Clinic and Hospital
888 S. King St.
Honolulu, HI 96813
808-522-4000
Teaching Specialties:
Surgery

IDAHO
Boise

St. Luke's Regional Medical Center
190 E. Bannock St.
Boise, ID 83712
208-386-2222
Teaching Specialties:
Internal Medicine-Geriatric Medicine

ILLINOIS
Alton

Southern Illinois University School of Dental Medicine
2800 College Ave.
Alton, IL 62002
618-474-7000
Teaching Specialties:
Dentistry

Anna

Choate Mental Health and Developmental Center
1000 N. Main St.
Anna, IL 62906
618-833-5161
Teaching Specialties:
Psychiatry

Berwyn

MacNeal Hospital
3249 S. Oak Park Ave.
Berwyn, IL 60402
708-795-9100
Teaching Specialties:
Internal Medicine, Internal Medicine-Cardiovascular Disease, Obstetrics/Gynecology, Surgery

Chicago

Columbus Hospital
2520 N. Lakeview Ave.
Chicago, IL 60614
773-883-7300
Teaching Specialties:
Internal Medicine, Obstetrics/Gynecology, Radiation Oncology, Surgery

Cook County Hospital
1835 W. Harrison St.
Chicago, IL 60612
773-633-6000
Teaching Specialties:
Anesthesiology, Colon and Rectal Surgery, Dentistry, Dermatology, Internal Medicine, Internal Medicine-Cardiovascular Disease, Internal Medicine-Endocrinology and Metabolism, Internal Medicine-Gastroenterology, Internal Medicine-Hematology, Internal Medicine-Infectious Diseases, Internal Medicine-Medical Oncology, Internal Medicine-Nephrology, Internal Medicine-Rheumatology, Neurological Surgery, Neurology, Obstetrics/Gynecology, Ophthalmology, Orthopedic Surgery, Otolaryngology, Psychiatry, Surgery, Thoracic Surgery, Urology

Edgewater Medical Center
5700 N. Ashland Ave.
Chicago, IL 60660
773-878-6000
Teaching Specialties:
Internal Medicine

Grant Hospital of Chicago
550 W. Webster Ave.
Chicago, IL 60614
773-883-2000
Teaching Specialties:
Internal Medicine

Grant Hospital of Chicago
Max Samter Institute of Allergy/Clinical Immunology
550 W. Webster Ave.
Chicago, IL 60614
312-883-2000 (Grant Hospital)
312-883-3655 (Institute)
Teaching Specialties:
Allergy/Immunology

Humana Hospital-Michael Reese
2929 S. Ellis
Chicago, IL 60616
312-791-2000
Teaching Specialties:
Anesthesiology, Internal Medicine, Internal Medicine-Cardiovascular Disease, Internal Medicine-Endocrinology and Metabolism, Internal Medicine-Gastroenterology, Internal Medicine-Infectious Diseases, Internal Medicine-Medical Oncology, Internal Medicine-Rheumatology, Neurology, Obstetrics/Gynecology, Orthopedic Surgery, Physical Medicine and Rehabilitation, Psychiatry, Radiation Oncology, Surgery, Urology

Hyde Park Hospital
5800 S. Stony Island Ave.
Chicago, IL 60637
312-643-9200
Teaching Specialties:
Surgery

Illinois Masonic Medical Center
836 W. Wellington Ave.
Chicago, IL 60657
312-975-1600
Teaching Specialties:
Anesthesiology, Dentistry, Internal Medicine, Internal Medicine-Cardiovascular Disease, Internal Medicine-Rheumatology, Obstetrics/Gynecology, Surgery

Louis A. Weiss Memorial Hospital
4646 N. Marine Dr.
Chicago, IL 60640
312-878-8700
Teaching Specialties:
Internal Medicine, Otolaryngology, Surgery

Mercy Hospital and Medical Center
Stevenson Expwy. & King Dr.
Chicago, IL 60619
312-567-2000
Teaching Specialties:
Internal Medicine, Internal Medicine-Rheumatology, Obstetrics/Gynecology, Radiation Oncology, Surgery

Mt. Sinai Hospital Medical Center of Chicago
1500 S. California Ave.
Chicago, IL 60608

312-542-2000

Teaching Specialties:
Dentistry, Internal Medicine, Internal Medicine-Cardiovascular Disease, Internal Medicine-Gastroenterology, Internal Medicine-Geriatric Medicine, Internal Medicine-Hematology, Internal Medicine-Infectious Diseases, Internal Medicine-Medical Oncology, Internal Medicine-Nephrology, Obstetrics/Gynecology, Physical Medicine and Rehabilitation, Psychiatry, Surgery

Northwestern Memorial Hospital
250 E. Superior St.
Chicago, IL 60611
312-908-2000

Teaching Specialties:
Allergy/Immunology, Anesthesiology, Dermatology, Internal Medicine, Internal Medicine-Cardiovascular Disease, Internal Medicine-Endocrinology and Metabolism, Internal Medicine-Gastroenterology, Internal Medicine-Geriatric Medicine, Internal Medicine-Hematology, Internal Medicine-Infectious Diseases, Internal Medicine-Medical Oncology, Internal Medicine-Nephrology, Internal Medicine-Rheumatology, Neurological Surgery, Neurology, Ophthalmology, Orthopedic Surgery, Otolaryngology, Physical Medicine and Rehabilitation, Psychiatry, Radiation Oncology, Surgery, Surgery-Vascular Surgery, Thoracic Surgery, Urology

Northwestern Memorial Hospital
Prentice Women's Hospital
333 E. Superior St.
Chicago, IL 60611
312-908-2000

Teaching Specialties:
Obstetrics/Gynecology

Northwestern University Dental School
240 E. Huron St.
Chicago, IL 60611-2972
312-503-6837

Teaching Specialties:
Dentistry

Ravenswood Hospital Medical Center
4550 N. Winchester Ave.
Chicago, IL 60640
312-878-4300

Teaching Specialties:
Dentistry, Internal Medicine, Orthopedic Surgery

Rehabilitation Institute of Chicago
345 E. Superior St.
Chicago, IL 60611
312-908-6000

Teaching Specialties:
Physical Medicine and Rehabilitation

Resurrection Medical Center
7435 W. Talcott Ave.
Chicago, IL 60631
773-774-8000

Teaching Specialties:
Anesthesiology, Obstetrics/Gynecology, Surgery

Rush-Presbyterian-St. Luke's Medical Center
1653 W. Congress Pkwy.
Chicago, IL 60612
312-942-5000

Teaching Specialties:
Anesthesiology, Dentistry, Dermatology, Internal Medicine, Internal Medicine-Cardiovascular Disease, Internal Medicine-Endocrinology and Metabolism, Internal Medicine-Gastroenterology, Internal Medicine-Geriatric Medicine, Internal Medicine-Hematology, Internal Medicine-Infectious Diseases, Internal Medicine-Medical Oncology, Internal Medicine-Nephrology, Internal Medicine-Rheumatology, Neurological Surgery, Neurology, Obstetrics/Gynecology, Ophthalmology, Orthopedic Surgery, Otolaryngology, Physical Medicine and Rehabilitation, Psychiatry, Radiation Oncology, Surgery, Surgery-Vascular Surgery, Thoracic Surgery, Urology

Schwab Rehabilitation Center
1401 S. California Blvd.
Chicago, IL 60608
312-522-2010

Teaching Specialties:
Physical Medicine and Rehabilitation

St. Cabrini Hospital
811 S. Lytle St.
Chicago, IL 60607
312-883-4300

Teaching Specialties:
Internal Medicine, Obstetrics/Gynecology, Radiation Oncology, Surgery

St. Joseph Hospital and Health Care Center
2900 N. Lake Shore Dr.
Chicago, IL 60657
312-665-3000

Teaching Specialties:
Internal Medicine, Obstetrics/Gynecology

University of Chicago Hospitals
PO Box 430
5841 S. Maryland Ave.
Chicago, IL 60637
312-702-1000

Teaching Specialties:
Anesthesiology, Dentistry, Dermatology, Internal Medicine, Internal Medicine-Cardiovascular Disease, Internal Medicine-Endocrinology and Metabolism, Internal Medicine-Gastroenterology, Internal

Medicine-Geriatric Medicine, Internal Medicine-Hematology, Internal Medicine-Infectious Diseases, Internal Medicine-Nephrology, Internal Medicine-Rheumatology, Neurological Surgery, Neurology, Obstetrics/Gynecology, Ophthalmology, Orthopedic Surgery, Otolaryngology, Psychiatry, Radiation Oncology, Surgery, Surgery-Vascular Surgery, Thoracic Surgery, Urology

University of Illinois at Chicago College of Dentistry
801 S. Paulina St.
Chicago, IL 60612
312-996-7520

Teaching Specialties:
Dentistry

University of Illinois Hospital and Clinics
1740 W. Taylor St.
Chicago, IL 60612
312-996-7000

Teaching Specialties:
Anesthesiology, Dermatology, Internal Medicine, Internal Medicine-Cardiovascular Disease, Internal Medicine-Endocrinology and Metabolism, Internal Medicine-Gastroenterology, Internal Medicine-Geriatric Medicine, Internal Medicine-Hematology, Internal Medicine-Infectious Diseases, Internal Medicine-Medical Oncology, Internal Medicine-Nephrology, Internal Medicine-Rheumatology, Neurological Surgery, Neurology, Obstetrics/Gynecology, Orthopedic Surgery, Otolaryngology, Physical Medicine and Rehabilitation, Psychiatry, Radiation Oncology, Surgery, Thoracic Surgery, Urology

University of Illinois Hospital and Clinics
Illinois Eye and Ear Infirmary
1855 W. Taylor St.
Chicago, IL 60612
312-996-6500

Teaching Specialties:
Ophthalmology, Otolaryngology

Decatur

Decatur Memorial Hospital
2300 N. Edward St.
Decatur, IL 62526
217-876-3000

Teaching Specialties:
Psychiatry

Evanston

Evanston Hospital
2650 Ridge Ave.
Evanston, IL 60201
847-570-2000

Teaching Specialties:
Anesthesiology, Dentistry, Internal Medicine, Internal Medicine-Gastroenterology, Internal

Medicine-Infectious Diseases, Neurological Surgery, Neurology, Obstetrics/Gynecology, Ophthalmology, Orthopedic Surgery, Otolaryngology, Psychiatry, Radiation Oncology, Surgery, Thoracic Surgery

St. Francis Hospital of Evanston
355 Ridge Ave.
Evanston, IL 60202
847-492-4000
Teaching Specialties:
Internal Medicine, Internal Medicine-Cardiovascular Disease, Internal Medicine-Hematology, Internal Medicine-Medical Oncology, Obstetrics/Gynecology, Orthopedic Surgery, Surgery

Evergreen Park

Little Company of Mary Hospital and Health Care Centers
2800 W. 95th St.
Evergreen Park, IL 60805
708-422-6200
Teaching Specialties:
Surgery

Glenview

Glenbrook Hospital
2100 Pfingsten Rd.
Glenview, IL 60025
847-657-5800
Teaching Specialties:
Internal Medicine-Infectious Diseases

Maywood

Loyola University of Chicago
Foster G. McGaw Hospital
2160 S. First Ave.
Maywood, IL 60153
708-216-3800
Teaching Specialties:
Anesthesiology, Dermatology, Internal Medicine, Internal Medicine-Cardiovascular Disease, Internal Medicine-Endocrinology and Metabolism, Internal Medicine-Gastroenterology, Internal Medicine-Geriatric Medicine, Internal Medicine-Hematology, Internal Medicine-Infectious Diseases, Internal Medicine-Nephrology, Internal Medicine-Rheumatology, Neurological Surgery, Neurology, Obstetrics/Gynecology, Ophthalmology, Orthopedic Surgery, Otolaryngology, Physical Medicine and Rehabilitation, Psychiatry, Surgery, Surgery-Vascular Surgery, Thoracic Surgery, Urology

Loyola University of Chicago School of Dentistry
2160 S. First Ave.
Maywood, IL 60153
708-216-4200
Teaching Specialties:
Dentistry

Oak Forest

Oak Forest Hospital of Cook County
15900 S. Cicero Ave.
Oak Forest, IL 60452
708-687-7200
Teaching Specialties:
Ophthalmology, Physical Medicine and Rehabilitation

Oak Lawn

Christ Hospital and Medical Center
4440 W. 95th St.
Oak Lawn, IL 60453
708-425-8000
Teaching Specialties:
Internal Medicine, Internal Medicine-Cardiovascular Disease, Neurology, Obstetrics/Gynecology, Orthopedic Surgery, Surgery

Oak Park

West Suburban Hospital Medical Center
Erie at Austin Blvd.
Oak Park, IL 60302
708-383-6200
Teaching Specialties:
Internal Medicine

Parkridge

Lutheran General Hospital
1775 W. Dempster St.
Parkridge, IL 60068
847-723-2210
Teaching Specialties:
Internal Medicine, Obstetrics/Gynecology, Orthopedic Surgery, Psychiatry, Surgery

Peoria

Methodist Medical Center of Illinois
221 N.E. Glen Oak Ave.
Peoria, IL 61636
309-672-5522
Teaching Specialties:
Neurological Surgery, Neurology

St. Francis Medical Center
530 N.E. Glen Oak Ave.
Peoria, IL 61637
309-655-2000
Teaching Specialties:
Internal Medicine, Neurological Surgery, Neurology, Obstetrics/Gynecology, Surgery

Springfield

Andrew McFarland Mental Health Center
901 Southwind Rd.
Springfield, IL 62703
217-786-6994
Teaching Specialties:
Psychiatry

Memorial Medical Center
800 N. Rutledge St.
Springfield, IL 62781
217-788-3000
Teaching Specialties:
Internal Medicine, Neurology, Obstetrics/Gynecology, Orthopedic Surgery, Otolaryngology, Psychiatry, Surgery, Surgery-Vascular Surgery, Urology

St. John's Hospital
800 E. Carpenter St.
Springfield, IL 62769
217-544-6464
Teaching Specialties:
Internal Medicine, Neurology, Obstetrics/Gynecology, Orthopedic Surgery, Otolaryngology, Psychiatry, Surgery, Surgery-Vascular Surgery, Urology

Urbana

Carle Foundation Hospital
611 W. Park St.
Urbana, IL 61801
217-383-3311
Teaching Specialties:
Colon and Rectal Surgery, Dentistry, Internal Medicine

Covenant Medical Center
1400 W. Park St.
Urbana, IL 61801
217-337-2500
Teaching Specialties:
Internal Medicine

Wheaton

Marianjoy Rehabilitation Center
26 W. 171 Roosevelt Rd.
Wheaton, IL 60187
630-462-4000
Teaching Specialties:
Physical Medicine and Rehabilitation

INDIANA
Fort Wayne

Lutheran Hospital of Indiana
7950 W. Jefferson Blvd
Fort Wayne, IN 46804
219-435-7001

Parkview Memorial Hospital
2200 Randallia Dr.
Fort Wayne, IN 46805
219-484-6636
Teaching Specialties:
Orthopedic Surgery

St. Joseph Medical Center
700 Broadway
Fort Wayne, IN 46802
219-425-3000
Teaching Specialties:
Orthopedic Surgery

Indianapolis

Indiana University Medical Center
550 N. University Blvd.
Indianapolis, IN 46202
317-274-5000
Teaching Specialties:
Anesthesiology, Dermatology, Internal
Medicine, Internal Medicine-Cardiovascular
Disease, Internal Medicine-Endocrinology
and Metabolism, Internal Medicine-Gastroen-
terology, Internal Medicine-Geriatric
Medicine, Internal Medicine-Hematology, In-
ternal Medicine-Infectious Diseases, Internal
Medicine-Medical Oncology, Internal
Medicine-Nephrology, Internal Medicine-
Rheumatology, Neurological Surgery, Neurol-
ogy, Obstetrics/Gynecology, Ophthalmology,
Orthopedic Surgery, Otolaryngology, Psychia-
try, Radiation Oncology, Surgery, Thoracic
Surgery, Urology

**Indiana University School
of Dentistry**
1121 W. Michigan St.
Indianapolis, IN 46202-5186
317-274-7957
Teaching Specialties:
Dentistry

Larue D. Carter Memorial Hospital
1315 W. 10th St.
Indianapolis, IN 46202
317-634-8401
Teaching Specialties:
Psychiatry

Methodist Hospital of Indiana
1701 N. Senate Blvd.
Indianapolis, IN 46202
317-929-2000
Teaching Specialties:
Internal Medicine, Internal Medicine-Cardiovascular Disease, Internal Medicine-Nephrology, Obstetrics/Gynecology, Ophthalmology,
Orthopedic Surgery, Surgery, Urology

**St. Vincent Hospital and Health
Care Center**
2001 W. 86th St.
Indianapolis, IN 46260
317-871-2945
Teaching Specialties:
Internal Medicine, Obstetrics/Gynecology,
Orthopedic Surgery

**William N. Wishard Memorial
Hospital**
1001 W. 10th St.
Indianapolis, IN 46202
317-630-7356
Teaching Specialties:
Anesthesiology, Dermatology, Internal
Medicine, Internal Medicine-Geriatric
Medicine, Neurological Surgery, Neurology,
Obstetrics/Gynecology, Ophthalmology, Or-
thopedic Surgery, Otolaryngology, Psychiatry,
Radiation Oncology, Surgery, Urology

Jeffersonville

Lifespring Mental Health Services
207 W. 13th St.
Jeffersonville, IN 47130
800-456-2117
Teaching Specialties:
Psychiatry

Muncie

Ball Memorial Hospital
2401 University Ave.
Muncie, IN 47303
317-747-3111
Teaching Specialties:
Internal Medicine

IOWA

Des Moines

Broadlawns Medical Center
1801 Hickman Rd.
Des Moines, IA 50314
515-282-2200
Teaching Specialties:
Surgery

Iowa Methodist Medical Center
1200 Pleasant St.
Des Moines, IA 50309
515-241-6212
Teaching Specialties:
Internal Medicine, Surgery

Mercy Hospital Medical Center
400 University Ave.
Des Moines, IA 50314

515-247-4278
Teaching Specialties:
Surgery

Iowa City

**University of Iowa College
of Dentistry**
100 Dental Science Bldg.
Iowa City, IA 52242
319-335-9650
Teaching Specialties:
Dentistry

**University of Iowa Hospitals
and Clinics**
200 Hawkins Dr.
Iowa City, IA 52242
319-356-1616
Teaching Specialties:
Allergy/Immunology, Anesthesiology, Der-
matology, Hand Surgery, Internal Medicine,
Internal Medicine-Cardiovascular Disease, In-
ternal Medicine-Endocrinology and
Metabolism, Internal Medicine-Gastroenterol-
ogy, Internal Medicine-Geriatric Medicine,
Internal Medicine-Hematology, Internal
Medicine-Infectious Diseases, Internal
Medicine-Medical Oncology, Internal
Medicine-Nephrology, Internal Medicine-
Rheumatology, Neurological Surgery, Neurol-
ogy, Obstetrics/Gynecology, Ophthalmology,
Orthopedic Surgery, Otolaryngology, Psychia-
try, Radiation Oncology, Surgery, Surgery-
Vascular Surgery, Thoracic Surgery, Urology

KANSAS

Kansas City

Bethany Medical Center
51 N. 12th St.
Kansas City, KS 66102
913-281-8400
Teaching Specialties:
Internal Medicine

University of Kansas Hospital
3901 Rainbow Blvd.
Kansas City, KS 66160
913-588-5000
Teaching Specialties:
Allergy/Immunology, Anesthesiology, Der-
matology, Internal Medicine, Internal
Medicine-Cardiovascular Disease, Internal
Medicine-Endocrinology and Metabolism, In-
ternal Medicine-Gastroenterology, Internal
Medicine-Geriatric Medicine, Internal
Medicine-Hematology, Internal Medicine-In-
fectious Diseases, Internal Medicine-Medical
Oncology, Internal Medicine-Nephrology, In-
ternal Medicine-Rheumatology, Neurological
Surgery, Neurology, Obstetrics/Gynecology,
Ophthalmology, Orthopedic Surgery, Oto-
laryngology, Physical Medicine and Rehabili-
tation, Psychiatry, Radiation Oncology,

Surgery, Surgery-Vascular Surgery, Thoracic Surgery, Urology

Topeka

C. F. Menninger Memorial Hospital
5800 S.W. Sixth Ave.
Topeka, KS 66606
913-273-7500
Teaching Specialties:
Psychiatry

Stormont-Vail Regional Medical Center
1500 S.W. 10th St.
Topeka, KS 66604-1353
913-354-6000
Teaching Specialties:
Internal Medicine

Topeka State Hospital
2700 S.W. Sixth St.
Topeka, KS 66606-1898
913-296-4596
Teaching Specialties:
Psychiatry

Wichita

HCA Wesley Medical Center
550 N. Hillside Ave.
Wichita, KS 67214
316-688-2097
Teaching Specialties:
Anesthesiology, Internal Medicine, Obstetrics/Gynecology, Orthopedic Surgery, Surgery

St. Francis Regional Medical Center
929 N. St. Francis Ave.
Wichita, KS 67214
316-268-5000
Teaching Specialties:
Anesthesiology, Internal Medicine, Orthopedic Surgery, Surgery

St. Joseph Medical Center
3600 E. Harry St.
Wichita, KS 67218
316-685-1111
Teaching Specialties:
Anesthesiology, Psychiatry

KENTUCKY

Lexington

Cardinal Hill Hospital
2050 Versailles Rd.
Lexington, KY 40504
606-254-5701
Teaching Specialties:
Physical Medicine and Rehabilitation

Central Baptist Hospital
1740 Nicholasville Rd.
Lexington, KY 40503
606-275-6100
Teaching Specialties:
Obstetrics/Gynecology

St. Joseph Hospital
1 St. Joseph Dr.
Lexington, KY 40504
606-278-3436
Teaching Specialties:
Urology

University of Kentucky College of Dentistry
800 Rose St.
Lexington, KY 40536
606-323-5850
Teaching Specialties:
Dentistry

University of Kentucky Hospital
Albert B. Chandler Medical Center
800 Rose St.
Lexington, KY 40536
606-323-5000
Teaching Specialties:
Anesthesiology, Internal Medicine, Internal Medicine-Cardiovascular Disease, Internal Medicine-Endocrinology and Metabolism, Internal Medicine-Gastroenterology, Internal Medicine-Geriatric Medicine, Internal Medicine-Hematology, Internal Medicine-Infectious Diseases, Internal Medicine-Medical Oncology, Internal Medicine-Nephrology, Internal Medicine-Rheumatology, Neurological Surgery, Neurology, Obstetrics/Gynecology, Ophthalmology, Orthopedic Surgery, Otolaryngology, Physical Medicine and Rehabilitation, Psychiatry, Radiation Oncology, Surgery, Surgery-Vascular Surgery, Thoracic Surgery, Urology

Louisville

Alliance Medical Pavilion
315 E. Broadway
Louisville, KY 40202
502-629-2000
Teaching Specialties:
Orthopedic Surgery

Frazier Rehabilitation Center
220 Abraham Flexner Way
Louisville, KY 40202
502-582-7400
Teaching Specialties:
Internal Medicine-Rheumatology, Physical Medicine and Rehabilitation

Humana Hospital-University of Louisville
545 S. Jackson St.
Louisville, KY 40202

502-562-3000
Teaching Specialties:
Anesthesiology, Dermatology, Internal Medicine, Internal Medicine-Cardiovascular Disease, Internal Medicine-Endocrinology and Metabolism, Internal Medicine-Gastroenterology, Internal Medicine-Infectious Diseases, Internal Medicine-Nephrology, Internal Medicine-Rheumatology, Neurological Surgery, Neurology, Obstetrics/Gynecology, Ophthalmology, Orthopedic Surgery, Otolaryngology, Psychiatry, Radiation Oncology, Surgery, Thoracic Surgery, Urology

Jewish Hospital
217 E. Chestnut St.
Louisville, KY 40202
502-587-4011
Teaching Specialties:
Orthopedic Surgery, Surgery, Thoracic Surgery, Urology

Norton Hospital
200 E. Chestnut St.
Louisville, KY 40202
502-629-8000
Teaching Specialties:
Allergy/Immunology, Neurological Surgery, Neurology, Obstetrics/Gynecology, Orthopedic Surgery, Otolaryngology, Psychiatry, Surgery, Urology

University of Louisville School of Dentistry
501 S. Preston St.
Louisville, KY 40292
502-852-5293
Teaching Specialties:
Dentistry

LOUISIANA

Baton Rouge

Earl K. Long Memorial Hospital
5825 Airline Hwy.
Baton Rouge, LA 70805
504-356-3361
Teaching Specialties:
Internal Medicine, Obstetrics/Gynecology, Orthopedic Surgery, Surgery

Houma

South Louisiana Medical Center
1978 Industrial Blvd.
Houma, LA 70360
504-873-2200
Teaching Specialties:
Internal Medicine, Obstetrics/Gynecology, Ophthalmology, Orthopedic Surgery, Surgery, Urology

Independence

Lallie Kemp Hospital
52579 Hwy. 51 South
Independence, LA 70443-8502
504-878-9421
Teaching Specialties:
Obstetrics/Gynecology

Lafayette

University Medical Center
2390 W. Congress St.
Lafayette, LA 70506-4016
318-261-6000
Teaching Specialties:
Internal Medicine, Obstetrics/Gynecology,
Orthopedic Surgery, Surgery

Lake Charles

**Dr. Walter Olin Moss Regional
Hospital**
1000 Walters St.
Lake Charles, LA 70607
318-475-8100
Teaching Specialties:
Obstetrics/Gynecology, Surgery

Monroe

E. A. Conway Memorial Hospital
4864 Jackson St.
Monroe, LA 71201
318-388-7000
Teaching Specialties:
Obstetrics/Gynecology, Ophthalmology,
Surgery

New Orleans

Eye, Ear, Nose and Throat Hospital
2626 Napoleon Ave.
New Orleans, LA 70115
504-896-1100
Teaching Specialties:
Ophthalmology, Otolaryngology

Jo Ellen Smith Medical Center
4444 General Meyer Ave.
New Orleans, LA 70131
504-363-7011
Teaching Specialties:
Urology

**Louisiana State University
Eye Center**
2020 Gravier St., Suite B
New Orleans, LA 70112
504-568-6700
Teaching Specialties:
Ophthalmology

**Louisiana State University School
of Dentistry**
1100 Florida Ave.
New Orleans, LA 70119
504-619-8700
Teaching Specialties:
Dentistry

**Medical Center of Louisiana
at New Orleans**
1532 Tulane Ave.
New Orleans, LA 70140
504-568-3201
Teaching Specialties:
Allergy/Immunology, Anesthesiology, Dentistry, Dermatology, Internal Medicine, Internal Medicine-Cardiovascular Disease, Internal Medicine-Endocrinology and Metabolism, Internal Medicine-Gastroenterology, Internal Medicine-Hematology, Internal Medicine-Infectious Diseases, Internal Medicine-Medical Oncology, Internal Medicine-Nephrology, Internal Medicine-Rheumatology, Neurological Surgery, Neurology, Obstetrics/Gynecology, Ophthalmology, Orthopedic Surgery, Otolaryngology, Physical Medicine and Rehabilitation, Psychiatry, Surgery, Surgery-Vascular Surgery, Thoracic Surgery, Urology

**Medical Center of Louisiana
at New Orleans**
Louisiana Rehabilitation Institute
1532 Tulane Ave., L&M Bldg.
New Orleans, LA 70140
504-568-2660
Teaching Specialties:
Physical Medicine and Rehabilitation

Ochsner Foundation Hospital
1516 Jefferson Hwy.
New Orleans, LA 70121
504-842-3306
Teaching Specialties:
Anesthesiology, Colon and Rectal Surgery, Dermatology, Internal Medicine, Internal Medicine-Cardiovascular Disease, Internal Medicine-Endocrinology and Metabolism, Internal Medicine-Gastroenterology, Internal Medicine-Infectious Diseases, Internal Medicine-Medical Oncology, Internal Medicine-Rheumatology, Neurology, Obstetrics/Gynecology, Ophthalmology, Orthopedic Surgery, Otolaryngology, Psychiatry, Surgery, Surgery-Vascular Surgery, Thoracic Surgery, Urology

River Oaks Psychiatric Hospital
1525 River Oaks Rd. West
New Orleans, LA 70123
504-733-2276
Teaching Specialties:
Psychiatry

Memorial Medical Center
2700 Napoleon Ave.
New Orleans, LA 70115
504-899-9311
Teaching Specialties:
Neurology

Touro Infirmary
1401 Foucher St.
New Orleans, LA 70115
504-897-7011
Teaching Specialties:
Orthopedic Surgery, Psychiatry, Surgery

**Tulane University Hospital
and Clinics**
1415 Tulane Ave.
New Orleans, LA 70112
504-588-5263
Teaching Specialties:
Allergy/Immunology, Anesthesiology, Dermatology, Internal Medicine, Internal Medicine-Cardiovascular Disease, Internal Medicine-Endocrinology and Metabolism, Internal Medicine-Gastroenterology, Internal Medicine-Hematology, Internal Medicine-Infectious Diseases, Internal Medicine-Nephrology, Internal Medicine-Rheumatology, Neurological Surgery, Neurology, Obstetrics/Gynecology, Ophthalmology, Orthopedic Surgery, Otolaryngology, Psychiatry, Surgery, Surgery-Vascular Surgery, Thoracic Surgery, Urology

University Hospital
2021 Perdido St.
New Orleans, LA 70112
504-588-3000
Teaching Specialties:
Internal Medicine-Gastroenterology, Internal Medicine-Infectious Diseases, Internal Medicine-Medical Oncology, Internal Medicine-Rheumatology, Neurology, Ophthalmology, Orthopedic Surgery, Surgery-Vascular Surgery, Urology

Pineville

**Huey P. Long Regional Medical
Center**
352 Hospital Blvd.
Pineville, LA 71360
318-448-0811
Teaching Specialties:
Obstetrics/Gynecology, Orthopedic Surgery,
Surgery, Urology

Shreveport

Louisiana State University Hospital
PO Box 33932
1541 Kings Hwy.
Shreveport, LA 71130
318-675-5000

Teaching Specialties:
Allergy/Immunology, Anesthesiology, Colon and Rectal Surgery, Internal Medicine, Internal Medicine-Cardiovascular Disease, Internal Medicine-Endocrinology and Metabolism, Internal Medicine-Gastroenterology, Internal Medicine-Hematology, Internal Medicine-Infectious Diseases, Internal Medicine-Medical Oncology, Internal Medicine-Nephrology, Internal Medicine-Rheumatology, Obstetrics/Gynecology, Ophthalmology, Orthopedic Surgery, Otolaryngology, Surgery, Urology

Schumpert Medical Center
1 St. Mary Pl.
Shreveport, LA 71101
318-227-4500
Teaching Specialties:
Colon and Rectal Surgery, Urology

MAINE
Portland

Maine Medical Center
22 Bramhall St.
Portland, ME 04102-3175
207-871-0111
Teaching Specialties:
Anesthesiology, Internal Medicine, Internal Medicine-Cardiovascular Disease, Internal Medicine-Endocrinology and Metabolism, Internal Medicine-Infectious Diseases, Internal Medicine-Nephrology, Obstetrics/Gynecology, Psychiatry, Surgery

MARYLAND
Baltimore

Francis Scott Key Medical Center
4940 Eastern Ave.
Baltimore, MD 21224
410-550-0289
Teaching Specialties:
Anesthesiology, Internal Medicine, Internal Medicine-Gastroenterology, Internal Medicine-Geriatric Medicine, Internal Medicine-Nephrology, Neurological Surgery, Neurology, Obstetrics/Gynecology, Orthopedic Surgery, Otolaryngology, Psychiatry, Surgery, Urology

Franklin Square Hospital Center
9000 Franklin Square
Baltimore, MD 21237
410-682-7000
Teaching Specialties:
Internal Medicine, Obstetrics/Gynecology, Psychiatry

Good Samaritan Hospital of Maryland
5601 Loch Raven Blvd.
Baltimore, MD 21239

410-532-8000
Teaching Specialties:
Allergy/Immunology, Dermatology, Internal Medicine, Orthopedic Surgery, Physical Medicine and Rehabilitation

Greater Baltimore Medical Center
6701 N. Charles St.
Baltimore, MD 21204
410-828-2000
Teaching Specialties:
Colon and Rectal Surgery, Internal Medicine, Obstetrics/Gynecology, Ophthalmology, Otolaryngology

Harbor Hospital Center
3001 S. Hanover St.
Baltimore, MD 21225
410-347-3200
Teaching Specialties:
Internal Medicine, Obstetrics/Gynecology

James Lawrence Kernan Hospital
2200 N. Forest Park Ave.
Baltimore, MD 21207
410-448-2500
Teaching Specialties:
Orthopedic Surgery

John Hopkins Medical Service
3100 Wyman Park Dr.
Baltimore, MD 21211
410-338-3000
Teaching Specialties:
Surgery

Johns Hopkins Hospital
600 N. Wolfe St.
Baltimore, MD 21287
410-955-5000
Teaching Specialties:
Allergy/Immunology, Anesthesiology, Dentistry, Dermatology, Internal Medicine, Internal Medicine-Cardiovascular Disease, Internal Medicine-Endocrinology and Metabolism, Internal Medicine-Gastroenterology, Internal Medicine-Geriatric Medicine, Internal Medicine-Hematology, Internal Medicine-Infectious Diseases, Internal Medicine-Medical Oncology, Internal Medicine-Nephrology, Internal Medicine-Rheumatology, Neurological Surgery, Neurology, Obstetrics/Gynecology, Orthopedic Surgery, Otolaryngology, Physical Medicine and Rehabilitation, Psychiatry, Radiation Oncology, Surgery, Thoracic Surgery, Urology

Johns Hopkins Hospital
Wilmer Eye Institute
600 N. Wolfe St.
Baltimore, MD 21287
410-955-6275
Teaching Specialties:
Ophthalmology

Maryland General Hospital
1531 S. Edgewood Rd., Suite D
Baltimore, MD 21227
410-646-5760
Teaching Specialties:
Internal Medicine, Obstetrics/Gynecology, Ophthalmology, Otolaryngology, Surgery

Mercy Medical Center
301 St. Paul Place
Baltimore, MD 21202
410-332-9000
Teaching Specialties:
Internal Medicine, Obstetrics/Gynecology, Surgery

Sheppard and Enoch Pratt Hospital
6501 N. Charles St.
Baltimore, MD 21204
410-938-3000
Teaching Specialties:
Psychiatry

Sinai Hospital of Baltimore
2401 W. Belvedere Ave.
Baltimore, MD 21215
410-601-9000
Teaching Specialties:
Internal Medicine, Obstetrics/Gynecology, Ophthalmology, Orthopedic Surgery, Otolaryngology, Physical Medicine and Rehabilitation, Surgery, Urology

St. Agnes Hospital of the City of Baltimore
900 Caton Ave.
Baltimore, MD 21229
410-368-6000
Teaching Specialties:
Internal Medicine, Orthopedic Surgery, Surgery

Union Memorial Hospital
201 E. University Pkwy.
Baltimore, MD 21218
410-554-2000
Teaching Specialties:
Internal Medicine, Obstetrics/Gynecology, Orthopedic Surgery, Surgery

University of Maryland at Baltimore
Baltimore College of Dentistry
Dental School
666 W. Baltimore St.
Baltimore, MD 21201
410-706-7460
Teaching Specialties:
Dentistry

University of Maryland Medical System
22 S. Greene St.

Baltimore, MD 21201
410-328-0199
Teaching Specialties:
Anesthesiology, Dermatology, Internal Medicine, Internal Medicine-Cardiovascular Disease, Internal Medicine-Endocrinology and Metabolism, Internal Medicine-Gastroenterology, Internal Medicine-Hematology, Internal Medicine-Infectious Diseases, Internal Medicine-Medical Oncology, Internal Medicine-Nephrology, Internal Medicine-Rheumatology, Neurological Surgery, Neurology, Obstetrics/Gynecology, Ophthalmology, Orthopedic Surgery, Otolaryngology, Psychiatry, Radiation Oncology, Surgery, Thoracic Surgery, Urology

Walter P. Carter Center
630 W. Fayette St.
Baltimore, MD 21201
410-209-6000
Teaching Specialties:
Psychiatry

Bethesda

Suburban Hospital
8600 Old Georgetown Rd.
Bethesda, MD 20814
301-530-3100
Teaching Specialties:
Colon and Rectal Surgery

Catonsville

Spring Grove Hospital Center
55 Wade Ave.
Catonsville, MD 21228
410-455-6000
Teaching Specialties:
Psychiatry

Cheverly

Prince George's Hospital Center
3001 Hospital Dr.
Cheverly, MD 20785
301-618-2000
Teaching Specialties:
Dentistry, Internal Medicine, Internal Medicine-Gastroenterology

Crownsville

Crownsville Hospital Center
1400 General's Hwy.
Crownsville, MD 21032
410-987-6200
Teaching Specialties:
Psychiatry

Silver Spring

Holy Cross Hospital of Silver Spring
1500 Forest Glen Rd.

Silver Spring, MD 20910
301-905-0100
Teaching Specialties:
Obstetrics/Gynecology, Surgery

Sykesville

Springfield Hospital Center
6655 Sykesville Rd.
Sykesville, MD 21784
410-795-2100
Teaching Specialties:
Psychiatry

MASSACHUSETTS

Belmont

McLean Hospital
115 Mill St.
Belmont, MA 02178
800-333-0338
617-855-2000
Teaching Specialties:
Psychiatry

Boston

Beth Israel Hospital
330 Brookline Ave.
Boston, MA 02215
617-735-3391
Teaching Specialties:
Anesthesiology, Dermatology, Internal Medicine, Internal Medicine-Cardiovascular Disease, Internal Medicine-Endocrinology and Metabolism, Internal Medicine-Gastroenterology, Internal Medicine-Geriatric Medicine, Internal Medicine-Hematology, Internal Medicine-Infectious Diseases, Internal Medicine-Medical Oncology, Internal Medicine-Nephrology, Neurological Surgery, Neurology, Obstetrics/Gynecology, Orthopedic Surgery, Otolaryngology, Psychiatry, Radiation Oncology, Surgery, Urology

Boston Medical Center
1 Boston Medical Center
Boston, MA 02118
617-534-5000
Teaching Specialties:
Anesthesiology, Dentistry, Dermatology, Internal Medicine, Internal Medicine-Cardiovascular Disease, Internal Medicine-Endocrinology and Metabolism, Internal Medicine-Gastroenterology, Internal Medicine-Hematology, Internal Medicine-Infectious Diseases, Internal Medicine-Medical Oncology, Internal Medicine-Nephrology, Internal Medicine-Rheumatology, Neurology, Obstetrics/Gynecology, Ophthalmology, Orthopedic Surgery, Otolaryngology, Psychiatry, Surgery, Surgery-Vascular Surgery, Thoracic Surgery, Urology

Boston University
Henry M. Goldman School of Graduate Dentistry
100 E. Newton St.
Boston, MA 02118
617-638-4700
Teaching Specialties:
Dentistry

Brigham and Women's Hospital
75 Francis St.
Boston, MA 02115
617-732-5500
Teaching Specialties:
Allergy/Immunology, Anesthesiology, Dentistry, Dermatology, Internal Medicine, Internal Medicine-Cardiovascular Disease, Internal Medicine-Endocrinology and Metabolism, Internal Medicine-Gastroenterology, Internal Medicine-Hematology, Internal Medicine-Infectious Diseases, Internal Medicine-Medical Oncology, Internal Medicine-Nephrology, Internal Medicine-Rheumatology, Neurological Surgery, Neurology, Obstetrics/Gynecology, Orthopedic Surgery, Radiation Oncology, Surgery, Surgery-Vascular Surgery, Thoracic Surgery, Urology

Carney Hospital
2100 Dorchester Ave.
Boston, MA 02124
617-296-4000
Teaching Specialties:
Internal Medicine, Orthopedic Surgery, Surgery

Dana-Farber Cancer Institute
44 Binney St.
Boston, MA 02115
617-632-3000
Teaching Specialties:
Radiation Oncology

Dr. Solomon Carter Fuller Mental Health Center
85 E. Newton St.
Boston, MA 02118
617-266-8800
Teaching Specialties:
Psychiatry

Erich Lindemann Mental Health Center
25 Staniford St.
Boston, MA 02114
617-727-7115
Teaching Specialties:
Psychiatry

Harvard School of Dental Medicine
188 Longwood Ave.
Boston, MA 02115

617-432-1405
Teaching Specialties:
Dentistry

Jewish Memorial Hospital
59 Townsend St.
Boston, MA 02119
617-442-8760
Teaching Specialties:
Internal Medicine-Geriatric Medicine

Joslin Diabetes Center, Inc.
1 Joslin Place
Boston, MA 02115
617-732-2440
Teaching Specialties:
Internal Medicine-Endocrinology and
Metabolism

**Massachusetts Eye and Ear
Infirmary**
243 Charles St.
Boston, MA 02114
617-523-7900
Teaching Specialties:
Ophthalmology, Otolaryngology

Massachusetts General Hospital
55 Fruit St.
Boston, MA 02114
617-726-2000
Teaching Specialties:
Allergy/Immunology, Anesthesiology, Dentistry, Dermatology, Internal Medicine, Internal Medicine-Cardiovascular Disease, Internal Medicine-Endocrinology and Metabolism, Internal Medicine-Gastroenterology, Internal Medicine-Hematology, Internal Medicine-Infectious Diseases, Internal Medicine-Medical Oncology, Internal Medicine-Nephrology, Internal Medicine-Rheumatology, Neurological Surgery, Neurology, Obstetrics/Gynecology, Orthopedic Surgery, Psychiatry, Radiation Oncology, Surgery, Surgery-Vascular Surgery, Thoracic Surgery, Urology

**Massachusetts Mental Health
Center**
74 Fenwood Rd.
Boston, MA 02115
617-734-1300
Teaching Specialties:
Psychiatry

New England Baptist Hospital
125 Parker Hill Ave.
Boston, MA 02120
617-754-5800
Teaching Specialties:
Orthopedic Surgery

New England Deaconess Hospital
1 Deaconess Rd.
Boston, MA 02215
617-732-7000
Teaching Specialties:
Internal Medicine, Internal Medicine-Cardiovascular Disease, Internal Medicine-Endocrinology and Metabolism, Internal Medicine-Gastroenterology, Internal Medicine-Hematology, Internal Medicine-Infectious Diseases, Internal Medicine-Medical Oncology, Neurology, Radiation Oncology, Surgery, Surgery-Vascular Surgery, Thoracic Surgery, Urology

New England Medical Center
750 Washington St.
Boston, MA 02111
617-636-5000
Teaching Specialties:
Anesthesiology, Dermatology, Internal Medicine, Internal Medicine-Cardiovascular Disease, Internal Medicine-Endocrinology and Metabolism, Internal Medicine-Gastroenterology, Internal Medicine-Hematology, Internal Medicine-Infectious Diseases, Internal Medicine-Medical Oncology, Internal Medicine-Nephrology, Internal Medicine-Rheumatology, Neurological Surgery, Neurology, Obstetrics/Gynecology, Ophthalmology, Orthopedic Surgery, Otolaryngology, Physical Medicine and Rehabilitation, Psychiatry, Radiation Oncology, Surgery, Surgery-Vascular Surgery, Thoracic Surgery, Urology

**Tufts University School of Dental
Medicine**
1 Kneeland St.
Boston, MA 02111
617-636-6638
Teaching Specialties:
Dentistry

University Hospital
88 E. Newton St.
Boston, MA 02118
617-638-8000
Teaching Specialties:
Anesthesiology, Dermatology, Internal Medicine, Internal Medicine-Cardiovascular Disease, Internal Medicine-Endocrinology and Metabolism, Internal Medicine-Gastroenterology, Internal Medicine-Geriatric Medicine, Internal Medicine-Hematology, Internal Medicine-Infectious Diseases, Internal Medicine-Medical Oncology, Internal Medicine-Nephrology, Internal Medicine-Rheumatology, Neurology, Ophthalmology, Orthopedic Surgery, Otolaryngology, Physical Medicine and Rehabilitation, Psychiatry, Surgery, Surgery-Vascular Surgery, Thoracic Surgery, Urology

Brighton

St. Elizabeth's Hospital
736 Cambridge St.
Brighton, MA 02135
617-789-3000
Teaching Specialties:
Anesthesiology, Internal Medicine, Internal Medicine-Cardiovascular Disease, Internal Medicine-Gastroenterology, Internal Medicine-Hematology, Internal Medicine-Medical Oncology, Neurological Surgery, Orthopedic Surgery, Psychiatry, Surgery, Thoracic Surgery, Urology

Brockton

Brockton Hospital
680 Centre St.
Brockton, MA 02402
508-941-7002
Teaching Specialties:
Surgery

Good Samaritan Medical Center
235 N. Pearl St.
Brockton, MA 02301
508-588-4000
Teaching Specialties:
Surgery

Burlington

Lahey Clinic Hospital
41 Mall Rd.
Burlington, MA 01805
617-273-5100
Teaching Specialties:
Colon and Rectal Surgery, Dermatology, Internal Medicine-Cardiovascular Disease, Internal Medicine-Endocrinology and Metabolism, Internal Medicine-Gastroenterology, Neurology, Orthopedic Surgery, Otolaryngology, Surgery, Thoracic Surgery, Urology

Cambridge

Cambridge Hospital
1493 Cambridge St.
Cambridge, MA 02139
617-498-1000
Teaching Specialties:
Internal Medicine, Psychiatry

Mt. Auburn Hospital
330 Mt. Auburn St.
Cambridge, MA 02138
617-492-3500
Teaching Specialties:
Internal Medicine, Surgery, Surgery-Vascular Surgery, Thoracic Surgery

Chelsea

Lawrence F. Quigley Memorial Hospital
91 Crest Ave.
Chelsea, MA 02150
617-884-5660
Teaching Specialties:
Urology

Dorchester

St. Mary's Women & Infant Center
90 Cushing Ave.
Dorchester, MA 02125
617-436-8600
Teaching Specialties:
Obstetrics/Gynecology

Framingham

Metrowest Medical Center
115 Lincoln St.
Framingham, MA 01702
508-383-1000
Teaching Specialties:
Internal Medicine, Obstetrics/Gynecology

Hyannis

Cape Cod Hospital
27 Park St.
Hyannis, MA 02601
508-771-1800
Teaching Specialties:
Surgery

Jamaica Plain

Faulkner Hospital
1153 Centre St.
Jamaica Plain, MA 02130
617-522-5800
Teaching Specialties:
Internal Medicine, Internal Medicine-Gastroenterology, Psychiatry, Surgery

Lemuel Shattuck Hospital
170 Morton St.
Jamaica Plain, MA 02130
617-522-8110
Teaching Specialties:
Internal Medicine-Gastroenterology, Psychiatry

Lemuel Shattuck Hospital
Bay Cove Mental Health Center
170 Morton St.
Jamaica Plain, MA 02130
617-522-8110
Teaching Specialties:
Psychiatry

Malden

Malden Hospital
100 Hospital Rd.
Malden, MA 02148
617-322-7560
Teaching Specialties:
Obstetrics/Gynecology

Newton

Newton-Wellesley Hospital
2014 Washington St.
Newton, MA 02162
617-243-6000
Teaching Specialties:
Internal Medicine, Orthopedic Surgery, Surgery

Pittsfield

Berkshire Medical Center
725 North St.
Pittsfield, MA 01201
413-447-2000
Teaching Specialties:
Dentistry, Internal Medicine, Obstetrics/Gynecology, Surgery

Roslindale

May Behavioral Health
780 American Legion Hwy.
Roslindale, MA 02131
617-325-6700
Teaching Specialties:
Psychiatry

Salem

Salem Hospital
81 Highland Ave.
Salem, MA 01970
508-741-1200
Teaching Specialties:
Internal Medicine

Springfield

Baystate Medical Center
759 Chestnut St.
Springfield, MA 01199
413-784-0000
Teaching Specialties:
Anesthesiology, Internal Medicine, Internal Medicine-Cardiovascular Disease, Internal Medicine-Endocrinology and Metabolism, Internal Medicine-Hematology, Internal Medicine-Infectious Diseases, Internal Medicine-Medical Oncology, Obstetrics/Gynecology, Orthopedic Surgery, Surgery

Stockbridge

Austen Riggs Center
25 Main St.

Stockbridge, MA 01262
413-298-5511
Teaching Specialties:
Psychiatry

Stoughton

New England Sinai Hospital and Rehabilitation Center
150 York St.
Stoughton, MA 2072
617-364-4850
Teaching Specialties:
Physical Medicine and Rehabilitation

Tewksbury

Tewksbury State Hospital
365 East St.
Tewksbury, MA 01876
617-727-4610
Teaching Specialties:
Psychiatry

Wellesley

Charles River Hospital
203 Grove St.
Wellesley, MA 02482-7413
781-235-8400
Teaching Specialties:
Psychiatry

Worcester

Medical Center of Central Massachusetts
119 Belmont St.
Worcester, MA 01605
508-793-6611
Teaching Specialties:
Internal Medicine, Internal Medicine-Geriatric Medicine, Obstetrics/Gynecology, Orthopedic Surgery, Surgery, Urology

St. Vincent Hospital
25 Winthrop St.
Worcester, MA 01604
508-798-1234
Teaching Specialties:
Internal Medicine, Internal Medicine-Cardiovascular Disease, Neurology, Obstetrics/Gynecology, Orthopedic Surgery, Surgery, Thoracic Surgery

University of Massachusetts Medical Center
55 Lake Ave. North
Worcester, MA 01655
508-856-0011
Teaching Specialties:
Anesthesiology, Internal Medicine, Internal Medicine-Cardiovascular Disease, Internal Medicine-Endocrinology and Metabolism, In-

ternal Medicine-Gastroenterology, Internal Medicine-Geriatric Medicine, Internal Medicine-Hematology, Internal Medicine-Infectious Diseases, Internal Medicine-Medical Oncology, Internal Medicine-Nephrology, Internal Medicine-Rheumatology, Neurology, Obstetrics/Gynecology, Orthopedic Surgery, Psychiatry, Surgery, Surgery-Vascular Surgery, Thoracic Surgery, Urology

Worcester Health and Hospitals Authority
26 Queen St.
Worcester, MA 01610
508-799-8200
Teaching Specialties:
Internal Medicine, Orthopedic Surgery, Surgery

Worcester State Hospital
305 Belmont St.
Worcester, MA 01604
508-752-4681
Teaching Specialties:
Psychiatry

MICHIGAN
Ann Arbor
University of Michigan Hospitals
1500 E. Medical Center Dr.
Ann Arbor, MI 48109
734-936-4000
Teaching Specialties:
Allergy/Immunology, Anesthesiology, Dermatology, Internal Medicine, Internal Medicine-Cardiovascular Disease, Internal Medicine-Endocrinology and Metabolism, Internal Medicine-Gastroenterology, Internal Medicine-Geriatric Medicine, Internal Medicine-Hematology, Internal Medicine-Infectious Diseases, Internal Medicine-Medical Oncology, Internal Medicine-Nephrology, Internal Medicine-Rheumatology, Neurological Surgery, Neurology, Obstetrics/Gynecology, Ophthalmology, Orthopedic Surgery, Otolaryngology, Physical Medicine and Rehabilitation, Psychiatry, Radiation Oncology, Surgery, Surgery-Vascular Surgery, Thoracic Surgery, Urology

University of Michigan School of Dentistry
1001 N. University Ave.
Ann Arbor, MI 48109-1078
734-763-6933
Teaching Specialties:
Dentistry

Dearborn
Oakwood Hospital
18101 Oakwood Blvd.
Dearborn, MI 48124
734-593-7000
Teaching Specialties:
Internal Medicine, Obstetrics/Gynecology, Orthopedic Surgery

Detroit
Detroit-Macomb Hospital Corporation
Oral and Maxillofacial Surgery
7733 E. Jefferson
Detroit, MI 48214-2598
313-499-4190
Teaching Specialties:
Dentistry

Detroit Psychiatric Institute
1151 Taylor St.
Detroit, MI 48202
313-874-7500
Teaching Specialties:
Psychiatry

Detroit Receiving Hospital and University Health Center
4201 St. Antoine Blvd.
Detroit, MI 48201
313-745-3000
Teaching Specialties:
Allergy/Immunology, Dentistry, Dermatology, Internal Medicine, Internal Medicine-Cardiovascular Disease, Internal Medicine-Endocrinology and Metabolism, Internal Medicine-Gastroenterology, Internal Medicine-Hematology, Internal Medicine-Infectious Diseases, Internal Medicine-Medical Oncology, Internal Medicine-Nephrology, Internal Medicine-Rheumatology, Neurological Surgery, Neurology, Obstetrics/Gynecology, Ophthalmology, Orthopedic Surgery, Otolaryngology, Radiation Oncology, Surgery, Thoracic Surgery

Grace Hospital
6071 W. Outer Dr.
Detroit, MI 48235
313-966-3300
Teaching Specialties:
Internal Medicine, Obstetrics/Gynecology, Ophthalmology, Orthopedic Surgery, Otolaryngology, Radiation Oncology, Surgery

Harper Hospital
3990 John R. St.
Detroit, MI 48201
313-745-8040
Teaching Specialties:
Allergy/Immunology, Dermatology, Internal Medicine, Internal Medicine-Cardiovascular Disease, Internal Medicine-Endocrinology and Metabolism, Internal Medicine-Gastroenterology, Internal Medicine-Hematology, Internal Medicine-Infectious Diseases, Internal Medicine-Medical Oncology, Internal Medicine-Nephrology, Internal Medicine-Rheumatology, Neurological Surgery, Neurology, Obstetrics/Gynecology, Ophthalmology, Orthopedic Surgery, Otolaryngology, Psychia-

try, Radiation Oncology, Surgery, Surgery-Vascular Surgery, Thoracic Surgery, Urology

Henry Ford Hospital
2799 W. Grand Blvd.
Detroit, MI 48202
313-876-2600
Teaching Specialties:
Allergy/Immunology, Anesthesiology, Colon and Rectal Surgery, Dentistry, Dermatology, Internal Medicine, Internal Medicine-Cardiovascular Disease, Internal Medicine-Endocrinology and Metabolism, Internal Medicine-Gastroenterology, Internal Medicine-Hematology, Internal Medicine-Infectious Diseases, Internal Medicine-Medical Oncology, Internal Medicine-Nephrology, Internal Medicine-Rheumatology, Neurological Surgery, Neurology, Obstetrics/Gynecology, Ophthalmology, Orthopedic Surgery, Otolaryngology, Psychiatry, Radiation Oncology, Surgery, Surgery-Vascular Surgery, Urology

Hutzel Hospital
4707 St. Antoine Blvd.
Detroit, MI 48201
313-745-7171
Teaching Specialties:
Internal Medicine-Rheumatology, Obstetrics/Gynecology, Otolaryngology, Surgery

Rehabilitation Institute of Michigan
261 Mack Ave.
Detroit, MI 48201
313-745-1203
Teaching Specialties:
Physical Medicine and Rehabilitation

Mercy Hospital
5555 Conner Ave.
Detroit, MI 48213
313-579-4000
Teaching Specialties:
Surgery

Sinai Hospital
6767 W. Outer Dr.
Detroit, MI 48235
313-493-6800
Teaching Specialties:
Anesthesiology, Dentistry, Internal Medicine, Internal Medicine-Cardiovascular Disease, Internal Medicine-Gastroenterology, Internal Medicine-Rheumatology, Obstetrics/Gynecology, Ophthalmology, Orthopedic Surgery, Physical Medicine and Rehabilitation, Psychiatry, Surgery

St. John Hospital and Medical Center
22101 Moross Rd.
Detroit, MI 48236
313-343-4000
Teaching Specialties:
Internal Medicine, Obstetrics/Gynecology, Surgery

507

University of Detroit
Mercy School of Dentistry
PO Box 19900
4001 W. McNichols Rd.
Detroit, MI 48219
313-494-6600
Teaching Specialties:
Dentistry

Flint

Hurley Medical Center
1 Hurley Plaza
Flint, MI 48503
810-257-9000
Teaching Specialties:
Internal Medicine, Obstetrics/Gynecology,
Orthopedic Surgery

McLaren Regional Medical Center
401 S. Ballenger Hwy.
Flint, MI 48532
810-762-2088
Teaching Specialties:
Internal Medicine, Orthopedic Surgery,
Surgery

Grand Rapids

Blodgett-Ferguson Campus
72 Sheldon Blvd., SE
Grand Rapids, MI 49503
616-356-4301
Teaching Specialties:
Colon and Rectal Surgery

Blodgett Memorial Medical Center
1840 Wealthy St., SE
Grand Rapids, MI 49506
616-774-7444
Teaching Specialties:
Internal Medicine, Obstetrics/Gynecology,
Orthopedic Surgery, Surgery

Butterworth Hospital
100 Michigan St., NE
Grand Rapids, MI 49503
800-968-1880
Teaching Specialties:
Internal Medicine, Obstetrics/Gynecology,
Orthopedic Surgery, Surgery

**Kent Community Hospital
Complex**
750 Fuller Ave., NE
Grand Rapids, MI 49503
616-336-3300
Teaching Specialties:
Psychiatry

Pine Rest Christian Hospital
300 68th St., SE
Grand Rapids, MI 49501-0165

616-455-5000
Teaching Specialties:
Psychiatry

St. Mary's Health Services
200 Jefferson St., SE
Grand Rapids, MI 49503
616-774-6090
Teaching Specialties:
Internal Medicine, Obstetrics/Gynecology,
Orthopedic Surgery, Psychiatry, Surgery

Grosse Pointe

Bon Secours Hospital
468 Cadieux Rd.
Grosse Pointe, MI 48230
313-343-1000
Teaching Specialties:
Internal Medicine

Kalamazoo

Borgess Medical Center
1521 Gull Rd.
Kalamazoo, MI 49001
616-383-7000
Teaching Specialties:
Internal Medicine, Orthopedic Surgery

Bronson Methodist Hospital
252 E. Lovell St.
Kalamazoo, MI 49007
616-341-7654
Teaching Specialties:
Internal Medicine, Orthopedic Surgery

Lansing

Michigan Capital Medical Center
401 W. Greenlawn Ave.
Lansing, MI 48910
517-334-2121
Teaching Specialties:
Internal Medicine, Internal Medicine-Gastroenterology, Surgery

Sparrow Hospital
1215 E. Michigan Ave.
Lansing, MI 48912
517-483-2700
Teaching Specialties:
Internal Medicine, Obstetrics/Gynecology

**St. Lawrence Hospital
and Healthcare Services**
1210 W. Saginaw St.
Lansing, MI 48915
517-372-3610
Teaching Specialties:
Internal Medicine, Internal Medicine-Hematology, Psychiatry, Surgery

Northville

Hawthorn Center
18471 Haggerty Rd.
Northville, MI 48167
313-349-3000
Teaching Specialties:
Psychiatry

**Northville Regional Psychiatric
Hospital**
41001 W. Seven Mile Rd.
Northville, MI 48167
313-349-1800
Teaching Specialties:
Psychiatry

Pontiac

North Oakland Medical Centers
461 W. Huron St.
Pontiac, MI 48341
248-857-7200
Teaching Specialties:
Obstetrics/Gynecology, Surgery

St. Joseph Mercy Hospital
900 Woodward Ave.
Pontiac, MI 48341
810-858-3000
Teaching Specialties:
Internal Medicine, Obstetrics/Gynecology,
Surgery

Royal Oak

William Beaumont Hospital
3601 W. 13 Mile Rd.
Royal Oak, MI 48073
248-551-5000
Teaching Specialties:
Colon and Rectal Surgery, Internal Medicine,
Internal Medicine-Cardiovascular Disease, In-
ternal Medicine-Gastroenterology, Internal
Medicine-Hematology, Internal Medicine-In-
fectious Diseases, Internal Medicine-Medical
Oncology, Obstetrics/Gynecology, Ophthal-
mology, Orthopedic Surgery, Physical
Medicine and Rehabilitation, Radiation On-
cology, Surgery, Urology

Saginaw

Saginaw General Hospital
1447 N. Harrison St.
Saginaw, MI 48602
517-771-4000
Teaching Specialties:
Internal Medicine, Obstetrics/Gynecology,
Surgery

St. Luke's Hospital
700 Cooper Ave.
Saginaw, MI 48602

517-771-6000
Teaching Specialties:
Internal Medicine, Surgery

St. Mary's Medical Center
830 S. Jefferson Ave.
Saginaw, MI 48601
517-776-8000
Teaching Specialties:
Internal Medicine

Southfield

Providence Hospital
16001 W. Nine Mile Rd.
Southfield, MI 48075
810-424-3000
Teaching Specialties:
Anesthesiology, Internal Medicine, Internal
Medicine-Cardiovascular Disease, Internal
Medicine-Gastroenterology, Obstetrics/Gyne-
cology, Orthopedic Surgery, Psychiatry, Radi-
ation Oncology, Surgery

Westland

Oakwood Healthcare Systems
2345 Merriman Rd.
Westland, MI 48186
313-467-2300
Teaching Specialties:
Ophthalmology

Ypsilanti

St. Joseph Mercy Hospital
5301 E. Huron River Dr.
Ypsilanti, MI 48197
313-712-3456
Teaching Specialties:
Internal Medicine, Neurological Surgery, Ob-
stetrics/Gynecology, Orthopedic Surgery,
Surgery, Urology

MINNESOTA

Minneapolis

Abbott-Northwestern Hospital
800 E. 28th St.
Minneapolis, MN 55407
612-863-4000
Teaching Specialties:
Colon and Rectal Surgery, Internal Medicine

Hennepin County Medical Center
701 Park Ave. South
Minneapolis, MN 55415
612-347-2121
Teaching Specialties:
Anesthesiology, Dentistry, Dermatology, Internal Medicine, Internal Medicine-Cardiovascular Disease, Internal Medicine-Geriatric

Medicine, Internal Medicine-Nephrology, Internal Medicine-Rheumatology, Neurological
Surgery, Neurology, Obstetrics/Gynecology,
Ophthalmology, Orthopedic Surgery, Otolaryngology, Psychiatry, Surgery

**University of Minnesota Hospital
and Clinic**
420 Delaware St., SE
Minneapolis, MN 55455
612-626-3000
Teaching Specialties:
Allergy/Immunology, Anesthesiology, Colon
and Rectal Surgery, Dermatology, Internal
Medicine, Internal Medicine-Cardiovascular
Disease, Internal Medicine-Endocrinology
and Metabolism, Internal Medicine-Gastroen-
terology, Internal Medicine-Geriatric
Medicine, Internal Medicine-Hematology, In-
ternal Medicine-Infectious Diseases, Internal
Medicine-Medical Oncology, Internal
Medicine-Nephrology, Internal Medicine-
Rheumatology, Neurological Surgery, Neurol-
ogy, Obstetrics/Gynecology, Ophthalmology,
Orthopedic Surgery, Otolaryngology, Physical
Medicine and Rehabilitation, Psychiatry, Ra-
diation Oncology, Surgery, Thoracic Surgery,
Urology

**University of Minnesota School
of Dentistry**
515 Delaware St., SE
Minneapolis, MN 55455
612-625-9982
Teaching Specialties:
Dentistry

Moorhead

**Lakeland Mental Health
Center, Inc.**
1010 32nd Ave. South
Moorhead, MN 56560
218-233-7524
Teaching Specialties:
Psychiatry

Rochester

Mayo Clinic
200 S.W. First St.
Rochester, MN 55905
507-284-2511
Teaching Specialties:
Allergy/Immunology, Anesthesiology, Colon
and Rectal Surgery, Dentistry, Dermatology,
Hand Surgery, Internal Medicine, Internal
Medicine-Cardiovascular Disease, Internal
Medicine-Endocrinology and Metabolism, In-
ternal Medicine-Gastroenterology, Internal
Medicine-Geriatric Medicine, Internal
Medicine-Hematology, Internal Medicine-In-
fectious Diseases, Internal Medicine-Medical
Oncology, Internal Medicine-Nephrology, In-
ternal Medicine-Rheumatology, Neurological
Surgery, Neurology, Obstetrics/Gynecology,
Ophthalmology, Orthopedic Surgery, Oto-

laryngology, Physical Medicine and Rehabilitation, Psychiatry, Surgery, Surgery-Vascular
Surgery, Thoracic Surgery, Urology

Rochester Methodist Hospital
201 W. Center St.
Rochester, MN 55902
507-266-7890
Teaching Specialties:
Allergy/Immunology, Anesthesiology, Colon
and Rectal Surgery, Dermatology, Internal
Medicine, Internal Medicine-Cardiovascular
Disease, Internal Medicine-Endocrinology
and Metabolism, Internal Medicine-Gastroen-
terology, Internal Medicine-Geriatric
Medicine, Internal Medicine-Hematology, In-
ternal Medicine-Infectious Diseases, Internal
Medicine-Medical Oncology, Neurology, Ob-
stetrics/Gynecology, Ophthalmology, Ortho-
pedic Surgery, Otolaryngology, Surgery,
Surgery-Vascular Surgery, Thoracic Surgery,
Urology

St. Mary's Hospital
1216 S.W. Second St.
Rochester, MN 55902
507-255-5123
Teaching Specialties:
Allergy/Immunology, Anesthesiology, Colon
and Rectal Surgery, Dermatology, Internal
Medicine, Internal Medicine-Cardiovascular
Disease, Internal Medicine-Endocrinology
and Metabolism, Internal Medicine-Gastroen-
terology, Internal Medicine-Geriatric
Medicine, Internal Medicine-Hematology, In-
ternal Medicine-Infectious Diseases, Internal
Medicine-Medical Oncology, Neurological
Surgery, Neurology, Obstetrics/Gynecology,
Ophthalmology, Orthopedic Surgery, Oto-
laryngology, Physical Medicine and Rehabili-
tation, Psychiatry, Surgery, Surgery-Vascular
Surgery, Thoracic Surgery, Urology

St. Paul

Regions Hospital
640 Jackson St.
St. Paul, MN 55101
612-221-3456
Teaching Specialties:
Dermatology, Internal Medicine, Internal
Medicine-Geriatric Medicine, Neurology, Ob-
stetrics/Gynecology, Ophthalmology, Oto-
laryngology, Psychiatry, Surgery, Thoracic
Surgery, Urology

MISSISSIPPI

Jackson

Mississippi Baptist Medical Center
1225 N. State St.
Jackson, MS 39202
601-968-1000
Teaching Specialties:
Urology

University of Mississippi Medical Center
University Hospitals and Clinics
2500 N. State St.
Jackson, MS 39216
601-984-1000
Teaching Specialties:
Anesthesiology, Internal Medicine, Internal Medicine-Cardiovascular Disease, Internal Medicine-Gastroenterology, Internal Medicine-Hematology, Internal Medicine-Infectious Diseases, Internal Medicine-Medical Oncology, Internal Medicine-Nephrology, Internal Medicine-Rheumatology, Neurological Surgery, Neurology, Obstetrics/Gynecology, Ophthalmology, Orthopedic Surgery, Otolaryngology, Psychiatry, Surgery, Thoracic Surgery, Urology

University of Mississippi School of Dentistry
2500 N. State St.
Jackson, MS 39216-4505
601-984-6000
Teaching Specialties:
Dentistry

Whitfield

Mississippi State Hospital
PO Box 157A
Whitfield, MS 39193
601-351-8000
Teaching Specialties:
Psychiatry

MISSOURI
Chesterfield

St. Luke's Hospital
232 S. Woods Mill Rd.
Chesterfield, MO 63017
314-434-1500
Teaching Specialties:
Internal Medicine, Internal Medicine-Cardiovascular Disease

Columbia

Boone Hospital Center
1600 E. Broadway
Columbia, MO 65201
314-875-4545
Teaching Specialties:
Neurological Surgery

Mid-Missouri Mental Health Center
3 Hospital Dr.
Columbia, MO 65201
314-449-2511
Teaching Specialties:
Psychiatry

University Hospital and Clinics
1 Hospital Dr.
Columbia, MO 65201
314-882-4141
Teaching Specialties:
Anesthesiology, Dermatology, Internal Medicine, Internal Medicine-Cardiovascular Disease, Internal Medicine-Endocrinology and Metabolism, Internal Medicine-Gastroenterology, Internal Medicine-Hematology, Internal Medicine-Infectious Diseases, Internal Medicine-Medical Oncology, Internal Medicine-Nephrology, Internal Medicine-Rheumatology, Neurological Surgery, Neurology, Obstetrics/Gynecology, Ophthalmology, Orthopedic Surgery, Otolaryngology, Physical Medicine and Rehabilitation, Psychiatry, Surgery, Surgery-Vascular Surgery, Thoracic Surgery, Urology

University Hospital and Clinics
Howard A. Rusk
Rehabilitation Center
315 Business Loop 70
Columbia, MO 65203
537-882-2121
Teaching Specialties:
Physical Medicine and Rehabilitation

Kansas City

Research Medical Center
2316 E. Meyer Blvd.
Kansas City, MO 64132
816-276-4000
Teaching Specialties:
Internal Medicine-Infectious Diseases

St. Luke's Hospital
4401 Wornall Rd.
Kansas City, MO 64111
816-932-2000
Teaching Specialties:
Anesthesiology, Internal Medicine, Obstetrics/Gynecology, Orthopedic Surgery, Surgery, Thoracic Surgery

Trinity Lutheran Hospital
3030 Baltimore Ave.
Kansas City, MO 64108
816-751-4600
Teaching Specialties:
Internal Medicine-Hematology, Internal Medicine-Medical Oncology

Truman Medical Center-West
2301 Holmes St.
Kansas City, MO 64108
816-556-3000
Teaching Specialties:
Internal Medicine, Internal Medicine-Cardiovascular Disease, Internal Medicine-Gastroenterology, Internal Medicine-Hematology, Internal Medicine-Infectious Diseases, Internal Medicine-Medical Oncology, Obstetrics/Gy-

necology, Ophthalmology, Orthopedic Surgery, Surgery

University of Missouri-Kansas City
School of Dentistry
650 E. 25th St.
Kansas City, MO 64108
816-235-2100
Teaching Specialties:
Dentistry

Western Missouri Mental Health Center
600 E. 22nd St.
Kansas City, MO 64108
816-471-3000
Teaching Specialties:
Psychiatry

Overland Park

Menorah Medical Center
5721 W. 119th Street
Overland Park, MO 66209
913-498-6000
Teaching Specialties:
Obstetrics/Gynecology, Surgery

Richmond Heights

St. Mary's Health Center
6420 Clayton Rd.
Richmond Heights, MO 63117
314-768-8000
Teaching Specialties:
Internal Medicine, Internal Medicine-Gastroenterology, Obstetrics/Gynecology, Orthopedic Surgery, Surgery, Urology

St. Louis

Anheuser-Busch Eye Institute
1755 S. Grand Blvd.
St. Louis, MO 63104
314-577-6038
Teaching Specialties:
Ophthalmology

Barnes-Jewish Hospital
1 Barnes Hospital Plaza
St. Louis, MO 63110
314-362-5000
Teaching Specialties:
Allergy/Immunology, Anesthesiology, Dermatology, Hand Surgery, Internal Medicine, Internal Medicine-Cardiovascular Disease, Internal Medicine-Endocrinology and Metabolism, Internal Medicine-Gastroenterology, Internal Medicine-Hematology, Internal Medicine-Infectious Diseases, Internal Medicine-Medical Oncology, Internal Medicine-Nephrology, Internal Medicine-Rheumatology, Neurological Surgery, Neurology, Obstetrics/Gynecology, Ophthalmology, Orthopedic Surgery, Otolaryngology, Psychia-

try, Radiation Oncology, Surgery, Surgery-Vascular Surgery, Thoracic Surgery, Urology

Deaconess Hospital
6150 Oakland Ave.
St. Louis, MO 63139
314-768-3000
Teaching Specialties:
Internal Medicine, Obstetrics/Gynecology

St. Louis Psyche Rehab Center
5300 Arsenal St.
St. Louis, MO 63139
314-644-8000
Teaching Specialties:
Psychiatry

Mallinckrodt Institute of Radiology
7425 Forsyth Blvd.
St. Louis, MO 63105
314-935-0799
Teaching Specialties:
Radiation Oncology

St. John's Mercy Medical Center
615 S. New Ballas Rd.
St. Louis, MO 63141
314-569-6000
Teaching Specialties:
Dentistry, Internal Medicine, Obstetrics/Gynecology, Surgery, Surgery-Vascular Surgery, Urology

St. Louis Regional Medical Center
5535 Delmar Blvd.
St. Louis, MO 63112
314-879-6308
Teaching Specialties:
Internal Medicine, Neurology, Obstetrics/Gynecology, Orthopedic Surgery, Otolaryngology

St. Louis University Medical Center
3635 Vista at Grand Blvd.
St. Louis, MO 63110-0250
314-577-8000
Teaching Specialties:
Allergy/Immunology, Anesthesiology, Internal Medicine, Internal Medicine-Cardiovascular Disease, Internal Medicine-Endocrinology and Metabolism, Internal Medicine-Gastroenterology, Internal Medicine-Hematology, Internal Medicine-Infectious Diseases, Internal Medicine-Medical Oncology, Internal Medicine-Nephrology, Internal Medicine-Rheumatology, Neurological Surgery, Neurology, Obstetrics/Gynecology, Orthopedic Surgery, Otolaryngology, Psychiatry, Surgery, Surgery-Vascular Surgery, Thoracic Surgery, Urology

St. Louis University Medical Center
Orthodontics Treatment
3320 Rutger St.
St. Louis, MO 63104

314-577-8181
Teaching Specialties:
Dentistry

NEBRASKA
Lincoln

University of Nebraska Medical Center
College of Dentistry
40th & Holdrege Sts.
Lincoln, NE 68583-0740
402-472-1344
Teaching Specialties:
Dentistry

Omaha

AMI St. Joseph Center for Mental Health
819 Dorcas St.
Omaha, NE 68108
402-449-4650
Teaching Specialties:
Psychiatry

AMI St. Joseph Hospital
601 N. 30th St.
Omaha, NE 68131
402-449-4000
Teaching Specialties:
Allergy/Immunology, Colon and Rectal Surgery, Internal Medicine, Internal Medicine-Cardiovascular Disease, Internal Medicine-Infectious Diseases, Neurology, Obstetrics/Gynecology, Orthopedic Surgery, Surgery, Urology

Bergan Mercy Medical Center
7500 Mercy Rd.
Omaha, NE 68124
402-398-6060
Teaching Specialties:
Obstetrics/Gynecology

Bishop Clarkson Memorial Hospital
44th St. & Dewey Ave.
Omaha, NE 68105
402-552-2000
Teaching Specialties:
Internal Medicine

Creighton University School of Dentistry
2500 California Plaza
Omaha, NE 68178
402-280-5060
Teaching Specialties:
Dentistry

Methodist Hospital
8303 Dodge St.
Omaha, NE 68114
402-331-1111
Teaching Specialties:
Urology

University of Nebraska Medical Center
600 S. 42nd St.
Omaha, NE 68198
402-559-4000
Teaching Specialties:
Anesthesiology, Internal Medicine, Internal Medicine-Cardiovascular Disease, Internal Medicine-Gastroenterology, Internal Medicine-Geriatric Medicine, Internal Medicine-Hematology, Internal Medicine-Medical Oncology, Neurology, Obstetrics/Gynecology, Ophthalmology, Orthopedic Surgery, Otolaryngology, Psychiatry, Surgery, Urology

NEVADA
Las Vegas

University Medical Center of Southern Nevada
1800 W. Charleston Blvd.
Las Vegas, NV 89102
702-383-2000
Teaching Specialties:
Internal Medicine, Obstetrics/Gynecology, Surgery

Women's Hospital
2127 W. Charleston Blvd.
Las Vegas, NV 89102
702-735-7106
Teaching Specialties:
Obstetrics/Gynecology

Reno

Washoe Medical Center
77 Pringle Way
Reno, NV 89520
702-328-4100
Teaching Specialties:
Internal Medicine

NEW HAMPSHIRE
Concord

New Hampshire Hospital
105 Pleasant St.
Concord, NH 03301
603-271-5200
Teaching Specialties:
Psychiatry

Lebanon

Dartmouth-Hitchcock Medical Center
1 Medical Center Dr.
Lebanon, NH 03756
603-650-5000
Teaching Specialties:
Anesthesiology, Dermatology, Internal Medicine, Internal Medicine-Cardiovascular Disease, Internal Medicine-Endocrinology and Metabolism, Internal Medicine-Gastroenterology, Internal Medicine-Hematology, Internal Medicine-Medical Oncology, Internal Medicine-Rheumatology, Neurological Surgery, Neurology, Orthopedic Surgery, Otolaryngology, Psychiatry, Surgery, Surgery-Vascular Surgery, Urology

NEW JERSEY

Atlantic City

Atlantic City Medical Center
1925 Pacific Ave.
Atlantic City, NJ 08401
609-344-4081
Teaching Specialties:
Internal Medicine, Orthopedic Surgery

Berlin

West Jersey Hospital-Berlin
100 Townsend Ave.
Berlin, NJ 08009
609-322-3200
Teaching Specialties:
Otolaryngology

Blackwood

Camden County Health Services Center
PO Box 1639
Woodbury Turnersville Rd.
Blackwood, NJ 08012
609-227-3000
Teaching Specialties:
Psychiatry

Browns Mills

Deborah Heart and Lung Center
200 Trenton Rd.
Browns Mills, NJ 08015
609-893-6611
Teaching Specialties:
Thoracic Surgery

Camden

Cooper Hospital-University Medical Center
1 Cooper Plaza
Camden, NJ 08103

609-342-2000
Teaching Specialties:
Internal Medicine, Internal Medicine-Cardiovascular Disease, Internal Medicine-Gastroenterology, Internal Medicine Hematology, Internal Medicine-Infectious Diseases, Internal Medicine-Medical Oncology, Internal Medicine-Nephrology, Internal Medicine-Rheumatology, Obstetrics/Gynecology, Ophthalmology, Psychiatry, Radiation Oncology, Surgery

West Jersey Hospital-Camden
1000 Atlantic Ave.
Camden, NJ 08104
609-246-
Teaching Specialties:
Otolaryngology

Edison

John F. Kennedy Medical Center
65 James St.
Edison, NJ 08818
732-321-7000
Teaching Specialties:
Colon and Rectal Surgery, Dentistry, Physical Medicine and Rehabilitation

Elizabeth

St. Elizabeth Hospital
225 Williamson St.
Elizabeth, NJ 07207
908-527-5000
Teaching Specialties:
Internal Medicine

Englewood

Englewood Hospital
350 Engle St.
Englewood, NJ 07631
201-894-3000
Teaching Specialties:
Dentistry, Internal Medicine, Obstetrics/Gynecology

Hackensack

Hackensack Medical Center
30 Prospect Ave.
Hackensack, NJ 07601
201-996-2000
Teaching Specialties:
Anesthesiology, Dentistry, Internal Medicine, Internal Medicine-Cardiovascular Disease, Internal Medicine-Infectious Diseases, Obstetrics/Gynecology, Orthopedic Surgery, Psychiatry, Surgery, Surgery-Vascular Surgery, Urology

Jersey City

Jersey City Medical Center
50 Baldwin Ave.

Jersey City, NJ 07304
201-915-2000
Teaching Specialties:
Dentistry, Internal Medicine, Internal Medicine-Cardiovascular Disease, Internal Medicine-Gastroenterology, Obstetrics/Gynecology, Ophthalmology, Orthopedic Surgery

Livingston

St. Barnabas Medical Center
94 Old Short Hills Rd.
Livingston, NJ 07039
201-533-5000
Teaching Specialties:
Anesthesiology, Internal Medicine, Internal Medicine-Nephrology, Neurological Surgery, Obstetrics/Gynecology, Psychiatry, Radiation Oncology, Surgery

Long Branch

Monmouth Medical Center
300 Second Ave.
Long Branch, NJ 07740
732-222-5200
Teaching Specialties:
Anesthesiology, Dentistry, Internal Medicine, Obstetrics/Gynecology, Orthopedic Surgery, Surgery

Marlton

West Jersey Hospital-Marlton
Route 73 & Brick Rd.
Marlton, NJ 08053
609-596-3500
Teaching Specialties:
Otolaryngology

Montclair

Mountainside Hospital
1 Bay Ave.
Montclair, NJ 07042
973-429-6000
Teaching Specialties:
Dentistry, Internal Medicine

Morristown

Morristown Memorial Hospital
100 Madison Ave.
Morristown, NJ 07960
973-971-5000
Teaching Specialties:
Dentistry, Internal Medicine, Obstetrics/Gynecology, Surgery

Neptune

Jersey Shore Medical Center
1945 Route 33
Neptune, NJ 07753
908-775-5500

Teaching Specialties:
Dentistry, Internal Medicine, Obstetrics/
Gynecology, Surgery

New Brunswick

Robert Wood Johnson University Hospital
1 Robert Wood Johnson Pl.
New Brunswick, NJ 08901
908-828-3000
Teaching Specialties:
Anesthesiology, Dentistry, Internal Medicine,
Internal Medicine-Cardiovascular Disease,
Internal Medicine-Endocrinology and
Metabolism, Internal Medicine-Gastroenterol-
ogy, Internal Medicine-Hematology, Internal
Medicine-Infectious Diseases, Internal
Medicine-Medical Oncology, Internal
Medicine-Nephrology, Internal Medicine-
Rheumatology, Neurology, Obstetrics/Gyne-
cology, Orthopedic Surgery, Surgery, Surgery-
Vascular Surgery, Thoracic Surgery, Urology

St. Peter's Medical Center
254 Easton Ave.
New Brunswick, NJ 08901
908-745-8600
Teaching Specialties:
Internal Medicine, Internal Medicine-Cardio-
vascular Disease, Internal Medicine-En-
docrinology and Metabolism, Internal
Medicine-Hematology, Internal Medicine-In-
fectious Diseases, Internal Medicine-Medical
Oncology, Internal Medicine-Nephrology,
Obstetrics/Gynecology, Orthopedic Surgery,
Thoracic Surgery

Newark

Newark Beth Israel Medical Center
201 Lyons Ave.
Newark, NJ 07112
973-926-7000
Teaching Specialties:
Dentistry, Internal Medicine, Internal
Medicine-Cardiovascular Disease, Internal
Medicine-Hematology, Internal Medicine-
Medical Oncology, Internal Medicine-
Nephrology, Internal Medicine-Rheumatolo-
gy, Obstetrics/Gynecology, Surgery,
Surgery-Vascular Surgery, Thoracic Surgery

St. James Hospital of Newark
155 Jefferson St.
Newark, NJ 07105
973-589-1300
Teaching Specialties:
Obstetrics/Gynecology

St. Michael's Medical Center
306 Dr. Martin Luther King Jr. Blvd.
Newark, NJ 07102
973-877-5000
Teaching Specialties:
Internal Medicine, Internal Medicine-Cardiovascular Disease, Internal Medicine-En-

docrinology and Metabolism, Internal
Medicine-Gastroenterology, Internal
Medicine-Hematology, Internal Medicine-In-
fectious Diseases, Internal Medicine-Medical
Oncology, Internal Medicine-Rheumatology,
Obstetrics/Gynecology, Surgery-Vascular
Surgery, Thoracic Surgery

United Hospitals Medical Center
15 S. Ninth St.
Newark, NJ 07107
201-268-8000
Teaching Specialties:
Internal Medicine, Internal Medicine-Hematology, Internal Medicine-Medical Oncology,
Ophthalmology, Orthopedic Surgery, Otolaryngology

United Hospitals Medical Center
Newark Eye and Ear Infirmary
15 S. Ninth St.
Newark, NJ 07107
201-268-8000
Teaching Specialties:
Ophthalmology, Otolaryngology

United Hospitals Medical Center
Orthopedic Unit
15 S. Ninth St.
Newark, NJ 07107
201-268-8000
Teaching Specialties:
Orthopedic Surgery

University of Medicine and Dentistry of New Jersey
University Hospital
150 Bergen St.
Newark, NJ 07103
973-982-4300
Teaching Specialties:
Allergy/Immunology, Anesthesiology, Der-
matology, Internal Medicine, Internal
Medicine-Cardiovascular Disease, Internal
Medicine-Endocrinology and Metabolism, In-
ternal Medicine-Gastroenterology, Internal
Medicine-Hematology, Internal Medicine-In-
fectious Diseases, Internal Medicine-Medical
Oncology, Internal Medicine-Nephrology, In-
ternal Medicine-Rheumatology, Neurological
Surgery, Neurology, Obstetrics/Gynecology,
Ophthalmology, Orthopedic Surgery, Oto-
laryngology, Physical Medicine and Rehabili-
tation, Psychiatry, Surgery, Surgery-Vascular
Surgery, Thoracic Surgery, Urology

University of Medicine and Dentistry of New Jersey
New Jersey Dental School
110 Bergen St.
Newark, NJ 07103-2400
973-972-4242
Teaching Specialties:
Dentistry

Orange

Hospital Center at Orange
188 S. Essex Ave.
Orange, NJ 07050
201-266-2020
Teaching Specialties:
Orthopedic Surgery

Paramus

Bergen Pines County Hospital
230 E. Ridgewood Ave.
Paramus, NJ 07652
201-967-4000
Teaching Specialties:
Internal Medicine, Psychiatry

Paterson

St. Joseph's Hospital and Medical Center
703 Main St.
Paterson, NJ 07503
201-977-2000
Teaching Specialties:
Anesthesiology, Dentistry, Internal Medicine,
Internal Medicine-Gastroenterology, Internal
Medicine-Hematology, Internal Medicine-
Medical Oncology, Obstetrics/Gynecology,
Orthopedic Surgery

Perth Amboy

Raritan Bay Medical Center
Perth Amboy Division
530 New Brunswick Ave.
Perth Amboy, NJ 08861
908-442-3700
Teaching Specialties:
Internal Medicine

Piscataway

University of Medicine and Dentistry of New Jersey
Community Mental Health Center
at Piscataway
671 Hoes Lane
Piscataway, NJ 08854
908-235-5500
Teaching Specialties:
Psychiatry

Plainfield

Muhlenberg Regional Medical Center
Park Ave. & Randolph Rd.
Plainfield, NJ 07061
908-668-2000
Teaching Specialties:
Colon and Rectal Surgery, Internal Medicine,
Obstetrics/Gynecology, Surgery

Princeton

Medical Center at Princeton
253 Witherspoon St.
Princeton, NJ 08540
609-497-4000
Teaching Specialties:
Internal Medicine, Surgery, Urology

Summit

Overlook Hospital
99 Beauvoir Ave.
Summit, NJ 07901
908-522-2000
Teaching Specialties:
Dentistry, Internal Medicine, Psychiatry, Surgery

Trenton

Greater Trenton Community Mental Health Center
132 N. Warren St.
Trenton, NJ 08607
609-396-6788
Teaching Specialties:
Psychiatry

Helene Fuld Medical Center
750 Brunswick Ave.
Trenton, NJ 08638
609-695-3627
Teaching Specialties:
Internal Medicine

St. Francis Medical Center
601 Hamilton Ave.
Trenton, NJ 08629
609-599-5000
Teaching Specialties:
Internal Medicine, Surgery

Trenton Psychiatric Hospital
PO Box 7500
Trenton, NJ 08628
609-633-1500
Teaching Specialties:
Psychiatry

Voorhees

West Jersey Hospital-Voorhees
101 Carnie Blvd.
Voorhees, NJ 08043
609-772-5000
Teaching Specialties:
Otolaryngology

West Orange

Kessler Institute for Rehabilitation
1199 Pleasant Valley Way
West Orange, NJ 07052

201-731-3600
Teaching Specialties:
Physical Medicine and Rehabilitation

Woodbury

Underwood-Memorial Hospital
509 N. Broad St.
Woodbury, NJ 08096
609-845-0100
Teaching Specialties:
Surgery

NEW MEXICO
Albuquerque

Lovelace Medical Center
5400 Gibson Blvd., SE
Albuquerque, NM 87108
505-262-7000
Teaching Specialties:
Otolaryngology, Surgery, Urology

University Hospital
2211 Lomas Blvd., NE
Albuquerque, NM 87106
505-843-2121
Teaching Specialties:
Dermatology, Internal Medicine, Internal Medicine-Cardiovascular Disease, Internal Medicine-Endocrinology and Metabolism, Internal Medicine-Gastroenterology, Internal Medicine-Hematology, Internal Medicine-Infectious Diseases, Internal Medicine-Medical Oncology, Internal Medicine-Nephrology, Internal Medicine-Rheumatology, Neurology, Obstetrics/Gynecology, Orthopedic Surgery, Otolaryngology, Psychiatry, Surgery, Thoracic Surgery, Urology

University of New Mexico Mental Health Center
2600 Marble Ave., NE
Albuquerque, NM 87131
505-843-2870
Teaching Specialties:
Psychiatry

NEW YORK
Albany

Albany Medical Center Hospital
43 New Scotland Ave.
Albany, NY 12208
518-262-3125
Teaching Specialties:
Anesthesiology, Dentistry, Internal Medicine, Internal Medicine-Cardiovascular Disease, Internal Medicine-Endocrinology and Metabolism, Internal Medicine-Gastroenterology, Internal Medicine-Geriatric Medicine, Internal Medicine-Hematology, Internal Medicine-Infectious Diseases, Internal

Medicine-Medical Oncology, Internal Medicine-Nephrology, Neurological Surgery, Neurology, Obstetrics/Gynecology, Ophthalmology, Orthopedic Surgery, Otolaryngology, Physical Medicine and Rehabilitation, Psychiatry, Surgery, Surgery-Vascular Surgery, Thoracic Surgery, Urology

Capital District Psychiatric Center
75 New Scotland Ave.
Albany, NY 12208
518-447-9611
Teaching Specialties:
Psychiatry

Child's Hospital
25 Hackett Blvd.
Albany, NY 12208
518-487-7200
Teaching Specialties:
Otolaryngology

St. Peter's Hospital
315 S. Manning Blvd.
Albany, NY 12208
518-525-1550
Teaching Specialties:
Dentistry, Internal Medicine, Obstetrics/Gynecology, Orthopedic Surgery, Otolaryngology, Physical Medicine and Rehabilitation, Surgery

Bronx

Bronx-Lebanon Hospital Center
1276 Fulton Ave.
Bronx, NY 10456
718-590-1800
Teaching Specialties:
Dentistry, Internal Medicine, Internal Medicine-Cardiovascular Disease, Internal Medicine-Gastroenterology, Internal Medicine-Hematology, Internal Medicine-Nephrology, Obstetrics/Gynecology, Ophthalmology, Orthopedic Surgery, Psychiatry, Surgery

Bronx Municipal Hospital Center
1400 Pelham Pkwy. South
Bronx, NY 10461
718-918-8141
Teaching Specialties:
Allergy/Immunology, Anesthesiology, Dentistry, Dermatology, Internal Medicine, Internal Medicine-Cardiovascular Disease, Internal Medicine-Endocrinology and Metabolism, Internal Medicine-Gastroenterology, Internal Medicine-Hematology, Internal Medicine-Infectious Diseases, Internal Medicine-Medical Oncology, Internal Medicine-Nephrology, Internal Medicine-Rheumatology, Neurological Surgery, Neurology, Obstetrics/Gynecology, Ophthalmology, Orthopedic Surgery, Otolaryngology, Physical Medicine and Rehabilitation, Psychiatry, Surgery, Surgery-Vascular Surgery, Thoracic Surgery, Urology

Bronx Psychiatric Center
1500 Waters Pl.
Bronx, NY 10461
718-931-0600
Teaching Specialties:
Psychiatry

Lincoln Medical and Mental Health Center
234 E. 149th St.
Bronx, NY 10451
718-579-5000
Teaching Specialties:
Anesthesiology, Dentistry, Dermatology, Internal Medicine, Internal Medicine-Cardiovascular Disease, Internal Medicine-Endocrinology and Metabolism, Internal Medicine-Gastroenterology, Internal Medicine-Hematology, Internal Medicine-Infectious Diseases, Neurology, Obstetrics/Gynecology, Ophthalmology, Orthopedic Surgery, Otolaryngology, Physical Medicine and Rehabilitation, Psychiatry, Surgery, Urology

Montefiore Medical Center
Henry and Lucy Moses Division
111 E. 210th St.
Bronx, NY 10467
718-920-4321
Teaching Specialties:
Anesthesiology, Dentistry, Dermatology, Internal Medicine, Internal Medicine-Cardiovascular Disease, Internal Medicine-Endocrinology and Metabolism, Internal Medicine-Gastroenterology, Internal Medicine-Geriatric Medicine, Internal Medicine-Hematology, Internal Medicine-Infectious Diseases, Internal Medicine-Medical Oncology, Internal Medicine-Nephrology, Internal Medicine-Rheumatology, Neurological Surgery, Neurology, Obstetrics/Gynecology, Ophthalmology, Orthopedic Surgery, Otolaryngology, Physical Medicine and Rehabilitation, Psychiatry, Radiation Oncology, Surgery, Surgery-Vascular Surgery, Thoracic Surgery, Urology

Montefiore Medical Center
Jack D. Weiler Hospital of the Albert Einstein College of Medicine
1825 Eastchester Rd.
Bronx, NY 10461
718-904-2000
Teaching Specialties:
Allergy/Immunology, Anesthesiology, Dermatology, Internal Medicine, Internal Medicine-Cardiovascular Disease, Internal Medicine-Endocrinology and Metabolism, Neurology, Obstetrics/Gynecology, Ophthalmology, Orthopedic Surgery, Otolaryngology, Physical Medicine and Rehabilitation, Radiation Oncology, Surgery, Surgery-Vascular Surgery, Thoracic Surgery, Urology

North Central Bronx Hospital
3424 Kossuth Ave.
Bronx, NY 10467
718-519-5000
Teaching Specialties:
Dermatology, Internal Medicine, Internal Medicine-Endocrinology and Metabolism, Obstetrics/Gynecology, Ophthalmology, Orthopedic Surgery, Physical Medicine and Rehabilitation, Surgery, Surgery-Vascular Surgery, Urology

Our Lady of Mercy Medical Center
600 E. 233rd St.
Bronx, NY 10466
718-920-9000
Teaching Specialties:
Dentistry, Internal Medicine, Internal Medicine-Cardiovascular Disease, Internal Medicine-Gastroenterology, Internal Medicine-Hematology, Internal Medicine-Nephrology, Obstetrics/Gynecology, Ophthalmology, Surgery, Urology

St. Barnabas Hospital
183rd St. & Third Ave.
Bronx, NY 10457
718-960-6107
Teaching Specialties:
Dentistry, Internal Medicine

Brooklyn

Brookdale Hospital Medical Center
Rockaway Pkwy. & Linden Blvd.
Brooklyn, NY 11212
718-240-5000
Teaching Specialties:
Anesthesiology, Dentistry, Internal Medicine, Internal Medicine-Endocrinology and Metabolism, Internal Medicine-Gastroenterology, Internal Medicine-Hematology, Internal Medicine-Medical Oncology, Internal Medicine-Nephrology, Obstetrics/Gynecology, Ophthalmology, Orthopedic Surgery, Otolaryngology, Psychiatry, Surgery, Urology

Brooklyn Hospital Center
121 DeKalb Ave.
Brooklyn, NY 11201
718-250-8000
Teaching Specialties:
Dentistry, Internal Medicine, Internal Medicine-Cardiovascular Disease, Internal Medicine-Gastroenterology, Internal Medicine-Hematology, Internal Medicine-Medical Oncology, Obstetrics/Gynecology, Ophthalmology, Physical Medicine and Rehabilitation, Surgery

Coney Island Hospital
2601 Ocean Pkwy.
Brooklyn, NY 11235
718-615-4000

Teaching Specialties:
Anesthesiology, Internal Medicine, Internal Medicine-Cardiovascular Disease, Internal Medicine-Endocrinology and Metabolism, Internal Medicine-Hematology, Internal Medicine-Rheumatology, Obstetrics/Gynecology, Ophthalmology, Orthopedic Surgery, Surgery, Urology

Interfaith Medical Center
555 Prospect Pl.
Brooklyn, NY 11238
718-935-7000
Teaching Specialties:
Dentistry, Internal Medicine, Internal Medicine-Cardiovascular Disease, Internal Medicine-Endocrinology and Metabolism, Internal Medicine-Gastroenterology, Internal Medicine-Hematology, Internal Medicine-Medical Oncology, Internal Medicine-Nephrology, Obstetrics/Gynecology, Ophthalmology

Kings County Hospital Center
451 Clarkson Ave.
Brooklyn, NY 11203
718-245-3131
Teaching Specialties:
Allergy/Immunology, Anesthesiology, Dentistry, Dermatology, Internal Medicine, Internal Medicine-Cardiovascular Disease, Internal Medicine-Endocrinology and Metabolism, Internal Medicine-Gastroenterology, Internal Medicine-Hematology, Internal Medicine-Infectious Diseases, Internal Medicine-Medical Oncology, Internal Medicine-Nephrology, Internal Medicine-Rheumatology, Neurological Surgery, Neurology, Obstetrics/Gynecology, Ophthalmology, Orthopedic Surgery, Otolaryngology, Physical Medicine and Rehabilitation, Psychiatry, Radiation Oncology, Surgery, Thoracic Surgery, Urology

Kingsboro Psychiatric Center
681 Clarkson Ave.
Brooklyn, NY 11203
718-221-7700
Teaching Specialties:
Psychiatry

Kingsbrook Jewish Medical Center
585 Schenectady Ave.
Brooklyn, NY 11203
718-604-5000
Teaching Specialties:
Internal Medicine, Orthopedic Surgery, Physical Medicine and Rehabilitation

Long Island College Hospital
339 Hicks St.
Brooklyn, NY 11201
718-780-4651
Teaching Specialties:
Allergy/Immunology, Dentistry, Internal Medicine, Internal Medicine-Cardiovascular Disease, Internal Medicine-Gastroenterology,

Internal Medicine-Hematology, Internal Medicine-Infectious Diseases, Internal Medicine-Medical Oncology, Internal Medicine-Nephrology, Internal Medicine-Rheumatology, Obstetrics/Gynecology, Ophthalmology, Orthopedic Surgery, Otolaryngology, Radiation Oncology, Surgery, Urology

Lutheran Medical Center
150 55th St.
Brooklyn, NY 11220
718-630-7000
Teaching Specialties:
Dentistry, Internal Medicine, Obstetrics/Gynecology, Radiation Oncology

Maimonides Medical Center
4802 10th Ave.
Brooklyn, NY 11219
718-283-6000
Teaching Specialties:
Anesthesiology, Dentistry, Internal Medicine, Internal Medicine-Cardiovascular Disease, Internal Medicine-Gastroenterology, Internal Medicine-Hematology, Internal Medicine-Infectious Diseases, Internal Medicine-Medical Oncology, Internal Medicine-Nephrology, Obstetrics/Gynecology, Ophthalmology, Orthopedic Surgery, Psychiatry, Surgery, Thoracic Surgery, Urology

Methodist Hospital of Brooklyn
506 Sixth St.
Brooklyn, NY 11215
718-780-3000
Teaching Specialties:
Anesthesiology, Internal Medicine, Internal Medicine-Cardiovascular Disease, Internal Medicine-Hematology, Internal Medicine-Medical Oncology, Radiation Oncology, Surgery

St. Mary's Hospital
170 Buffalo Ave.
Brooklyn, NY 11213
718-221-3000
Teaching Specialties:
Internal Medicine, Internal Medicine-Hematology, Internal Medicine-Medical Oncology, Obstetrics/Gynecology, Orthopedic Surgery, Surgery

State University of New York Health Science Center at Brooklyn
University Hospital of Brooklyn
450 Clarkson Ave.
Brooklyn, NY 11203
718-270-1000
Teaching Specialties:
Allergy/Immunology, Dermatology, Internal Medicine, Internal Medicine-Cardiovascular Disease, Internal Medicine-Endocrinology and Metabolism, Internal Medicine-Gastroenterology, Internal Medicine-Hematology, Internal Medicine-Infectious Diseases, Internal Medicine-Medical Oncology, Internal Medicine-Nephrology, Internal Medicine-Rheumatology, Neurological Surgery, Neurology, Obstetrics/Gynecology, Ophthalmology, Orthopedic Surgery, Otolaryngology, Psychiatry, Surgery, Thoracic Surgery, Urology

Woodhull Medical and Mental Health Center
760 Broadway
Brooklyn, NY 11206
718-963-8000
Teaching Specialties:
Dentistry, Internal Medicine, Internal Medicine-Hematology, Internal Medicine-Medical Oncology, Surgery

Wyckoff Heights Medical Center
374 Stockholm St.
Brooklyn, NY 11237
718-963-7102
Teaching Specialties:
Dentistry, Internal Medicine

Buffalo

Buffalo General Hospital
100 High St.
Buffalo, NY 14203
716-845-5600
Teaching Specialties:
Allergy/Immunology, Anesthesiology, Colon and Rectal Surgery, Dermatology, Internal Medicine, Internal Medicine-Cardiovascular Disease, Internal Medicine-Gastroenterology, Internal Medicine-Hematology, Neurological Surgery, Obstetrics/Gynecology, Ophthalmology, Orthopedic Surgery, Physical Medicine and Rehabilitation, Surgery, Thoracic Surgery, Urology

Erie County Medical Center
462 Grider St.
Buffalo, NY 14215
716-898-3000
Teaching Specialties:
Anesthesiology, Dentistry, Dermatology, Hand Surgery, Internal Medicine, Internal Medicine-Cardiovascular Disease, Internal Medicine-Endocrinology and Metabolism, Internal Medicine-Gastroenterology, Internal Medicine-Hematology, Internal Medicine-Infectious Diseases, Internal Medicine-Nephrology, Internal Medicine-Rheumatology, Neurological Surgery, Neurology, Obstetrics/Gynecology, Ophthalmology, Orthopedic Surgery, Otolaryngology, Physical Medicine and Rehabilitation, Psychiatry, Surgery, Urology

Mercy Hospital
565 Abbott Rd.
Buffalo, NY 14220
716-826-7000
Teaching Specialties:
Internal Medicine

Millard Fillmore Hospitals
3 Gates Circle
Buffalo, NY 14209
716-887-4600
Teaching Specialties:
Anesthesiology, Dentistry, Hand Surgery, Internal Medicine, Internal Medicine-Cardiovascular Disease, Neurological Surgery, Obstetrics/Gynecology, Ophthalmology, Surgery, Thoracic Surgery

Millard Fillmore Hospitals
Dent Neurological Institute
3 Gates Circle
Buffalo, NY 14209
716-887-4793
Teaching Specialties:
Neurology

Roswell Park Cancer Institute
Elm & Carlton Sts.
Buffalo, NY 14263
716-845-2300
Teaching Specialties:
Dentistry, Internal Medicine-Gastroenterology, Internal Medicine-Medical Oncology, Thoracic Surgery, Urology

Sisters of Charity Hospital of Buffalo
2157 Main St.
Buffalo, NY 14214
716-862-2000
Teaching Specialties:
Internal Medicine, Obstetrics/Gynecology, Otolaryngology

State University of New York at Buffalo
School of Dental Medicine
325 Squire Hall
Buffalo, NY 14214
716-829-2383 (Clinical Affairs)
Teaching Specialties:
Dentistry

Camden

Our Lady of Lourdes Medical Center
1600 Haddon Ave.
Camden, NY 08103
609-757-3500
Teaching Specialties:
Obstetrics/Gynecology

Cooperstown

Mary Imogene Bassett Hospital
1 Atwell Rd.
Cooperstown, NY 13326
607-547-3100

Teaching Specialties:
Internal Medicine, Surgery

East Meadow

Nassau County Medical Center
2201 Hempstead Tpk.
East Meadow, NY 11554
516-572-0123
Teaching Specialties:
Allergy/Immunology, Anesthesiology, Dentistry, Internal Medicine, Internal Medicine-Cardiovascular Disease, Internal Medicine-Endocrinology and Metabolism, Internal Medicine-Gastroenterology, Internal Medicine-Hematology, Internal Medicine-Infectious Diseases, Internal Medicine-Medical Oncology, Internal Medicine-Nephrology, Neurology, Obstetrics/Gynecology, Ophthalmology, Orthopedic Surgery, Physical Medicine and Rehabilitation, Psychiatry, Surgery

Elmhurst

Elmhurst Hospital Center
79-01 Broadway
Elmhurst, NY 11373
718-334-4000
Teaching Specialties:
Anesthesiology, Dermatology, Internal Medicine, Internal Medicine-Cardiovascular Disease, Internal Medicine-Gastroenterology, Neurological Surgery, Obstetrics/Gynecology, Ophthalmology, Orthopedic Surgery, Otolaryngology, Physical Medicine and Rehabilitation, Psychiatry, Surgery, Surgery-Vascular Surgery, Urology

St. John's Queens Hospital
90-02 Queens Blvd.
Elmhurst, NY 11373
718-457-1300
Teaching Specialties:
Internal Medicine, Obstetrics/Gynecology, Orthopedic Surgery

Far Rockaway

Peninsula Hospital Center
51-15 Beach Channel Dr.
Far Rockaway, NY 11691-1074
718-945-7100
Teaching Specialties:
Dentistry

St. John's Episcopal Hospital-South Shore
327 Beach 19th St.
Far Rockaway, NY 11691
718-869-7000
Teaching Specialties:
Internal Medicine, Obstetrics/Gynecology

Flushing

Flushing Hospital Medical Center
45th Ave. & Parsons Blvd.
Flushing, NY 11355
718-670-5000
Teaching Specialties:
Dentistry, Internal Medicine, Obstetrics/Gynecology, Surgery

New York Hospital Medical Center of Queens
56-45 Main St.
Flushing, NY 11355
718-670-1021
Teaching Specialties:
Dentistry, Internal Medicine, Internal Medicine-Gastroenterology, Internal Medicine-Infectious Diseases, Internal Medicine-Nephrology, Obstetrics/Gynecology, Surgery

Forest Hills

La Guardia Hospital
102-01 66th Rd.
Forest Hills, NY 11375
718-830-4000
Teaching Specialties:
Internal Medicine, Surgery, Urology

Harrison

St. Vincent's Hospital and Medical Center of New York
Westchester Branch
275 North St.
Harrison, NY 10528
914-967-6500
Teaching Specialties:
Psychiatry

Huntington

Huntington Hospital
270 Park Ave.
Huntington, NY 11743
516-351-2000
Teaching Specialties:
Surgery

Jamaica

Catholic Medical Center of Brooklyn and Queens
88-25 153rd St.
Jamaica, NY 11432
718-558-6900
Teaching Specialties:
Dentistry

Jamaica Hospital
8900 Van Wyck Expwy.
Jamaica, NY 11418
718-206-6000

Teaching Specialties:
Dentistry, Internal Medicine, Internal Medicine-Cardiovascular Disease, Internal Medicine-Gastroenterology, Internal Medicine-Hematology, Obstetrics/Gynecology, Surgery

Mary Immaculate Hospital
152-11 89th Ave.
Jamaica, NY 11432
718-291-3300
Teaching Specialties:
Internal Medicine, Internal Medicine-Cardiovascular Disease, Internal Medicine-Gastroenterology, Internal Medicine-Hematology, Internal Medicine-Infectious Diseases, Internal Medicine-Medical Oncology, Obstetrics/Gynecology, Ophthalmology, Orthopedic Surgery, Surgery

Queens Hospital Center
82-68 164th St.
Jamaica, NY 11432
718-883-3000
Teaching Specialties:
Internal Medicine, Internal Medicine-Endocrinology and Metabolism, Neurology, Obstetrics/Gynecology, Ophthalmology, Orthopedic Surgery, Otolaryngology, Physical Medicine and Rehabilitation, Psychiatry, Surgery, Urology

Johnson City

Wilson Memorial Hospital
33-57 Harrison St.
Johnson City, NY 13790
607-763-6060
Teaching Specialties:
Internal Medicine

Manhasset

North Shore University Hospital
300 Community Dr.
Manhasset, NY 11030
516-562-0100
Teaching Specialties:
Allergy/Immunology, Dentistry, Internal Medicine, Internal Medicine-Cardiovascular Disease, Internal Medicine-Gastroenterology, Internal Medicine-Geriatric Medicine, Internal Medicine-Hematology, Internal Medicine-Infectious Diseases, Internal Medicine-Medical Oncology, Internal Medicine-Nephrology, Internal Medicine-Rheumatology, Neurology, Obstetrics/Gynecology, Ophthalmology, Psychiatry, Surgery

Middletown

Middletown Psychiatric Center
141 Monhagen Ave.
Middletown, NY 10940
914-342-5511
Teaching Specialties:
Psychiatry

Mineola

Winthrop-University Hospital
259 First St.
Mineola, NY 11501
516-663-0333
Teaching Specialties:
Internal Medicine, Internal Medicine-Cardio-
vascular Disease, Internal Medicine-En-
docrinology and Metabolism, Internal
Medicine-Gastroenterology, Internal
Medicine-Hematology, Internal Medicine-In-
fectious Diseases, Internal Medicine-Medical
Oncology, Internal Medicine-Nephrology,
Obstetrics/Gynecology, Surgery

New Hyde Park

**Parker Jewish Institute for Health
Care and Rehabilitation**
271-11 76th Ave.
New Hyde Park, NY 11040
718-289-2160
Teaching Specialties:
Physical Medicine and Rehabilitation

Long Island Jewish Medical Center
270-05 76th Ave.
New Hyde Park, NY 11040
718-470-7000
Teaching Specialties:
Allergy/Immunology, Anesthesiology, Den-
tistry, Internal Medicine, Internal Medicine-
Cardiovascular Disease, Internal Medicine-
Endocrinology and Metabolism, Internal
Medicine-Gastroenterology, Internal
Medicine-Geriatric Medicine, Internal
Medicine-Hematology, Internal Medicine-In-
fectious Diseases, Internal Medicine-Medical
Oncology, Internal Medicine-Nephrology, In-
ternal Medicine-Rheumatology, Neurology,
Obstetrics/Gynecology, Ophthalmology, Or-
thopedic Surgery, Otolaryngology, Physical
Medicine and Rehabilitation, Psychiatry,
Surgery, Surgery-Vascular Surgery, Thoracic
Surgery, Urology

Long Island Jewish Medical Center
Hillside Hospital
270-05 76th Ave.
New Hyde Park, NY 11040
516-470-7000
Teaching Specialties:
Psychiatry

New Rochelle

**New Rochelle Hospital Medical
Center**
16 Guion Pl.
New Rochelle, NY 10801
914-632-5000
Teaching Specialties:
Internal Medicine, Surgery

New York

Bellevue Hospital Center
462 First Ave. & 27th St.
New York, NY 10016
212-562-4141
Teaching Specialties:
Anesthesiology, Dermatology, Internal
Medicine, Internal Medicine-Cardiovascular
Disease, Internal Medicine-Endocrinology
and Metabolism, Internal Medicine-Gastroen-
terology, Internal Medicine-Hematology, In-
ternal Medicine-Infectious Diseases, Internal
Medicine-Medical Oncology, Internal
Medicine-Nephrology, Internal Medicine-
Rheumatology, Neurological Surgery, Neurol-
ogy, Obstetrics/Gynecology, Ophthalmology,
Orthopedic Surgery, Otolaryngology, Physical
Medicine and Rehabilitation, Psychiatry, Ra-
diation Oncology, Surgery, Surgery-Vascular
Surgery, Thoracic Surgery, Urology

Beth Israel Medical Center
First Ave. & 16th St.
New York, NY 10003
212-420-2000
Teaching Specialties:
Anesthesiology, Dentistry, Dermatology, In-
ternal Medicine, Internal Medicine-Cardio-
vascular Disease, Internal Medicine-En-
docrinology and Metabolism, Internal
Medicine-Gastroenterology, Internal
Medicine-Hematology, Internal Medicine-In-
fectious Diseases, Internal Medicine-Medical
Oncology, Internal Medicine-Nephrology,
Obstetrics/Gynecology, Ophthalmology,
Physical Medicine and Rehabilitation, Psychi-
atry, Radiation Oncology, Surgery, Urology

Cabrini Medical Center
227 E. 19th St.
New York, NY 10003
212-995-6000
Teaching Specialties:
Internal Medicine, Internal Medicine-Cardio-
vascular Disease, Internal Medicine-Gastroen-
terology, Internal Medicine-Hematology, In-
ternal Medicine-Infectious Diseases, Internal
Medicine-Medical Oncology, Internal
Medicine-Rheumatology, Ophthalmology,
Psychiatry, Surgery, Urology

Coler Memorial Hospital
Franklin D. Roosevelt Island
New York, NY 10044
212-848-6000
Teaching Specialties:
Dentistry

**Columbia University School
of Dental and Oral Surgery**
Columbia-Presbyterian
Medical Center
622 W. 168th St.
New York, NY 10032
212-305-2500

Teaching Specialties:
Dentistry

Goldwater Memorial Hospital
Franklin D. Roosevelt Island
New York, NY 10044
212-318-8000
Teaching Specialties:
Dentistry, Physical Medicine and Rehabilita-
tion

Harlem Hospital Center
506 Lenox Ave.
New York, NY 10037
212-939-1000
Teaching Specialties:
Dentistry, Internal Medicine, Internal
Medicine-Cardiovascular Disease, Internal
Medicine-Gastroenterology, Internal
Medicine-Hematology, Internal Medicine-In-
fectious Diseases, Internal Medicine-Medical
Oncology, Internal Medicine-Nephrology,
Neurology, Obstetrics/Gynecology, Ophthal-
mology, Orthopedic Surgery, Psychiatry,
Surgery

**Hospital for Joint Diseases
Orthopedic Institute**
301 E. 17th St.
New York, NY 10003
212-598-6000
Teaching Specialties:
Internal Medicine-Rheumatology, Orthopedic Surgery, Physical Medicine and Rehabilitation

Hospital for Special Surgery
535 E. 70th St.
New York, NY 10021
212-606-1000
Teaching Specialties:
Hand Surgery, Orthopedic Surgery

Lenox Hill Hospital
100 E. 77th St.
New York, NY 10021
212-434-2000
Teaching Specialties:
Dentistry, Internal Medicine, Internal
Medicine-Cardiovascular Disease, Internal
Medicine-Gastroenterology, Internal
Medicine-Hematology, Internal Medicine-In-
fectious Diseases, Internal Medicine-Medical
Oncology, Internal Medicine-Nephrology,
Obstetrics/Gynecology, Ophthalmology, Or-
thopedic Surgery, Surgery, Urology

**Manhattan Eye, Ear and Throat
Hospital**
210 E. 64th St.
New York, NY 10021
212-838-9200
Teaching Specialties:
Ophthalmology, Otolaryngology

Manhattan Psychiatric Center-Ward's Island
600 E. 125th St.
New York, NY 10035
212-369-0500
Teaching Specialties:
Psychiatry

Memorial Sloan-Kettering Cancer Center
1275 York Ave.
New York, NY 10021
800-525-2225
212-639-2000
Teaching Specialties:
Anesthesiology, Dentistry, Internal Medicine, Internal Medicine-Cardiovascular Disease, Internal Medicine-Gastroenterology, Internal Medicine-Hematology, Internal Medicine-Infectious Diseases, Internal Medicine-Medical Oncology, Neurology, Otolaryngology, Physical Medicine and Rehabilitation, Radiation Oncology, Surgery, Thoracic Surgery, Urology

Metropolitan Hospital Center
1901 First Ave.
New York, NY 10029
212-423-6262
Teaching Specialties:
Anesthesiology, Dentistry, Dermatology, Internal Medicine, Internal Medicine-Cardiovascular Disease, Internal Medicine-Gastroenterology, Internal Medicine-Hematology, Internal Medicine-Infectious Diseases, Internal Medicine-Nephrology, Internal Medicine-Rheumatology, Neurology, Obstetrics/Gynecology, Ophthalmology, Orthopedic Surgery, Physical Medicine and Rehabilitation, Psychiatry, Surgery, Urology

Mt. Sinai Medical Center
1 Gustave Levy Pl.
New York, NY 10029
212-241-6500
Teaching Specialties:
Allergy/Immunology, Anesthesiology, Dentistry, Dermatology, Internal Medicine, Internal Medicine-Cardiovascular Disease, Internal Medicine-Endocrinology and Metabolism, Internal Medicine-Gastroenterology, Internal Medicine-Geriatric Medicine, Internal Medicine-Hematology, Internal Medicine-Infectious Diseases, Internal Medicine-Medical Oncology, Internal Medicine-Nephrology, Internal Medicine-Rheumatology, Neurological Surgery, Neurology, Obstetrics/Gynecology, Ophthalmology, Orthopedic Surgery, Otolaryngology, Physical Medicine and Rehabilitation, Psychiatry, Surgery, Surgery-Vascular Surgery, Thoracic Surgery, Urology

New York Eye and Ear Infirmary
310 E. 14th St.
New York, NY 10003
212-979-4000
Teaching Specialties:
Ophthalmology, Otolaryngology

New York Hospital-Cornell Medical Center
525 E. 68th St.
New York, NY 10021
212-746-5000
Teaching Specialties:
Allergy/Immunology, Anesthesiology, Dentistry, Dermatology, Hand Surgery, Internal Medicine, Internal Medicine-Cardiovascular Disease, Internal Medicine-Endocrinology and Metabolism, Internal Medicine-Gastroenterology, Internal Medicine-Hematology, Internal Medicine-Infectious Diseases, Internal Medicine-Medical Oncology, Internal Medicine-Nephrology, Internal Medicine-Rheumatology, Neurological Surgery, Neurology, Obstetrics/Gynecology, Ophthalmology, Orthopedic Surgery, Otolaryngology, Physical Medicine and Rehabilitation, Psychiatry, Surgery, Thoracic Surgery, Urology

New York Hospital
Payne Whitney Psychiatric Clinic
525 E. 68th St.
New York, NY 10021
212-746-5454
Teaching Specialties:
Psychiatry

New York Infirmary-Beekman Downtown Hospital
170 William St.
New York, NY 10038
212-312-5000
Teaching Specialties:
Internal Medicine, Obstetrics/Gynecology

New York State Psychiatric Institute
722 W. 168th St.
New York, NY 10032
212-960-2200
Teaching Specialties:
Psychiatry

New York University College of Dentistry
345 E. 24th St.
New York, NY 10010-4099
212-998-9800
Teaching Specialties:
Dentistry

New York University Medical Center
560 First Ave.
New York, NY 10016
212-263-7300
Teaching Specialties:
Anesthesiology, Dermatology, Internal Medicine, Neurological Surgery, Neurology, Obstetrics/Gynecology, Ophthalmology, Orthopedic Surgery, Otolaryngology, Psychiatry, Radiation Oncology, Surgery-Vascular Surgery, Thoracic Surgery, Urology

New York University Medical Center
Rusk Institute
400 E. 34th St.
New York, NY 10016
212-263-6030
Teaching Specialties:
Physical Medicine and Rehabilitation

North General Hospital
1879 Madison Ave.
New York, NY 10035
212-423-4000
Teaching Specialties:
Internal Medicine, Ophthalmology, Surgery

Presbyterian Hospital in the City of New York
Columbia-Presbyterian Medical Center
622 W. 168th St.
New York, NY 10032
212-305-2500
Teaching Specialties:
Allergy/Immunology, Anesthesiology, Dermatology, Internal Medicine, Internal Medicine-Cardiovascular Disease, Internal Medicine-Endocrinology and Metabolism, Internal Medicine-Gastroenterology, Internal Medicine-Hematology, Internal Medicine-Infectious Diseases, Internal Medicine-Medical Oncology, Internal Medicine-Nephrology, Internal Medicine-Rheumatology, Neurological Surgery, Neurology, Obstetrics/Gynecology, Ophthalmology, Orthopedic Surgery, Otolaryngology, Physical Medicine and Rehabilitation, Psychiatry, Radiation Oncology, Surgery, Thoracic Surgery, Urology

St. Luke's-Roosevelt Hospital Center
Roosevelt Division
1000 10th Avenue
New York, NY 10019
212-523-4000
Teaching Specialties:
Allergy/Immunology, Colon and Rectal Surgery, Internal Medicine, Internal Medicine-Gastroenterology, Internal Medicine-Hematology, Internal Medicine-Medical Oncology, Obstetrics/Gynecology, Otolaryngology, Surgery, Urology

St. Luke's-Roosevelt Hospital Center
St. Luke's Division
1111 Amsterdam Ave.
New York, NY 10025
212-523-4000

Teaching Specialties:
Anesthesiology, Dentistry, Dermatology, Hand Surgery, Internal Medicine, Internal Medicine-Cardiovascular Disease, Internal Medicine-Endocrinology and Metabolism, Internal Medicine-Gastroenterology, Internal Medicine-Hematology, Internal Medicine-Infectious Diseases, Internal Medicine-Medical Oncology, Internal Medicine-Nephrology, Internal Medicine-Rheumatology, Obstetrics/Gynecology, Ophthalmology, Orthopedic Surgery, Otolaryngology, Psychiatry, Urology

St. Vincent's Hospital and Medical Center of New York
153 W. 11th St.
New York, NY 10011
212-604-7000
Teaching Specialties:
Anesthesiology, Internal Medicine, Internal Medicine-Cardiovascular Disease, Internal Medicine-Gastroenterology, Internal Medicine-Hematology, Internal Medicine-Infectious Diseases, Internal Medicine-Medical Oncology, Internal Medicine-Nephrology, Internal Medicine-Rheumatology, Neurology, Obstetrics/Gynecology, Ophthalmology, Orthopedic Surgery, Otolaryngology, Physical Medicine and Rehabilitation, Psychiatry, Surgery

Oceanside

South Nassau Communities Hospital
2445 Oceanside Rd.
Oceanside, NY 11572
516-763-2030
Teaching Specialties:
Surgery

Port Jefferson

St. Charles Hospital and Rehabilitation Center
200 Belle Terre Rd.
Port Jefferson, NY 11777
516-474-6000
Teaching Specialties:
Dentistry, Orthopedic Surgery

Queens Village

Creedmoor Psychiatric Center
80-45 Winchester Blvd.
Queens Village, NY 11427
718-464-7500
Teaching Specialties:
Psychiatry

Rochester

Eastman Dental Center
625 Elmwood Ave.
Rochester, NY 14620
716-275-5051

Teaching Specialties:
Dentistry

Genesee Hospital
224 Alexander St.
Rochester, NY 14607
716-263-6000
Teaching Specialties:
Dentistry, Internal Medicine, Obstetrics/Gynecology, Orthopedic Surgery, Otolaryngology, Surgery, Surgery-Vascular Surgery, Urology

Highland Hospital of Rochester
1000 South Ave.
Rochester, NY 14620
716-473-2200
Teaching Specialties:
Internal Medicine, Obstetrics/Gynecology, Orthopedic Surgery, Surgery

Monroe Community Hospital
435 E. Henrietta Rd.
Rochester, NY 14620
716-274-7100
Teaching Specialties:
Internal Medicine-Rheumatology, Physical Medicine and Rehabilitation

Rochester General Hospital
1425 Portland Ave.
Rochester, NY 14621
716-338-4000
Teaching Specialties:
Internal Medicine, Internal Medicine-Hematology, Internal Medicine-Medical Oncology, Obstetrics/Gynecology, Orthopedic Surgery, Otolaryngology, Surgery, Surgery-Vascular Surgery, Thoracic Surgery, Urology

St. Mary's Hospital
89 Genesee St.
Rochester, NY 14611
716-464-3000
Teaching Specialties:
Internal Medicine, Internal Medicine-Gastroenterology, Ophthalmology, Surgery

Strong Memorial Hospital of the University of Rochester
601 Elmwood Ave.
Rochester, NY 14642
716-275-2121
Teaching Specialties:
Allergy/Immunology, Anesthesiology, Dentistry, Dermatology, Hand Surgery, Internal Medicine, Internal Medicine-Cardiovascular Disease, Internal Medicine-Endocrinology and Metabolism, Internal Medicine-Gastroenterology, Internal Medicine-Hematology, Internal Medicine-Infectious Diseases, Internal Medicine-Medical Oncology, Internal Medicine-Nephrology, Internal Medicine-Rheumatology, Neurological Surgery, Neurology, Obstetrics/Gynecology, Ophthalmology,

Orthopedic Surgery, Otolaryngology, Physical Medicine and Rehabilitation, Psychiatry, Radiation Oncology, Surgery, Surgery-Vascular Surgery, Thoracic Surgery, Urology

Rockville Centre

Mercy Hospital
1000 N. Village Ave.
Rockville Centre, NY 11570
516-255-0111
Teaching Specialties:
Obstetrics/Gynecology

Schenectady

Ellis Hospital
1101 Nott St.
Schenectady, NY 12308
518-382-4124
Teaching Specialties:
Internal Medicine, Orthopedic Surgery

St. Clare's Hospital of Schenectady
600 McClellan St.
Schenectady, NY 12304
518-382-2000
Teaching Specialties:
Dentistry

Sunnyview Hospital and Rehabilitation Center
1270 Belmont Ave.
Schenectady, NY 12308
518-382-4523
Teaching Specialties:
Physical Medicine and Rehabilitation

Staten Island

Bayley Seton Hospital
75 Vanderbilt Ave.
Staten Island, NY 10304
718-390-6000
Teaching Specialties:
Dermatology, Ophthalmology

St. Vincent's Medical Center of Richmond
355 Bard Ave.
Staten Island, NY 10310
718-876-1234
Teaching Specialties:
Internal Medicine, Internal Medicine-Cardiovascular Disease, Obstetrics/Gynecology, Psychiatry, Surgery

Staten Island University Hospital
475 Seaview Ave.
Staten Island, NY 10305
718-226-9000
Teaching Specialties:
Dentistry, Internal Medicine, Obstetrics/Gynecology, Surgery

Stony Brook

State University of New York at Stony Brook
School of Dental Medicine
Health Sciences Center
Stony Brook, NY 11790
516-632-8989
Teaching Specialties:
Dentistry

State University of New York at Stony Brook University Hospital
Health Sciences Center
Stony Brook, NY 11794
516-689-8333
Teaching Specialties:
Allergy/Immunology, Anesthesiology, Dermatology, Internal Medicine, Internal Medicine-Cardiovascular Disease, Internal Medicine-Endocrinology and Metabolism, Internal Medicine-Gastroenterology, Internal Medicine-Hematology, Internal Medicine-Infectious Diseases, Internal Medicine-Medical Oncology, Internal Medicine-Nephrology, Internal Medicine-Rheumatology, Neurology, Obstetrics/Gynecology, Orthopedic Surgery, Psychiatry, Surgery, Surgery-Vascular Surgery

Syracuse

Community-General Hospital of Greater Syracuse
Broad Rd.
Syracuse, NY 13215
315-492-5011
Teaching Specialties:
Otolaryngology, Surgery

Crouse-Irving Memorial Hospital
736 Irving Ave.
Syracuse, NY 13210
315-470-7111
Teaching Specialties:
Anesthesiology, Internal Medicine, Internal Medicine-Infectious Diseases, Neurological Surgery, Neurology, Obstetrics/Gynecology, Ophthalmology, Orthopedic Surgery, Otolaryngology, Surgery, Thoracic Surgery, Urology

Richard H. Hutchings Psychiatric Center
620 Madison St.
Syracuse, NY 13210
315-473-4980
Teaching Specialties:
Psychiatry

St. Camillus Health and Rehabilitation Center
813 Fay Rd.
Syracuse, NY 13219-3098
315-488-2951

Teaching Specialties:
Physical Medicine and Rehabilitation

St. Joseph's Hospital Health Center
301 Prospect Ave.
Syracuse, NY 13203
315-448-5111
Teaching Specialties:
Anesthesiology, Dentistry, Obstetrics/Gynecology, Otolaryngology, Urology

State University of New York Health Science Center
University Hospital
750 E. Adams St.
Syracuse, NY 13210
315-464-5540
Teaching Specialties:
Anesthesiology, Dentistry, Internal Medicine, Internal Medicine-Cardiovascular Disease, Internal Medicine-Endocrinology and Metabolism, Internal Medicine-Gastroenterology, Internal Medicine-Hematology, Internal Medicine-Infectious Diseases, Internal Medicine-Medical Oncology, Internal Medicine-Nephrology, Internal Medicine-Rheumatology, Neurological Surgery, Neurology, Obstetrics/Gynecology, Ophthalmology, Orthopedic Surgery, Otolaryngology, Physical Medicine and Rehabilitation, Psychiatry, Radiation Oncology, Surgery, Thoracic Surgery, Urology

Utica

St. Luke's Memorial Hospital Center
PO Box 479
Utica, NY 13503
315-798-6000
Teaching Specialties:
Dentistry

Valhalla

Westchester County Medical Center
Valhalla Campus
Valhalla, NY 10595
914-285-7000
Teaching Specialties:
Anesthesiology, Dentistry, Dermatology, Internal Medicine, Internal Medicine-Cardiovascular Disease, Internal Medicine-Endocrinology and Metabolism, Internal Medicine-Gastroenterology, Internal Medicine-Geriatric Medicine, Internal Medicine-Hematology, Internal Medicine-Infectious Diseases, Internal Medicine-Medical Oncology, Internal Medicine-Nephrology, Internal Medicine-Rheumatology, Neurology, Obstetrics/Gynecology, Ophthalmology, Orthopedic Surgery, Physical Medicine and Rehabilitation, Psychiatry, Surgery, Urology

West Haverstraw

Helen Hayes Hospital
Route 9W
West Haverstraw, NY 10993
914-947-3000
Teaching Specialties:
Orthopedic Surgery

White Plains

New York Hospital
Westchester Division
21 Bloomingdale Rd.
White Plains, NY 10605
914-682-9100
Teaching Specialties:
Psychiatry

NORTH CAROLINA
Chapel Hill

University of North Carolina at Chapel Hill
School of Dentistry
CB 7450, Tarrson Hall
Chapel Hill, NC 27599-7450
919-966-1161
Teaching Specialties:
Dentistry

University of North Carolina Hospitals
101 Manning Dr.
Chapel Hill, NC 27514
919-966-4131
Teaching Specialties:
Anesthesiology, Dermatology, Internal Medicine, Internal Medicine-Cardiovascular Disease, Internal Medicine-Endocrinology and Metabolism, Internal Medicine-Gastroenterology, Internal Medicine-Geriatric Medicine, Internal Medicine-Hematology, Internal Medicine-Infectious Diseases, Internal Medicine-Medical Oncology, Internal Medicine-Nephrology, Internal Medicine-Rheumatology, Neurological Surgery, Neurology, Obstetrics/Gynecology, Ophthalmology, Orthopedic Surgery, Otolaryngology, Psychiatry, Radiation Oncology, Surgery, Surgery-Vascular Surgery, Thoracic Surgery, Urology

Charlotte

Carolinas Medical Center
1000 Blythe Blvd.
Charlotte, NC 28203
704-355-2000
Teaching Specialties:
Dentistry, Internal Medicine, Obstetrics/Gynecology, Orthopedic Surgery, Surgery, Surgery-Vascular Surgery, Thoracic Surgery

Orthopaedic Hospital of Charlotte
1901 Randolph Rd.
Charlotte, NC 28207
704-375-6792
Teaching Specialties:
Orthopedic Surgery

Durham

Duke University Medical Center
Erwin Road
Durham, NC 27710
919-684-8111
Teaching Specialties:
Anesthesiology, Dermatology, Internal Medicine, Internal Medicine-Cardiovascular Disease, Internal Medicine-Endocrinology and Metabolism, Internal Medicine-Gastroenterology, Internal Medicine-Geriatric Medicine, Internal Medicine-Hematology, Internal Medicine-Infectious Diseases, Internal Medicine-Medical Oncology, Internal Medicine-Nephrology, Internal Medicine-Rheumatology, Neurological Surgery, Neurology, Obstetrics/Gynecology, Ophthalmology, Orthopedic Surgery, Otolaryngology, Psychiatry, Radiation Oncology, Surgery, Thoracic Surgery, Urology

Durham County General Hospital
3643 N. Roxboro St.
Durham, NC 27704
919-470-4000
Teaching Specialties:
Neurological Surgery, Orthopedic Surgery, Surgery

North Carolina Eye & Ear Hospital & Clinic
1110 W. Main St.
Durham, NC 27701
919-682-9341
Teaching Specialties:
Ophthalmology

Goldsboro

Cherry Hospital
Caller Box 8000
Goldsboro, NC 27533
919-731-3200
Teaching Specialties:
Psychiatry

Greensboro

Moses H. Cone Memorial Hospital
1200 N. Elm St.
Greensboro, NC 27401
910-574-7000
Teaching Specialties:
Internal Medicine

Greenville

East Carolina University School of Medicine
Family Practice Center,
Department of Dentistry
600 Moie Blvd.
Greenville, NC 27858
919-816-4618
Teaching Specialties:
Dentistry

Pitt County Memorial Hospital
2100 Stantonsburg Rd.
Greenville, NC 27834
919-816-4100
Teaching Specialties:
Allergy/Immunology, Internal Medicine, Internal Medicine-Cardiovascular Disease, Internal Medicine-Endocrinology and Metabolism, Internal Medicine-Nephrology, Obstetrics/Gynecology, Psychiatry, Surgery

Pitt County Mental Health Center
203 Government Circle
Greenville, NC 27834
919-413-1600
Teaching Specialties:
Psychiatry

Raleigh

Dorothea Dix Hospital
820 S. Boylan Ave.
Raleigh, NC 27603
919-733-5324
Teaching Specialties:
Psychiatry

Wake Medical Center
3000 New Bern Ave.
Raleigh, NC 27610
919-250-8000
Teaching Specialties:
Obstetrics/Gynecology, Orthopedic Surgery, Surgery, Urology

Wilmington

New Hanover Regional Medical Center
2131 S. 17th St.
Wilmington, NC 28402
919-343-7000
Teaching Specialties:
Internal Medicine, Obstetrics/Gynecology, Surgery

Winston-Salem

Bowman Gray School of Medicine
Department of Dentistry
Medical Center Blvd.
Winston-Salem, NC 27157

910-716-2011
Teaching Specialties:
Dentistry

Forsyth Memorial Hospital
3333 Silas Creek Pkwy.
Winston-Salem, NC 27103
910-718-5000
Teaching Specialties:
Obstetrics/Gynecology, Surgery, Urology

North Carolina Baptist Hospital
Medical Center Blvd.
Winston-Salem, NC 27157
910-716-2011
Teaching Specialties:
Allergy/Immunology, Anesthesiology, Dermatology, Internal Medicine, Internal Medicine-Cardiovascular Disease, Internal Medicine-Gastroenterology, Internal Medicine-Geriatric Medicine, Internal Medicine-Infectious Diseases, Internal Medicine-Medical Oncology, Internal Medicine-Nephrology, Internal Medicine-Rheumatology, Neurological Surgery, Neurology, Obstetrics/Gynecology, Ophthalmology, Orthopedic Surgery, Otolaryngology, Psychiatry, Radiation Oncology, Surgery, Thoracic Surgery, Urology

NORTH DAKOTA

Fargo

Dakota Hospital
1720 S. University Dr.
Fargo, ND 58103
701-280-4100
Teaching Specialties:
Internal Medicine

Southeast Human Services Center
2624 Ninth Ave., SW
Fargo, ND 58103-2350
701-298-4500
Teaching Specialties:
Psychiatry

St. Luke's Hospitals-Meritcare
720 Fourth St. North
Fargo, ND 58122
701-234-6000
Teaching Specialties:
Internal Medicine, Psychiatry, Surgery

Grand Forks

United Hospital
1200 S. Columbia Rd.
Grand Forks, ND 58201
701-780-5000
Teaching Specialties:
Surgery

OHIO

Akron

Akron City Hospital
525 Market St.
Akron, OH 44309
330-375-3000
Teaching Specialties:
Internal Medicine, Obstetrics/Gynecology, Ophthalmology, Orthopedic Surgery, Surgery, Urology

Akron General Medical Center
400 Wabash Ave.
Akron, OH 44307
330-384-6000
Teaching Specialties:
Internal Medicine, Obstetrics/Gynecology, Orthopedic Surgery, Psychiatry, Surgery, Urology

St. Thomas Medical Center
444 N. Main St.
Akron, OH 44310
330-375-3000
Teaching Specialties:
Internal Medicine, Psychiatry

Canton

Aultman Hospital
2600 Sixth St., SW
Canton, OH 44710
330-452-9911
Teaching Specialties:
Internal Medicine, Obstetrics/Gynecology

Timken Mercy Medical Center
1320 Timken Mercy Dr., NW
Canton, OH 44708
330-489-1000
Teaching Specialties:
Internal Medicine

Cincinnati

Bethesda Oak Hospital
619 Oak St.
Cincinnati, OH 45206
513-569-6111
Teaching Specialties:
Hand Surgery, Obstetrics/Gynecology, Orthopedic Surgery

Christ Hospital
2139 Auburn Ave.
Cincinnati, OH 45219
513-369-2000
Teaching Specialties:
Internal Medicine, Neurological Surgery, Obstetrics/Gynecology, Surgery

Good Samaritan Hospital
375 Dicksmith Ave.
Cincinnati, OH 45220
513-872-1400
Teaching Specialties:
Internal Medicine, Neurological Surgery, Obstetrics/Gynecology, Orthopedic Surgery, Surgery, Surgery-Vascular Surgery

Jewish Hospital of Cincinnati
3200 Burnet Ave.
Cincinnati, OH 45229
513-569-2000
Teaching Specialties:
Internal Medicine, Surgery

Providence Hospital
2446 Kipling Ave.
Cincinnati, OH 45239
513-853-5000
Teaching Specialties:
Surgery

University of Cincinnati Hospital
234 Goodman St.
Cincinnati, OH 45267
513-558-1000
Teaching Specialties:
Allergy/Immunology, Anesthesiology, Dentistry, Dermatology, Hand Surgery, Internal Medicine, Internal Medicine-Cardiovascular Disease, Internal Medicine-Endocrinology and Metabolism, Internal Medicine-Gastroenterology, Internal Medicine-Hematology, Internal Medicine-Infectious Diseases, Internal Medicine-Medical Oncology, Internal Medicine-Nephrology, Internal Medicine-Rheumatology, Neurological Surgery, Neurology, Obstetrics/Gynecology, Ophthalmology, Orthopedic Surgery, Otolaryngology, Physical Medicine and Rehabilitation, Psychiatry, Radiation Oncology, Surgery, Urology

Cleveland

Case Western Reserve University School of Dentistry
2123 Abington Rd.
Cleveland, OH 44106-4905
216-368-3200
Teaching Specialties:
Dentistry

Cleveland Clinic
1 Clinical Center
9500 Euclid Ave.
Cleveland, OH 44195
800-223-2273
216-444-2200
Teaching Specialties:
Allergy/Immunology, Anesthesiology, Colon and Rectal Surgery, Dentistry, Dermatology, Internal Medicine, Internal Medicine-Cardiovascular Disease, Internal Medicine-Endocrinology and Metabolism, Internal Medicine-Gastroenterology, Internal Medicine-Geriatric Medicine, Internal Medicine-Hematology, Internal Medicine-Infectious Diseases, Internal Medicine-Medical Oncology, Internal Medicine-Nephrology, Internal Medicine-Rheumatology, Neurological Surgery, Neurology, Ophthalmology, Orthopedic Surgery, Otolaryngology, Psychiatry, Radiation Oncology, Surgery, Surgery-Vascular Surgery, Thoracic Surgery, Urology

Cleveland Psychiatric Institute
1708 Southpoint Dr.
Cleveland, OH 44109
216-787-0500
Teaching Specialties:
Psychiatry

Cleveland Psychoanalytic Institute
11328 Euclid Ave.
Cleveland, OH 44106
216-229-5959
Teaching Specialties:
Psychiatry

Fairview General Hospital
18101 Lorain Ave.
Cleveland, OH 44111
216-476-7000
Teaching Specialties:
Surgery

Lutheran Medical Center
2609 Franklin Blvd.
Cleveland, OH 44113
216-696-4300
Teaching Specialties:
Internal Medicine, Surgery

Meridia Huron Hospital
13951 Terrace Rd.
Cleveland, OH 44112
216-761-3300
Teaching Specialties:
Anesthesiology, Internal Medicine, Surgery

MetroHealth Center for Rehabilitation
2500 MetroHealth Dr.
Cleveland, OH 44109
216-459-3473
216-459-4166
Teaching Specialties:
Internal Medicine-Endocrinology and Metabolism, Physical Medicine and Rehabilitation

MetroHealth Medical Center
2500 MetroHealth Dr.
Cleveland, OH 44109
216-398-6000
Teaching Specialties:
Anesthesiology, Dentistry, Dermatology, Internal Medicine, Internal Medicine-Cardiovascular Disease, Internal Medicine-Endocrinology and Metabolism, Internal

Medicine-Gastroenterology, Internal Medicine-Geriatric Medicine, Internal Medicine-Hematology, Internal Medicine-Infectious Diseases, Internal Medicine-Medical Oncology, Internal Medicine-Rheumatology, Neurological Surgery, Neurology, Obstetrics/Gynecology, Ophthalmology, Orthopedic Surgery, Otolaryngology, Physical Medicine and Rehabilitation, Psychiatry, Surgery, Thoracic Surgery, Urology

Mt. Sinai Medical Center
1 Mt. Sinai Dr.
Cleveland, OH 44106
216-421-4000
Teaching Specialties:
Dentistry, Internal Medicine, Obstetrics/Gynecology, Ophthalmology, Orthopedic Surgery, Psychiatry, Surgery

St. Luke's Hospital
11311 Shaker Blvd.
Cleveland, OH 44104
216-368-7000
Teaching Specialties:
Dentistry, Internal Medicine, Obstetrics/Gynecology, Ophthalmology, Orthopedic Surgery, Surgery

St. Vincent Charity Hospital and Health Center
2351 E. 22nd St.
Cleveland, OH 44115
216-861-6200
Teaching Specialties:
Internal Medicine, Ophthalmology

University Hospitals of Cleveland
11100 Euclid Ave.
Cleveland, OH 44106
216-844-1000
Teaching Specialties:
Anesthesiology, Dermatology, Internal Medicine, Internal Medicine-Cardiovascular Disease, Internal Medicine-Endocrinology and Metabolism, Internal Medicine-Gastroenterology, Internal Medicine-Geriatric Medicine, Internal Medicine-Hematology, Internal Medicine-Infectious Diseases, Internal Medicine-Medical Oncology, Internal Medicine-Nephrology, Internal Medicine-Rheumatology, Neurological Surgery, Neurology, Obstetrics/Gynecology, Ophthalmology, Orthopedic Surgery, Otolaryngology, Psychiatry, Radiation Oncology, Surgery, Thoracic Surgery, Urology

Columbus

Grant Medical Center
111 S. Grant Ave.
Columbus, OH 43215
614-461-3232
Teaching Specialties:
Colon and Rectal Surgery, Internal Medicine-Gastroenterology, Obstetrics/Gynecology,

Physical Medicine and Rehabilitation, Psychiatry, Surgery

Mt. Carmel East Hospital
6001 E. Broad St.
Columbus, OH 43213
614-234-6000
Teaching Specialties:
Surgery

Mt. Carmel Medical Center
793 W. State St.
Columbus, OH 43222
614-225-5000
Teaching Specialties:
Internal Medicine, Internal Medicine-Cardiovascular Disease, Obstetrics/Gynecology, Orthopedic Surgery, Physical Medicine and Rehabilitation, Psychiatry, Surgery

Ohio State University College of Dentistry
305 W. 12th Ave.
Columbus, OH 43210-1241
614-292-2401
Teaching Specialties:
Dentistry

Ohio State University Hospitals
450 W. 10th Ave.
Columbus, OH 43210
614-293-8000
Teaching Specialties:
Anesthesiology, Dermatology, Hand Surgery, Internal Medicine, Internal Medicine-Cardiovascular Disease, Internal Medicine-Endocrinology and Metabolism, Internal Medicine-Gastroenterology, Internal Medicine-Hematology, Internal Medicine-Infectious Diseases, Internal Medicine-Medical Oncology, Internal Medicine-Nephrology, Neurological Surgery, Neurology, Obstetrics/Gynecology, Ophthalmology, Orthopedic Surgery, Otolaryngology, Physical Medicine and Rehabilitation, Psychiatry, Radiation Oncology, Surgery, Surgery-Vascular Surgery, Thoracic Surgery, Urology

Riverside Methodist Hospitals
3535 Olentangy River Rd.
Columbus, OH 43214
614-261-5000
Teaching Specialties:
Hand Surgery, Internal Medicine, Neurological Surgery, Neurology, Obstetrics/Gynecology, Orthopedic Surgery, Physical Medicine and Rehabilitation, Psychiatry, Surgery, Urology

Dayton

Good Samaritan Hospital and Health Center
2222 Philadelphia Dr.
Dayton, OH 45406

937-278-2612
Teaching Specialties:
Dermatology, Internal Medicine, Internal Medicine-Cardiovascular Disease, Psychiatry, Surgery

Miami Valley Hospital
1 Wyoming St.
Dayton, OH 45409
937-223-6192
Teaching Specialties:
Dentistry, Internal Medicine, Obstetrics/Gynecology, Orthopedic Surgery, Surgery

Franciscan Medical Center
1 Franciscan Way
Dayton, OH 45408
937-229-6000
Teaching Specialties:
Dermatology, Surgery

Kettering

Kettering Medical Center
3535 Southern Blvd.
Kettering, OH 45429
937-298-4331
Teaching Specialties:
Internal Medicine, Psychiatry, Surgery

Ravenna

Robinson Memorial Hospital
6847 N. Chestnut St.
Ravenna, OH 44266
330-297-0811
Teaching Specialties:
Surgery

Toledo

Medical College of Ohio Hospital
3000 Arlington Ave.
Toledo, OH 43614
419-381-4172
Teaching Specialties:
Anesthesiology, Dentistry, Internal Medicine, Internal Medicine-Cardiovascular Disease, Internal Medicine-Endocrinology and Metabolism, Internal Medicine-Hematology, Internal Medicine-Infectious Diseases, Internal Medicine-Medical Oncology, Internal Medicine-Nephrology, Obstetrics/Gynecology, Orthopedic Surgery, Physical Medicine and Rehabilitation, Psychiatry, Surgery, Urology

Mercy Hospital
2200 Jefferson Ave.
Toledo, OH 43624
419-259-1500
Teaching Specialties:
Internal Medicine-Endocrinology and Metabolism

St. Vincent Medical Center
2213 Cherry St.
Toledo, OH 43608
419-321-3232
Teaching Specialties:
Internal Medicine, Internal Medicine-Hematology, Internal Medicine-Medical Oncology, Obstetrics/Gynecology, Orthopedic Surgery, Physical Medicine and Rehabilitation, Psychiatry, Surgery, Urology

Toledo Hospital
2142 N. Cove Blvd.
Toledo, OH 43606
419-471-4218
Teaching Specialties:
Anesthesiology, Internal Medicine, Internal Medicine-Cardiovascular Disease, Obstetrics/Gynecology, Orthopedic Surgery, Physical Medicine and Rehabilitation, Surgery, Urology

Toledo Mental Health Center
930 S. Detroit Ave.
Toledo, OH 43614-2701
419-381-1881
Teaching Specialties:
Psychiatry

Westerville

St. Ann's Hospital of Columbus
500 S. Cleveland Ave.
Westerville, OH 43081
614-898-4000
Teaching Specialties:
Obstetrics/Gynecology

Worthington

Harding Hospital
445 E. Granville Rd.
Worthington, OH 43085
614-885-5381
Teaching Specialties:
Psychiatry

Youngstown

St. Elizabeth Hospital Medical Center
1044 Belmont Ave.
Youngstown, OH 44501
330-746-7211
Teaching Specialties:
Dentistry, Internal Medicine, Obstetrics/Gynecology, Surgery

Western Reserve Care System-Northside Medical Center
500 Gypsy Lane
Youngstown, OH 44501
330-747-1444
Teaching Specialties:
Anesthesiology, Internal Medicine, Surgery

Western Reserve Care System-Southside Medical Center
345 Oak Hill Ave.
Youngstown, OH 44501
330-747-0777
Teaching Specialties:
Anesthesiology, Dentistry, Internal Medicine, Surgery

OKLAHOMA
Norman

Griffin Memorial Hospital
900 E. Main St.
Norman, OK 73070
405-321-4880
Teaching Specialties:
Psychiatry

Oklahoma City

Baptist Medical Center of Oklahoma
3300 N.W. Expressway
Oklahoma City, OK 73112
405-949-3011
Teaching Specialties:
Otolaryngology

Bone and Joint Hospital
1111 N. Dewey Ave.
Oklahoma City, OK 73103
405-272-9671
Teaching Specialties:
Orthopedic Surgery

Oklahoma Medical Center
940 N.E. 13th St.
Oklahoma City, OK 73104
405-271-4700
Teaching Specialties:
Anesthesiology, Dentistry, Dermatology, Internal Medicine, Internal Medicine-Cardiovascular Disease, Internal Medicine-Endocrinology and Metabolism, Internal Medicine-Gastroenterology, Internal Medicine-Hematology, Internal Medicine-Infectious Diseases, Internal Medicine-Medical Oncology, Internal Medicine-Nephrology, Internal Medicine-Rheumatology, Neurological Surgery, Obstetrics/Gynecology, Ophthalmology, Orthopedic Surgery, Otolaryngology, Psychiatry, Radiation Oncology, Surgery, Thoracic Surgery, Urology

Presbyterian Hospital
700 N.E. 13th St.
Oklahoma City, OK 73104-5070
405-271-5100

Teaching Specialties:
Orthopedic Surgery, Surgery

St. Anthony Hospital
1000 N. Lee St.
Oklahoma City, OK 73101
405-272-7000
Teaching Specialties:
Dentistry, Neurological Surgery

University of Oklahoma College of Dentistry
1001 N.E. Stanton L. Young Blvd.
Oklahoma City, OK 73117
405-271-6326
Teaching Specialties:
Dentistry

Tulsa

Hillcrest Medical Center
1124 S. Utica Ave.
Tulsa, OK 74124
918-584-1351
Teaching Specialties:
Internal Medicine, Obstetrics/Gynecology, Psychiatry, Surgery

St. Francis Hospital
6161 S. Yale Ave.
Tulsa, OK 74136
918-494-2200
Teaching Specialties:
Internal Medicine, Obstetrics/Gynecology, Surgery

St. John Medical Center
1923 S. Utica Ave.
Tulsa, OK 74104-6502
918-744-2345
Teaching Specialties:
Internal Medicine, Obstetrics/Gynecology, Surgery

Tulsa Psychiatric Center
1620 E. 12th St.
Tulsa, OK 74120
918-582-2131
Teaching Specialties:
Psychiatry

OREGON
Clackamas

Kaiser Sunnyside Medical Center
10180 S.E. Sunnyside Rd.
Clackamas, OR 97015
503-652-2880
Teaching Specialties:
Neurological Surgery

Portland

Emanuel Hospital and Health Center
2801 N. Gantenbein Ave.
Portland, OR 97227
503-280-3200
Teaching Specialties:
Internal Medicine, Obstetrics/Gynecology, Orthopedic Surgery, Surgery

Good Samaritan Hospital and Medical Center
1015 N.W. 22nd Ave.
Portland, OR 97210
503-229-7711
Teaching Specialties:
Internal Medicine, Neurology, Obstetrics/Gynecology, Ophthalmology, Surgery

Oregon Health Sciences University
School of Dentistry
611 S.W. Campus Dr.
Portland, OR 97201
503-494-8867
Teaching Specialties:
Dentistry

Oregon Health Sciences University
University Hospital
3181 S.W. Sam Jackson Park Rd.
Portland, OR 97201
503-494-8311
Teaching Specialties:
Anesthesiology, Dermatology, Internal Medicine, Internal Medicine-Cardiovascular Disease, Internal Medicine-Endocrinology and Metabolism, Internal Medicine-Gastroenterology, Internal Medicine-Geriatric Medicine, Internal Medicine-Hematology, Internal Medicine-Infectious Diseases, Internal Medicine-Medical Oncology, Internal Medicine-Nephrology, Internal Medicine-Rheumatology, Neurological Surgery, Neurology, Obstetrics/Gynecology, Ophthalmology, Orthopedic Surgery, Otolaryngology, Psychiatry, Radiation Oncology, Surgery, Surgery-Vascular Surgery, Thoracic Surgery, Urology

Providence Medical Center
4805 N.E. Glisan St.
Portland, OR 97213
503-230-1111
Teaching Specialties:
Internal Medicine

St. Vincent Hospital and Medical Center
9205 S.W. Barnes Rd.
Portland, OR 97225
503-297-4411
Teaching Specialties:
Internal Medicine, Surgery

PENNSYLVANIA

Scranton

Community Medical Center
1822 Mulberry St.
Scranton, PA 18510
717-969-8000
Teaching Specialties:
Internal Medicine

Abington

Abington Memorial Hospital
1200 Old York Rd.
Abington, PA 19001
215-576-2000
Teaching Specialties:
Dentistry, Internal Medicine, Obstetrics/Gynecology, Orthopedic Surgery, Psychiatry, Surgery, Urology

Allentown

The Allentown Hospital-Lehigh Valley Hospital Center
1200 S. Cedarcrest Blvd.
Allentown, PA 18103
610-402-8000
Teaching Specialties:
Colon and Rectal Surgery, Dentistry, Internal Medicine-Cardiovascular Disease, Obstetrics/Gynecology, Surgery

Sacred Heart Hospital
421 Chew St.
Allentown, PA 18102
610-776-4500
Teaching Specialties:
Dentistry

Bethlehem

Muhlenberg Hospital Center
2545 Schoenersville Rd.
Bethlehem, PA 18017-7384
610-861-2200
Teaching Specialties:
Dentistry

St. Luke's Hospital
801 Ostrum St.
Bethlehem, PA 18015
610-954-4000
Teaching Specialties:
Internal Medicine, Obstetrics/Gynecology

Bristol

Lower Bucks Hospital
501 Bath Rd.
Bristol, PA 19007
215-785-9200
Teaching Specialties:
Obstetrics/Gynecology

Bryn Mawr

Bryn Mawr Hospital
130 S. Bryn Mawr Ave.
Bryn Mawr, PA 19010
610-526-3000
Teaching Specialties:
Internal Medicine, Orthopedic Surgery, Surgery, Urology

Danville

Geisinger Medical Center
100 N. Academy Ave.
Danville, PA 17822
717-271-6211
Teaching Specialties:
Anesthesiology, Dermatology, Internal Medicine, Internal Medicine-Cardiovascular Disease, Internal Medicine-Rheumatology, Obstetrics/Gynecology, Ophthalmology, Orthopedic Surgery, Otolaryngology, Surgery, Urology

Darby

Mercy Catholic Medical Center
Fitzgerald Mercy Division
1500 Lansdowne Ave.
Darby, PA 19023
610-237-4000
Teaching Specialties:
Hand Surgery, Internal Medicine, Psychiatry, Surgery

Drexel Hill

Delaware County Memorial Hospital
501 N. Lansdowne Ave.
Drexel Hill, PA 19026
610-284-8100
Teaching Specialties:
Orthopedic Surgery

Easton

Easton Hospital
250 S. 21st St.
Easton, PA 18042-3892
610-250-4000
Teaching Specialties:
Internal Medicine, Surgery

Erie

Hamot Medical Center
201 State St.
Erie, PA 16550
814-877-6000
Teaching Specialties:
Colon and Rectal Surgery, Orthopedic Surgery

St. Vincent Health Center
232 W. 25th St.
Erie, PA 16544
814-452-5000
Teaching Specialties:
Colon and Rectal Surgery

Fort Washington

Northwestern Institute
450 Bethlehem Pike
Fort Washington, PA 19034
215-641-5300
Teaching Specialties:
Psychiatry

Harrisburg

Harrisburg Hospital
111 S. Front St.
Harrisburg, PA 17101
717-782-3131
Teaching Specialties:
Internal Medicine, Obstetrics/Gynecology,
Orthopedic Surgery, Surgery

**Polyclinic Medical Center
of Harrisburg**
2601 N. Third St.
Harrisburg, PA 17110
717-782-4141
Teaching Specialties:
Internal Medicine, Orthopedic Surgery,
Surgery

Hershey

Penn State University Hospital
Elizabethtown Hospital
500 University Dr.
Hershey, PA 17033
717-531-7320
Teaching Specialties:
Orthopedic Surgery

Penn State University Hospital
The Milton S. Hershey Medical
Center
500 University Dr.
Hershey, PA 17033
717-531-8521
Teaching Specialties:
Anesthesiology, Dermatology, Internal
Medicine, Internal Medicine-Cardiovascular
Disease, Internal Medicine-Endocrinology
and Metabolism, Internal Medicine-Gastroen-
terology, Internal Medicine-Hematology, In-
ternal Medicine-Infectious Diseases, Internal
Medicine-Medical Oncology, Internal
Medicine-Nephrology, Neurology, Obstet-
rics/Gynecology, Ophthalmology, Orthope-
dic Surgery, Otolaryngology, Psychiatry,
Surgery, Surgery-Vascular Surgery, Thoracic
Surgery, Urology

Johnstown

**Conemaugh Valley Memorial
Hospital**
1086 Franklin St.
Johnstown, PA 15905
814-533-9000
Teaching Specialties:
Internal Medicine, Surgery

Lancaster

Lancaster General Hospital
555 N. Duke St.
Lancaster, PA 17601-3555
717-299-5511
Teaching Specialties:
Urology

McKeesport

McKeesport Hospital
1500 Fifth Ave.
McKeesport, PA 15132
412-664-2000
Teaching Specialties:
Internal Medicine, Surgery

Norristown

Norristown State Hospital
1001 Sterigere St.
Norristown, PA 19401
610-270-1000
Teaching Specialties:
Psychiatry

Philadelphia

Albert Einstein Medical Center
5501 Old York Rd.
Philadelphia, PA 19141
215-456-7890
Teaching Specialties:
Anesthesiology, Dentistry, Internal Medicine,
Internal Medicine-Cardiovascular Disease, In-
ternal Medicine-Gastroenterology, Internal
Medicine-Geriatric Medicine, Internal
Medicine-Nephrology, Internal Medicine-
Rheumatology, Neurology, Obstetrics/Gyne-
cology, Orthopedic Surgery, Physical
Medicine and Rehabilitation, Psychiatry, Ra-
diation Oncology, Surgery

**American Oncologic Hospital-
Fox Chase Cancer Center**
7701 Burholme Ave.
Philadelphia, PA 19111
215-728-6900
Teaching Specialties:
Internal Medicine-Hematology, Internal
Medicine-Medical Oncology, Radiation On-
cology, Surgery

Chestnut Hill Hospital
8835 Germantown Ave.
Philadelphia, PA 19118
215-248-8200
Teaching Specialties:
Obstetrics/Gynecology

Episcopal Hospital
100 E. Lehigh Ave.
Philadelphia, PA 19125-1098
215-427-7000
Teaching Specialties:
Internal Medicine, Internal Medicine-Cardiovascular Disease, Otolaryngology, Surgery

**Frankford Hospital of the City
of Philadelphia**
Knights & Red Lion Rds.
Philadelphia, PA 19114
215-612-4000
Teaching Specialties:
Obstetrics/Gynecology, Surgery

Friends Hospital
4641 Roosevelt Blvd.
Philadelphia, PA 19124
215-831-4600
Teaching Specialties:
Psychiatry

**Germantown Hospital and Medical
Center**
1 Penn Blvd.
Philadelphia, PA 19144-1498
215-951-8000
Teaching Specialties:
Internal Medicine, Obstetrics/Gynecology

Graduate Hospital
1 Graduate Plaza
Philadelphia, PA 19146
215-893-2000
Teaching Specialties:
Dentistry, Dermatology, Internal Medicine,
Internal Medicine-Cardiovascular Disease, In-
ternal Medicine-Gastroenterology, Physical
Medicine and Rehabilitation, Surgery

Hahnemann University Hospital
Broad & Vine Sts.
Philadelphia, PA 19102
215-762-7000
Teaching Specialties:
Anesthesiology, Dentistry, Dermatology, In-
ternal Medicine, Internal Medicine-Cardio-
vascular Disease, Internal Medicine-En-
docrinology and Metabolism, Internal
Medicine-Gastroenterology, Internal
Medicine-Hematology, Internal Medicine-In-
fectious Diseases, Internal Medicine-Medical
Oncology, Internal Medicine-Nephrology, In-
ternal Medicine-Rheumatology, Neurological
Surgery, Neurology, Obstetrics/Gynecology,
Ophthalmology, Orthopedic Surgery, Oto-

laryngology, Psychiatry, Radiation Oncology, Surgery, Surgery-Vascular Surgery, Thoracic Surgery

Hospital of the Medical College of Pennsylvania
3300 Henry Ave.
Philadelphia, PA 19129
215-842-6000
Teaching Specialties:
Dentistry, Internal Medicine, Internal Medicine-Cardiovascular Disease, Internal Medicine-Endocrinology and Metabolism, Internal Medicine-Gastroenterology, Internal Medicine-Hematology, Internal Medicine-Infectious Diseases, Internal Medicine-Medical Oncology, Internal Medicine-Nephrology, Internal Medicine-Rheumatology, Neurology, Obstetrics/Gynecology, Orthopedic Surgery, Psychiatry, Surgery, Urology

Hospital of the University of Pennsylvania
3400 Spruce St.
Philadelphia, PA 19104
215-662-4000
Teaching Specialties:
Allergy/Immunology, Anesthesiology, Dermatology, Hand Surgery, Internal Medicine, Internal Medicine-Cardiovascular Disease, Internal Medicine-Endocrinology and Metabolism, Internal Medicine-Gastroenterology, Internal Medicine-Geriatric Medicine, Internal Medicine-Hematology, Internal Medicine-Infectious Diseases, Internal Medicine-Medical Oncology, Internal Medicine-Nephrology, Internal Medicine-Rheumatology, Neurological Surgery, Neurology, Obstetrics/Gynecology, Orthopedic Surgery, Otolaryngology, Physical Medicine and Rehabilitation, Psychiatry, Radiation Oncology, Surgery, Surgery-Vascular Surgery, Thoracic Surgery, Urology

Mercy Catholic Medical Center
Misericordia Division
5301 Cedar Ave.
Philadelphia, PA 19143
215-748-9000
Teaching Specialties:
Internal Medicine, Internal Medicine-Gastroenterology, Surgery

Methodist Hospital
2301 S. Broad St.
Philadelphia, PA 19148
215-952-9000
Teaching Specialties:
Obstetrics/Gynecology, Orthopedic Surgery

Moss Rehabilitation Hospital
1200 W. Tabor Rd.
Philadelphia, PA 19141
215-456-9900
Teaching Specialties:
Internal Medicine-Rheumatology, Orthope-

dic Surgery, Physical Medicine and Rehabilitation

Pennsylvania Hospital
800 Spruce St.
Philadelphia, PA 19107
215-829-3000
Teaching Specialties:
Dermatology, Internal Medicine, Internal Medicine-Infectious Diseases, Neurological Surgery, Neurology, Obstetrics/Gynecology, Orthopedic Surgery, Otolaryngology, Psychiatry, Surgery, Urology

Presbyterian Medical Center of Philadelphia
39th & Market Sts.
Philadelphia, PA 19104
215-662-8000
Teaching Specialties:
Internal Medicine, Internal Medicine-Cardiovascular Disease, Internal Medicine-Gastroenterology, Ophthalmology

Scheie Eye Institute
51 N. 39th St.
Philadelphia, PA 19104
215-662-8100
Teaching Specialties:
Ophthalmology

Temple University Hospital
3401 N. Broad St.
Philadelphia, PA 19140
215-707-2000
Teaching Specialties:
Anesthesiology, Internal Medicine, Internal Medicine-Cardiovascular Disease, Internal Medicine-Endocrinology and Metabolism, Internal Medicine-Gastroenterology, Internal Medicine-Hematology, Internal Medicine-Infectious Diseases, Internal Medicine-Medical Oncology, Internal Medicine-Nephrology, Internal Medicine-Rheumatology, Neurological Surgery, Neurology, Obstetrics/Gynecology, Ophthalmology, Orthopedic Surgery, Otolaryngology, Physical Medicine and Rehabilitation, Psychiatry, Surgery, Surgery-Vascular Surgery, Urology

Temple University School of Dentistry
3223 N. Broad St.
Philadelphia, PA 19140
215-707-2803
Teaching Specialties:
Dentistry

Thomas Jefferson University Hospital
111 S. 11th St.
Philadelphia, PA 19107
215-955-6000
Teaching Specialties:
Allergy/Immunology, Anesthesiology, Colon

and Rectal Surgery, Dentistry, Dermatology, Hand Surgery, Internal Medicine, Internal Medicine-Cardiovascular Disease, Internal Medicine-Gastroenterology, Internal Medicine-Hematology, Internal Medicine-Infectious Diseases, Internal Medicine-Medical Oncology, Internal Medicine-Nephrology, Internal Medicine-Rheumatology, Neurological Surgery, Neurology, Obstetrics/Gynecology, Orthopedic Surgery, Otolaryngology, Physical Medicine and Rehabilitation, Psychiatry, Radiation Oncology, Surgery, Thoracic Surgery, Urology

University of Pennsylvania School of Dental Medicine
4001 Spruce St.
Philadelphia, PA 19104
215-898-8961
Teaching Specialties:
Dentistry

Wills Eye Hospital
900 Walnut St.
Philadelphia, PA 19107
215-928-3000
Teaching Specialties:
Ophthalmology

Pittsburgh

Allegheny General Hospital
320 E. North Ave.
Pittsburgh, PA 15212
412-359-3131
Teaching Specialties:
Anesthesiology, Dentistry, Internal Medicine, Internal Medicine-Cardiovascular Disease, Internal Medicine-Gastroenterology, Internal Medicine-Medical Oncology, Obstetrics/Gynecology, Otolaryngology, Radiation Oncology, Surgery, Thoracic Surgery, Urology

Harmarville Rehabilitation Center
PO Box 11460
Pittsburgh, PA 15238
412-781-5700
Teaching Specialties:
Physical Medicine and Rehabilitation

Magee-Womens Hospital
300 Halket St.
Pittsburgh, PA 15213-3180
412-641-1000
Teaching Specialties:
Anesthesiology, Obstetrics/Gynecology

Mercy Hospital of Pittsburgh
1400 Locust St.
Pittsburgh, PA 15219
412-232-8111
Teaching Specialties:
Anesthesiology, Internal Medicine, Orthopedic Surgery, Physical Medicine and Rehabilitation, Surgery

Montefiore University Hospital
3459 Fifth Ave.
Pittsburgh, PA 15213
412-648-6000
Teaching Specialties:
Anesthesiology, Dentistry, Internal Medicine, Internal Medicine-Cardiovascular Disease, Internal Medicine-Endocrinology and Metabolism, Internal Medicine-Gastroenterology, Internal Medicine-Hematology, Internal Medicine-Infectious Diseases, Internal Medicine-Medical Oncology, Internal Medicine-Nephrology, Neurological Surgery, Neurology, Orthopedic Surgery, Psychiatry, Surgery, Thoracic Surgery, Urology

Montefiore University Hospital
Eye and Ear Hospital of Pittsburgh
200 Lothrop St.
Pittsburgh, PA 15213
412-648-6336
Teaching Specialties:
Otolaryngology

Presbyterian University Hospital
200 Lothrop St.
Pittsburgh, PA 15213
412-647-3325
Teaching Specialties:
Anesthesiology, Dermatology, Internal Medicine, Internal Medicine-Cardiovascular Disease, Internal Medicine-Endocrinology and Metabolism, Internal Medicine-Gastroenterology, Internal Medicine-Geriatric Medicine, Internal Medicine-Hematology, Internal Medicine-Infectious Diseases, Internal Medicine-Medical Oncology, Internal Medicine-Nephrology, Internal Medicine-Rheumatology, Neurological Surgery, Neurology, Orthopedic Surgery, Physical Medicine and Rehabilitation, Psychiatry, Surgery, Thoracic Surgery, Urology

Shadyside Hospital
5230 Centre Ave.
Pittsburgh, PA 15232
412-623-2121
Teaching Specialties:
Internal Medicine, Internal Medicine-Cardiovascular Disease, Internal Medicine-Endocrinology and Metabolism, Internal Medicine-Gastroenterology, Internal Medicine-Geriatric Medicine

St. Francis Medical Center
400 45th St.
Pittsburgh, PA 15201
412-622-4343
Teaching Specialties:
Dentistry, Internal Medicine, Internal Medicine-Cardiovascular Disease, Ophthalmology, Physical Medicine and Rehabilitation, Psychiatry

St. Margaret Memorial Hospital
815 Freeport Rd.

Pittsburgh, PA 15215
412-784-4000
Teaching Specialties:
Internal Medicine-Cardiovascular Disease, Orthopedic Surgery, Physical Medicine and Rehabilitation

University of Pittsburgh School of Dental Medicine
C-333 Salk Hall
3501 Terrace St.
Pittsburgh, PA 15261
412-648-8760
Teaching Specialties:
Dentistry

Western Pennsylvania Hospital
4800 Friendship Ave.
Pittsburgh, PA 15224
412-578-5000
Teaching Specialties:
Anesthesiology, Internal Medicine, Internal Medicine-Cardiovascular Disease, Internal Medicine-Gastroenterology, Obstetrics/Gynecology, Surgery

Western Psychiatric Institute and Clinic
3811 O'Hara St.
Pittsburgh, PA 15213
412-624-2100
Teaching Specialties:
Psychiatry

Reading

Community General Hospital
145 N. Sixth St.
Reading, PA 19601
610-376-1900
Teaching Specialties:
Dentistry

St. Joseph Hospital
12th & Walnut Sts.
Reading, PA 19603
610-378-2000
Teaching Specialties:
Dentistry

Sayre

Robert Packer Hospital
Guthrie Square
Sayre, PA 18840
717-888-6666
Teaching Specialties:
Internal Medicine, Internal Medicine-Gastroenterology, Surgery

Scranton

Mercy Hospital of Scranton
746 Jefferson Ave.

Scranton, PA 18510
717-348-7100
Teaching Specialties:
Internal Medicine, Internal Medicine-Gastroenterology

Moses Taylor Hospital
700 Quincy Ave.
Scranton, PA 18510
717-963-2100
Teaching Specialties:
Internal Medicine

Upland

Crozer-Chester Medical Center
1 Medical Center Blvd.
Upland, PA 19013
610-447-2000
Teaching Specialties:
Internal Medicine, Internal Medicine-Gastroenterology, Neurological Surgery, Obstetrics/Gynecology, Psychiatry, Surgery

West Reading

Reading Hospital and Medical Center
Sixth Ave. & Spruce St.
West Reading, PA 19612
610-378-6000
Teaching Specialties:
Internal Medicine, Obstetrics/Gynecology, Surgery

Wynnewood

Lankenau Hospital
100 Lancaster Ave.
Wynnewood, PA 19096
610-645-2000
Teaching Specialties:
Internal Medicine, Internal Medicine-Cardiovascular Disease, Internal Medicine-Gastroenterology, Internal Medicine-Hematology, Internal Medicine-Nephrology, Obstetrics/Gynecology, Orthopedic Surgery, Surgery

York

York Hospital
1001 S. George St.
York, PA 17403
717-851-2345
Teaching Specialties:
Dentistry, Internal Medicine, Obstetrics/Gynecology, Surgery

PUERTO RICO
Bayamon

Hospital Universitario Dr. Ramon Ruiz Arnau
Ave. Laurel Santa Juanita

Bayamon, PR 00966
787-787-5151
Teaching Specialties:
Internal Medicine

Caguas

Caguas Regional Hospital
Carratera Caguas A Cidra
Caguas, PR 00626
787-744-2500
Teaching Specialties:
Internal Medicine, Obstetrics/Gynecology

Carolina

Hospital Dr. Federico Trilla
PO Box 3869
Carolina, PR 00984
787-757-1800
Teaching Specialties:
Internal Medicine-Geriatric Medicine

Mayaguez

Dr. Ramon E. Betances Hospital-Mayaguez Medical Center Branch
Mayaguez, PR 00708
787-834-8686
Teaching Specialties:
Internal Medicine, Obstetrics/Gynecology, Surgery

Ponce

Hospital de Damas
2225 Ponce by Pass
Edif Parra 407
Ponce, PR 00731
787-840-8686
Teaching Specialties:
Internal Medicine, Internal Medicine-Cardiovascular Disease, Surgery

Hospital Oncologico Andres Grillasca
Centro Medico de Ponce
Ponce, PR 00733
787-848-0800
Teaching Specialties:
Surgery

Hospital San Lucas
Guadalupe St.
Ponce, PR 00731
787-840-4545
Teaching Specialties:
Internal Medicine, Internal Medicine-Cardiovascular Disease

Ponce Regional Hospital
Barrio Machuelo
Ponce, PR 00731
787-844-2080

Teaching Specialties:
Internal Medicine, Obstetrics/Gynecology, Surgery

Rio Piedras

San Juan Municipal Hospital
Apartado 21405
Rio Piedras, PR 00928
787-765-6728
Teaching Specialties:
Anesthesiology, Internal Medicine, Internal Medicine-Cardiovascular Disease, Internal Medicine-Endocrinology and Metabolism, Internal Medicine-Gastroenterology, Internal Medicine-Hematology, Internal Medicine-Medical Oncology, Internal Medicine-Rheumatology, Neurological Surgery, Neurology, Obstetrics/Gynecology, Ophthalmology, Orthopedic Surgery, Otolaryngology

San German

Hospital de la Concepción
41 Luna St.
San German, PR 00753
787-892-1860
Teaching Specialties:
Internal Medicine

San Juan

Fundación Hospital Metropolitan
PO Box 11981
San Juan, PR 00922
787-793-6200
Teaching Specialties:
Radiation Oncology

Industrial Hospital
Puerto Rico Medical Center
San Juan, PR 00936
787-754-2500
Teaching Specialties:
Anesthesiology

Puerto Rico Rehabilitation Center
Puerto Rico Medical Center
San Juan, PR 00935
787-765-3522
Teaching Specialties:
Physical Medicine and Rehabilitation

University Hospital
Puerto Rico Medical Center
Rio Piedras Station
San Juan, PR 00935
787-754-3654
Teaching Specialties:
Anesthesiology, Dermatology, Internal Medicine, Internal Medicine-Cardiovascular Disease, Internal Medicine-Endocrinology and Metabolism, Internal Medicine-Gastroenterology, Internal Medicine-Geriatric Medicine, Internal Medicine-Hematology, In-

ternal Medicine-Infectious Diseases, Internal Medicine-Medical Oncology, Internal Medicine-Nephrology, Internal Medicine-Rheumatology, Neurological Surgery, Neurology, Obstetrics/Gynecology, Ophthalmology, Orthopedic Surgery, Otolaryngology, Physical Medicine and Rehabilitation, Psychiatry, Radiation Oncology, Surgery, Urology

University of Puerto Rico School of Dentistry
GPO Box 5067
Medical Sciences Campus
San Juan, PR 00936
787-758-2525
Teaching Specialties:
Dentistry

RHODE ISLAND

East Providence

Emma Pendleton Bradley Hospital
1011 Veterans Memorial Pkwy.
East Providence, RI 02915
401-432-1000
Teaching Specialties:
Psychiatry

Pawtucket

Memorial Hospital of Rhode Island
111 Brewster St.
Pawtucket, RI 02860
401-729-2000
Teaching Specialties:
Dermatology, Internal Medicine, Internal Medicine-Cardiovascular Disease, Internal Medicine-Geriatric Medicine, Internal Medicine-Hematology, Internal Medicine-Infectious Diseases, Internal Medicine-Medical Oncology

Providence

Butler Hospital
345 Blackstone Blvd.
Providence, RI 02906
401-455-6200
Teaching Specialties:
Psychiatry

Miriam Hospital
164 Summit Ave.
Providence, RI 02906
401-331-8500
Teaching Specialties:
Internal Medicine, Internal Medicine-Cardiovascular Disease, Internal Medicine-Hematology, Internal Medicine-Infectious Diseases, Internal Medicine-Medical Oncology, Psychiatry, Surgery

Providence Center for Counseling and Psychiatric Services
520 Hope St.
Providence, RI 02906
401-276-4000
Teaching Specialties:
Psychiatry

Rhode Island Hospital
593 Eddy St.
Providence, RI 02903
401-444-4000
Teaching Specialties:
Allergy/Immunology, Dermatology, Internal Medicine, Internal Medicine-Cardiovascular Disease, Internal Medicine-Endocrinology and Metabolism, Internal Medicine-Gastroenterology, Internal Medicine-Hematology, Internal Medicine-Infectious Diseases, Internal Medicine-Nephrology, Internal Medicine-Rheumatology, Neurological Surgery, Neurology, Obstetrics/Gynecology, Ophthalmology, Orthopedic Surgery, Psychiatry, Surgery, Urology

Roger Williams Hospital
825 Chalkstone Ave.
Providence, RI 02908
401-456-2000
Teaching Specialties:
Dermatology, Internal Medicine, Internal Medicine-Cardiovascular Disease, Internal Medicine-Endocrinology and Metabolism, Internal Medicine-Gastroenterology, Internal Medicine-Geriatric Medicine, Internal Medicine-Hematology, Internal Medicine-Infectious Diseases, Internal Medicine-Medical Oncology, Internal Medicine-Nephrology, Internal Medicine-Rheumatology, Urology

Women and Infants Hospital of Rhode Island
101 Dudley St.
Providence, RI 02905
401-274-1100
Teaching Specialties:
Obstetrics/Gynecology

SOUTH CAROLINA
Charleston

Charleston Memorial Hospital
326 Calhoun St.
Charleston, SC 29401
803-577-0600
Teaching Specialties:
Internal Medicine, Internal Medicine-Nephrology, Obstetrics/Gynecology, Otolaryngology, Psychiatry, Surgery, Thoracic Surgery, Urology

Medical University of South Carolina
College of Dental Medicine

500 MUSC Complex
Charleston, SC 29425
803-792-3811
Teaching Specialties:
Dentistry

Medical University of South Carolina
Medical Center of Medical University of South Carolina
171 Ashley Ave.
Charleston, SC 29425
803-792-3897
Teaching Specialties:
Anesthesiology, Dermatology, Internal Medicine, Internal Medicine-Cardiovascular Disease, Internal Medicine-Endocrinology and Metabolism, Internal Medicine-Gastroenterology, Internal Medicine-Hematology, Internal Medicine-Infectious Diseases, Internal Medicine-Medical Oncology, Internal Medicine-Nephrology, Internal Medicine-Rheumatology, Neurological Surgery, Neurology, Obstetrics/Gynecology, Ophthalmology, Orthopedic Surgery, Otolaryngology, Psychiatry, Radiation Oncology, Surgery, Thoracic Surgery, Urology

Columbia

Richland Memorial Hospital
5 Richland Medical Park
Columbia, SC 29203
803-434-7000
Teaching Specialties:
Anesthesiology, Dentistry, Internal Medicine, Internal Medicine-Cardiovascular Disease, Internal Medicine-Endocrinology and Metabolism, Internal Medicine-Medical Oncology, Obstetrics/Gynecology, Ophthalmology, Orthopedic Surgery, Surgery

William S. Hall Psychiatric Institute
1800 Colonial Dr.
Columbia, SC 29202
803-734-7113
Teaching Specialties:
Psychiatry

Greenville

Greenville Memorial Hospital
701 Grove Rd.
Greenville, SC 29605
803-455-7000
Teaching Specialties:
Internal Medicine, Obstetrics/Gynecology, Orthopedic Surgery, Surgery

Spartanburg

Spartanburg Regional Medical Center
101 E. Wood St.

Spartanburg, SC 29303
864-560-6107
Teaching Specialties:
Surgery

SOUTH DAKOTA
Sioux Falls

McKennan Hospital
800 E. 21st St.
Sioux Falls, SD 57105
605-339-8000
Teaching Specialties:
Internal Medicine, Psychiatry

Sioux Valley Hospital
1100 S. Euclid Ave.
Sioux Falls, SD 57117-5039
605-333-1000
Teaching Specialties:
Internal Medicine

Southeastern Mental Health Center
2000 S. Summit Ave.
Sioux Falls, SD 57105
605-336-0510
Teaching Specialties:
Psychiatry

TENNESSEE
Bristol

Bristol Regional Medical Center
1 Medical Park Blvd.
Bristol, TN 37620
423-844-1121
Teaching Specialties:
Internal Medicine

Chattanooga

Erlanger Medical Center
975 E. Third St.
Chattanooga, TN 37403
423-778-7000
Teaching Specialties:
Internal Medicine, Obstetrics/Gynecology, Ophthalmology, Orthopedic Surgery, Surgery

Willie D. Miller Eye Center
975 E. Third St.
Chattanooga, TN 37403
423-778-6000
Teaching Specialties:
Ophthalmology

Johnson City

Johnson City Medical Center Hospital
400 N. State of Franklin Rd.

Johnson City, TN 37604-6904
423-431-6111
Teaching Specialties:
Internal Medicine, Internal Medicine-Cardiovascular Disease, Internal Medicine-Gastroenterology, Internal Medicine Medical Oncology, Psychiatry, Surgery

Watauga Area Mental Health Center
109 W. Watauga Ave.
Johnson City, TN 37601
423-928-6545
Teaching Specialties:
Psychiatry

Woodridge Hospital
403 State of Franklin Rd.
Johnson City, TN 37604
423-928-7111
Teaching Specialties:
Psychiatry

Kingsport

Holston Valley Hospital and Medical Center
130 W. Ravine St.
Kingsport, TN 37662
423-224-4000
Teaching Specialties:
Internal Medicine, Surgery

Knoxville

University of Tennessee Memorial Hospital
1924 Alcoa Hwy.
Knoxville, TN 37920
423-544-9000
Teaching Specialties:
Anesthesiology, Dentistry, Internal Medicine, Obstetrics/Gynecology, Surgery

Memphis

Baptist Memorial Hospital
899 Madison Ave.
Memphis, TN 38146
901-227-2727
Teaching Specialties:
Allergy/Immunology, Dermatology, Internal Medicine, Internal Medicine-Endocrinology and Metabolism, Internal Medicine-Hematology, Internal Medicine-Medical Oncology, Internal Medicine-Rheumatology, Neurological Surgery, Neurology, Orthopedic Surgery, Surgery, Surgery-Vascular Surgery, Thoracic Surgery, Urology

Memphis Mental Health Institute
865 Poplar Ave.
Memphis, TN 38174
901-524-1201

Teaching Specialties:
Psychiatry

Methodist Hospitals of Memphis
Central Unit
1265 Union Ave.
Memphis, TN 38104
901-726-7000
Teaching Specialties:
Internal Medicine, Neurological Surgery, Ophthalmology, Otolaryngology, Surgery, Urology

Regional Medical Center at Memphis
877 Jefferson Ave.
Memphis, TN 38103
901-545-7100
Teaching Specialties:
Anesthesiology, Dermatology, Internal Medicine, Internal Medicine-Cardiovascular Disease, Internal Medicine-Endocrinology and Metabolism, Internal Medicine-Gastroenterology, Internal Medicine-Geriatric Medicine, Internal Medicine-Hematology, Internal Medicine-Infectious Diseases, Internal Medicine-Medical Oncology, Internal Medicine-Nephrology, Internal Medicine-Rheumatology, Neurological Surgery, Neurology, Obstetrics/Gynecology, Ophthalmology, Orthopedic Surgery, Otolaryngology, Psychiatry, Surgery, Thoracic Surgery, Urology

University of Tennessee College of Dentistry
875 Union Ave.
Memphis, TN 38163
901-448-6241
Teaching Specialties:
Dentistry

University of Tennessee Medical Center
62 S. Dunlap St.
Memphis, TN 38163
901-448-5544
Teaching Specialties:
Allergy/Immunology, Anesthesiology, Dermatology, Internal Medicine, Neurology, Obstetrics/Gynecology, Otolaryngology, Psychiatry, Surgery, Thoracic Surgery

Nashville

Baptist Hospital
2000 Church St.
Nashville, TN 37236
615-329-5555
Teaching Specialties:
Internal Medicine, Neurological Surgery, Obstetrics/Gynecology, Otolaryngology, Urology

George W. Hubbard Hospital of Meharry Medical College
1005 D. B. Todd Blvd.

Nashville, TN 37208
615-327-5831
Teaching Specialties:
Internal Medicine, Psychiatry

Meharry Medical College School of Dentistry
1005 D. B. Todd Blvd.
Nashville, TN 37208
615-327-6489
Teaching Specialties:
Dentistry

Metropolitan Nashville General Hospital
72 Hermitage Ave.
Nashville, TN 37210
615-862-4490
Teaching Specialties:
Dermatology, Internal Medicine, Neurology, Obstetrics/Gynecology, Orthopedic Surgery, Otolaryngology, Surgery, Urology

Middle Tennessee Mental Health Institute
221 Stewart's Ferry Pike
Nashville, TN 37214
615-902-7400
Teaching Specialties:
Psychiatry

St. Thomas Hospital
4220 Harding Rd.
Nashville, TN 37205
615-222-2111
Teaching Specialties:
Internal Medicine-Gastroenterology, Internal Medicine-Infectious Diseases, Internal Medicine-Medical Oncology, Internal Medicine-Rheumatology, Neurological Surgery, Surgery, Surgery-Vascular Surgery

Vanderbilt University Hospital and Clinic
1161 21st Ave. South
Nashville, TN 37232
615-322-2415
Teaching Specialties:
Allergy/Immunology, Anesthesiology, Dentistry, Dermatology, Internal Medicine, Internal Medicine-Cardiovascular Disease, Internal Medicine-Endocrinology and Metabolism, Internal Medicine-Gastroenterology, Internal Medicine-Hematology, Internal Medicine-Infectious Diseases, Internal Medicine-Medical Oncology, Internal Medicine-Nephrology, Internal Medicine-Rheumatology, Neurological Surgery, Neurology, Obstetrics/Gynecology, Ophthalmology, Orthopedic Surgery, Otolaryngology, Psychiatry, Surgery, Surgery-Vascular Surgery, Thoracic Surgery, Urology

TEXAS

Amarillo

Harrington Cancer Center
1500 Wallace Blvd.
Amarillo, TX 79106
800-274-4673
806-359-4673
Teaching Specialties:
Internal Medicine-Medical Oncology

High Plains Baptist Hospital
1600 Wallace Blvd.
Amarillo, TX 79106
806-358-3151
Teaching Specialties:
Internal Medicine, Internal Medicine-Medical Oncology, Obstetrics/Gynecology

Northwest Texas Hospital
1501 Coulter Dr.
Amarillo, TX 79175
806-354-1000
Teaching Specialties:
Internal Medicine, Internal Medicine-Medical Oncology, Obstetrics/Gynecology

St. Anthony's Hospital
200 N.W. Seventh St.
Amarillo, TX 79107
806-376-4411
Teaching Specialties:
Internal Medicine

Austin

Austin State Hospital
4110 Guadalupe St.
Austin, TX 78751
512-452-0381
Teaching Specialties:
Psychiatry

Austin-Travis County Mental Health Center
1430 Collier St.
Austin, TX 78704
512-447-4141
Teaching Specialties:
Psychiatry

Brackenridge Hospital
601 E. 15th St.
Austin, TX 78701
512-476-6461
Teaching Specialties:
Internal Medicine, Obstetrics/Gynecology, Psychiatry

Dallas

Baylor College of Dentistry
3302 Gaston Ave.
Dallas, TX 75246
214-828-8100
Teaching Specialties:
Dentistry

Baylor Institute for Rehabilitation
3505 Gaston Ave.
Dallas, TX 75246
800-422-9567
214-826-7030
Teaching Specialties:
Physical Medicine and Rehabilitation

Baylor University Medical Center
3500 Gaston Ave.
Dallas, TX 75246
214-820-0111
Teaching Specialties:
Colon and Rectal Surgery, Internal Medicine, Internal Medicine-Cardiovascular Disease, Internal Medicine-Gastroenterology, Internal Medicine-Infectious Diseases, Internal Medicine-Medical Oncology, Internal Medicine-Nephrology, Obstetrics/Gynecology, Orthopedic Surgery, Physical Medicine and Rehabilitation, Psychiatry, Surgery, Surgery-Vascular Surgery, Urology

Dallas County Hospital District
Parkland Memorial Hospital
5201 Harry Hines Blvd.
Dallas, TX 75235
214-590-8000
Teaching Specialties:
Allergy/Immunology, Anesthesiology, Colon and Rectal Surgery, Dentistry, Dermatology, Internal Medicine, Internal Medicine-Cardiovascular Disease, Internal Medicine-Endocrinology and Metabolism, Internal Medicine-Gastroenterology, Internal Medicine-Hematology, Internal Medicine-Infectious Diseases, Internal Medicine-Medical Oncology, Internal Medicine-Nephrology, Internal Medicine-Rheumatology, Neurological Surgery, Neurology, Obstetrics/Gynecology, Ophthalmology, Orthopedic Surgery, Otolaryngology, Physical Medicine and Rehabilitation, Psychiatry, Surgery, Surgery-Vascular Surgery, Thoracic Surgery, Urology

Methodist Medical Center
1441 N. Beckley Ave.
Dallas, TX 75203
214-947-8181
Teaching Specialties:
Internal Medicine, Obstetrics/Gynecology, Surgery

Presbyterian Hospital of Dallas
8200 Walnut Hill Lane
Dallas, TX 75231
214-369-4111
Teaching Specialties:
Colon and Rectal Surgery, Internal Medicine, Psychiatry

St. Paul Medical Center
5909 Harry Hines Blvd.
Dallas, TX 75235
214-879-1000
Teaching Specialties:
Internal Medicine, Neurological Surgery, Obstetrics/Gynecology, Otolaryngology, Surgery

Timberlawn Psychiatric Hospital
4600 Samuell Blvd.
Dallas, TX 75228
214-381-7181
Teaching Specialties:
Psychiatry

Zale-Lipshy University Hospital
5151 Harry Hines Blvd.
Dallas, TX 75235
214-590-3000
Teaching Specialties:
Dermatology, Neurological Surgery, Otolaryngology

El Paso

R. E. Thomason General Hospital
4815 Alameda Ave.
El Paso, TX 79905
915-544-1200
Teaching Specialties:
Anesthesiology, Internal Medicine, Obstetrics/Gynecology, Orthopedic Surgery, Psychiatry, Surgery

Fort Worth

Harris Methodist Fort Worth
1301 Pennsylvania Ave.
Fort Worth, TX 76104
817-882-2000
Teaching Specialties:
Obstetrics/Gynecology, Orthopedic Surgery

Tarrant County Hospital District
John Peter Smith Hospital
1500 S. Main St.
Fort Worth, TX 76104
817-921-3431
Teaching Specialties:
Obstetrics/Gynecology, Orthopedic Surgery, Otolaryngology, Surgery

Galveston

University of Texas Medical Branch Hospitals
301 University Blvd.
Galveston, TX 77555
409-772-1011
Teaching Specialties:
Allergy/Immunology, Anesthesiology, Dentistry, Dermatology, Internal Medicine, Internal Medicine-Cardiovascular Disease, Internal Medicine-Gastroenterology, Internal

Medicine-Infectious Diseases, Internal Medicine-Medical Oncology, Internal Medicine-Nephrology, Internal Medicine-Rheumatology, Neurological Surgery, Neurology, Obstetrics/Gynecology, Ophthalmology, Orthopedic Surgery, Otolaryngology, Psychiatry, Radiation Oncology, Surgery, Thoracic Surgery, Urology

Houston

Harris County Hospital District

Ben Taub General Hospital
1504 Taub Loop
Houston, TX 77030
713-793-2000
Teaching Specialties:
Anesthesiology, Dermatology, Internal Medicine, Internal Medicine-Cardiovascular Disease, Internal Medicine-Endocrinology and Metabolism, Internal Medicine-Gastroenterology, Internal Medicine-Hematology, Internal Medicine-Infectious Diseases, Internal Medicine-Medical Oncology, Internal Medicine-Nephrology, Internal Medicine-Rheumatology, Neurological Surgery, Neurology, Obstetrics/Gynecology, Ophthalmology, Orthopedic Surgery, Otolaryngology, Physical Medicine and Rehabilitation, Psychiatry, Radiation Oncology, Surgery, Surgery-Vascular Surgery, Thoracic Surgery, Urology

Harris County Hospital District

Lyndon B. Johnson General Hospital
5656 Kelley St.
Houston, TX 77026
713-636-5000
Teaching Specialties:
Dermatology, Internal Medicine, Obstetrics/Gynecology, Otolaryngology, Physical Medicine and Rehabilitation, Surgery

Harris County Psychiatric Center

2800 S. MacGregor Way
Houston, TX 77021
713-741-5000
Teaching Specialties:
Psychiatry

Hermann Hospital

6411 Fannin St.
Houston, TX 77030
713-704-4000
Teaching Specialties:
Anesthesiology, Colon and Rectal Surgery, Dermatology, Internal Medicine, Internal Medicine-Cardiovascular Disease, Internal Medicine-Endocrinology and Metabolism, Internal Medicine-Gastroenterology, Internal Medicine-Hematology, Internal Medicine-Infectious Diseases, Internal Medicine-Nephrology, Internal Medicine-Rheumatology, Neurology, Obstetrics/Gynecology, Ophthalmology, Orthopedic Surgery, Otolaryngology, Psychiatry, Surgery, Thoracic Surgery, Urology

The Institute for Rehabilitation and Research

1333 Moursund Ave.
Houston, TX 77030
800-447-3422
713-799-5000
Teaching Specialties:
Physical Medicine and Rehabilitation

Methodist Hospital

6565 Fannin St.
Houston, TX 77030
713-790-3311
Teaching Specialties:
Anesthesiology, Dermatology, Internal Medicine, Internal Medicine-Cardiovascular Disease, Internal Medicine-Endocrinology and Metabolism, Internal Medicine-Gastroenterology, Internal Medicine-Hematology, Internal Medicine-Infectious Diseases, Internal Medicine-Medical Oncology, Internal Medicine-Nephrology, Neurological Surgery, Neurology, Ophthalmology, Orthopedic Surgery, Otolaryngology, Physical Medicine and Rehabilitation, Psychiatry, Radiation Oncology, Surgery, Surgery-Vascular Surgery, Thoracic Surgery, Urology

St. Joseph Hospital

1919 LaBranch St.
Houston, TX 77002
713-757-1000
Teaching Specialties:
Internal Medicine, Obstetrics/Gynecology, Orthopedic Surgery, Surgery, Urology

St. Luke's Episcopal Hospital

6720 Bertner Ave.
Houston, TX 77030
713-791-2011
Teaching Specialties:
Internal Medicine, Internal Medicine-Cardiovascular Disease, Ophthalmology, Physical Medicine and Rehabilitation, Surgery, Thoracic Surgery, Urology

University of Texas Health Science Center at Houston

Dental Branch
PO Box 20068
Houston, TX 77225-0068
713-500-4000
Teaching Specialties:
Dentistry

University of Texas M. D. Anderson Cancer Center

1515 Holcombe Blvd.
Houston, TX 77030
713-792-2121
Teaching Specialties:
Dentistry, Dermatology, Internal Medicine-Rheumatology, Neurological Surgery, Psychiatry, Radiation Oncology, Surgery, Thoracic Surgery, Urology

Lubbock

St. Mary of the Plains Hospital

4000 24th St.
Lubbock, TX 79410
806-796-6000
Teaching Specialties:
Orthopedic Surgery, Psychiatry

University Medical Center

602 Indiana Ave.
Lubbock, TX 79415
806-743-3111
Teaching Specialties:
Anesthesiology, Dermatology, Internal Medicine, Internal Medicine-Cardiovascular Disease, Internal Medicine-Gastroenterology, Internal Medicine-Medical Oncology, Internal Medicine-Nephrology, Neurology, Obstetrics/Gynecology, Ophthalmology, Psychiatry, Surgery

Odessa

Medical Center Hospital

500 W. Fourth St.
Odessa, TX 79760
915-333-7111
Teaching Specialties:
Obstetrics/Gynecology

San Antonio

Bexar County Hospital District

Medical Center Hospital
4502 Medical Dr.
San Antonio, TX 78229
210-616-4000
Teaching Specialties:
Anesthesiology, Dermatology, Internal Medicine, Internal Medicine-Cardiovascular Disease, Internal Medicine-Endocrinology and Metabolism, Internal Medicine-Gastroenterology, Internal Medicine-Geriatric Medicine, Internal Medicine-Hematology, Internal Medicine-Infectious Diseases, Internal Medicine-Medical Oncology, Internal Medicine-Nephrology, Internal Medicine-Rheumatology, Neurological Surgery, Neurology, Obstetrics/Gynecology, Ophthalmology, Orthopedic Surgery, Otolaryngology, Physical Medicine and Rehabilitation, Psychiatry, Radiation Oncology, Surgery, Thoracic Surgery, Urology

Cancer Therapy and Research Center

4450 Medical Dr.
San Antonio, TX 78229
210-616-5500
Teaching Specialties:
Radiation Oncology

Humana Hospital-San Antonio
8026 Floyd Curl Dr.
San Antonio, TX 78229
210-692-8110
Teaching Specialties:
Urology

University of Texas Health Science Center at San Antonio
Dental School
7703 Floyd Curl Dr.
San Antonio, TX 78284-7906
210-567-3160
Teaching Specialties:
Dentistry

Temple

Scott and White Memorial Hospital
2401 S. 31st St.
Temple, TX 76508
817-724-2111
Teaching Specialties:
Anesthesiology, Internal Medicine, Internal Medicine-Cardiovascular Disease, Internal Medicine-Endocrinology and Metabolism, Internal Medicine-Gastroenterology, Obstetrics/Gynecology, Ophthalmology, Orthopedic Surgery, Surgery, Urology

Terrell

Terrell State Hospital
1200 E. Brin St.
Terrell, TX 75160
214-563-6452
Teaching Specialties:
Psychiatry

UTAH

Salt Lake City

Holy Cross Hospital
1050 E. South Temple
Salt Lake City, UT 84102
801-350-4111
Teaching Specialties:
Orthopedic Surgery, Otolaryngology, Surgery

LDS Hospital
Eighth Ave. & C St.
Salt Lake City, UT 84143
801-321-1100
Teaching Specialties:
Internal Medicine, Obstetrics/Gynecology, Orthopedic Surgery, Radiation Oncology, Surgery, Thoracic Surgery, Urology

Salt Lake Valley Mental Health
450 S. 300 East
Salt Lake City, UT 84111
801-535-5767

Teaching Specialties:
Psychiatry

University of Utah Hospital and Clinics
50 N. Medical Dr.
Salt Lake City, UT 84132
801-581-2121
Teaching Specialties:
Anesthesiology, Dentistry, Dermatology, Internal Medicine, Internal Medicine-Cardiovascular Disease, Internal Medicine-Endocrinology and Metabolism, Internal Medicine-Gastroenterology, Internal Medicine-Geriatric Medicine, Internal Medicine-Hematology, Internal Medicine-Infectious Diseases, Internal Medicine-Medical Oncology, Internal Medicine-Nephrology, Internal Medicine-Rheumatology, Neurological Surgery, Neurology, Obstetrics/Gynecology, Ophthalmology, Orthopedic Surgery, Otolaryngology, Physical Medicine and Rehabilitation, Psychiatry, Radiation Oncology, Surgery, Thoracic Surgery, Urology

Western Institute of Neuropsychiatry
501 Chipeta Way
Salt Lake City, UT 84108
801-583-2500
Teaching Specialties:
Psychiatry

VERMONT

Brattleboro

Brattleboro Retreat
75 Linden St.
Brattleboro, VT 05301
802-257-7785
Teaching Specialties:
Psychiatry

Burlington

Fletcher Allen Healthcare MCHV Campus
111 Colchester Ave.
Burlington, VT 05401
802-656-2345
Teaching Specialties:
Anesthesiology, Dentistry, Internal Medicine, Internal Medicine-Cardiovascular Disease, Internal Medicine-Endocrinology and Metabolism, Internal Medicine-Gastroenterology, Internal Medicine-Hematology, Internal Medicine-Infectious Diseases, Internal Medicine-Medical Oncology, Internal Medicine-Nephrology, Internal Medicine-Rheumatology, Neurological Surgery, Neurology, Obstetrics/Gynecology, Orthopedic Surgery, Otolaryngology, Psychiatry, Surgery, Urology

Colchester

Fanny Allen Hospital
101 College Pkwy.
Colchester, VT 05446
802-654-1115
Teaching Specialties:
Urology

VIRGINIA

Alexandria

Mt. Vernon Hospital
2501 Parker's Lane
Alexandria, VA 22306
703-664-7000
Teaching Specialties:
Internal Medicine, Physical Medicine and Rehabilitation

Arlington

Arlington Hospital
1701 N. George Mason Dr.
Arlington, VA 22205
703-558-5000
Teaching Specialties:
Internal Medicine-Nephrology, Orthopedic Surgery, Surgery

Charlottesville

University of Virginia Medical Center
PO Box 466
Charlottesville, VA 22908
804-924-0211
Teaching Specialties:
Allergy/Immunology, Anesthesiology, Dentistry, Dermatology, Internal Medicine, Internal Medicine-Cardiovascular Disease, Internal Medicine-Endocrinology and Metabolism, Internal Medicine-Gastroenterology, Internal Medicine-Geriatric Medicine, Internal Medicine-Hematology, Internal Medicine-Infectious Diseases, Internal Medicine-Medical Oncology, Internal Medicine-Nephrology, Internal Medicine-Rheumatology, Neurological Surgery, Neurology, Obstetrics/Gynecology, Ophthalmology, Orthopedic Surgery, Otolaryngology, Physical Medicine and Rehabilitation, Psychiatry, Radiation Oncology, Surgery, Thoracic Surgery, Urology

Danville

Memorial Hospital of Danville
142 S. Main St.
Danville, VA 24541
804-799-2100
Teaching Specialties:
Urology

Falls Church

Fairfax Hospital
3300 Gallows Rd.
Falls Church, VA 22042
703-698-1110
Teaching Specialties:
Obstetrics/Gynecology, Orthopedic Surgery,
Physical Medicine and Rehabilitation, Psychiatry, Surgery, Urology

Newport News

Riverside Regional Medical Center
500 J. Clyde Morris Blvd.
Newport News, VA 23601
757-594-2000
Teaching Specialties:
Obstetrics/Gynecology

Norfolk

**Department of Psychiatry
and Behavioral Sciences**
825 Fairfax Ave., Suite 710
Norfolk, VA 23507
757-446-5888
Teaching Specialties:
Psychiatry

Depaul Medical Center
150 Kingsley Lane
Norfolk, VA 23505
757-889-5000
Teaching Specialties:
Internal Medicine, Obstetrics/Gynecology,
Surgery

Sentara Leigh Hospital
830 Kempsville Rd.
Norfolk, VA 23502
757-466-6000
Teaching Specialties:
Internal Medicine, Orthopedic Surgery,
Surgery, Urology

Sentara Norfolk General Hospital
600 Gresham Dr.
Norfolk, VA 23507
757-668-3000
Teaching Specialties:
Internal Medicine, Neurological Surgery, Obstetrics/Gynecology, Ophthalmology, Orthopedic Surgery, Otolaryngology, Physical
Medicine and Rehabilitation, Psychiatry, Radiation Oncology, Surgery, Surgery-Vascular
Surgery, Urology

Portsmouth

Maryview Medical Center
3636 High St.
Portsmouth, VA 23707
757-398-2200

Teaching Specialties:
Radiation Oncology

Portsmouth General Hospital
850 Crawford Pkwy.
Portsmouth, VA 23704
757-398-4000
Teaching Specialties:
Obstetrics/Gynecology

Richmond

**Sheltering Arms Rehabilitation
Hospital**
1311 Palmyra Ave.
Richmond, VA 23227
804-342-4100
Teaching Specialties:
Physical Medicine and Rehabilitation

Virginia Commonwealth University
Medical College of Virginia
Hospitals
110 N. 12th St.
Richmond, VA 23298
804-828-0100
Teaching Specialties:
Allergy/Immunology, Anesthesiology, Dermatology, Internal Medicine, Internal
Medicine-Cardiovascular Disease, Internal
Medicine-Endocrinology and Metabolism, Internal Medicine-Gastroenterology, Internal
Medicine-Geriatric Medicine, Internal
Medicine-Hematology, Internal Medicine-Infectious Diseases, Internal Medicine-Medical
Oncology, Internal Medicine-Nephrology, Internal Medicine-Rheumatology, Neurological
Surgery, Neurology, Obstetrics/Gynecology,
Ophthalmology, Orthopedic Surgery, Otolaryngology, Physical Medicine and Rehabilitation, Psychiatry, Radiation Oncology,
Surgery, Surgery-Vascular Surgery, Thoracic
Surgery, Urology

Virginia Commonwealth University
Medical College of Virginia
School of Dentistry
Box 980598
Richmond, VA 23298
804-828-9903
Teaching Specialties:
Dentistry

Roanoke

**Community Hospital of Roanoke
Valley**
101 Elm Ave., SE
Roanoke, VA 24013
703-985-8000
Teaching Specialties:
Internal Medicine

Roanoke Memorial Hospitals
1722 S. Jefferson St.

Roanoke, VA 24014
703-981-7000
Teaching Specialties:
Internal Medicine, Internal Medicine-Cardiovascular Disease, Internal Medicine-Infectious
Diseases, Obstetrics/Gynecology, Orthopedic
Surgery, Otolaryngology, Surgery

Virginia Beach

Virginia Beach General Hospital
1060 First Colonial Rd.
Virginia Beach, VA 23454
757-481-8000
Teaching Specialties:
Radiation Oncology

WASHINGTON

Seattle

**Fred Hutchinson Cancer Research
Center**
1124 Columbia St.
Seattle, WA 98104
206-667-5000
Teaching Specialties:
Internal Medicine-Medical Oncology

Harborview Medical Center
325 Ninth Ave.
Seattle, WA 98104
206-223-3000
Teaching Specialties:
Allergy/Immunology, Anesthesiology, Internal Medicine, Internal Medicine-Geriatric
Medicine, Neurological Surgery, Neurology,
Ophthalmology, Orthopedic Surgery, Physical Medicine and Rehabilitation, Psychiatry,
Surgery, Thoracic Surgery, Urology

Pacific Medical Center
1200 12th Ave. South
Seattle, WA 98144
206-326-4000
Teaching Specialties:
Internal Medicine, Surgery

Providence Medical Center
500 17th Ave.
Seattle, WA 98122
206-320-2000
Teaching Specialties:
Internal Medicine, Surgery

Swedish Hospital Medical Center
747 Broadway Ave.
Seattle, WA 98122
206-386-6000
Teaching Specialties:
Internal Medicine, Obstetrics/Gynecology,
Orthopedic Surgery, Surgery

University of Washington Medical Center
1959 N.E. Pacific St.
Seattle, WA 98195
206-548-3300
Teaching Specialties:
Allergy/Immunology, Anesthesiology, Dermatology, Internal Medicine, Internal Medicine-Cardiovascular Disease, Internal Medicine-Endocrinology and Metabolism, Internal Medicine-Gastroenterology, Internal Medicine-Hematology, Internal Medicine-Infectious Diseases, Internal Medicine-Medical Oncology, Internal Medicine-Nephrology, Internal Medicine-Rheumatology, Neurological Surgery, Neurology, Obstetrics/Gynecology, Ophthalmology, Orthopedic Surgery, Otolaryngology, Physical Medicine and Rehabilitation, Psychiatry, Radiation Oncology, Surgery, Surgery-Vascular Surgery, Thoracic Surgery, Urology

University of Washington School of Dentistry
1959 N.E. Pacific St., D322
Seattle, WA 98195
206-543-7072
Teaching Specialties:
Dentistry

Virginia Mason Medical Center
925 Seneca St.
Seattle, WA 98101
206-624-1144
Teaching Specialties:
Allergy/Immunology, Anesthesiology, Internal Medicine, Orthopedic Surgery, Surgery, Urology

Spokane

Deaconess Medical Center-Spokane
800 W. Fifth Ave.
Spokane, WA 99204
509-458-5800
Teaching Specialties:
Internal Medicine

Sacred Heart Medical Center
101 W. Eighth Ave.
Spokane, WA 99204
509-455-3131
Teaching Specialties:
Internal Medicine

WEST VIRGINIA
Charleston

Charleston Area Medical Center
3200 MacCorkle Ave., SE
Charleston, WV 25304
304-348-5432

Teaching Specialties:
Psychiatry

Charleston Area Medical Center
Memorial Division
3200 MacCorkle Ave., SE
Charleston, WV 25304
304-348-5432
Teaching Specialties:
Dentistry, Internal Medicine, Surgery

Charleston Area Medical Center
Women and Children's Hospital of West Virginia
800 Pennsylvania Ave.
Charleston, WV 25302
304-348-5432
Teaching Specialties:
Obstetrics/Gynecology

Huntington

Cabell Huntington Hospital
1340 Hal Greer Blvd.
Huntington, WV 25701
304-526-2000
Teaching Specialties:
Internal Medicine, Internal Medicine-Cardiovascular Disease, Internal Medicine-Endocrinology and Metabolism, Internal Medicine-Infectious Diseases, Surgery

St. Mary's Hospital
2900 First Ave.
Huntington, WV 25702
304-526-1234
Teaching Specialties:
Internal Medicine, Surgery

Morgantown

Monongalia General Hospital
1200 J. D. Anderson Dr.
Morgantown, WV 26505
304-598-1200
Teaching Specialties:
Orthopedic Surgery, Thoracic Surgery

West Virginia University Hospitals
Stadium Dr.
Morgantown, WV 26506
304-598-4000
Teaching Specialties:
Anesthesiology, Dermatology, Internal Medicine, Internal Medicine-Cardiovascular Disease, Internal Medicine-Gastroenterology, Internal Medicine-Nephrology, Neurological Surgery, Neurology, Obstetrics/Gynecology, Ophthalmology, Orthopedic Surgery, Otolaryngology, Psychiatry, Surgery, Thoracic Surgery, Urology

West Virginia University School of Dentistry
Department of Oral Diagnosis and Radiology
Morgantown, WV 26505
304-293-2459
Teaching Specialties:
Dentistry

Wheeling

Ohio Valley Medical Center
2000 Eoff St.
Wheeling, WV 26003
304-234-0123
Teaching Specialties:
Internal Medicine, Obstetrics/Gynecology, Urology

Wheeling Hospital
1 Medical Park
Wheeling, WV 26003
304-243-3000
Teaching Specialties:
Obstetrics/Gynecology

WISCONSIN
La Crosse

Lutheran Hospital-La Crosse
1910 South Ave.
La Crosse, WI 54601
608-785-0530
Teaching Specialties:
Dentistry, Internal Medicine, Surgery, Urology

Madison

Meriter Hospital
202 S. Park St.
Madison, WI 53715
608-267-6000
Teaching Specialties:
Dentistry, Neurological Surgery, Obstetrics/Gynecology, Orthopedic Surgery, Psychiatry, Surgery

St. Marys Hospital Medical Center
707 S. Mills St.
Madison, WI 53715
608-251-6100
Teaching Specialties:
Obstetrics/Gynecology, Orthopedic Surgery, Surgery

University of Wisconsin Hospital and Clinics
600 Highland Ave.
Madison, WI 53792
608-263-6400
Teaching Specialties:
Allergy/Immunology, Anesthesiology, Der-

matology, Internal Medicine, Internal Medicine-Cardiovascular Disease, Internal Medicine-Endocrinology and Metabolism, Internal Medicine-Gastroenterology, Internal Medicine-Geriatric Medicine, Internal Medicine-Hematology, Internal Medicine-Infectious Diseases, Internal Medicine-Medical Oncology, Internal Medicine-Nephrology, Internal Medicine-Rheumatology, Neurological Surgery, Neurology, Obstetrics/Gynecology, Ophthalmology, Otolaryngology, Physical Medicine and Rehabilitation, Psychiatry, Radiation Oncology, Surgery, Thoracic Surgery, Urology

Marshfield

St. Joseph's Hospital
611 St. Joseph Ave.
Marshfield, WI 54449
715-387-1713
Teaching Specialties:
Dermatology, Internal Medicine, Surgery

Milwaukee

Columbia Hospital
2025 E. Newport Ave.
Milwaukee, WI 53211
414-961-3300
Teaching Specialties:
Orthopedic Surgery, Psychiatry

Curative Rehabilitation Center
1000 N. 92nd St.
Milwaukee, WI 53226
414-259-1414
Teaching Specialties:
Physical Medicine and Rehabilitation

Froedtert Memorial Lutheran Hospital
9200 W. Wisconsin Ave.
Milwaukee, WI 53226
414-259-3000
Teaching Specialties:
Allergy/Immunology, Dermatology, Internal Medicine, Internal Medicine-Gastroenterology, Internal Medicine-Infectious Diseases, Internal Medicine-Nephrology, Internal

Medicine-Rheumatology, Neurological Surgery, Neurology, Orthopedic Surgery, Physical Medicine and Rehabilitation, Psychiatry, Surgery, Urology

John L. Doyne Hospital
8700 W. Wisconsin Ave.
Milwaukee, WI 53226
414-257-7996
Teaching Specialties:
Allergy/Immunology, Anesthesiology, Dermatology, Internal Medicine, Internal Medicine-Cardiovascular Disease, Internal Medicine-Endocrinology and Metabolism, Internal Medicine-Gastroenterology, Internal Medicine-Hematology, Internal Medicine-Infectious Diseases, Internal Medicine-Medical Oncology, Internal Medicine-Nephrology, Internal Medicine-Rheumatology, Neurological Surgery, Neurology, Obstetrics/Gynecology, Ophthalmology, Orthopedic Surgery, Otolaryngology, Physical Medicine and Rehabilitation, Psychiatry, Radiation Oncology, Surgery, Surgery-Vascular Surgery, Thoracic Surgery, Urology

Marquette University School of Dentistry
604 N. 16th St.
Milwaukee, WI 53233
414-288-3532
Teaching Specialties:
Dentistry

Medical College of Wisconsin
Department of Oral and Maxillofacial Surgery
9200 W. Wisconsin Ave.
Milwaukee, WI 53226
414-454-5760
Teaching Specialties:
Dentistry

Milwaukee Psychiatric Hospital
1220 Dewey Ave.
Milwaukee, WI 53213
414-454-6600
Teaching Specialties:
Psychiatry

Sinai Samaritan Medical Center-Mt. Sinai Campus
945 N. 12th St.
Milwaukee, WI 53201
414-345-3400
Teaching Specialties:
Internal Medicine, Internal Medicine-Cardiovascular Disease, Obstetrics/Gynecology, Orthopedic Surgery, Psychiatry

St. Joseph's Hospital
5000 W. Chambers St.
Milwaukee, WI 53210
414-447-2000
Teaching Specialties:
Orthopedic Surgery

St. Luke's Medical Center
2900 W. Oklahoma Ave.
Milwaukee, WI 53215
414-649-6000
Teaching Specialties:
Otolaryngology, Physical Medicine and Rehabilitation, Thoracic Surgery

Oshkosh

Mercy Medical Center
631 Hazel St.
Oshkosh, WI 54901
414-236-2000
Teaching Specialties:
Psychiatry

Winnebago

Winnebago Mental Health Institute
PO Box 9
Winnebago, WI 54985
920-236-2904
Teaching Specialties:
Psychiatry

To find a hospital with a teaching specialty of interest to you, turn to the appropriate disorder and look for your state. Because any number of teaching specialties could qualify a hospital for inclusion under one of these disorders, check the list of teaching specialties under the Teaching Hospitals by State and City listing (page 486) to see if the hospital has the specific specialty that you need.

Bold type indicates an Academic Medical Center Hospital.

Bold type with an asterisk indicates a private Academic Medical Center Hospital.

A ▼ or † or ■ indicates a hospital associated with a National Institutes of Health research center.

Italic type indicates Medicare-approved heart and liver transplant centers in The Heart and Blood Vessels and The Digestive System sections only.

Cancer

▼ indicates National Cancer Institute: Comprehensive, Clinical, or Consortium Cancer Center

ALABAMA

▼University of Alabama Hospitals, Birmingham

University of South Alabama Medical Center, Mobile

ARIZONA

▼*University Medical Center, Tucson

ARKANSAS

University Hospital of Arkansas, Little Rock

CALIFORNIA

California Medical Center-Los Angeles, Los Angeles

Cedars-Sinai Medical Center, Los Angeles

▼City of Hope National Medical Center, Duarte

Green Hospital of Scripps Clinic, La Jolla

Kaiser Foundation Hospital, Los Angeles

*Loma Linda University Medical Center, Loma Linda

Long Beach Memorial Medical Center, Long Beach

Los Angeles County Harbor-University of California, Los Angeles Medical Center, Torrance

Los Angeles County-University of Southern California Medical Center, Los Angeles

Mt. Zion Medical Center of University of California, San Francisco, San Francisco

San Francisco General Hospital and Medical Center, San Francisco

Seton Medical Center, Daly City

St. Joseph Hospital, Orange

St. Mary's Hospital and Medical Center, San Francisco

*Stanford University Hospital, Stanford

▼University of California, Los Angeles Medical Center, Los Angeles

University of California, Davis Medical Center, Sacramento

University of California, Irvine Medical Center, Orange

▼University of California, San Diego Medical Center, San Diego

University of California, San Francisco Medical Center, San Francisco

▼University of Southern California The Kenneth Norris Jr. Cancer Hospital, Los Angeles

COLORADO

Denver Health and Hospitals, Denver

Presbyterian-St. Luke's Medical Center, Denver

▼University of Colorado Health Sciences Center University Hospital, Denver

CONNECTICUT

Hospital of St. Raphael, New Haven

University of Connecticut Health Center John Dempsey Hospital, Farmington

University of Connecticut Health Center Uncas on Thames Hospital, Norwich

▼***Yale-New Haven Hospital, New Haven**

DISTRICT OF COLUMBIA

District of Columbia General Hospital, Washington

***George Washington University Hospital, Washington**

▼***Georgetown University Hospital, Washington**

***Howard University Hospital, Washington**

Washington Hospital Center, Washington

FLORIDA

Jackson Memorial Hospital, Miami

***Shands Hospital at the University of Florida, Gainesville**

University of South Florida H. Lee Moffitt Cancer Center, Tampa

GEORGIA

***Emory University Hospital, Atlanta**

Grady Memorial Hospital, Atlanta

Medical College of Georgia Georgia Radiation Therapy Center at Augusta, Augusta

Medical College of Georgia Hospital and Clinics, Augusta

ILLINOIS

Columbus Hospital, Chicago

Cook County Hospital, Chicago

Evanston Hospital, Evanston

Humana Hospital-Michael Reese, Chicago

Mercy Hospital and Medical Center, Chicago

Mt. Sinai Hospital Medical Center of Chicago, Chicago

▼***Northwestern Memorial Hospital, Chicago**

▼***Rush-Presbyterian-St. Luke's Medical Center, Chicago**

St. Cabrini Hospital, Chicago

St. Francis Hospital of Evanston, Evanston

▼***University of Chicago Hospitals, Chicago**

▼**University of Illinois Hospital and Clinics, Chicago**

INDIANA

Indiana University Medical Center, Indianapolis

William N. Wishard Memorial Hospital, Indianapolis

IOWA

University of Iowa Hospitals and Clinics, Iowa City

KANSAS

University of Kansas Hospital, Kansas City

KENTUCKY

Humana Hospital-University of Louisville, Louisville

University of Kentucky Hospital Albert B. Chandler Medical Center, Lexington

LOUISIANA

University Hospital, New Orleans

Louisiana State University Hospital, Shreveport

Medical Center of Louisiana at New Orleans, New Orleans

Ochsner Foundation Hospital, New Orleans

MARYLAND

▼***Johns Hopkins Hospital, Baltimore**

***University of Maryland Medical System, Baltimore**

MASSACHUSETTS

Baystate Medical Center, Springfield

***Beth Israel Hospital, Boston**

Boston Medical Center, Boston

***Brigham and Women's Hospital, Boston**

▼Dana-Farber Cancer Institute, Boston

***Massachusetts General Hospital, Boston**

New England Deaconess Hospital, Boston

***New England Medical Center, Boston**

St. Elizabeth's Hospital, Boston

***University Hospital, Boston**

University of Massachusetts Medical Center, Worcester

MICHIGAN

Detroit Receiving Hospital and University Health Center, Detroit

***Grace Hospital, Detroit**

▼***Harper Hospital, Detroit**

Henry Ford Hospital, Detroit

Providence Hospital, Southfield

▼**University of Michigan Hospitals, Ann Arbor**

William Beaumont Hospital, Royal Oak

MINNESOTA

▼Mayo Clinic, Rochester

Rochester Methodist Hospital, Rochester

***St. Mary's Hospital, Rochester**

University of Minnesota Hospital and Clinic, Minneapolis

MISSISSIPPI

University of Mississippi Medical Center University Hospitals and Clinics, Jackson

MISSOURI

***Barnes-Jewish Hospital, St. Louis**

Mallinckrodt Institute of Radiology, St. Louis

***St. Louis University Medical Center, St. Louis**

Trinity Lutheran Hospital,
Kansas City

**Truman Medical Center-West,
Kansas City**

**University Hospital and Clinics,
Columbia**

NEBRASKA

**University of Nebraska Medical
Center, Omaha**

NEW HAMPSHIRE

▼Dartmouth-Hitchcock Medical
Center, Hanover

NEW JERSEY

Cooper Hospital-University Medical
Center, Camden

Newark Beth Israel Medical Center,
Newark

***Robert Wood Johnson University
Hospital, New Brunswick**

St. Barnabas Medical Center,
Livingston

St. Joseph's Hospital and Medical
Center, Paterson

St. Michael's Medical Center,
Newark

St. Peter's Medical Center,
New Brunswick

United Hospitals Medical Center,
Newark

**University of Medicine and
Dentistry of New Jersey University
Hospital, Newark**

NEW MEXICO

University Hospital, Albuquerque

NEW YORK

***Albany Medical Center Hospital,
Albany**

**Bellevue Hospital Center,
New York**

Beth Israel Medical Center,
New York

Bronx Municipal Hospital Center,
Bronx

Brookdale Hospital Medical
Center, Brooklyn

Brooklyn Hospital Center,
Brooklyn

Cabrini Medical Center, New York

Harlem Hospital Center, New York

Interfaith Medical Center,
Brooklyn

**Kings County Hospital Center,
Brooklyn**

Lenox Hill Hospital, New York

Long Island College Hospital,
Brooklyn

Long Island Jewish Medical Center,
New Hyde Park

Lutheran Medical Center, Brooklyn

Maimonides Medical Center,
Brooklyn

Mary Immaculate Hospital, Jamaica

▼Memorial Sloan-Kettering Cancer
Center, New York

Methodist Hospital of Brooklyn,
Brooklyn

***Montefiore Medical Center Henry
and Lucy Moses Division, Bronx**

▼Montefiore Medical Center Jack
D. Weiler Hospital of the Albert
Einstein College of Medicine,
Bronx

***Mt. Sinai Medical Center,
New York**

Nassau County Medical Center,
East Meadow

***New York Hospital-Cornell
Medical Center, New York**

**▼*New York University Medical
Center, New York**

North Shore University Hospital,
Manhasset

**▼*Presbyterian Hospital in the City
of New York Columbia-
Presbyterian Medical Center, New
York**

▼Rochester General Hospital,
Rochester

▼Roswell Park Cancer Institute,
Buffalo

St. Luke's-Roosevelt Hospital
Center Roosevelt Division,
New York

St. Luke's-Roosevelt Hospital
Center St. Luke's Division,
New York

St. Mary's Hospital, Brooklyn

St. Vincent's Hospital and Medical
Center of New York, New York

**State University of New York at
Stony Brook University Hospital,
Stony Brook**

**State University of New York
Health Science Center University
Hospital, Syracuse**

**State University of New York
Health Science Center at Brooklyn
University Hospital of Brooklyn,
Brooklyn**

**▼*Strong Memorial Hospital of the
University of Rochester, Rochester**

**Westchester County Medical
Center, Valhalla**

Winthrop-University Hospital,
Mineola

Woodhull Medical and Mental
Health Center, Brooklyn

NORTH CAROLINA

**▼*Duke University Medical Center,
Durham**

**▼*North Carolina Baptist Hospital,
Winston-Salem**

**▼University of North Carolina
Hospitals, Chapel Hill**

OHIO

Cleveland Clinic, Cleveland

**Medical College of Ohio Hospital,
Toledo**

**MetroHealth Medical Center,
Cleveland**

**▼Ohio State University Hospitals,
Columbus**

St. Vincent Medical Center, Toledo

**▼*University Hospitals of
Cleveland, Cleveland**

**University of Cincinnati Hospital,
Cincinnati**

OKLAHOMA

**Oklahoma Medical Center,
Oklahoma City**

OREGON

**Oregon Health Sciences University
University Hospital, Portland**

PENNSYLVANIA

Albert Einstein Medical Center, Philadelphia

*Allegheny General Hospital, Pittsburgh

▼American Oncologic Hospital-Fox Chase Cancer Center, Philadelphia

*Hahnemann University Hospital, Philadelphia

*Hospital of the Medical College of Pennsylvania, Philadelphia

▼*Hospital of the University of Pennsylvania, Philadelphia

▼Montefiore University Hospital, Pittsburgh

Penn State University Hospital The Milton S. Hershey Medical Center, Hershey

▼*Presbyterian University Hospital, Pittsburgh

*Temple University Hospital, Philadelphia

*Thomas Jefferson University Hospital, Philadelphia

PUERTO RICO

Fundación Hospital Metropolitan, San Juan

San Juan Municipal Hospital, Rio Piedras

University Hospital, San Juan

RHODE ISLAND

Memorial Hospital of Rhode Island, Pawtucket

Miriam Hospital, Providence

▼Roger Williams Hospital, Providence

SOUTH CAROLINA

Medical Center of Medical University of South Carolina, Charleston

Richland Memorial Hospital, Columbia

TENNESSEE

Baptist Memorial Hospital, Memphis

Johnson City Medical Center Hospital, Johnson City

Regional Medical Center at Memphis, Memphis

St. Thomas Hospital, Nashville

*Vanderbilt University Hospital and Clinic, Nashville

TEXAS

Baylor University Medical Center, Dallas

Bexar County Hospital District Medical Center Hospital, San Antonio

▼Cancer Therapy and Research Center, San Antonio

Dallas County Hospital District Parkland Memorial Hospital, Dallas

Harrington Cancer Center, Amarillo

Harris County Hospital District Ben Taub General Hospital, Houston

High Plains Baptist Hospital, Amarillo

*Methodist Hospital, Houston

Northwest Texas Hospital, Amarillo

University Medical Center, Lubbock

▼University of Texas M. D. Anderson Cancer Center, Houston

University of Texas Medical Branch Hospitals, Galveston

UTAH

LDS Hospital, Salt Lake City

▼University of Utah Hospital and Clinics, Salt Lake City

VERMONT

▼*Fletcher Allen Healthcare MCHV Campus, Burlington

VIRGINIA

Maryview Medical Center, Portsmouth

Sentara Norfolk General Hospital, Norfolk

University of Virginia Medical Center, Charlottesville

Virginia Beach General Hospital, Virginia Beach

▼Virginia Commonwealth University Medical College of Virginia Hospitals, Richmond

WASHINGTON

▼Fred Hutchinson Cancer Research Center, Seattle

University of Washington Medical Center, Seattle

WISCONSIN

John L. Doyne Hospital, Milwaukee

▼University of Wisconsin Hospital and Clinics, Madison

The Blood

ALABAMA

University of Alabama Hospitals, Birmingham

▼University of South Alabama Medical Center, Mobile

ARIZONA

*University Medical Center, Tucson

ARKANSAS

University Hospital of Arkansas, Little Rock

CALIFORNIA

Cedars-Sinai Medical Center, Los Angeles

Green Hospital of Scripps Clinic, La Jolla

Kaiser Foundation Hospital, Los Angeles

Los Angeles County Harbor-University of California, Los Angeles Medical Center, Torrance

Los Angeles County-University of Southern California Medical Center, Los Angeles

Olive View Medical Center, Sylmar

▼San Francisco General Hospital and Medical Center, San Francisco

*Stanford University Hospital, Stanford

University of California, Los Angeles Medical Center, Los Angeles

University of California, Davis Medical Center, Sacramento

University of California, Irvine Medical Center, Orange

University of California, San Diego Medical Center, San Diego

University of California, San Francisco Medical Center, San Francisco

COLORADO

Denver Health and Hospitals, Denver

University of Colorado Health Sciences Center University Hospital, Denver

CONNECTICUT

University of Connecticut Health Center John Dempsey Hospital, Farmington

*Yale-New Haven Hospital, New Haven

DISTRICT OF COLUMBIA

District of Columbia General Hospital, Washington

*George Washington University Hospital, Washington

*Georgetown University Hospital, Washington

*Howard University Hospital, Washington

FLORIDA

Jackson Memorial Hospital, Miami

*Shands Hospital at the University of Florida, Gainesville

University Medical Center, Jacksonville

GEORGIA

*Emory University Hospital, Atlanta

Grady Memorial Hospital, Atlanta

Medical College of Georgia Hospital and Clinics, Augusta

ILLINOIS

Cook County Hospital, Chicago

*Loyola University of Chicago Foster G. McGaw Hospital, Maywood

Mt. Sinai Hospital Medical Center of Chicago, Chicago

*Northwestern Memorial Hospital, Chicago

*Rush-Presbyterian-St. Luke's Medical Center, Chicago

St. Francis Hospital of Evanston, Evanston

*University of Chicago Hospitals, Chicago

University of Illinois Hospital and Clinics, Chicago

INDIANA

Indiana University Medical Center, Indianapolis

IOWA

University of Iowa Hospitals and Clinics, Iowa City

KANSAS

University of Kansas Hospital, Kansas City

KENTUCKY

University of Kentucky Hospital Albert B. Chandler Medical Center, Lexington

LOUISIANA

Louisiana State University Hospital, Shreveport

Medical Center of Louisiana at New Orleans, New Orleans

*Tulane University Hospital and Clinics, New Orleans

MARYLAND

*Johns Hopkins Hospital, Baltimore

*University of Maryland Medical System, Baltimore

MASSACHUSETTS

Baystate Medical Center, Springfield

*Beth Israel Hospital, Boston

▼Boston Medical Center, Boston

*Brigham and Women's Hospital, Boston

*Massachusetts General Hospital, Boston

New England Deaconess Hospital, Boston

*New England Medical Center, Boston

St. Elizabeth's Hospital, Boston

*University Hospital, Boston

University of Massachusetts Medical Center, Worcester

MICHIGAN

Detroit Receiving Hospital and University Health Center, Detroit

*Harper Hospital, Detroit

Henry Ford Hospital, Detroit

St. Lawrence Hospital and Healthcare Services, Lansing

University of Michigan Hospitals, Ann Arbor

William Beaumont Hospital, Royal Oak

MINNESOTA

Mayo Clinic, Rochester

Rochester Methodist Hospital, Rochester

*St. Mary's Hospital, Rochester

University of Minnesota Hospital and Clinic, Minneapolis

MISSISSIPPI

University of Mississippi Medical Center University Hospitals and Clinics, Jackson

MISSOURI

*Barnes-Jewish Hospital, St. Louis

*St. Louis University Medical Center, St. Louis

Trinity Lutheran Hospital, Kansas City

Truman Medical Center-West, Kansas City

University Hospital and Clinics, Columbia

NEBRASKA

University of Nebraska Medical Center, Omaha

NEW HAMPSHIRE

Dartmouth-Hitchcock Medical Center, Hanover

NEW JERSEY

Cooper Hospital-University Medical Center, Camden

Newark Beth Israel Medical Center, Newark

*Robert Wood Johnson University Hospital, New Brunswick

St. Joseph's Hospital and Medical Center, Paterson

St. Michael's Medical Center, Newark

St. Peter's Medical Center, New Brunswick

United Hospitals Medical Center, Newark

University of Medicine and Dentistry of New Jersey University Hospital, Newark

NEW MEXICO

University Hospital, Albuquerque

NEW YORK

*Albany Medical Center Hospital, Albany

Bellevue Hospital Center, New York

Beth Israel Medical Center, New York

Bronx-Lebanon Hospital Center, Bronx

Bronx Municipal Hospital Center, Bronx

Brookdale Hospital Medical Center, Brooklyn

Brooklyn Hospital Center, Brooklyn

*Buffalo General Hospital, Buffalo

Cabrini Medical Center, New York

Coney Island Hospital, Brooklyn

Erie County Medical Center, Buffalo

Harlem Hospital Center, New York

Interfaith Medical Center, Brooklyn

Jamaica Hospital, Jamaica

Kings County Hospital Center, Brooklyn

Lenox Hill Hospital, New York

Lincoln Medical and Mental Health Center, Bronx

Long Island College Hospital, Brooklyn

Long Island Jewish Medical Center, New Hyde Park

Maimonides Medical Center, Brooklyn

Mary Immaculate Hospital, Jamaica

Memorial Sloan-Kettering Cancer Center, New York

Methodist Hospital of Brooklyn, Brooklyn

Metropolitan Hospital Center, New York

▼*Montefiore Medical Center Henry and Lucy Moses Division, Bronx

*Mt. Sinai Medical Center, New York

Nassau County Medical Center, East Meadow

*New York Hospital-Cornell Medical Center, New York

North Shore University Hospital, Manhasset

Our Lady of Mercy Medical Center, Bronx

▼*Presbyterian Hospital in the City of New York Columbia-Presbyterian Medical Center, New York

Rochester General Hospital, Rochester

St. Luke's-Roosevelt Hospital Center Roosevelt Division, New York

St. Luke's-Roosevelt Hospital Center St. Luke's Division, New York

St. Mary's Hospital, Brooklyn

St. Vincent's Hospital and Medical Center of New York, New York

State University of New York at Stony Brook University Hospital, Stony Brook

State University of New York Health Science Center University Hospital, Syracuse

State University of New York Health Science Center at Brooklyn University Hospital of Brooklyn, Brooklyn

*Strong Memorial Hospital of the University of Rochester, Rochester

Westchester County Medical Center, Valhalla

Winthrop-University Hospital, Mineola

Woodhull Medical and Mental Health Center, Brooklyn

NORTH CAROLINA

▼*Duke University Medical Center, Durham

University of North Carolina Hospitals, Chapel Hill

OHIO

Cleveland Clinic, Cleveland

Medical College of Ohio Hospital, Toledo

MetroHealth Medical Center, Cleveland

Ohio State University Hospitals, Columbus

St. Vincent Medical Center, Toledo

*University Hospitals of Cleveland, Cleveland

University of Cincinnati Hospital, Cincinnati

OKLAHOMA

Oklahoma Medical Center, Oklahoma City

OREGON

Oregon Health Sciences University University Hospital, Portland

PENNSYLVANIA

American Oncologic Hospital-Fox Chase Cancer Center, Philadelphia

*Hahnemann University Hospital, Philadelphia

*Hospital of the Medical College of Pennsylvania, Philadelphia

*Hospital of the University of Pennsylvania, Philadelphia

Lankenau Hospital, Wynnewood

Montefiore University Hospital, Pittsburgh

Penn State University Hospital The Milton S. Hershey Medical Center, Hershey

*Presbyterian University Hospital, Pittsburgh

*Temple University Hospital, Philadelphia

*Thomas Jefferson University Hospital, Philadelphia

PUERTO RICO

San Juan Municipal Hospital, Rio Piedras

University Hospital, San Juan

RHODE ISLAND

Memorial Hospital of Rhode Island, Pawtucket

Miriam Hospital, Providence

*Rhode Island Hospital, Providence

Roger Williams Hospital, Providence

SOUTH CAROLINA

Medical Center of Medical University of South Carolina, Charleston

TENNESSEE

Baptist Memorial Hospital, Memphis

Regional Medical Center at Memphis, Memphis

*Vanderbilt University Hospital and Clinic, Nashville

TEXAS

Bexar County Hospital District Medical Center Hospital, San Antonio

Dallas County Hospital District Parkland Memorial Hospital, Dallas

Harris County Hospital District Ben Taub General Hospital, Houston

*Hermann Hospital, Houston

*Methodist Hospital, Houston

UTAH

University of Utah Hospital and Clinics, Salt Lake City

VERMONT

*Fletcher Allen Healthcare MCHV Campus, Burlington

VIRGINIA

University of Virginia Medical Center, Charlottesville

Virginia Commonwealth University Medical College of Virginia Hospitals, Richmond

WASHINGTON

University of Washington Medical Center, Seattle

WISCONSIN

John L. Doyne Hospital, Milwaukee

University of Wisconsin Hospital and Clinics, Madison

The Brain and Nervous System

▼ indicates National Institute on Aging: Alzheimer's Disease Center

† indicates National Institute of Neurological Disorders and Stroke: Epilepsy Clinical Research Center

■ indicates National Institute of Neurological Disorders and Stroke: Neuromuscular Clinical Research Center

ALABAMA

University of Alabama Hospitals, Birmingham

University of South Alabama Medical Center, Mobile

ARIZONA

Maricopa Medical Center, Phoenix

St. Joseph's Hospital and Medical Center Barrow Neurological Institute, Phoenix

Tucson Medical Center, Tucson

*University Medical Center, Tucson

ARKANSAS

University Hospital of Arkansas, Little Rock

CALIFORNIA

Highland General Hospital, Oakland

Huntington Memorial Hospital, Pasadena

Kaiser Foundation Hospital, Los Angeles

Kaiser Foundation Hospital, Sacramento

Kaiser Foundation Hospital, San Diego

*Loma Linda University Medical Center, Loma Linda

Los Angeles County Harbor-University of California, Los Angeles Medical Center, Torrance

▼Los Angeles County-University of Southern California Medical Center, Los Angeles

Riverside General Hospital University Medical Center, Riverside

San Francisco General Hospital and Medical Center, San Francisco

Santa Clara Valley Medical Center, San Jose

†*Stanford University Hospital, Stanford

†University of California, Los Angeles Medical Center, Los Angeles

University of California, Davis Medical Center, Sacramento

University of California, Irvine Medical Center, Orange

▼University of California, San Diego Medical Center, San Diego

University of California, San Francisco Medical Center, San Francisco

COLORADO
Denver Health and Hospitals, Denver

University of Colorado Health Sciences Center University Hospital, Denver

CONNECTICUT
Hartford Hospital, Hartford

University of Connecticut Health Center John Dempsey Hospital, Farmington

†*Yale-New Haven Hospital, New Haven

DELAWARE
Medical Center of Delaware, Wilmington

DISTRICT OF COLUMBIA
District of Columbia General Hospital, Washington

*George Washington University Hospital, Washington

*Georgetown University Hospital, Washington

*Howard University Hospital, Washington

Washington Hospital Center, Washington

FLORIDA
Jackson Memorial Hospital, Miami

Mt. Sinai Medical Center, Miami Beach

*Shands Hospital at the University of Florida, Gainesville

Tampa General Hospital, Tampa

GEORGIA
*Crawford Long Hospital of Emory University, Atlanta

*Emory University Hospital, Atlanta

Grady Memorial Hospital, Atlanta

Medical College of Georgia Hospital and Clinics, Augusta

University Hospital, Augusta

ILLINOIS
Christ Hospital and Medical Center, Oak Lawn

Cook County Hospital, Chicago

Evanston Hospital, Evanston

Humana Hospital-Michael Reese, Chicago

*Loyola University of Chicago Foster G. McGaw Hospital, Maywood

▼Memorial Medical Center, Springfield

Methodist Medical Center of Illinois, Peoria

*Northwestern Memorial Hospital, Chicago

*Rush-Presbyterian-St. Luke's Medical Center, Chicago

St. Francis Medical Center, Peoria

▼St. John's Hospital, Springfield

*University of Chicago Hospitals, Chicago

University of Illinois Hospital and Clinics, Chicago

INDIANA
Indiana University Medical Center, Indianapolis

William N. Wishard Memorial Hospital, Indianapolis

IOWA
University of Iowa Hospitals and Clinics, Iowa City

KANSAS
University of Kansas Hospital, Kansas City

KENTUCKY
Humana Hospital-University of Louisville, Louisville

Norton Hospital, Louisville

▼University of Kentucky Hospital Albert B. Chandler Medical Center, Lexington

LOUISIANA
University Hospital, New Orleans

Medical Center of Louisiana at New Orleans, New Orleans

Ochsner Foundation Hospital, New Orleans

Memorial Medical Center, New Orleans

*Tulane University Hospital and Clinics, New Orleans

MARYLAND
Francis Scott Key Medical Center, Baltimore

▼*Johns Hopkins Hospital, Baltimore

*University of Maryland Medical System, Baltimore

MASSACHUSETTS
*Beth Israel Hospital, Boston

Boston Medical Center, Boston

*Brigham and Women's Hospital, Boston

Lahey Clinic Hospital, Burlington

▼*Massachusetts General Hospital, Boston

New England Deaconess Hospital, Boston

*New England Medical Center, Boston

St. Elizabeth's Hospital, Boston

St. Vincent Hospital, Worcester

*University Hospital, Boston

University of Massachusetts Medical Center, Worcester

MICHIGAN
Detroit Receiving Hospital and University Health Center, Detroit

*Harper Hospital, Detroit

Henry Ford Hospital, Detroit

St. Joseph Mercy Hospital, Ann Arbor

▼University of Michigan Hospitals, Ann Arbor

MINNESOTA
Hennepin County Medical Center, Minneapolis

▼Mayo Clinic, Rochester

THE BRAIN AND NERVOUS SYSTEM

Rochester Methodist Hospital, Rochester

*St. Mary's Hospital, Rochester

Regions Hospital, St. Paul

†University of Minnesota Hospital and Clinic, Minneapolis

MISSISSIPPI

University of Mississippi Medical Center University Hospitals and Clinics, Jackson

MISSOURI

▼†*Barnes-Jewish Hospital, St. Louis

Boone Hospital Center, Columbia

St. Louis Regional Medical Center, St. Louis

*St. Louis University Medical Center, St. Louis

University Hospital and Clinics, Columbia

NEBRASKA

AMI St. Joseph Hospital, Omaha

University of Nebraska Medical Center, Omaha

NEW HAMPSHIRE

Dartmouth-Hitchcock Medical Center, Hanover

NEW JERSEY

*Robert Wood Johnson University Hospital, New Brunswick

St. Barnabas Medical Center, Livingston

University of Medicine and Dentistry of New Jersey University Hospital, Newark

NEW MEXICO

University Hospital, Albuquerque

NEW YORK

*Albany Medical Center Hospital, Albany

Bellevue Hospital Center, New York

Bronx Municipal Hospital Center, Bronx

*Buffalo General Hospital, Buffalo

Crouse-Irving Memorial Hospital, Syracuse

Elmhurst Hospital Center, Flushing

Erie County Medical Center, Buffalo

Harlem Hospital Center, New York

Kings County Hospital Center, Brooklyn

Lincoln Medical and Mental Health Center, Bronx

Long Island Jewish Medical Center, New Hyde Park

Memorial Sloan-Kettering Cancer Center, New York

Metropolitan Hospital Center, New York

Millard Fillmore Hospitals, Buffalo

Millard Fillmore Hospitals Dent Neurological Institute, Buffalo

*Montefiore Medical Center Henry and Lucy Moses Division, Bronx

Montefiore Medical Center Jack D. Weiler Hospital of the Albert Einstein College of Medicine, Bronx

*Mt. Sinai Medical Center, New York

Nassau County Medical Center, East Meadow

*New York Hospital-Cornell Medical Center, New York

▼*New York University Medical Center, New York

North Shore University Hospital, Manhasset

▼■*Presbyterian Hospital in the City of New York Columbia-Presbyterian Medical Center, New York

Queens Hospital Center, Jamaica

St. Vincent's Hospital and Medical Center of New York, New York

State University of New York at Stony Brook University Hospital, Stony Brook

State University of New York Health Science Center University Hospital, Syracuse

State University of New York Health Science Center at Brooklyn University Hospital of Brooklyn, Brooklyn

▼*Strong Memorial Hospital of the University of Rochester, Rochester

Westchester County Medical Center, Valhalla

NORTH CAROLINA

▼†*Duke University Medical Center, Durham

Durham County General Hospital, Durham

*North Carolina Baptist Hospital, Winston-Salem

University of North Carolina Hospitals, Chapel Hill

OHIO

Christ Hospital, Cincinnati

Cleveland Clinic, Cleveland

Good Samaritan Hospital, Cincinnati

MetroHealth Medical Center, Cleveland

Ohio State University Hospitals, Columbus

Riverside Methodist Hospitals, Columbus

▼*University Hospitals of Cleveland, Cleveland

University of Cincinnati Hospital, Cincinnati

OKLAHOMA

Oklahoma Medical Center, Oklahoma City

St. Anthony Hospital, Oklahoma City

OREGON

Good Samaritan Hospital and Medical Center, Portland

Kaiser Sunnyside Medical Center, Clackamas

▼Oregon Health Sciences University University Hospital, Portland

PENNSYLVANIA

Albert Einstein Medical Center, Philadelphia

Crozer-Chester Medical Center, Upland

*Hahnemann University Hospital, Philadelphia

*Hospital of the Medical College of Pennsylvania, Philadelphia

■*Hospital of the University of Pennsylvania, Philadelphia

▼Montefiore University Hospital, Pittsburgh

Penn State University Hospital The Milton S. Hershey Medical Center, Hershey

Pennsylvania Hospital, Philadelphia

▼*Presbyterian University Hospital, Pittsburgh

*Temple University Hospital, Philadelphia

*Thomas Jefferson University Hospital, Philadelphia

PUERTO RICO

San Juan Municipal Hospital, Rio Piedras

University Hospital, San Juan

RHODE ISLAND

*Rhode Island Hospital, Providence

SOUTH CAROLINA

Medical Center of Medical University of South Carolina, Charleston

TENNESSEE

Baptist Hospital, Nashville

Baptist Memorial Hospital, Memphis

Methodist Hospitals of Memphis Central Unit, Memphis

Metropolitan Nashville General Hospital, Nashville

Regional Medical Center at Memphis, Memphis

St. Thomas Hospital, Nashville

University of Tennessee Medical Center, Memphis

*Vanderbilt University Hospital and Clinic, Nashville

TEXAS

Bexar County Hospital District Medical Center Hospital, San Antonio

Dallas County Hospital District Parkland Memorial Hospital, Dallas

†Harris County Hospital District Ben Taub General Hospital, Houston

*Hermann Hospital, Houston

†*Methodist Hospital, Houston

St. Paul Medical Center, Dallas

University Medical Center, Lubbock

University of Texas M. D. Anderson Cancer Center, Houston

University of Texas Medical Branch Hospitals, Galveston

Zale-Lipshy University Hospital, Dallas

UTAH

University of Utah Hospital and Clinics, Salt Lake City

VERMONT

*Fletcher Allen Healthcare MCHV Campus, Burlington

VIRGINIA

Sentara Norfolk General Hospital, Norfolk

University of Virginia Medical Center, Charlottesville

†Virginia Commonwealth University Medical College of Virginia Hospitals, Richmond

WASHINGTON

Harborview Medical Center, Seattle

†University of Washington Medical Center, Seattle

WEST VIRGINIA

*West Virginia University Hospitals, Morgantown

WISCONSIN

*Froedtert Memorial Lutheran Hospital, Milwaukee

Meriter Hospital, Madison

John L. Doyne Hospital, Milwaukee

University of Wisconsin Hospital and Clinics, Madison

Dental and Oral Disorders

ALABAMA

University of Alabama School of Dentistry, Birmingham

CALIFORNIA

Cedars-Sinai Medical Center, Los Angeles

Highland General Hospital, Oakland

Loma Linda University School of Dentistry, Loma Linda

Los Angeles County Harbor-University of California, Los Angeles Medical Center, Torrance

Los Angeles County-King-Drew Medical Center, Los Angeles

Los Angeles County-University of Southern California Medical Center, Los Angeles

University of California, Los Angeles School of Dentistry Center for the Health Sciences, Los Angeles

University of California, San Francisco School of Dentistry, San Francisco

University of Southern California School of Dentistry, Los Angeles

University of the Pacific School of Dentistry, San Francisco

Valley Medical Center of Fresno, Fresno

COLORADO

Denver Health and Hospitals, Denver

St. Joseph Hospital, Denver

University of Colorado School
of Dentistry, Denver

CONNECTICUT

Danbury Hospital, Danbury

Hartford Hospital, Hartford

Hospital of St. Raphael, New Haven

Mt. Sinai Hospital, Hartford

Southbury Training School,
Southbury

St. Francis Hospital and Medical
Center, Hartford

St. Mary's Hospital, Waterbury

University of Connecticut School
of Dental Medicine, Farmington

Waterbury Hospital, Waterbury

***Yale-New Haven Hospital, New
Haven**

DELAWARE

Medical Center of Delaware,
Wilmington

DISTRICT OF COLUMBIA

***Georgetown University Hospital,
Washington**

Howard University College
of Dentistry, Washington

St. Elizabeths Hospital DC
Commission on Mental Health
Services, Washington

Washington Hospital Center,
Washington

FLORIDA

Dade County Dental Research
Clinic, Miami

Jackson Memorial Hospital, Miami

Mt. Sinai Medical Center,
Miami Beach

University Medical Center,
Jacksonville

University of Florida College
of Dentistry, Gainesville

GEORGIA

Emory University School
of Medicine, Atlanta

Medical College of Georgia School
of Dentistry, Augusta

HAWAII

Queen's Medical Center, Honolulu

ILLINOIS

Carle Foundation Hospital, Urbana

Cook County Hospital, Chicago

Evanston Hospital, Evanston

Illinois Masonic Medical Center,
Chicago

Loyola University of Chicago
School of Dentistry, Maywood

Mt. Sinai Hospital Medical Center
of Chicago, Chicago

Northwestern University Dental
School, Chicago

Ravenswood Hospital Medical
Center, Chicago

***Rush-Presbyterian-St. Luke's
Medical Center, Chicago**

Southern Illinois University School
of Dental Medicine, Alton

***University of Chicago Hospitals,
Chicago**

University of Illinois at Chicago
College of Dentistry, Chicago

INDIANA

Indiana University School
of Dentistry, Indianapolis

IOWA

University of Iowa College
of Dentistry, Iowa City

KENTUCKY

University of Kentucky College
of Dentistry, Lexington

University of Louisville School
of Dentistry, Louisville

LOUISIANA

Louisiana State University School
of Dentistry, New Orleans

**Medical Center of Louisiana
at New Orleans, New Orleans**

MARYLAND

***Johns Hopkins Hospital,
Baltimore**

Prince George's Hospital Center,
Cheverly

University of Maryland at Baltimore
Baltimore College of Dentistry
Dental School, Baltimore

MASSACHUSETTS

Berkshire Medical Center, Pittsfield

Boston Medical Center, Boston

Boston University Henry M.
Goldman School of Graduate
Dentistry, Boston

***Brigham and Women's Hospital,
Boston**

Harvard School of Dental
Medicine, Boston

***Massachusetts General Hospital,
Boston**

Tufts University School of Dental
Medicine, Boston

MICHIGAN

Detroit-Macomb Hospital
Corporation Oral and Maxillofacial
Surgery, Detroit

Detroit Receiving Hospital and
University Health Center, Detroit

Henry Ford Hospital, Detroit

Sinai Hospital, Detroit

University of Detroit Mercy School
of Dentistry, Detroit

University of Michigan School
of Dentistry, Ann Arbor

MINNESOTA

Hennepin County Medical Center,
Minneapolis

Mayo Clinic, Rochester

University of Minnesota School
of Dentistry, Minneapolis

MISSISSIPPI

University of Mississippi School
of Dentistry, Jackson

MISSOURI

St. John's Mercy Medical Center, St. Louis

St. Louis University Medical Center Orthodontics Treatment, St. Louis

University of Missouri-Kansas City School of Dentistry, Kansas City

NEBRASKA

Creighton University School of Dentistry, Omaha

University of Nebraska Medical Center College of Dentistry, Lincoln

NEW JERSEY

Englewood Hospital, Englewood

Hackensack Medical Center, Hackensack

Jersey City Medical Center, Jersey City

Jersey Shore Medical Center, Neptune

John F. Kennedy Medical Center, Edison

Monmouth Medical Center, Long Branch

Morristown Memorial Hospital, Morristown

Mountainside Hospital, Montclair

Newark Beth Israel Medical Center, Newark

Overlook Hospital, Summit

*Robert Wood Johnson University Hospital, New Brunswick

St. Joseph's Hospital and Medical Center, Paterson

University of Medicine and Dentistry of New Jersey New Jersey Dental School, Newark

NEW YORK

*Albany Medical Center Hospital, Albany

Beth Israel Medical Center, New York

New York Hospital Medical Center of Queens, Flushing

Bronx-Lebanon Hospital Center, Bronx

Bronx Municipal Hospital Center, Bronx

Brookdale Hospital Medical Center, Brooklyn

Brooklyn Hospital Center, Brooklyn

Catholic Medical Center of Brooklyn and Queens, Jamaica

Coler Memorial Hospital, New York

Columbia University School of Dental and Oral Surgery Columbia Presbyterian Medical Center, New York

Eastman Dental Center, Rochester

Erie County Medical Center, Buffalo

Flushing Hospital Medical Center, Flushing

Genesee Hospital, Rochester

Goldwater Memorial Hospital, New York

Harlem Hospital Center, New York

Interfaith Medical Center, Brooklyn

Jamaica Hospital, Jamaica

Kings County Hospital Center, Brooklyn

Lenox Hill Hospital, New York

Lincoln Medical and Mental Health Center, Bronx

Long Island College Hospital, Brooklyn

Long Island Jewish Medical Center, New Hyde Park

Lutheran Medical Center, Brooklyn

Maimonides Medical Center, Brooklyn

Memorial Sloan-Kettering Cancer Center, New York

Metropolitan Hospital Center, New York

Millard Fillmore Hospitals, Buffalo

*Montefiore Medical Center Henry and Lucy Moses Division, Bronx

*Mt. Sinai Medical Center, New York

Nassau County Medical Center, East Meadow

*New York Hospital-Cornell Medical Center, New York

New York University College of Dentistry, New York

North Shore University Hospital, Manhasset

Our Lady of Mercy Medical Center, Bronx

Peninsula Hospital Center, Far Rockaway

Roswell Park Cancer Institute, Buffalo

St. Barnabas Hospital, Bronx

St. Charles Hospital and Rehabilitation Center, Port Jefferson

St. Clare's Hospital of Schenectady, Schenectady

St. Joseph's Hospital Health Center, Syracuse

St. Luke's Memorial Hospital Center, Utica

St. Luke's-Roosevelt Hospital Center St. Luke's Division, New York

St. Peter's Hospital, Albany

State University of New York at Buffalo School of Dental Medicine, Buffalo

State University of New York at Stony Brook School of Dental Medicine, Stony Brook

State University of New York Health Science Center University Hospital, Syracuse

Staten Island University Hospital, Staten Island

*Strong Memorial Hospital of the University of Rochester, Rochester

Westchester County Medical Center, Valhalla

Woodhull Medical and Mental Health Center, Brooklyn

Wyckoff Heights Medical Center, Brooklyn

NORTH CAROLINA

Bowman Gray School of Medicine Department of Dentistry, Winston-Salem

Carolinas Medical Center, Charlotte

East Carolina University School of
Medicine Family Practice Center,
Department of Dentistry,
Greenville

University of North Carolina at
Chapel Hill School of Dentistry,
Chapel Hill

OHIO

Case Western Reserve University
School of Dentistry, Cleveland

Cleveland Clinic, Cleveland

**Medical College of Ohio Hospital,
Toledo**

**MetroHealth Medical Center,
Cleveland**

Miami Valley Hospital, Dayton

Mt. Sinai Medical Center,
Cleveland

Ohio State University College
of Dentistry, Columbus

St. Elizabeth Hospital Medical
Center, Youngstown

St. Luke's Hospital, Cleveland

**University of Cincinnati Hospital,
Cincinnati**

Western Reserve Care System-
Southside Medical Center,
Youngstown

OKLAHOMA

**Oklahoma Medical Center,
Oklahoma City**

St. Anthony Hospital,
Oklahoma City

University of Oklahoma College
of Dentistry, Oklahoma City

OREGON

Oregon Health Sciences University
School of Dentistry, Portland

PENNSYLVANIA

Abington Memorial Hospital,
Abington

Albert Einstein Medical Center,
Philadelphia

***Allegheny General Hospital,
Pittsburgh**

The Allentown Hospital-Lehigh
Valley Hospital Center, Allentown

Community General Hospital,
Reading

Graduate Hospital, Philadelphia

***Hahnemann University Hospital,
Philadelphia**

***Hospital of the Medical College
of Pennsylvania, Philadelphia**

Montefiore University Hospital,
Pittsburgh

Muhlenberg Hospital Center,
Bethlehem

Sacred Heart Hospital, Allentown

St. Francis Medical Center,
Pittsburgh

St. Joseph Hospital, Reading

Temple University School
of Dentistry, Philadelphia

***Thomas Jefferson University
Hospital, Philadelphia**

University of Pennsylvania School
of Dental Medicine, Philadelphia

University of Pittsburgh School
of Dental Medicine, Pittsburgh

York Hospital, York

PUERTO RICO

University of Puerto Rico School
of Dentistry, San Juan

SOUTH CAROLINA

Medical University of South
Carolina College of Dental
Medicine, Charleston

Richland Memorial Hospital,
Columbia

TENNESSEE

Meharry Medical College School
of Dentistry, Nashville

University of Tennessee College
of Dentistry, Memphis

University of Tennessee Memorial
Hospital, Knoxville

***Vanderbilt University Hospital
and Clinic, Nashville**

TEXAS

Baylor College of Dentistry, Dallas

**Dallas County Hospital District
Parkland Memorial Hospital,
Dallas**

University of Texas Health Science
Center at Houston Dental Branch,
Houston

University of Texas Health Science
Center at San Antonio Dental
School, San Antonio

University of Texas M. D. Anderson
Cancer Center, Houston

**University of Texas Medical Branch
Hospitals, Galveston**

UTAH

**University of Utah Hospital
and Clinics, Salt Lake City**

VERMONT

***Fletcher Allen Healthcare
MCHV Campus, Burlington**

VIRGINIA

**University of Virginia Medical
Center, Charlottesville**

Virginia Commonwealth University
Medical College of Virginia School
of Dentistry, Richmond

WASHINGTON

University of Washington School
of Dentistry, Seattle

WEST VIRGINIA

Charleston Area Medical Center
Memorial Division, Charleston

West Virginia University School
of Dentistry, Morgantown

WISCONSIN

Lutheran Hospital-La Crosse,
La Crosse

Marquette University School
of Dentistry, Milwaukee

Medical College of Wisconsin
Department of Oral and
Maxillofacial Surgery, Milwaukee

Meriter Hospital, Madison

The Digestive System

Italic type indicates Health Care Financing Administration: Medicare Liver Transplant Center

ALABAMA
University of Alabama Hospitals, Birmingham

ARIZONA
Kino Community Hospital, Tucson
*University Medical Center, Tucson

ARKANSAS
University Hospital of Arkansas, Little Rock

CALIFORNIA
California-Pacific Medical Center, San Francisco

Cedars-Sinai Medical Center, Los Angeles

Green Hospital of Scripps Clinic, La Jolla

Kaiser Foundation Hospital, Los Angeles

*Loma Linda University Medical Center, Loma Linda

Los Angeles County Harbor-University of California, Los Angeles Medical Center, Torrance

Los Angeles County-King-Drew Medical Center, Los Angeles

Los Angeles County-University of Southern California Medical Center, Los Angeles

San Francisco General Hospital and Medical Center, San Francisco

Sansum Medical Clinic, Santa Barbara

Santa Barbara Cottage Hospital, Santa Barbara

Santa Clara Valley Medical Center, San Jose

*Stanford University Hospital, Stanford

University of California, Los Angeles Medical Center, Los Angeles

University of California, Davis Medical Center, Sacramento

University of California, Irvine Medical Center, Orange

University of California, San Diego Medical Center, San Diego

University of California, San Francisco Medical Center, San Francisco

COLORADO
Denver Health and Hospitals, Denver

University of Colorado Health Sciences Center University Hospital, Denver

CONNECTICUT
Bridgeport Hospital, Bridgeport

Griffin Hospital, Derby

Hospital of St. Raphael, New Haven

Norwalk Hospital, Norwalk

St. Francis Hospital and Medical Center, Hartford

University of Connecticut Health Center John Dempsey Hospital, Farmington

Waterbury Hospital, Waterbury

*Yale-New Haven Hospital, New Haven

DISTRICT OF COLUMBIA
District of Columbia General Hospital, Washington

*George Washington University Hospital, Washington

*Georgetown University Hospital, Washington

*Howard University Hospital, Washington

FLORIDA
Florida Hospital Medical Center, Orlando

Jackson Memorial Hospital, Miami

Mt. Sinai Medical Center, Miami Beach

Cleveland Clinic Hospital, Fort Lauderdale

Orlando Regional Medical Center, Orlando

*Shands Hospital at the University of Florida, Gainesville

University Medical Center, Jacksonville

GEORGIA
*Emory University Hospital, Atlanta

Grady Memorial Hospital, Atlanta

Medical College of Georgia Hospital and Clinics, Augusta

ILLINOIS
Carle Foundation Hospital, Urbana

Cook County Hospital, Chicago

Evanston Hospital, Evanston

Humana Hospital-Michael Reese, Chicago

*Loyola University of Chicago Foster G. McGaw Hospital, Maywood

Mt. Sinai Hospital Medical Center of Chicago, Chicago

*Northwestern Memorial Hospital, Chicago

*Rush-Presbyterian-St. Luke's Medical Center, Chicago

*University of Chicago Hospitals, Chicago

University of Illinois Hospital and Clinics, Chicago

INDIANA
Indiana University Medical Center, Indianapolis

IOWA
University of Iowa Hospitals and Clinics, Iowa City

KANSAS
University of Kansas Hospital, Kansas City

KENTUCKY
Humana Hospital-University of Louisville, Louisville

University of Kentucky Hospital Albert B. Chandler Medical Center, Lexington

LOUISIANA
University Hospital, New Orleans

Louisiana State University Hospital, Shreveport

Medical Center of Louisiana at New Orleans, New Orleans

Ochsner Foundation Hospital, New Orleans

Schumpert Medical Center, Shreveport

*Tulane University Hospital and Clinics, New Orleans

MARYLAND

Francis Scott Key Medical Center, Baltimore

Greater Baltimore Medical Center, Baltimore

*Johns Hopkins Hospital, Baltimore

Prince George's Hospital Center, Cheverly

Suburban Hospital, Bethesda

*University of Maryland Medical System, Baltimore

MASSACHUSETTS

*Beth Israel Hospital, Boston

Boston Medical Center, Boston

*Brigham and Women's Hospital, Boston

Faulkner Hospital, Boston

Lahey Clinic Hospital, Burlington

Lemuel Shattuck Hospital, Boston

*Massachusetts General Hospital, Boston

New England Deaconess Hospital, Boston

*New England Medical Center, Boston

St. Elizabeth's Hospital, Boston

*University Hospital, Boston

University of Massachusetts Medical Center, Worcester

MICHIGAN

Detroit Receiving Hospital and University Health Center, Detroit

Blodgett-Ferguson Campus, Grand Rapids

*Harper Hospital, Detroit

Henry Ford Hospital, Detroit

Michigan Capital Medical Center, Lansing

Providence Hospital, Southfield

Sinai Hospital, Detroit

University of Michigan Hospitals, Ann Arbor

William Beaumont Hospital, Royal Oak

MINNESOTA

Abbott-Northwestern Hospital, Minneapolis

Mayo Clinic, Rochester

Rochester Methodist Hospital, Rochester

*St. Mary's Hospital, Rochester

University of Minnesota Hospital and Clinic, Minneapolis

MISSISSIPPI

University of Mississippi Medical Center University Hospitals and Clinics, Jackson

MISSOURI

*Barnes-Jewish Hospital, St. Louis

*St. Louis University Medical Center, St. Louis

St. Mary's Health Center, St. Louis

Truman Medical Center-West, Kansas City

University Hospital and Clinics, Columbia

NEBRASKA

AMI St. Joseph Hospital, Omaha

University of Nebraska Medical Center, Omaha

NEW HAMPSHIRE

Dartmouth-Hitchcock Medical Center, Hanover

NEW JERSEY

Cooper Hospital-University Medical Center, Camden

Jersey City Medical Center, Jersey City

John F. Kennedy Medical Center, Edison

Muhlenberg Regional Medical Center, Plainfield

*Robert Wood Johnson University Hospital, New Brunswick

St. Joseph's Hospital and Medical Center, Paterson

St. Michael's Medical Center, Newark

University of Medicine and Dentistry of New Jersey University Hospital, Newark

NEW MEXICO

University Hospital, Albuquerque

NEW YORK

*Albany Medical Center Hospital, Albany

Bellevue Hospital Center, New York

Beth Israel Medical Center, New York

New York Hospital Medical Center of Queens, Flushing

Bronx-Lebanon Hospital Center, Bronx

Bronx Municipal Hospital Center, Bronx

Brookdale Hospital Medical Center, Brooklyn

Brooklyn Hospital Center, Brooklyn

*Buffalo General Hospital, Buffalo

Cabrini Medical Center, New York

Elmhurst Hospital Center, Flushing

Erie County Medical Center, Buffalo

Harlem Hospital Center, New York

Interfaith Medical Center, Brooklyn

Jamaica Hospital, Jamaica

Kings County Hospital Center, Brooklyn

Lenox Hill Hospital, New York

Lincoln Medical and Mental Health Center, Bronx

Long Island College Hospital, Brooklyn

Long Island Jewish Medical Center, New Hyde Park

Maimonides Medical Center, Brooklyn

Mary Immaculate Hospital, Jamaica

Memorial Sloan-Kettering Cancer Center, New York

Metropolitan Hospital Center, New York

*Montefiore Medical Center Henry and Lucy Moses Division, Bronx

*Mt. Sinai Medical Center, New York

Nassau County Medical Center, East Meadow

*New York Hospital-Cornell Medical Center, New York

North Shore University Hospital, Manhasset

Our Lady of Mercy Medical Center, Bronx

*Presbyterian Hospital in the City of New York Columbia-Presbyterian Medical Center, New York

Roswell Park Cancer Institute, Buffalo

St. Luke's-Roosevelt Hospital Center Roosevelt Division, New York

St. Luke's-Roosevelt Hospital Center St. Luke's Division, New York

St. Mary's Hospital, Rochester

St. Vincent's Hospital and Medical Center of New York, New York

State University of New York at Stony Brook University Hospital, Stony Brook

State University of New York Health Science Center University Hospital, Syracuse

State University of New York Health Science Center at Brooklyn University Hospital of Brooklyn, Brooklyn

*Strong Memorial Hospital of the University of Rochester, Rochester

Westchester County Medical Center, Valhalla

Winthrop-University Hospital, Mineola

NORTH CAROLINA

*Duke University Medical Center, Durham

*North Carolina Baptist Hospital, Winston-Salem

University of North Carolina Hospitals, Chapel Hill

OHIO

Cleveland Clinic, Cleveland

Grant Medical Center, Columbus

MetroHealth Medical Center, Cleveland

Ohio State University Hospitals, Columbus

*University Hospitals of Cleveland, Cleveland

University of Cincinnati Hospital, Cincinnati

OKLAHOMA

Oklahoma Medical Center, Oklahoma City

OREGON

Oregon Health Sciences University University Hospital, Portland

PENNSYLVANIA

Albert Einstein Medical Center, Philadelphia

*Allegheny General Hospital, Pittsburgh

The Allentown Hospital-Lehigh Valley Hospital Center, Allentown

Crozer-Chester Medical Center, Upland

Graduate Hospital, Philadelphia

*Hahnemann University Hospital, Philadelphia

Hamot Medical Center, Erie

*Hospital of the Medical College of Pennsylvania, Philadelphia

*Hospital of the University of Pennsylvania, Philadelphia

Lankenau Hospital, Wynnewood

Mercy Catholic Medical Center Misericordia Division, Philadelphia

Mercy Hospital of Scranton, Scranton

Montefiore University Hospital, Pittsburgh

Penn State University Hospital The Milton S. Hershey Medical Center, Hershey

Presbyterian Medical Center of Philadelphia, Philadelphia

*Presbyterian University Hospital, Pittsburgh

Robert Packer Hospital, Sayre

Shadyside Hospital, Pittsburgh

St. Vincent Health Center, Erie

*Temple University Hospital, Philadelphia

*Thomas Jefferson University Hospital, Philadelphia

Western Pennsylvania Hospital, Pittsburgh

PUERTO RICO

San Juan Municipal Hospital, Rio Piedras

University Hospital, San Juan

RHODE ISLAND

*Rhode Island Hospital, Providence

Roger Williams Hospital, Providence

SOUTH CAROLINA

Medical Center of Medical University of South Carolina, Charleston

Richland Memorial Hospital, Columbia

TENNESSEE

Johnson City Medical Center Hospital, Johnson City

Regional Medical Center at Memphis, Memphis

St. Thomas Hospital, Nashville

*Vanderbilt University Hospital and Clinic, Nashville

TEXAS

Baylor University Medical Center, Dallas

Bexar County Hospital District Medical Center Hospital, San Antonio

Dallas County Hospital District Parkland Memorial Hospital, Dallas

Harris County Hospital District Ben Taub General Hospital, Houston

*Hermann Hospital, Houston

*Methodist Hospital, Houston

Presbyterian Hospital of Dallas, Dallas

*Scott and White Memorial Hospital, Temple

University Medical Center, Lubbock

University of Texas Medical Branch Hospitals, Galveston

UTAH
University of Utah Hospital and Clinics, Salt Lake City

VERMONT
*Fletcher Allen Healthcare MCHV Campus, Burlington

VIRGINIA
University of Virginia Medical Center, Charlottesville

Virginia Commonwealth University Medical College of Virginia Hospitals, Richmond

WASHINGTON
University of Washington Medical Center, Seattle

WEST VIRGINIA
*West Virginia University Hospitals, Morgantown

WISCONSIN
*Froedtert Memorial Lutheran Hospital, Milwaukee

John L. Doyne Hospital, Milwaukee

University of Wisconsin Hospital and Clinics, Madison

The Ears, Nose, and Throat

ALABAMA
University of Alabama Hospitals, Birmingham

ARKANSAS
University Hospital of Arkansas, Little Rock

CALIFORNIA
Kaiser Foundation Hospital, Anaheim

Kaiser Foundation Hospital, Oakland

Kaiser Foundation Hospital, San Diego

Kaiser Foundation Hospital, San Francisco

Kaiser Foundation Hospital, Santa Clara

*Loma Linda University Medical Center, Loma Linda

Los Angeles County-King-Drew Medical Center, Los Angeles

Los Angeles County-Rancho Los Amigos Medical Center, Downey

Los Angeles County-University of Southern California Medical Center, Los Angeles

Olive View Medical Center, Sylmar

Riverside General Hospital University Medical Center, Riverside

San Bernardino County Medical Center, San Bernardino

San Francisco General Hospital and Medical Center, San Francisco

Santa Clara Valley Medical Center, San Jose

*Stanford University Hospital, Stanford

University of California, Los Angeles Medical Center, Los Angeles

University of California, Davis Medical Center, Sacramento

University of California, Irvine Medical Center, Orange

University of California, San Diego Medical Center, San Diego

University of California, San Francisco Medical Center, San Francisco

COLORADO
Denver Health and Hospitals, Denver

St. Joseph Hospital, Denver

University of Colorado Health Sciences Center University Hospital, Denver

CONNECTICUT
Hartford Hospital, Hartford

Hospital of St. Raphael, New Haven

New Britain General Hospital, New Britain

St. Francis Hospital and Medical Center, Hartford

University of Connecticut Health Center John Dempsey Hospital, Farmington

*Yale-New Haven Hospital, New Haven

DISTRICT OF COLUMBIA
*Georgetown University Hospital, Washington

Washington Hospital Center, Washington

FLORIDA
Jackson Memorial Hospital, Miami

*Shands Hospital at the University of Florida, Gainesville

Tampa General Hospital, Tampa

GEORGIA
*Emory University Hospital, Atlanta

Grady Memorial Hospital, Atlanta

Medical College of Georgia Hospital and Clinics, Augusta

ILLINOIS
Cook County Hospital, Chicago

Evanston Hospital, Evanston

Louis A. Weiss Memorial Hospital, Chicago

*Loyola University of Chicago Foster G. McGaw Hospital, Maywood

Memorial Medical Center, Springfield

*Northwestern Memorial Hospital, Chicago

*Rush-Presbyterian-St. Luke's Medical Center, Chicago

St. John's Hospital, Springfield

*University of Chicago Hospitals, Chicago

University of Illinois Hospital and Clinics, Chicago

University of Illinois Hospital and Clinics Illinois Eye and Ear Infirmary, Chicago

INDIANA

Indiana University Medical Center, Indianapolis

William N. Wishard Memorial Hospital, Indianapolis

IOWA

University of Iowa Hospitals and Clinics, Iowa City

KANSAS

University of Kansas Hospital, Kansas City

KENTUCKY

Humana Hospital-University of Louisville, Louisville

Norton Hospital, Louisville

University of Kentucky Hospital Albert B. Chandler Medical Center, Lexington

LOUISIANA

Eye, Ear, Nose and Throat Hospital, New Orleans

Louisiana State University Hospital, Shreveport

Medical Center of Louisiana at New Orleans, New Orleans

Ochsner Foundation Hospital, New Orleans

*Tulane University Hospital and Clinics, New Orleans

MARYLAND

Francis Scott Key Medical Center, Baltimore

Greater Baltimore Medical Center, Baltimore

*Johns Hopkins Hospital, Baltimore

Maryland General Hospital, Baltimore

Sinai Hospital of Baltimore, Baltimore

*University of Maryland Medical System, Baltimore

MASSACHUSETTS

*Beth Israel Hospital, Boston

Boston Medical Center, Boston

Lahey Clinic Hospital, Burlington

Massachusetts Eye and Ear Infirmary, Boston

*New England Medical Center, Boston

*University Hospital, Boston

MICHIGAN

Detroit Receiving Hospital and University Health Center, Detroit

*Grace Hospital, Detroit

*Harper Hospital, Detroit

Henry Ford Hospital, Detroit

Hutzel Hospital, Detroit

University of Michigan Hospitals, Ann Arbor

MINNESOTA

Hennepin County Medical Center, Minneapolis

Mayo Clinic, Rochester

Rochester Methodist Hospital, Rochester

*St. Mary's Hospital, Rochester

Regions Hospital, St. Paul

University of Minnesota Hospital and Clinic, Minneapolis

MISSISSIPPI

University of Mississippi Medical Center University Hospitals and Clinics, Jackson

MISSOURI

*Barnes-Jewish Hospital, St. Louis

St. Louis Regional Medical Center, St. Louis

*St. Louis University Medical Center, St. Louis

University Hospital and Clinics, Columbia

NEBRASKA

University of Nebraska Medical Center, Omaha

NEW HAMPSHIRE

Dartmouth-Hitchcock Medical Center, Hanover

NEW JERSEY

United Hospitals Medical Center, Newark

United Hospitals Medical Center Newark Eye and Ear Infirmary, Newark

University of Medicine and Dentistry of New Jersey University Hospital, Newark

West Jersey Hospital-Berlin, Berlin

West Jersey Hospital-Camden, Camden

West Jersey Hospital-Marlton, Marlton

West Jersey Hospital-Voorhees, Voorhees

NEW MEXICO

Lovelace Medical Center, Albuquerque

University Hospital, Albuquerque

NEW YORK

*Albany Medical Center Hospital, Albany

Bellevue Hospital Center, New York

Bronx Municipal Hospital Center, Bronx

Brookdale Hospital Medical Center, Brooklyn

Child's Hospital, Albany

Community-General Hospital of Greater Syracuse, Syracuse

Crouse-Irving Memorial Hospital, Syracuse

Elmhurst Hospital Center, Flushing

Erie County Medical Center, Buffalo

Genesee Hospital, Rochester

Kings County Hospital Center, Brooklyn

Lincoln Medical and Mental Health Center, Bronx

Long Island College Hospital, Brooklyn

Long Island Jewish Medical Center, New Hyde Park

Manhattan Eye, Ear and Throat Hospital, New York

Memorial Sloan-Kettering Cancer Center, New York

*Montefiore Medical Center Henry and Lucy Moses Division, Bronx

Montefiore Medical Center Jack D. Weiler Hospital of the Albert Einstein College of Medicine, Bronx

*Mt. Sinai Medical Center, New York

New York Eye and Ear Infirmary, New York

*New York Hospital-Cornell Medical Center, New York

*New York University Medical Center, New York

*Presbyterian Hospital in the City of New York Columbia-Presbyterian Medical Center, New York

Queens Hospital Center, Jamaica

Rochester General Hospital, Rochester

Sisters of Charity Hospital of Buffalo, Buffalo

St. Joseph's Hospital Health Center, Syracuse

St. Luke's-Roosevelt Hospital Center Roosevelt Division, New York

St. Luke's-Roosevelt Hospital Center St. Luke's Division, New York

St. Peter's Hospital, Albany

St. Vincent's Hospital and Medical Center of New York, New York

State University of New York Health Science Center University Hospital, Syracuse

State University of New York Health Science Center at Brooklyn University Hospital of Brooklyn, Brooklyn

*Strong Memorial Hospital of the University of Rochester, Rochester

NORTH CAROLINA

*Duke University Medical Center, Durham

*North Carolina Baptist Hospital, Winston-Salem

University of North Carolina Hospitals, Chapel Hill

OHIO

Cleveland Clinic, Cleveland

MetroHealth Medical Center, Cleveland

Ohio State University Hospitals, Columbus

*University Hospitals of Cleveland, Cleveland

University of Cincinnati Hospital, Cincinnati

OKLAHOMA

Baptist Medical Center of Oklahoma, Oklahoma City

Oklahoma Medical Center, Oklahoma City

OREGON

Oregon Health Sciences University University Hospital, Portland

PENNSYLVANIA

*Allegheny General Hospital, Pittsburgh

Episcopal Hospital, Philadelphia

Geisinger Medical Center, Danville

*Hahnemann University Hospital, Philadelphia

*Hospital of the University of Pennsylvania, Philadelphia

Montefiore University Hospital Eye and Ear Hospital of Pittsburgh, Pittsburgh

Penn State University Hospital The Milton S. Hershey Medical Center, Hershey

Pennsylvania Hospital, Philadelphia

*Temple University Hospital, Philadelphia

*Thomas Jefferson University Hospital, Philadelphia

PUERTO RICO

San Juan Municipal Hospital, Rio Piedras

University Hospital, San Juan

SOUTH CAROLINA

Charleston Memorial Hospital, Charleston

Medical Center of Medical University of South Carolina, Charleston

TENNESSEE

Baptist Hospital, Nashville

Methodist Hospitals of Memphis Central Unit, Memphis

Metropolitan Nashville General Hospital, Nashville

Regional Medical Center at Memphis, Memphis

University of Tennessee Medical Center, Memphis

*Vanderbilt University Hospital and Clinic, Nashville

TEXAS

Bexar County Hospital District Medical Center Hospital, San Antonio

Dallas County Hospital District Parkland Memorial Hospital, Dallas

Harris County Hospital District Ben Taub General Hospital, Houston

Harris County Hospital District Lyndon B. Johnson General Hospital, Houston

*Hermann Hospital, Houston

*Methodist Hospital, Houston

St. Paul Medical Center, Dallas

Tarrant County Hospital District
John Peter Smith Hospital,
Fort Worth

**University of Texas Medical Branch
Hospitals, Galveston**

Zale-Lipshy University Hospital,
Dallas

UTAH

Holy Cross Hospital, Salt Lake City

**University of Utah Hospital
and Clinics, Salt Lake City**

VERMONT

***Fletcher Allen Healthcare
MCHV Campus, Burlington**

VIRGINIA

Roanoke Memorial Hospitals,
Roanoke

Sentara Norfolk General Hospital,
Norfolk

**University of Virginia Medical
Center, Charlottesville**

**Virginia Commonwealth University
Medical College of Virginia
Hospitals, Richmond**

WASHINGTON

**University of Washington Medical
Center, Seattle**

WEST VIRGINIA

***West Virginia University
Hospitals, Morgantown**

WISCONSIN

John L. Doyne Hospital, Milwaukee

St. Luke's Medical Center,
Milwaukee

**University of Wisconsin Hospital
and Clinics, Madison**

The Endocrine System

■ indicates National Institute of Diabetes and
Digestive and Kidney Diseases: Diabetes
Control and Complications Trial Center

ALABAMA

**University of Alabama Hospitals,
Birmingham**

ARIZONA

Kino Community Hospital, Tucson

***University Medical Center, Tucson**

ARKANSAS

**University Hospital of Arkansas,
Little Rock**

CALIFORNIA

Cedars-Sinai Medical Center,
Los Angeles

Green Hospital of Scripps Clinic,
La Jolla

**Los Angeles County Harbor-
University of California, Los
Angeles Medical Center, Torrance**

**Los Angeles County-University
of Southern California Medical
Center, Los Angeles**

Olive View Medical Center, Sylmar

Santa Clara Valley Medical Center,
San Jose

***Stanford University Hospital,
Stanford**

**University of California, Los
Angeles Medical Center,
Los Angeles**

**University of California, Davis
Medical Center, Sacramento**

**University of California, Irvine
Medical Center, Orange**

**▼University of California, San
Diego Medical Center, San Diego**

**University of California, San
Francisco Medical Center,
San Francisco**

COLORADO

Denver Health and Hospitals,
Denver

**University of Colorado Health
Sciences Center University
Hospital, Denver**

CONNECTICUT

**University of Connecticut Health
Center John Dempsey Hospital,
Farmington**

**▼*Yale-New Haven Hospital,
New Haven**

DISTRICT OF COLUMBIA

District of Columbia General
Hospital, Washington

***George Washington University
Hospital, Washington**

***Georgetown University Hospital,
Washington**

***Howard University Hospital,
Washington**

FLORIDA

Jackson Memorial Hospital, Miami

***Shands Hospital at the University
of Florida, Gainesville**

University Medical Center,
Jacksonville

University of South Florida H. Lee
Moffitt Cancer Center, Tampa

GEORGIA

***Emory University Hospital,
Atlanta**

Grady Memorial Hospital, Atlanta

**Medical College of Georgia
Hospital and Clinics, Augusta**

ILLINOIS

Cook County Hospital, Chicago

Humana Hospital-Michael Reese,
Chicago

***Loyola University of Chicago
Foster G. McGaw Hospital,
Maywood**

**▼*Northwestern Memorial
Hospital, Chicago**

***Rush-Presbyterian-St. Luke's
Medical Center, Chicago**

***University of Chicago Hospitals,
Chicago**

**University of Illinois Hospital
and Clinics, Chicago**

INDIANA

**Indiana University Medical Center,
Indianapolis**

IOWA

**▼University of Iowa Hospitals
and Clinics, Iowa City**

KANSAS

University of Kansas Hospital, Kansas City

KENTUCKY

Humana Hospital-University of Louisville, Louisville

University of Kentucky Hospital Albert B. Chandler Medical Center, Lexington

LOUISIANA

Louisiana State University Hospital, Shreveport

Medical Center of Louisiana at New Orleans, New Orleans

Ochsner Foundation Hospital, New Orleans

*Tulane University Hospital and Clinics, New Orleans

MAINE

Maine Medical Center, Portland

MARYLAND

*Johns Hopkins Hospital, Baltimore

▼*University of Maryland Medical System, Baltimore

MASSACHUSETTS

Baystate Medical Center, Springfield

*Beth Israel Hospital, Boston

Boston Medical Center, Boston

*Brigham and Women's Hospital, Boston

▼Joslin Diabetes Center, Inc., Boston

Lahey Clinic Hospital, Burlington

▼*Massachusetts General Hospital, Boston

New England Deaconess Hospital, Boston

*New England Medical Center, Boston

*University Hospital, Boston

University of Massachusetts Medical Center, Worcester

MICHIGAN

Detroit Receiving Hospital and University Health Center, Detroit

*Harper Hospital, Detroit

▼Henry Ford Hospital, Detroit

▼University of Michigan Hospitals, Ann Arbor

MINNESOTA

▼Mayo Clinic, Rochester

Rochester Methodist Hospital, Rochester

*St. Mary's Hospital, Rochester

▼University of Minnesota Hospital and Clinic, Minneapolis

MISSOURI

*Barnes-Jewish Hospital, St. Louis

*St. Louis University Medical Center, St. Louis

▼University Hospital and Clinics, Columbia

NEW HAMPSHIRE

Dartmouth-Hitchcock Medical Center, Hanover

NEW JERSEY

*Robert Wood Johnson University Hospital, New Brunswick

St. Michael's Medical Center, Newark

St. Peter's Medical Center, New Brunswick

University of Medicine and Dentistry of New Jersey University Hospital, Newark

NEW MEXICO

▼University Hospital, Albuquerque

NEW YORK

*Albany Medical Center Hospital, Albany

Bellevue Hospital Center, New York

Beth Israel Medical Center, New York

Bronx Municipal Hospital Center, Bronx

Brookdale Hospital Medical Center, Brooklyn

Coney Island Hospital, Brooklyn

Erie County Medical Center, Buffalo

Interfaith Medical Center, Brooklyn

Kings County Hospital Center, Brooklyn

Lincoln Medical and Mental Health Center, Bronx

Long Island Jewish Medical Center, New Hyde Park

*Montefiore Medical Center Henry and Lucy Moses Division, Bronx

Montefiore Medical Center Jack D. Weiler Hospital of the Albert Einstein College of Medicine, Bronx

*Mt. Sinai Medical Center, New York

Nassau County Medical Center, East Meadow

▼*New York Hospital-Cornell Medical Center, New York

North Central Bronx Hospital, Bronx

*Presbyterian Hospital in the City of New York Columbia-Presbyterian Medical Center, New York

Queens Hospital Center, Jamaica

St. Luke's-Roosevelt Hospital Center St. Luke's Division, New York

State University of New York at Stony Brook University Hospital, Stony Brook

State University of New York Health Science Center University Hospital, Syracuse

State University of New York Health Science Center at Brooklyn University Hospital of Brooklyn, Brooklyn

*Strong Memorial Hospital of the University of Rochester, Rochester

Westchester County Medical Center, Valhalla

Winthrop-University Hospital, Mineola

NORTH CAROLINA

*Duke University Medical Center, Durham

Pitt County Memorial Hospital, Greenville

University of North Carolina Hospitals, Chapel Hill

OHIO

Cleveland Clinic, Cleveland

Medical College of Ohio Hospital, Toledo

Mercy Hospital, Toledo

MetroHealth Center for Rehabilitation, Cleveland

MetroHealth Medical Center, Cleveland

Ohio State University Hospitals, Columbus

*University Hospitals of Cleveland, Cleveland

University of Cincinnati Hospital, Cincinnati

OKLAHOMA

Oklahoma Medical Center, Oklahoma City

OREGON

Oregon Health Sciences University University Hospital, Portland

PENNSYLVANIA

*Hahnemann University Hospital, Philadelphia

*Hospital of the Medical College of Pennsylvania, Philadelphia

*Hospital of the University of Pennsylvania, Philadelphia

Montefiore University Hospital, Pittsburgh

Penn State University Hospital The Milton S. Hershey Medical Center, Hershey

*Presbyterian University Hospital, Pittsburgh

Shadyside Hospital, Pittsburgh

*Temple University Hospital, Philadelphia

PUERTO RICO

San Juan Municipal Hospital, Rio Piedras

University Hospital, San Juan

RHODE ISLAND

*Rhode Island Hospital, Providence

Roger Williams Hospital, Providence

SOUTH CAROLINA

▼Medical University of South Carolina Medical Center of Medical University of South Carolina, Charleston

Richland Memorial Hospital, Columbia

TENNESSEE

Baptist Memorial Hospital, Memphis

Regional Medical Center at Memphis, Memphis

▼*Vanderbilt University Hospital and Clinic, Nashville

TEXAS

Bexar County Hospital District Medical Center Hospital, San Antonio

▼Dallas County Hospital District Parkland Memorial Hospital, Dallas

Harris County Hospital District Ben Taub General Hospital, Houston

*Hermann Hospital, Houston

*Methodist Hospital, Houston

*Scott and White Memorial Hospital, Temple

UTAH

University of Utah Hospital and Clinics, Salt Lake City

VERMONT

*Fletcher Allen Healthcare MCHV Campus, Burlington

VIRGINIA

University of Virginia Medical Center, Charlottesville

Virginia Commonwealth University Medical College of Virginia Hospitals, Richmond

WASHINGTON

University of Washington Medical Center, Seattle

WEST VIRGINIA

Cabell Huntington Hospital, Huntington

WISCONSIN

John L. Doyne Hospital, Milwaukee

University of Wisconsin Hospital and Clinics, Madison

The Eyes

ALABAMA

Cooper Green Hospital, Birmingham

Eye Foundation Hospital, Birmingham

University of Alabama Hospitals, Birmingham

University of South Alabama Medical Center, Mobile

ARIZONA

Carondelet St. Joseph's Hospital, Tucson

Kino Community Hospital, Tucson

*University Medical Center, Tucson

ARKANSAS

University Hospital of Arkansas, Little Rock

CALIFORNIA

California-Pacific Medical Center, San Francisco

Highland General Hospital, Oakland

*Loma Linda University Medical Center, Loma Linda

Long Beach Memorial Medical Center, Long Beach

Los Angeles County Harbor-University of California, Los Angeles Medical Center, Torrance

Los Angeles County-King-Drew Medical Center, Los Angeles

Los Angeles County-University of Southern California Medical Center, Los Angeles

Riverside General Hospital University Medical Center, Riverside

San Francisco General Hospital and Medical Center, San Francisco

Santa Clara Valley Medical Center, San Jose

*Stanford University Hospital, Stanford

University of California, Los Angeles Medical Center Jules Stein Eye Institute, Los Angeles

University of California, Davis Medical Center, Sacramento

University of California, Irvine Medical Center, Orange

University of California, San Diego Medical Center, San Diego

University of California, San Francisco Medical Center, San Francisco

White Memorial Medical Center, Los Angeles

COLORADO

Denver Health and Hospitals, Denver

University of Colorado Health Sciences Center University Hospital, Denver

CONNECTICUT

*Yale-New Haven Hospital, New Haven

DISTRICT OF COLUMBIA

District of Columbia General Hospital, Washington

*George Washington University Hospital, Washington

*Georgetown University Hospital, Washington

*Howard University Hospital, Washington

Washington Hospital Center, Washington

FLORIDA

Bascom Palmer Eye Institute-Anne Bates Leach Eye Hospital, Miami

Jackson Memorial Hospital, Miami

*Shands Hospital at the University of Florida, Gainesville

Tampa General Hospital, Tampa

GEORGIA

*Emory University Hospital, Atlanta

Grady Memorial Hospital, Atlanta

Medical College of Georgia Hospital and Clinics, Augusta

ILLINOIS

Cook County Hospital, Chicago

Evanston Hospital, Evanston

*Loyola University of Chicago Foster G. McGaw Hospital, Maywood

*Northwestern Memorial Hospital, Chicago

Oak Forest Hospital of Cook County, Oak Forest

*Rush-Presbyterian-St. Luke's Medical Center, Chicago

*University of Chicago Hospitals, Chicago

University of Illinois Hospital and Clinics Illinois Eye and Ear Infirmary, Chicago

INDIANA

Indiana University Medical Center, Indianapolis

Methodist Hospital of Indiana, Indianapolis

William N. Wishard Memorial Hospital, Indianapolis

IOWA

University of Iowa Hospitals and Clinics, Iowa City

KANSAS

University of Kansas Hospital, Kansas City

KENTUCKY

Humana Hospital-University of Louisville, Louisville

University of Kentucky Hospital Albert B. Chandler Medical Center, Lexington

LOUISIANA

E. A. Conway Memorial Hospital, Monroe

Eye, Ear, Nose and Throat Hospital, New Orleans

University Hospital, New Orleans

Louisiana State University Eye Center, New Orleans

Louisiana State University Hospital, Shreveport

Medical Center of Louisiana at New Orleans, New Orleans

Ochsner Foundation Hospital, New Orleans

South Louisiana Medical Center, Houma

*Tulane University Hospital and Clinics, New Orleans

MARYLAND

Greater Baltimore Medical Center, Baltimore

Johns Hopkins Hospital Wilmer Eye Institute, Baltimore

Maryland General Hospital, Baltimore

Sinai Hospital of Baltimore, Baltimore

*University of Maryland Medical System, Baltimore

MASSACHUSETTS

Boston Medical Center, Boston

Massachusetts Eye and Ear Infirmary, Boston

*New England Medical Center, Boston

*University Hospital, Boston

MICHIGAN

Detroit Receiving Hospital and University Health Center, Detroit

*Grace Hospital, Detroit

*Harper Hospital, Detroit

Henry Ford Hospital, Detroit

Sinai Hospital, Detroit

University of Michigan Hospitals, Ann Arbor

Oakwood Healthcare Systems, Westland

William Beaumont Hospital, Royal Oak

MINNESOTA

Hennepin County Medical Center, Minneapolis

Mayo Clinic, Rochester

Rochester Methodist Hospital, Rochester

*St. Mary's Hospital, Rochester

Regions Hospital, St. Paul

University of Minnesota Hospital and Clinic, Minneapolis

MISSISSIPPI

University of Mississippi Medical Center University Hospitals and Clinics, Jackson

MISSOURI

*Barnes-Jewish Hospital, St. Louis

Anheuser-Busch Eye Institute, St. Louis

Truman Medical Center-West, Kansas City

University Hospital and Clinics, Columbia

NEBRASKA

University of Nebraska Medical Center, Omaha

NEW JERSEY

Cooper Hospital-University Medical Center, Camden

Jersey City Medical Center, Jersey City

United Hospitals Medical Center, Newark

United Hospitals Medical Center Newark Eye and Ear Infirmary, Newark

University of Medicine and Dentistry of New Jersey University Hospital, Newark

NEW YORK

*Albany Medical Center Hospital, Albany

Bayley Seton Hospital, Staten Island

Bellevue Hospital Center, New York

Beth Israel Medical Center, New York

Bronx-Lebanon Hospital Center, Bronx

Bronx Municipal Hospital Center, Bronx

Brookdale Hospital Medical Center, Brooklyn

Brooklyn Hospital Center, Brooklyn

*Buffalo General Hospital, Buffalo

Cabrini Medical Center, New York

Coney Island Hospital, Brooklyn

Crouse-Irving Memorial Hospital, Syracuse

Elmhurst Hospital Center, Flushing

Erie County Medical Center, Buffalo

Harlem Hospital Center, New York

Interfaith Medical Center, Brooklyn

Kings County Hospital Center, Brooklyn

Lenox Hill Hospital, New York

Lincoln Medical and Mental Health Center, Bronx

Long Island College Hospital, Brooklyn

Long Island Jewish Medical Center, New Hyde Park

Maimonides Medical Center, Brooklyn

Manhattan Eye, Ear and Throat Hospital, New York

Mary Immaculate Hospital, Jamaica

Metropolitan Hospital Center, New York

Millard Fillmore Hospitals, Buffalo

*Montefiore Medical Center Henry and Lucy Moses Division, Bronx

Montefiore Medical Center Jack D. Weiler Hospital of the Albert Einstein College of Medicine, Bronx

*Mt. Sinai Medical Center, New York

Nassau County Medical Center, East Meadow

New York Eye and Ear Infirmary, New York

*New York Hospital-Cornell Medical Center, New York

*New York University Medical Center, New York

North Central Bronx Hospital, Bronx

North General Hospital, New York

North Shore University Hospital, Manhasset

Our Lady of Mercy Medical Center, Bronx

*Presbyterian Hospital in the City of New York Columbia-Presbyterian Medical Center, New York

Queens Hospital Center, Jamaica

St. Luke's-Roosevelt Hospital Center St. Luke's Division, New York

St. Mary's Hospital, Rochester

St. Vincent's Hospital and Medical Center of New York, New York

State University of New York Health Science Center University Hospital, Syracuse

*Strong Memorial Hospital of the University of Rochester, Rochester

Westchester County Medical Center, Valhalla

NORTH CAROLINA

*Duke University Medical Center, Durham

North Carolina Eye & Ear Hospital & Clinic, Durham

*North Carolina Baptist Hospital, Winston-Salem

University of North Carolina
Hospitals, Chapel Hill

OHIO
Akron City Hospital, Akron

Cleveland Clinic, Cleveland

MetroHealth Medical Center, Cleveland

Mt. Sinai Medical Center, Cleveland

Ohio State University Hospitals, Columbus

St. Luke's Hospital, Cleveland

St. Vincent Charity Hospital and Health Center, Cleveland

*University Hospitals of Cleveland, Cleveland

University of Cincinnati Hospital, Cincinnati

OKLAHOMA
Oklahoma Medical Center, Oklahoma City

OREGON
Good Samaritan Hospital and Medical Center, Portland

Oregon Health Sciences University University Hospital, Portland

PENNSYLVANIA
Geisinger Medical Center, Danville

*Hahnemann University Hospital, Philadelphia

Penn State University Hospital The Milton S. Hershey Medical Center, Hershey

Presbyterian Medical Center of Philadelphia, Philadelphia

Scheie Eye Institute, Philadelphia

St. Francis Medical Center, Pittsburgh

*Temple University Hospital, Philadelphia

Wills Eye Hospital, Philadelphia

PUERTO RICO
San Juan Municipal Hospital, Rio Piedras

University Hospital, San Juan

RHODE ISLAND
*Rhode Island Hospital, Providence

SOUTH CAROLINA
Medical Center of Medical University of South Carolina, Charleston

Richland Memorial Hospital, Columbia

TENNESSEE
Erlanger Medical Center, Chattanooga

Methodist Hospitals of Memphis Central Unit, Memphis

Regional Medical Center at Memphis, Memphis

*Vanderbilt University Hospital and Clinic, Nashville

Willie D. Miller Eye Center, Chattanooga

TEXAS
Bexar County Hospital District Medical Center Hospital, San Antonio

Dallas County Hospital District Parkland Memorial Hospital, Dallas

Harris County Hospital District Ben Taub General Hospital, Houston

*Hermann Hospital, Houston

*Methodist Hospital, Houston

*Scott and White Memorial Hospital, Temple

St. Luke's Episcopal Hospital, Houston

University Medical Center, Lubbock

University of Texas Medical Branch Hospitals, Galveston

UTAH
University of Utah Hospital and Clinics, Salt Lake City

VIRGINIA
Sentara Norfolk General Hospital, Norfolk

University of Virginia Medical Center, Charlottesville

Virginia Commonwealth University Medical College of Virginia Hospitals, Richmond

WASHINGTON
Harborview Medical Center, Seattle

University of Washington Medical Center, Seattle

WEST VIRGINIA
*West Virginia University Hospitals, Morgantown

WISCONSIN
John L. Doyne Hospital, Milwaukee

University of Wisconsin Hospital and Clinics, Madison

The Heart and Blood Vessels

Italic type indicates Health Care Financing Administration: Medicare Heart Transplant Center

▼ indicates National Institute of Neurological Disorders and Stroke: Stroke Clinical Research Center

ALABAMA
University of Alabama Hospitals, Birmingham

University of South Alabama Medical Center, Mobile

ARIZONA
Good Samaritan Regional Medical Center, Phoenix

*University Medical Center, Tucson

ARKANSAS
University Hospital of Arkansas, Little Rock

CALIFORNIA
California-Pacific Medical Center, San Francisco

Cedars-Sinai Medical Center, Los Angeles

Green Hospital of Scripps Clinic, La Jolla

Kaiser Foundation Hospital,
Los Angeles

***Loma Linda University Medical
Center, Loma Linda**

Long Beach Memorial Medical
Center, Long Beach

**Los Angeles County Harbor-
University of California, Los
Angeles Medical Center, Torrance**

Los Angeles County-King-Drew
Medical Center, Los Angeles

**Los Angeles County-University
of Southern California Medical
Center, Los Angeles**

Mercy Hospital and Medical
Center, San Diego

▼Mt. Zion Medical Center of
University of California, San
Francisco, San Francisco

Sharp Memorial Hospital, San Diego

St. Mary Medical Center,
Long Beach

St. Mary's Hospital and Medical
Center, San Francisco

St. Vincent Medical Center,
Los Angeles

**Stanford University Hospital,
Stanford*

▼*University of California, Los Angeles
Medical Center, Los Angeles*

**University of California, Davis
Medical Center, Sacramento**

**University of California, Irvine
Medical Center, Orange**

**University of California, San Diego
Medical Center, San Diego**

▼**University of California, San
Francisco Medical Center,
San Francisco**

Valley Medical Center of Fresno,
Fresno

COLORADO

Denver Health and Hospitals,
Denver

**University of Colorado Health
Sciences Center University
Hospital, Denver**

CONNECTICUT

Bridgeport Hospital, Bridgeport

Hartford Hospital, Hartford

Hospital of St. Raphael, New Haven

Mt. Sinai Hospital, Hartford

Norwalk Hospital, Norwalk

St. Vincent's Medical Center,
Bridgeport

**University of Connecticut Health
Center John Dempsey Hospital,
Farmington**

**Yale-New Haven Hospital,
New Haven*

DISTRICT OF COLUMBIA

District of Columbia General
Hospital, Washington

***George Washington University
Hospital, Washington**

***Georgetown University Hospital,
Washington**

***Howard University Hospital,
Washington**

Washington Hospital Center,
Washington

FLORIDA

▼**Jackson Memorial Hospital,
Miami**

Mt. Sinai Medical Center,
Miami Beach

**Shands Hospital at the University
of Florida, Gainesville*

Tampa General Hospital, Tampa

University Medical Center,
Jacksonville

GEORGIA

*Emory University Hospital, Atlanta

Grady Memorial Hospital, Atlanta

**Medical College of Georgia
Hospital and Clinics, Augusta**

ILLINOIS

Christ Hospital and Medical
Center, Oak Lawn

Cook County Hospital, Chicago

Humana Hospital-Michael Reese,
Chicago

Illinois Masonic Medical Center,
Chicago

**Loyola University of Chicago Foster
G. McGaw Hospital, Maywood*

MacNeal Hospital, Berwyn

Memorial Medical Center,
Springfield

Mt. Sinai Hospital Medical Center
of Chicago, Chicago

***Northwestern Memorial Hospital,
Chicago**

***Rush-Presbyterian-St. Luke's
Medical Center, Chicago**

St. Francis Hospital of Evanston,
Evanston

St. John's Hospital, Springfield

***University of Chicago Hospitals,
Chicago**

**University of Illinois Hospital
and Clinics, Chicago**

INDIANA

*Indiana University Medical Center,
Indianapolis*

*Methodist Hospital of Indiana,
Indianapolis*

IOWA

▼**University of Iowa Hospitals
and Clinics, Iowa City**

KANSAS

**University of Kansas Hospital,
Kansas City**

KENTUCKY

**Humana Hospital-University
of Louisville, Louisville**

**University of Kentucky Hospital
Albert B. Chandler Medical Center,
Lexington**

LOUISIANA

University Hospital, New Orleans

**Louisiana State University
Hospital, Shreveport**

**Medical Center of Louisiana
at New Orleans, New Orleans**

*Ochsner Foundation Hospital,
New Orleans*

***Tulane University Hospital
and Clinics, New Orleans**

MAINE

Maine Medical Center, Portland

MARYLAND

▼*Johns Hopkins Hospital, Baltimore

▼*University of Maryland Medical System, Baltimore

MASSACHUSETTS

Baystate Medical Center, Springfield

*Beth Israel Hospital, Boston

Boston Medical Center, Boston

*Brigham and Women's Hospital, Boston

Lahey Clinic Hospital, Burlington

▼*Massachusetts General Hospital, Boston

Mt. Auburn Hospital, Cambridge

New England Deaconess Hospital, Boston

*New England Medical Center, Boston

St. Elizabeth's Hospital, Boston

St. Vincent Hospital, Worcester

*University Hospital, Boston

University of Massachusetts Medical Center, Worcester

MICHIGAN

Detroit Receiving Hospital and University Health Center, Detroit

*Harper Hospital, Detroit

▼Henry Ford Hospital, Detroit

Providence Hospital, Southfield

Sinai Hospital, Detroit

University of Michigan Hospitals, Ann Arbor

William Beaumont Hospital, Royal Oak

MINNESOTA

Hennepin County Medical Center, Minneapolis

▼Mayo Clinic, Rochester

Rochester Methodist Hospital, Rochester

*St. Mary's Hospital, Rochester

University of Minnesota Hospital and Clinic, Minneapolis

MISSISSIPPI

University of Mississippi Medical Center University Hospitals and Clinics, Jackson

MISSOURI

▼*Barnes-Jewish Hospital, St. Louis

St. John's Mercy Medical Center, St. Louis

*St. Louis University Medical Center, St. Louis

St. Luke's Hospital, Chesterfield

Truman Medical Center-West, Kansas City

University Hospital and Clinics, Columbia

NEBRASKA

AMI St. Joseph Hospital, Omaha

University of Nebraska Medical Center, Omaha

NEW HAMPSHIRE

Dartmouth-Hitchcock Medical Center, Hanover

NEW JERSEY

Cooper Hospital-University Medical Center, Camden

Hackensack Medical Center, Hackensack

Jersey City Medical Center, Jersey City

Newark Beth Israel Medical Center, Newark

*Robert Wood Johnson University Hospital, New Brunswick

St. Michael's Medical Center, Newark

St. Peter's Medical Center, New Brunswick

University of Medicine and Dentistry of New Jersey University Hospital, Newark

NEW MEXICO

University Hospital, Albuquerque

NEW YORK

*Albany Medical Center Hospital, Albany

Bellevue Hospital Center, New York

Beth Israel Medical Center, New York

Bronx-Lebanon Hospital Center, Bronx

Bronx Municipal Hospital Center, Bronx

Brooklyn Hospital Center, Brooklyn

*Buffalo General Hospital, Buffalo

Cabrini Medical Center, New York

Coney Island Hospital, Brooklyn

Elmhurst Hospital Center, Flushing

Erie County Medical Center, Buffalo

Genesee Hospital, Rochester

Harlem Hospital Center, New York

Interfaith Medical Center, Brooklyn

Jamaica Hospital, Jamaica

Kings County Hospital Center, Brooklyn

Lenox Hill Hospital, New York

Lincoln Medical and Mental Health Center, Bronx

Long Island College Hospital, Brooklyn

Long Island Jewish Medical Center, New Hyde Park

Maimonides Medical Center, Brooklyn

Mary Immaculate Hospital, Jamaica

Memorial Sloan-Kettering Cancer Center, New York

Methodist Hospital of Brooklyn, Brooklyn

Metropolitan Hospital Center, New York

Millard Fillmore Hospitals, Buffalo

*Montefiore Medical Center Henry and Lucy Moses Division, Bronx

Montefiore Medical Center Jack D. Weiler Hospital of the Albert Einstein College of Medicine, Bronx

*Mt. Sinai Medical Center, New York

Nassau County Medical Center, East Meadow

▼*New York Hospital-Cornell Medical Center, New York

*New York University Medical Center, New York

North Central Bronx Hospital, Bronx

North Shore University Hospital, Manhasset

Our Lady of Mercy Medical Center, Bronx

*Presbyterian Hospital in the City of New York Columbia-Presbyterian Medical Center, New York

Rochester General Hospital, Rochester

St. Luke's-Roosevelt Hospital Center St. Luke's Division, New York

St. Vincent's Hospital and Medical Center of New York, New York

St. Vincent's Medical Center of Richmond, Staten Island

State University of New York at Stony Brook University Hospital, Stony Brook

State University of New York Health Science Center University Hospital, Syracuse

State University of New York Health Science Center at Brooklyn University Hospital of Brooklyn, Brooklyn

*Strong Memorial Hospital of the University of Rochester, Rochester

Westchester County Medical Center, Valhalla

Winthrop-University Hospital, Mineola

NORTH CAROLINA

Carolinas Medical Center, Charlotte

▼*Duke University Medical Center, Durham

▼*North Carolina Baptist Hospital, Winston-Salem

Pitt County Memorial Hospital, Greenville

University of North Carolina Hospitals, Chapel Hill

OHIO

Cleveland Clinic, Cleveland

Good Samaritan Hospital, Cincinnati

Good Samaritan Hospital and Health Center, Dayton

Medical College of Ohio Hospital, Toledo

MetroHealth Medical Center, Cleveland

Mt. Carmel Medical Center, Columbus

Ohio State University Hospitals, Columbus

Toledo Hospital, Toledo

*University Hospitals of Cleveland, Cleveland

University of Cincinnati Hospital, Cincinnati

OKLAHOMA

Oklahoma Medical Center, Oklahoma City

OREGON

▼Oregon Health Sciences University University Hospital, Portland

PENNSYLVANIA

Albert Einstein Medical Center, Philadelphia

*Allegheny General Hospital, Pittsburgh

The Allentown Hospital-Lehigh Valley Hospital Center, Allentown

Episcopal Hospital, Philadelphia

Geisinger Medical Center, Danville

Graduate Hospital, Philadelphia

*Hahnemann University Hospital, Philadelphia

*Hospital of the Medical College of Pennsylvania, Philadelphia

▼*Hospital of the University of Pennsylvania, Philadelphia

Lankenau Hospital, Wynnewood

Montefiore University Hospital, Pittsburgh

Penn State University Hospital The Milton S. Hershey Medical Center, Hershey

Presbyterian Medical Center of Philadelphia, Philadelphia

*Presbyterian University Hospital, Pittsburgh

Shadyside Hospital, Pittsburgh

St. Francis Medical Center, Pittsburgh

St. Margaret Memorial Hospital, Pittsburgh

*Temple University Hospital, Philadelphia

*Thomas Jefferson University Hospital, Philadelphia

Western Pennsylvania Hospital, Pittsburgh

PUERTO RICO

Hospital de Damas, Ponce

Hospital San Lucas, Ponce

San Juan Municipal Hospital, Rio Piedras

University Hospital, San Juan

RHODE ISLAND

Memorial Hospital of Rhode Island, Pawtucket

Miriam Hospital, Providence

*Rhode Island Hospital, Providence

Roger Williams Hospital, Providence

SOUTH CAROLINA

Medical Center of Medical University of South Carolina, Charleston

Richland Memorial Hospital, Columbia

TENNESSEE

Baptist Memorial Hospital, Memphis

Johnson City Medical Center Hospital, Johnson City

Regional Medical Center at Memphis, Memphis

St. Thomas Hospital, Nashville

*Vanderbilt University Hospital and Clinic, Nashville

TEXAS

Baylor University Medical Center,
Dallas

**Bexar County Hospital District
Medical Center Hospital,
San Antonio**

**Dallas County Hospital District
Parkland Memorial Hospital,
Dallas**

Harris County Hospital District Ben
Taub General Hospital, Houston

▼*Hermann Hospital, Houston

*Methodist Hospital, Houston

*Scott and White Memorial
Hospital, Temple

St. Luke's Episcopal Hospital, Houston

University Medical Center,
Lubbock

**University of Texas Medical Branch
Hospitals, Galveston**

UTAH

University of Utah Hospital
and Clinics, Salt Lake City

VERMONT

**Fletcher Allen Healthcare
MCHV Campus, Burlington**

VIRGINIA

Roanoke Memorial Hospitals,
Roanoke

Sentara Norfolk General Hospital,
Norfolk

**University of Virginia Medical
Center, Charlottesville**

Virginia Commonwealth University
Medical College of Virginia Hospitals,
Richmond

WASHINGTON

University of Washington Medical
Center, Seattle

WEST VIRGINIA

Cabell Huntington Hospital,
Huntington

**West Virginia University
Hospitals, Morgantown**

WISCONSIN

John L. Doyne Hospital, Milwaukee

Sinai Samaritan Medical Center-
Mt. Sinai Campus, Milwaukee

University of Wisconsin Hospital
and Clinics, Madison

The Kidneys and Urinary Tract

ALABAMA

Cooper Green Hospital,
Birmingham

**University of Alabama Hospitals,
Birmingham**

ARIZONA

University Medical Center, Tucson

ARKANSAS

**University Hospital of Arkansas,
Little Rock**

CALIFORNIA

Cedars-Sinai Medical Center,
Los Angeles

Kaiser Foundation Hospital,
Hayward

Kaiser Foundation Hospital,
Los Angeles

Kaiser Foundation Hospital,
Sacramento

Kaiser Permanente Medical Center,
Walnut Creek

**Loma Linda University Medical
Center, Loma Linda**

**Los Angeles County Harbor-
University of California, Los
Angeles Medical Center, Torrance**

**Los Angeles County-University
of Southern California Medical
Center, Los Angeles**

Mercy Hospital and Medical
Center, San Diego

Olive View Medical Center, Sylmar

San Bernardino County Medical
Center, San Bernardino

**San Francisco General Hospital
and Medical Center, San Francisco**

Santa Clara Valley Medical Center,
San Jose

St. Vincent Medical Center,
Los Angeles

**Stanford University Hospital,
Stanford**

**University of California, Los
Angeles Medical Center,
Los Angeles**

**University of California, Davis
Medical Center, Sacramento**

**University of California, Irvine
Medical Center, Orange**

**University of California, San Diego
Medical Center, San Diego**

**University of California, San
Francisco Medical Center,
San Francisco**

University of Southern California
The Kenneth Norris Jr. Cancer
Hospital, Los Angeles

White Memorial Medical Center,
Los Angeles

COLORADO

Denver Health and Hospitals,
Denver

**University of Colorado Health
Sciences Center University
Hospital, Denver**

CONNECTICUT

Hartford Hospital, Hartford

Hospital of St. Raphael, New Haven

New Britain General Hospital,
New Britain

St. Francis Hospital and Medical
Center, Hartford

**University of Connecticut Health
Center John Dempsey Hospital,
Farmington**

Waterbury Hospital, Waterbury

**Yale-New Haven Hospital,
New Haven**

DELAWARE

Alfred I. Dupont Institute,
Wilmington

DISTRICT OF COLUMBIA

District of Columbia General
Hospital, Washington

*George Washington University
Hospital, Washington

*Georgetown University Hospital,
Washington

*Howard University Hospital,
Washington

Sibley Memorial Hospital,
Washington

Washington Hospital Center,
Washington

FLORIDA

Jackson Memorial Hospital, Miami

*Shands Hospital at the University
of Florida, Gainesville

Tampa General Hospital, Tampa

University of South Florida H. Lee
Moffitt Cancer Center, Tampa

GEORGIA

*Emory University Hospital,
Atlanta

Grady Memorial Hospital, Atlanta

Medical College of Georgia
Hospital and Clinics, Augusta

University Hospital, Augusta

ILLINOIS

Cook County Hospital, Chicago

Humana Hospital-Michael Reese,
Chicago

*Loyola University of Chicago
Foster G. McGaw Hospital,
Maywood

Memorial Medical Center,
Springfield

Mt. Sinai Hospital Medical Center
of Chicago, Chicago

*Northwestern Memorial Hospital,
Chicago

*Rush-Presbyterian-St. Luke's
Medical Center, Chicago

St. John's Hospital, Springfield

*University of Chicago Hospitals,
Chicago

University of Illinois Hospital
and Clinics, Chicago

INDIANA

Indiana University Medical Center,
Indianapolis

Methodist Hospital of Indiana,
Indianapolis

William N. Wishard Memorial
Hospital, Indianapolis

IOWA

University of Iowa Hospitals
and Clinics, Iowa City

KANSAS

University of Kansas Hospital,
Kansas City

KENTUCKY

Humana Hospital-University
of Louisville, Louisville

Jewish Hospital, Louisville

Norton Hospital, Louisville

St. Joseph Hospital, Lexington

University of Kentucky Hospital
Albert B. Chandler Medical Center,
Lexington

LOUISIANA

University Hospital, New Orleans

Huey P. Long Regional Medical
Center, Pineville

Jo Ellen Smith Medical Center,
New Orleans

Louisiana State University
Hospital, Shreveport

Medical Center of Louisiana
at New Orleans, New Orleans

Ochsner Foundation Hospital,
New Orleans

Schumpert Medical Center,
Shreveport

South Louisiana Medical Center,
Houma

*Tulane University Hospital
and Clinics, New Orleans

MAINE

Maine Medical Center, Portland

MARYLAND

Francis Scott Key Medical Center,
Baltimore

*Johns Hopkins Hospital,
Baltimore

Sinai Hospital of Baltimore,
Baltimore

*University of Maryland Medical
System, Baltimore

MASSACHUSETTS

*Beth Israel Hospital, Boston

Boston Medical Center, Boston

*Brigham and Women's Hospital,
Boston

Lahey Clinic Hospital, Burlington

Lawrence F. Quigley Memorial
Hospital, Chelsea

*Massachusetts General Hospital,
Boston

Medical Center of Central
Massachusetts, Worcester

New England Deaconess Hospital,
Boston

*New England Medical Center,
Boston

St. Elizabeth's Hospital, Boston

*University Hospital, Boston

University of Massachusetts
Medical Center, Worcester

MICHIGAN

Detroit Receiving Hospital and
University Health Center, Detroit

*Harper Hospital, Detroit

Henry Ford Hospital, Detroit

St. Joseph Mercy Hospital,
Ann Arbor

University of Michigan Hospitals,
Ann Arbor

William Beaumont Hospital,
Royal Oak

MINNESOTA

Hennepin County Medical Center,
Minneapolis

Mayo Clinic, Rochester

Rochester Methodist Hospital,
Rochester

*St. Mary's Hospital, Rochester

Regions Hospital, St. Paul

University of Minnesota Hospital
and Clinic, Minneapolis

MISSISSIPPI

Mississippi Baptist Medical Center, Jackson

University of Mississippi Medical Center University Hospitals and Clinics, Jackson

MISSOURI

*Barnes-Jewish Hospital, St. Louis

St. John's Mercy Medical Center, St. Louis

*St. Louis University Medical Center, St. Louis

St. Mary's Health Center, St. Louis

University Hospital and Clinics, Columbia

NEBRASKA

AMI St. Joseph Hospital, Omaha

Methodist Hospital, Omaha

University of Nebraska Medical Center, Omaha

NEW HAMPSHIRE

Dartmouth-Hitchcock Medical Center, Hanover

NEW JERSEY

Cooper Hospital-University Medical Center, Camden

Hackensack Medical Center, Hackensack

Medical Center at Princeton, Princeton

Newark Beth Israel Medical Center, Newark

*Robert Wood Johnson University Hospital, New Brunswick

St. Barnabas Medical Center, Livingston

St. Peter's Medical Center, New Brunswick

University of Medicine and Dentistry of New Jersey University Hospital, Newark

NEW MEXICO

Lovelace Medical Center, Albuquerque

University Hospital, Albuquerque

NEW YORK

*Albany Medical Center Hospital, Albany

Bellevue Hospital Center, New York

Beth Israel Medical Center, New York

New York Hospital Medical Center of Queens, Flushing

Bronx-Lebanon Hospital Center, Bronx

Bronx Municipal Hospital Center, Bronx

Brookdale Hospital Medical Center, Brooklyn

*Buffalo General Hospital, Buffalo

Cabrini Medical Center, New York

Coney Island Hospital, Brooklyn

Crouse-Irving Memorial Hospital, Syracuse

Elmhurst Hospital Center, Flushing

Erie County Medical Center, Buffalo

Genesee Hospital, Rochester

Harlem Hospital Center, New York

Interfaith Medical Center, Brooklyn

Kings County Hospital Center, Brooklyn

La Guardia Hospital, Forest Hills

Lenox Hill Hospital, New York

Lincoln Medical and Mental Health Center, Bronx

Long Island College Hospital, Brooklyn

Long Island Jewish Medical Center, New Hyde Park

Maimonides Medical Center, Brooklyn

Memorial Sloan-Kettering Cancer Center, New York

Metropolitan Hospital Center, New York

*Montefiore Medical Center Henry and Lucy Moses Division, Bronx

Montefiore Medical Center Jack D. Weiler Hospital of the Albert Einstein College of Medicine, Bronx

*Mt. Sinai Medical Center, New York

Nassau County Medical Center, East Meadow

*New York Hospital-Cornell Medical Center, New York

*New York University Medical Center, New York

North Central Bronx Hospital, Bronx

North Shore University Hospital, Manhasset

Our Lady of Mercy Medical Center, Bronx

*Presbyterian Hospital in the City of New York Columbia-Presbyterian Medical Center, New York

Queens Hospital Center, Jamaica

Rochester General Hospital, Rochester

Roswell Park Cancer Institute, Buffalo

St. Joseph's Hospital Health Center, Syracuse

St. Luke's-Roosevelt Hospital Center Roosevelt Division, New York

St. Luke's-Roosevelt Hospital Center St. Luke's Division, New York

St. Vincent's Hospital and Medical Center of New York, New York

State University of New York at Stony Brook University Hospital, Stony Brook

State University of New York Health Science Center University Hospital, Syracuse

State University of New York Health Science Center at Brooklyn University Hospital of Brooklyn, Brooklyn

*Strong Memorial Hospital of the University of Rochester, Rochester

Westchester County Medical Center, Valhalla

Winthrop-University Hospital, Mineola

NORTH CAROLINA

*Duke University Medical Center, Durham

Forsyth Memorial Hospital, Winston-Salem

*North Carolina Baptist Hospital, Winston-Salem

Pitt County Memorial Hospital, Greenville

University of North Carolina Hospitals, Chapel Hill

Wake Medical Center, Raleigh

OHIO

Akron City Hospital, Akron

Akron General Medical Center, Akron

Cleveland Clinic, Cleveland

Medical College of Ohio Hospital, Toledo

MetroHealth Medical Center, Cleveland

Ohio State University Hospitals, Columbus

Riverside Methodist Hospitals, Columbus

St. Vincent Medical Center, Toledo

Toledo Hospital, Toledo

*University Hospitals of Cleveland, Cleveland

University of Cincinnati Hospital, Cincinnati

OKLAHOMA

Oklahoma Medical Center, Oklahoma City

OREGON

Oregon Health Sciences University University Hospital, Portland

PENNSYLVANIA

Abington Memorial Hospital, Abington

Albert Einstein Medical Center, Philadelphia

*Allegheny General Hospital, Pittsburgh

Bryn Mawr Hospital, Bryn Mawr

Geisinger Medical Center, Danville

*Hahnemann University Hospital, Philadelphia

*Hospital of the Medical College of Pennsylvania, Philadelphia

*Hospital of the University of Pennsylvania, Philadelphia

Lancaster General Hospital, Lancaster

Lankenau Hospital, Wynnewood

Montefiore University Hospital, Pittsburgh

Penn State University Hospital The Milton S. Hershey Medical Center, Hershey

Pennsylvania Hospital, Philadelphia

*Presbyterian University Hospital, Pittsburgh

*Temple University Hospital, Philadelphia

*Thomas Jefferson University Hospital, Philadelphia

PUERTO RICO

University Hospital, San Juan

RHODE ISLAND

*Rhode Island Hospital, Providence

Roger Williams Hospital, Providence

SOUTH CAROLINA

Charleston Memorial Hospital, Charleston

Medical Center of Medical University of South Carolina, Charleston

TENNESSEE

Baptist Hospital, Nashville

Baptist Memorial Hospital, Memphis

Methodist Hospitals of Memphis Central Unit, Memphis

Metropolitan Nashville General Hospital, Nashville

Regional Medical Center at Memphis, Memphis

*Vanderbilt University Hospital and Clinic, Nashville

TEXAS

Baylor University Medical Center, Dallas

Bexar County Hospital District Medical Center Hospital, San Antonio

Dallas County Hospital District Parkland Memorial Hospital, Dallas

Harris County Hospital District Ben Taub General Hospital, Houston

*Hermann Hospital, Houston

Humana Hospital-San Antonio, San Antonio

*Methodist Hospital, Houston

*Scott and White Memorial Hospital, Temple

St. Joseph Hospital, Houston

St. Luke's Episcopal Hospital, Houston

University Medical Center, Lubbock

University of Texas M. D. Anderson Cancer Center, Houston

University of Texas Medical Branch Hospitals, Galveston

UTAH

LDS Hospital, Salt Lake City

University of Utah Hospital and Clinics, Salt Lake City

VERMONT

Fanny Allen Hospital, Colchester

*Fletcher Allen Healthcare MCHV Campus, Burlington

VIRGINIA

Arlington Hospital, Arlington

Fairfax Hospital, Falls Church

Memorial Hospital of Danville, Danville

Sentara Leigh Hospital, Norfolk

Sentara Norfolk General Hospital, Norfolk

University of Virginia Medical Center, Charlottesville

Virginia Commonwealth University Medical College of Virginia Hospitals, Richmond

WASHINGTON

Harborview Medical Center, Seattle

University of Washington Medical Center, Seattle

Virginia Mason Medical Center, Seattle

WEST VIRGINIA

Ohio Valley Medical Center, Wheeling

*West Virginia University Hospitals, Morgantown

WISCONSIN

*Froedtert Memorial Lutheran Hospital, Milwaukee

Lutheran Hospital-La Crosse, La Crosse

John L. Doyne Hospital, Milwaukee

University of Wisconsin Hospital and Clinics, Madison

The Lungs and Respiratory System

ALABAMA

University of Alabama Hospitals, Birmingham

University of South Alabama Medical Center, Mobile

ARIZONA

Good Samaritan Regional Medical Center, Phoenix

*University Medical Center, Tucson

ARKANSAS

University Hospital of Arkansas, Little Rock

CALIFORNIA

Barlow Respiratory Hospital, Los Angeles

California-Pacific Medical Center, San Francisco

Cedars-Sinai Medical Center, Los Angeles

Hospital of the Good Samaritan, Los Angeles

Kaiser Foundation Hospital, Fontana

*Loma Linda University Medical Center, Loma Linda

Los Angeles County Harbor-University of California, Los Angeles Medical Center, Torrance

Los Angeles County-King-Drew Medical Center, Los Angeles

Los Angeles County-University of Southern California Medical Center, Los Angeles

Olive View Medical Center, Sylmar

Santa Clara Valley Medical Center, San Jose

Sharp Memorial Hospital, San Diego

St. Joseph Hospital, Orange

*Stanford University Hospital, Stanford

University of California, Los Angeles Medical Center, Los Angeles

University of California, Davis Medical Center, Sacramento

University of California, Irvine Medical Center, Orange

University of California, San Diego Medical Center, San Diego

University of California, San Francisco Medical Center, San Francisco

COLORADO

Denver Health and Hospitals, Denver

University of Colorado Health Sciences Center University Hospital, Denver

CONNECTICUT

Mt. Sinai Hospital, Hartford

Norwalk Hospital, Norwalk

University of Connecticut Health Center John Dempsey Hospital, Farmington

*Yale-New Haven Hospital, New Haven

DELAWARE

Medical Center of Delaware, Wilmington

DISTRICT OF COLUMBIA

District of Columbia General Hospital, Washington

*George Washington University Hospital, Washington

*Georgetown University Hospital, Washington

*Howard University Hospital, Washington

Washington Hospital Center, Washington

FLORIDA

Jackson Memorial Hospital, Miami

Mt. Sinai Medical Center, Miami Beach

*Shands Hospital at the University of Florida, Gainesville

Tampa General Hospital, Tampa

University of South Florida H. Lee Moffitt Cancer Center, Tampa

GEORGIA

*Crawford Long Hospital of Emory University, Atlanta

*Emory University Hospital, Atlanta

Grady Memorial Hospital, Atlanta

Medical College of Georgia Hospital and Clinics, Augusta

ILLINOIS

Cook County Hospital, Chicago

Evanston Hospital, Evanston

Humana Hospital-Michael Reese, Chicago

*Loyola University of Chicago Foster G. McGaw Hospital, Maywood

Mt. Sinai Hospital Medical Center of Chicago, Chicago

*Northwestern Memorial Hospital, Chicago

*Rush-Presbyterian-St. Luke's Medical Center, Chicago

*University of Chicago Hospitals, Chicago

University of Illinois Hospital and Clinics, Chicago

INDIANA

Indiana University Medical Center, Indianapolis

Methodist Hospital of Indiana, Indianapolis

IOWA

University of Iowa Hospitals and Clinics, Iowa City

KANSAS

University of Kansas Hospital, Kansas City

KENTUCKY

Humana Hospital-University of Louisville, Louisville

Jewish Hospital, Louisville

University of Kentucky Hospital Albert B. Chandler Medical Center, Lexington

LOUISIANA

University Hospital, New Orleans

Louisiana State University Hospital, Shreveport

Medical Center of Louisiana at New Orleans, New Orleans

Ochsner Foundation Hospital, New Orleans

Memorial Medical Center, New Orleans

Touro Infirmary, New Orleans

*Tulane University Hospital and Clinics, New Orleans

MAINE

Maine Medical Center, Portland

MARYLAND

Francis Scott Key Medical Center, Baltimore

*Johns Hopkins Hospital, Baltimore

*University of Maryland Medical System, Baltimore

MASSACHUSETTS

Boston Medical Center, Boston

*Brigham and Women's Hospital, Boston

Lahey Clinic Hospital, Burlington

*Massachusetts General Hospital, Boston

Mt. Auburn Hospital, Cambridge

New England Deaconess Hospital, Boston

*New England Medical Center, Boston

St. Elizabeth's Hospital, Boston

St. Vincent Hospital, Worcester

*University Hospital, Boston

University of Massachusetts Medical Center, Worcester

MICHIGAN

Detroit Receiving Hospital and University Health Center, Detroit

*Harper Hospital, Detroit

Henry Ford Hospital, Detroit

Michigan Capital Medical Center, Lansing

Sinai Hospital, Detroit

University of Michigan Hospitals, Ann Arbor

MINNESOTA

Mayo Clinic, Rochester

Rochester Methodist Hospital, Rochester

*St. Mary's Hospital, Rochester

Regions Hospital, St. Paul

University of Minnesota Hospital and Clinic, Minneapolis

MISSISSIPPI

University of Mississippi Medical Center University Hospitals and Clinics, Jackson

MISSOURI

*Barnes-Jewish Hospital, St. Louis

*St. Louis University Medical Center, St. Louis

St. Luke's Hospital, Kansas City

St. Mary's Health Center, St. Louis

Truman Medical Center-West, Kansas City

University Hospital and Clinics, Columbia

NEBRASKA

AMI St. Joseph Hospital, Omaha

University of Nebraska Medical Center, Omaha

NEW HAMPSHIRE

Dartmouth-Hitchcock Medical Center, Hanover

NEW JERSEY

Community Medical Center, Scranton

Cooper Hospital-University Medical Center, Camden

Deborah Heart and Lung Center, Browns Mills

Hackensack Medical Center, Hackensack

Newark Beth Israel Medical Center, Newark

*Robert Wood Johnson University Hospital, New Brunswick

St. Michael's Medical Center, Newark

St. Peter's Medical Center, New Brunswick

United Hospitals Medical Center, Newark

University of Medicine and Dentistry of New Jersey University Hospital, Newark

NEW MEXICO

University Hospital, Albuquerque

NEW YORK

*Albany Medical Center Hospital, Albany

Bellevue Hospital Center, New York

Beth Israel Medical Center, New York

New York Hospital Medical Center of Queens, Flushing

Bronx-Lebanon Hospital Center, Bronx

Bronx Municipal Hospital Center, Bronx

Brookdale Hospital Medical Center, Brooklyn

Brooklyn Hospital Center, Brooklyn

*Buffalo General Hospital, Buffalo

Cabrini Medical Center, New York

Coney Island Hospital, Brooklyn

Crouse-Irving Memorial Hospital, Syracuse

Elmhurst Hospital Center, Flushing

Erie County Medical Center, Buffalo

Harlem Hospital Center, New York

Interfaith Medical Center, Brooklyn

Kings County Hospital Center, Brooklyn

Lenox Hill Hospital, New York

Lincoln Medical and Mental Health Center, Bronx

Long Island College Hospital, Brooklyn

Long Island Jewish Medical Center, New Hyde Park

Maimonides Medical Center, Brooklyn

Mary Immaculate Hospital, Jamaica

Memorial Sloan-Kettering Cancer Center, New York

Methodist Hospital of Brooklyn, Brooklyn

Metropolitan Hospital Center, New York

Millard Fillmore Hospitals, Buffalo

*Montefiore Medical Center Henry and Lucy Moses Division, Bronx

Montefiore Medical Center Jack D. Weiler Hospital of the Albert Einstein College of Medicine, Bronx

*Mt. Sinai Medical Center, New York

Nassau County Medical Center, East Meadow

*New York Hospital-Cornell Medical Center, New York

*New York University Medical Center, New York

North Shore University Hospital, Manhasset

*Presbyterian Hospital in the City of New York Columbia-Presbyterian Medical Center, New York

Rochester General Hospital, Rochester

Roswell Park Cancer Institute, Buffalo

St. Luke's-Roosevelt Hospital Center Roosevelt Division, New York

St. Luke's-Roosevelt Hospital Center St. Luke's Division, New York

St. Vincent's Hospital and Medical Center of New York, New York

State University of New York at Stony Brook University Hospital, Stony Brook

State University of New York Health Science Center University Hospital, Syracuse

State University of New York Health Science Center at Brooklyn University Hospital of Brooklyn, Brooklyn

*Strong Memorial Hospital of the University of Rochester, Rochester

Westchester County Medical Center, Valhalla

Winthrop-University Hospital, Mineola

NORTH CAROLINA

Carolinas Medical Center, Charlotte

*Duke University Medical Center, Durham

*North Carolina Baptist Hospital, Winston-Salem

Pitt County Memorial Hospital, Greenville

University of North Carolina Hospitals, Chapel Hill

OHIO

Cleveland Clinic, Cleveland

Medical College of Ohio Hospital, Toledo

MetroHealth Medical Center, Cleveland

Ohio State University Hospitals, Columbus

St. Vincent Medical Center, Toledo

Toledo Hospital, Toledo

*University Hospitals of Cleveland, Cleveland

University of Cincinnati Hospital, Cincinnati

OKLAHOMA

Oklahoma Medical Center, Oklahoma City

OREGON

Oregon Health Sciences University University Hospital, Portland

PENNSYLVANIA

Albert Einstein Medical Center, Philadelphia

*Allegheny General Hospital, Pittsburgh

Crozer-Chester Medical Center, Upland

Geisinger Medical Center, Danville

Graduate Hospital, Philadelphia

*Hahnemann University Hospital, Philadelphia

*Hospital of the Medical College of Pennsylvania, Philadelphia

*Hospital of the University of Pennsylvania, Philadelphia

Montefiore University Hospital, Pittsburgh

Penn State University Hospital The Milton S. Hershey Medical Center, Hershey

Presbyterian Medical Center of Philadelphia, Philadelphia

*Presbyterian University Hospital, Pittsburgh

*Temple University Hospital, Philadelphia

*Thomas Jefferson University Hospital, Philadelphia

Western Pennsylvania Hospital, Pittsburgh

PUERTO RICO

San Juan Municipal Hospital, Rio Piedras

University Hospital, San Juan

RHODE ISLAND

Memorial Hospital of Rhode Island, Pawtuckct

Roger Williams Hospital, Providence

SOUTH CAROLINA

Charleston Memorial Hospital, Charleston

Medical Center of Medical University of South Carolina, Charleston

Richland Memorial Hospital, Columbia

TENNESSEE

Baptist Memorial Hospital, Memphis

Johnson City Medical Center Hospital, Johnson City

Regional Medical Center at Memphis, Memphis

University of Tennessee Medical Center, Memphis

*Vanderbilt University Hospital and Clinic, Nashville

TEXAS

Bexar County Hospital District Medical Center Hospital, San Antonio

Dallas County Hospital District Parkland Memorial Hospital, Dallas

Harris County Hospital District Ben Taub General Hospital, Houston

*Hermann Hospital, Houston

*Methodist Hospital, Houston

*Scott and White Memorial Hospital, Temple

St. Luke's Episcopal Hospital, Houston

University of Texas M. D. Anderson Cancer Center, Houston

University of Texas Medical Branch Hospitals, Galveston

UTAH

LDS Hospital, Salt Lake City

University of Utah Hospital and Clinics, Salt Lake City

VERMONT

*Fletcher Allen Healthcare MCHV Campus, Burlington

VIRGINIA

Roanoke Memorial Hospitals, Roanoke

University of Virginia Medical Center, Charlottesville

Virginia Commonwealth University Medical College of Virginia Hospitals, Richmond

WASHINGTON

Harborview Medical Center, Seattle

University of Washington Medical Center, Seattle

WEST VIRGINIA

Cabell Huntington Hospital, Huntington

Monongalia General Hospital, Morgantown

St. Mary's Hospital, Huntington

*West Virginia University Hospitals, Morgantown

WISCONSIN

*Froedtert Memorial Lutheran Hospital, Milwaukee

John L. Doyne Hospital, Milwaukee

St. Luke's Medical Center, Milwaukee

University of Wisconsin Hospital and Clinics, Madison

The Muscles and Bones

▼ indicates National Institute of Arthritis and Musculoskeletal and Skin Diseases: Multipurpose Arthritis and Musculoskeletal Diseases Center

ALABAMA

Cooper Green Hospital, Birmingham

▼University of Alabama Hospitals, Birmingham

University of South Alabama Medical Center, Mobile

ARIZONA

Maricopa Medical Center, Phoenix

*University Medical Center, Tucson

ARKANSAS

University Hospital of Arkansas, Little Rock

CALIFORNIA

Cedars-Sinai Medical Center, Los Angeles

Centinela Hospital Medical Center, Inglewood

Century City Hospital, Los Angeles

▼Green Hospital of Scripps Clinic, La Jolla

Highland General Hospital, Oakland

Kaiser Foundation Hospital, Sacramento

Kaiser Foundation Hospital, San Francisco

*Loma Linda University Medical Center, Loma Linda

Los Angeles County Harbor-University of California, Los Angeles Medical Center, Torrance

Los Angeles County-King-Drew Medical Center, Los Angeles

Los Angeles County-Rancho Los Amigos Medical Center, Downey

Los Angeles County-University of Southern California Medical Center, Los Angeles

Mt. Zion Medical Center of University of California, San Francisco, San Francisco

Orthopaedic Hospital, Los Angeles

San Bernardino County Medical Center, San Bernardino

San Francisco General Hospital and Medical Center, San Francisco

Santa Clara Valley Medical Center, San Jose

Seton Medical Center, Daly City

St. Mary's Hospital and Medical Center, San Francisco

▼*Stanford University Hospital, Stanford

▼University of California, Los Angeles Medical Center, Los Angeles

University of California, Davis Medical Center, Sacramento

University of California, Irvine Medical Center, Orange

University of California, San Diego Medical Center, San Diego

University of California, San Francisco Medical Center, San Francisco

COLORADO

Denver Health and Hospitals, Denver

University of Colorado Health Sciences Center University Hospital, Denver

CONNECTICUT

Hartford Hospital, Hartford

Hospital of St. Raphael, New Haven

St. Francis Hospital and Medical Center, Hartford

▼University of Connecticut Health Center John Dempsey Hospital, Farmington

*Yale-New Haven Hospital, New Haven

DELAWARE

Alfred I. Dupont Institute, Wilmington

DISTRICT OF COLUMBIA

District of Columbia General Hospital, Washington

*George Washington University Hospital, Washington

*Georgetown University Hospital, Washington

Greater Southeast Community Hospital, Washington

*Howard University Hospital, Washington

Providence Hospital, Washington

Sibley Memorial Hospital, Washington

Washington Hospital Center, Washington

FLORIDA

Doctors' Hospital, Coral Gables

Jackson Memorial Hospital, Miami

Orlando Regional Medical Center, Orlando

*Shands Hospital at the University of Florida, Gainesville

Tampa General Hospital, Tampa

University Medical Center, Jacksonville

GEORGIA

*Crawford Long Hospital of Emory University, Atlanta

*Emory University Hospital, Atlanta

Georgia Baptist Medical Center, Atlanta

Grady Memorial Hospital, Atlanta

Hughston Sports Medicine Hospital, Columbus

Medical College of Georgia Hospital and Clinics, Augusta

University Hospital, Augusta

HAWAII

Queen's Medical Center, Honolulu

ILLINOIS

Christ Hospital and Medical Center, Oak Lawn

Cook County Hospital, Chicago

Evanston Hospital, Evanston

Humana Hospital-Michael Reese, Chicago

Illinois Masonic Medical Center, Chicago

*Loyola University of Chicago Foster G. McGaw Hospital, Maywood

Lutheran General Hospital, Chicago

Memorial Medical Center, Springfield

Mercy Hospital and Medical Center, Chicago

▼*Northwestern Memorial Hospital, Chicago

Ravenswood Hospital Medical Center, Chicago

*Rush-Presbyterian-St. Luke's Medical Center, Chicago

St. Francis Hospital of Evanston, Evanston

St. John's Hospital, Springfield

*University of Chicago Hospitals, Chicago

University of Illinois Hospital and Clinics, Chicago

INDIANA

▼Indiana University Medical Center, Indianapolis

Lutheran Hospital of Indiana, Fort Wayne

Methodist Hospital of Indiana, Indianapolis

Parkview Memorial Hospital, Fort Wayne

St. Joseph Medical Center, Fort Wayne

St. Vincent Hospital and Health Care Center, Indianapolis

William N. Wishard Memorial Hospital, Indianapolis

IOWA

University of Iowa Hospitals and Clinics, Iowa City

KANSAS

HCA Wesley Medical Center, Wichita

St. Francis Regional Medical Center, Wichita

University of Kansas Hospital, Kansas City

KENTUCKY

Frazier Rehabilitation Center, Louisville

Humana Hospital-University of Louisville, Louisville

Jewish Hospital, Louisville

Alliance Medical Pavilion,
Louisville

Norton Hospital, Louisville

**University of Kentucky Hospital
Albert B. Chandler Medical Center,
Lexington**

LOUISIANA

Earl K. Long Memorial Hospital,
Baton Rouge

University Hospital, New Orleans

Huey P. Long Regional Medical
Center, Pineville

**Louisiana State University
Hospital, Shreveport**

**Medical Center of Louisiana
at New Orleans, New Orleans**

Ochsner Foundation Hospital,
New Orleans

South Louisiana Medical Center,
Houma

Touro Infirmary, New Orleans

***Tulane University Hospital
and Clinics, New Orleans**

University Medical Center,
Lafayette

MARYLAND

Francis Scott Key Medical Center,
Baltimore

Good Samaritan Hospital
of Maryland, Baltimore

James Lawrence Kernan Hospital,
Baltimore

***Johns Hopkins Hospital,
Baltimore**

Sinai Hospital of Baltimore,
Baltimore

St. Agnes Hospital of the City
of Baltimore, Baltimore

Union Memorial Hospital,
Baltimore

***University of Maryland Medical
System, Baltimore**

MASSACHUSETTS

Baystate Medical Center,
Springfield

*Beth Israel Hospital, Boston

▼Boston Medical Center, Boston

▼***Brigham and Women's Hospital,
Boston**

Carney Hospital, Boston

Lahey Clinic Hospital, Burlington

***Massachusetts General Hospital,
Boston**

Medical Center of Central
Massachusetts, Worcester

New England Baptist Hospital,
Boston

***New England Medical Center,
Boston**

Newton-Wellesley Hospital, Newton

St. Elizabeth's Hospital, Boston

St. Vincent Hospital, Worcester

▼***University Hospital, Boston**

**University of Massachusetts
Medical Center, Worcester**

Worcester Health and Hospitals
Authority, Worcester

MICHIGAN

Blodgett Memorial Medical Center,
Grand Rapids

Borgess Medical Center, Kalamazoo

Bronson Methodist Hospital,
Kalamazoo

Butterworth Hospital,
Grand Rapids

Detroit Receiving Hospital and
University Health Center, Detroit

*Grace Hospital, Detroit

*Harper Hospital, Detroit

Henry Ford Hospital, Detroit

Hurley Medical Center, Flint

Hutzel Hospital, Detroit

McLaren Regional Medical Center,
Flint

Oakwood Hospital, Dearborn

Providence Hospital, Southfield

Sinai Hospital, Detroit

St. Joseph Mercy Hospital,
Ann Arbor

St. Mary's Health Services,
Grand Rapids

▼**University of Michigan Hospitals,
Ann Arbor**

William Beaumont Hospital,
Royal Oak

MINNESOTA

Hennepin County Medical Center,
Minneapolis

Mayo Clinic, Rochester

Rochester Methodist Hospital,
Rochester

*St. Mary's Hospital, Rochester

**University of Minnesota Hospital
and Clinic, Minneapolis**

MISSISSIPPI

**University of Mississippi Medical
Center University Hospitals and
Clinics, Jackson**

MISSOURI

*Barnes-Jewish Hospital, St. Louis

St. Louis Regional Medical Center,
St. Louis

***St. Louis University Medical
Center, St. Louis**

St. Luke's Hospital, Kansas City

St. Mary's Health Center, St. Louis

**Truman Medical Center-West,
Kansas City**

**University Hospital and Clinics,
Columbia**

NEBRASKA

AMI St. Joseph Hospital, Omaha

**University of Nebraska Medical
Center, Omaha**

NEW HAMPSHIRE

Dartmouth-Hitchcock Medical
Center, Hanover

NEW JERSEY

Atlantic City Medical Center,
Atlantic City

Cooper Hospital-University Medical
Center, Camden

Hackensack Medical Center,
Hackensack

Hospital Center at Orange, Orange

Jersey City Medical Center,
Jersey City

Monmouth Medical Center,
Long Branch

Newark Beth Israel Medical Center, Newark

*Robert Wood Johnson University Hospital, New Brunswick

St. Joseph's Hospital and Medical Center, Paterson

St. Michael's Medical Center, Newark

St. Peter's Medical Center, New Brunswick

United Hospitals Medical Center, Newark

United Hospitals Medical Center Orthopedic Unit, Newark

University of Medicine and Dentistry of New Jersey University Hospital, Newark

NEW MEXICO

University Hospital, Albuquerque

NEW YORK

*Albany Medical Center Hospital, Albany

Bellevue Hospital Center, New York

Bronx-Lebanon Hospital Center, Bronx

Bronx Municipal Hospital Center, Bronx

Brookdale Hospital Medical Center, Brooklyn

*Buffalo General Hospital, Buffalo

Cabrini Medical Center, New York

Coney Island Hospital, Brooklyn

Crouse-Irving Memorial Hospital, Syracuse

Ellis Hospital, Schenectady

Elmhurst Hospital Center, Flushing

Erie County Medical Center, Buffalo

Genesee Hospital, Rochester

Harlem Hospital Center, New York

Helen Hayes Hospital, West Haverstraw

Highland Hospital of Rochester, Rochester

Hospital for Joint Diseases Orthopedic Institute, New York

Hospital for Special Surgery, New York

Kings County Hospital Center, Brooklyn

Kingsbrook Jewish Medical Center, Brooklyn

Lenox Hill Hospital, New York

Lincoln Medical and Mental Health Center, Bronx

Long Island College Hospital, Brooklyn

Long Island Jewish Medical Center, New Hyde Park

Maimonides Medical Center, Brooklyn

Mary Immaculate Hospital, Jamaica

Metropolitan Hospital Center, New York

Millard Fillmore Hospitals, Buffalo

Monroe Community Hospital, Rochester

*Montefiore Medical Center Henry and Lucy Moses Division, Bronx

Montefiore Medical Center Jack D. Weiler Hospital of the Albert Einstein College of Medicine, Bronx

*Mt. Sinai Medical Center, New York

Nassau County Medical Center, East Meadow

▼*New York Hospital-Cornell Medical Center, New York

*New York University Medical Center, New York

North Central Bronx Hospital, Bronx

North Shore University Hospital, Manhasset

*Presbyterian Hospital in the City of New York Columbia-Presbyterian Medical Center, New York

Queens Hospital Center, Jamaica

Rochester General Hospital, Rochester

St. Charles Hospital and Rehabilitation Center, Port Jefferson

St. John's Queens Hospital, Elmhurst

St. Luke's-Roosevelt Hospital Center St. Luke's Division, New York

St. Mary's Hospital, Brooklyn

St. Peter's Hospital, Albany

St. Vincent's Hospital and Medical Center of New York, New York

State University of New York at Stony Brook University Hospital, Stony Brook

State University of New York Health Science Center University Hospital, Syracuse

State University of New York Health Science Center at Brooklyn University Hospital of Brooklyn, Brooklyn

*Strong Memorial Hospital of the University of Rochester, Rochester

Westchester County Medical Center, Valhalla

NORTH CAROLINA

Carolinas Medical Center, Charlotte

*Duke University Medical Center, Durham

Durham County General Hospital, Durham

*North Carolina Baptist Hospital, Winston-Salem

Orthopaedic Hospital of Charlotte, Charlotte

▼University of North Carolina Hospitals, Chapel Hill

Wake Medical Center, Raleigh

OHIO

Akron City Hospital, Akron

Akron General Medical Center, Akron

Bethesda Oak Hospital, Cincinnati

Cleveland Clinic, Cleveland

Good Samaritan Hospital, Cincinnati

Medical College of Ohio Hospital, Toledo

MetroHealth Medical Center, Cleveland

Miami Valley Hospital, Dayton

Mt. Carmel Medical Center, Columbus

577

Mt. Sinai Medical Center, Cleveland

Ohio State University Hospitals, Columbus

Riverside Methodist Hospitals, Columbus

St. Luke's Hospital, Cleveland

St. Vincent Medical Center, Toledo

Toledo Hospital, Toledo

▼***University Hospitals of Cleveland, Cleveland**

University of Cincinnati Hospital, Cincinnati

OKLAHOMA

Bone and Joint Hospital, Oklahoma City

Oklahoma Medical Center, Oklahoma City

Presbyterian Hospital, Oklahoma City

OREGON

Emanuel Hospital and Health Center, Portland

Oregon Health Sciences University University Hospital, Portland

PENNSYLVANIA

Abington Memorial Hospital, Abington

Albert Einstein Medical Center, Philadelphia

Bryn Mawr Hospital, Bryn Mawr

Delaware County Memorial Hospital, Drexel Hill

Geisinger Medical Center, Danville

*Hahnemann University Hospital, Philadelphia

Hamot Medical Center, Erie

Harrisburg Hospital, Harrisburg

*Hospital of the Medical College of Pennsylvania, Philadelphia

*Hospital of the University of Pennsylvania, Philadelphia

Lankenau Hospital, Wynnewood

Mercy Catholic Medical Center Fitzgerald Mercy Division, Philadelphia

Mercy Hospital of Pittsburgh, Pittsburgh

Methodist Hospital, Philadelphia

Montefiore University Hospital, Pittsburgh

Moss Rehabilitation Hospital, Philadelphia

Penn State University Hospital Elizabethtown Hospital, Hershey

Penn State University Hospital The Milton S. Hershey Medical Center, Hershey

Pennsylvania Hospital, Philadelphia

Polyclinic Medical Center of Harrisburg, Harrisburg

*Presbyterian University Hospital, Pittsburgh

St. Margaret Memorial Hospital, Pittsburgh

*Temple University Hospital, Philadelphia

*Thomas Jefferson University Hospital, Philadelphia

PUERTO RICO

San Juan Municipal Hospital, Rio Piedras

University Hospital, San Juan

RHODE ISLAND

*Rhode Island Hospital, Providence

Roger Williams Hospital, Providence

SOUTH CAROLINA

Greenville Memorial Hospital, Greenville

Medical Center of Medical University of South Carolina, Charleston

Richland Memorial Hospital, Columbia

TENNESSEE

Baptist Memorial Hospital, Memphis

Erlanger Medical Center, Chattanooga

Metropolitan Nashville General Hospital, Nashville

Regional Medical Center at Memphis, Memphis

St. Thomas Hospital, Nashville

*Vanderbilt University Hospital and Clinic, Nashville

TEXAS

Baylor University Medical Center, Dallas

Bexar County Hospital District Medical Center Hospital, San Antonio

Dallas County Hospital District Parkland Memorial Hospital, Dallas

Harris County Hospital District Ben Taub General Hospital, Houston

Harris Methodist Fort Worth, Fort Worth

*Hermann Hospital, Houston

*Methodist Hospital, Houston

R. E. Thomason General Hospital, El Paso

*Scott and White Memorial Hospital, Temple

St. Joseph Hospital, Houston

St. Mary of the Plains Hospital, Lubbock

Tarrant County Hospital District John Peter Smith Hospital, Fort Worth

University of Texas M. D. Anderson Cancer Center, Houston

University of Texas Medical Branch Hospitals, Galveston

UTAH

Holy Cross Hospital, Salt Lake City

LDS Hospital, Salt Lake City

University of Utah Hospital and Clinics, Salt Lake City

VERMONT

*Fletcher Allen Healthcare MCHV Campus, Burlington

VIRGINIA

Arlington Hospital, Arlington

Fairfax Hospital, Falls Church

Roanoke Memorial Hospitals, Roanoke

Sentara Leigh Hospital, Norfolk

Sentara Norfolk General Hospital, Norfolk

University of Virginia Medical Center, Charlottesville

Virginia Commonwealth University Medical College of Virginia Hospitals, Richmond

WASHINGTON

Harborview Medical Center, Seattle

Swedish Hospital Medical Center, Seattle

University of Washington Medical Center, Seattle

Virginia Mason Medical Center, Seattle

WEST VIRGINIA

Monongalia General Hospital, Morgantown

*West Virginia University Hospitals, Morgantown

WISCONSIN

Columbia Hospital, Milwaukee

*Froedtert Memorial Lutheran Hospital, Milwaukee

Meriter Hospital, Madison

John L. Doyne Hospital, Milwaukee

Sinai Samaritan Medical Center-Mt. Sinai Campus, Milwaukee

St. Joseph's Hospital, Milwaukee

St. Marys Hospital Medical Center, Madison

University of Wisconsin Hospital and Clinics, Madison

The Skin

ALABAMA

University of Alabama Hospitals, Birmingham

ARIZONA

Kino Community Hospital, Tucson

*University Medical Center, Tucson

ARKANSAS

University Hospital of Arkansas, Little Rock

CALIFORNIA

*Loma Linda University Medical Center, Loma Linda

Los Angeles County Harbor-University of California, Los Angeles Medical Center, Torrance

Los Angeles County-King-Drew Medical Center, Los Angeles

Los Angeles County-University of Southern California Medical Center, Los Angeles

San Francisco General Hospital and Medical Center, San Francisco

Santa Clara Valley Medical Center, San Jose

*Stanford University Hospital, Stanford

University of California, Los Angeles Medical Center, Los Angeles

University of California, Davis Medical Center, Sacramento

University of California, Irvine Medical Center, Orange

University of California, San Diego Medical Center, San Diego

University of California, San Francisco Medical Center, San Francisco

COLORADO

Denver Health and Hospitals, Denver

University of Colorado Health Sciences Center University Hospital, Denver

CONNECTICUT

*Yale-New Haven Hospital, New Haven

DISTRICT OF COLUMBIA

*George Washington University Hospital, Washington

*Howard University Hospital, Washington

Washington Hospital Center, Washington

FLORIDA

Jackson Memorial Hospital, Miami

Mt. Sinai Medical Center, Miami Beach

Tampa General Hospital, Tampa

GEORGIA

*Emory University Hospital, Atlanta

Grady Memorial Hospital, Atlanta

Medical College of Georgia Hospital and Clinics, Augusta

University Hospital, Augusta

ILLINOIS

Cook County Hospital, Chicago

*Loyola University of Chicago Foster G. McGaw Hospital, Maywood

*Northwestern Memorial Hospital, Chicago

*Rush-Presbyterian-St. Luke's Medical Center, Chicago

*University of Chicago Hospitals, Chicago

University of Illinois Hospital and Clinics, Chicago

INDIANA

Indiana University Medical Center, Indianapolis

William N. Wishard Memorial Hospital, Indianapolis

IOWA

University of Iowa Hospitals and Clinics, Iowa City

KANSAS

University of Kansas Hospital, Kansas City

KENTUCKY

Humana Hospital-University of Louisville, Louisville

LOUISIANA

Medical Center of Louisiana at New Orleans, New Orleans

Ochsner Foundation Hospital, New Orleans

*Tulane University Hospital
and Clinics, New Orleans

MARYLAND

Good Samaritan Hospital
of Maryland, Baltimore

*Johns Hopkins Hospital,
Baltimore

*University of Maryland Medical
System, Baltimore

MASSACHUSETTS

*Beth Israel Hospital, Boston

Boston Medical Center, Boston

*Brigham and Women's Hospital,
Boston

Lahey Clinic Hospital, Burlington

*Massachusetts General Hospital,
Boston

*New England Medical Center,
Boston

*University Hospital, Boston

MICHIGAN

Detroit Receiving Hospital and
University Health Center, Detroit

*Harper Hospital, Detroit

Henry Ford Hospital, Detroit

University of Michigan Hospitals,
Ann Arbor

MINNESOTA

Hennepin County Medical Center,
Minneapolis

Mayo Clinic, Rochester

Rochester Methodist Hospital,
Rochester

*St. Mary's Hospital, Rochester

Regions Hospital, St. Paul

University of Minnesota Hospital
and Clinic, Minneapolis

MISSOURI

*Barnes-Jewish Hospital, St. Louis

University Hospital and Clinics,
Columbia

NEW HAMPSHIRE

Dartmouth-Hitchcock Medical
Center, Hanover

NEW JERSEY

University of Medicine and
Dentistry of New Jersey University
Hospital, Newark

NEW MEXICO

University Hospital, Albuquerque

NEW YORK

Bayley Seton Hospital,
Staten Island

Bellevue Hospital Center,
New York

Beth Israel Medical Center,
New York

Bronx Municipal Hospital Center,
Bronx

*Buffalo General Hospital, Buffalo

Elmhurst Hospital Center, Flushing

Erie County Medical Center,
Buffalo

Kings County Hospital Center,
Brooklyn

Lincoln Medical and Mental
Health Center, Bronx

Metropolitan Hospital Center,
New York

*Montefiore Medical Center Henry
and Lucy Moses Division, Bronx

Montefiore Medical Center Jack D.
Weiler Hospital of the Albert
Einstein College of Medicine,
Bronx

*Mt. Sinai Medical Center,
New York

*New York Hospital-Cornell
Medical Center, New York

*New York University Medical
Center, New York

North Central Bronx Hospital,
Bronx

*Presbyterian Hospital in the City
of New York Columbia-
Presbyterian Medical Center,
New York

St. Luke's-Roosevelt Hospital
Center St. Luke's Division,
New York

State University of New York at
Stony Brook University Hospital,
Stony Brook

State University of New York
Health Science Center at Brooklyn
University Hospital of Brooklyn,
Brooklyn

*Strong Memorial Hospital of the
University of Rochester, Rochester

Westchester County Medical
Center, Valhalla

NORTH CAROLINA

*Duke University Medical Center,
Durham

*North Carolina Baptist Hospital,
Winston-Salem

University of North Carolina
Hospitals, Chapel Hill

OHIO

Cleveland Clinic, Cleveland

Good Samaritan Hospital
and Health Center, Dayton

MetroHealth Medical Center,
Cleveland

Ohio State University Hospitals,
Columbus

Franciscan Medical Center, Dayton

*University Hospitals of Cleveland,
Cleveland

University of Cincinnati Hospital,
Cincinnati

OKLAHOMA

Oklahoma Medical Center,
Oklahoma City

OREGON

Oregon Health Sciences University
University Hospital, Portland

PENNSYLVANIA

Geisinger Medical Center, Danville

Graduate Hospital, Philadelphia

*Hahnemann University Hospital,
Philadelphia

*Hospital of the University
of Pennsylvania, Philadelphia

Penn State University Hospital The Milton S. Hershey Medical Center, Hershey

Pennsylvania Hospital, Philadelphia

*Presbyterian University Hospital, Pittsburgh

*Thomas Jefferson University Hospital, Philadelphia

PUERTO RICO

University Hospital, San Juan

RHODE ISLAND

Memorial Hospital of Rhode Island, Pawtucket

*Rhode Island Hospital, Providence

Roger Williams Hospital, Providence

SOUTH CAROLINA

Medical Center of Medical University of South Carolina, Charleston

TENNESSEE

Baptist Memorial Hospital, Memphis

Metropolitan Nashville General Hospital, Nashville

Regional Medical Center at Memphis, Memphis

University of Tennessee Medical Center, Memphis

*Vanderbilt University Hospital and Clinic, Nashville

TEXAS

Bexar County Hospital District Medical Center Hospital, San Antonio

Dallas County Hospital District Parkland Memorial Hospital, Dallas

Harris County Hospital District Ben Taub General Hospital, Houston

Harris County Hospital District Lyndon B. Johnson General Hospital, Houston

*Hermann Hospital, Houston

*Methodist Hospital, Houston

University Medical Center, Lubbock

University of Texas M. D. Anderson Cancer Center, Houston

University of Texas Medical Branch Hospitals, Galveston

Zale-Lipshy University Hospital, Dallas

UTAH

University of Utah Hospital and Clinics, Salt Lake City

VIRGINIA

University of Virginia Medical Center, Charlottesville

Virginia Commonwealth University Medical College of Virginia Hospitals, Richmond

WASHINGTON

University of Washington Medical Center, Seattle

WEST VIRGINIA

*West Virginia University Hospitals, Morgantown

WISCONSIN

*Froedtert Memorial Lutheran Hospital, Milwaukee

John L. Doyne Hospital, Milwaukee

St. Joseph's Hospital, Marshfield

University of Wisconsin Hospital and Clinics, Madison

Health Problems of Men

ALABAMA

Cooper Green Hospital, Birmingham

University of Alabama Hospitals, Birmingham

ARIZONA

*University Medical Center, Tucson

ARKANSAS

University Hospital of Arkansas, Little Rock

CALIFORNIA

Kaiser Foundation Hospital, Hayward

Kaiser Foundation Hospital, Los Angeles

Kaiser Foundation Hospital, Sacramento

Kaiser Permanente Medical Center, Walnut Creek

*Loma Linda University Medical Center, Loma Linda

Los Angeles County Harbor-University of California, Los Angeles Medical Center, Torrance

Los Angeles County-University of Southern California Medical Center, Los Angeles

Mercy Hospital and Medical Center, San Diego

Olive View Medical Center, Sylmar

San Bernardino County Medical Center, San Bernardino

San Francisco General Hospital and Medical Center, San Francisco

Santa Clara Valley Medical Center, San Jose

*Stanford University Hospital, Stanford

University of California, Los Angeles Medical Center, Los Angeles

University of California, Davis Medical Center, Sacramento

University of California, Irvine Medical Center, Orange

University of California, San Diego Medical Center, San Diego

University of California, San Francisco Medical Center, San Francisco

University of Southern California The Kenneth Norris Jr. Cancer Hospital, Los Angeles

White Memorial Medical Center, Los Angeles

COLORADO

Denver Health and Hospitals, Denver

University of Colorado Health Sciences Center University Hospital, Denver

CONNECTICUT

Hartford Hospital, Hartford

New Britain General Hospital, New Britain

St. Francis Hospital and Medical Center, Hartford

University of Connecticut Health Center John Dempsey Hospital, Farmington

Waterbury Hospital, Waterbury

*Yale-New Haven Hospital, New Haven

DELAWARE

Alfred I. Dupont Institute, Wilmington

DISTRICT OF COLUMBIA

District of Columbia General Hospital, Washington

*George Washington University Hospital, Washington

*Georgetown University Hospital, Washington

*Howard University Hospital, Washington

Sibley Memorial Hospital, Washington

Washington Hospital Center, Washington

FLORIDA

Jackson Memorial Hospital, Miami

*Shands Hospital at the University of Florida, Gainesville

Tampa General Hospital, Tampa

University of South Florida H. Lee Moffitt Cancer Center, Tampa

GEORGIA

*Emory University Hospital, Atlanta

Grady Memorial Hospital, Atlanta

Medical College of Georgia Hospital and Clinics, Augusta

University Hospital, Augusta

ILLINOIS

Cook County Hospital, Chicago

Humana Hospital-Michael Reese, Chicago

*Loyola University of Chicago Foster G. McGaw Hospital, Maywood

Memorial Medical Center, Springfield

*Northwestern Memorial Hospital, Chicago

*Rush-Presbyterian-St. Luke's Medical Center, Chicago

St. John's Hospital, Springfield

*University of Chicago Hospitals, Chicago

University of Illinois Hospital and Clinics, Chicago

INDIANA

Indiana University Medical Center, Indianapolis

Methodist Hospital of Indiana, Indianapolis

William N. Wishard Memorial Hospital, Indianapolis

IOWA

University of Iowa Hospitals and Clinics, Iowa City

KANSAS

University of Kansas Hospital, Kansas City

KENTUCKY

Humana Hospital-University of Louisville, Louisville

Jewish Hospital, Louisville

Norton Hospital, Louisville

St. Joseph Hospital, Lexington

University of Kentucky Hospital Albert B. Chandler Medical Center, Lexington

LOUISIANA

University Hospital, New Orleans

Huey P. Long Regional Medical Center, Pineville

Jo Ellen Smith Medical Center, New Orleans

Louisiana State University Hospital, Shreveport

Medical Center of Louisiana at New Orleans, New Orleans

Ochsner Foundation Hospital, New Orleans

Schumpert Medical Center, Shreveport

South Louisiana Medical Center, Houma

*Tulane University Hospital and Clinics, New Orleans

MARYLAND

Francis Scott Key Medical Center, Baltimore

*Johns Hopkins Hospital, Baltimore

Sinai Hospital of Baltimore, Baltimore

*University of Maryland Medical System, Baltimore

MASSACHUSETTS

*Beth Israel Hospital, Boston

Boston Medical Center, Boston

*Brigham and Women's Hospital, Boston

Lahey Clinic Hospital, Burlington

Lawrence F. Quigley Memorial Hospital, Chelsea

*Massachusetts General Hospital, Boston

Medical Center of Central Massachusetts, Worcester

New England Deaconess Hospital, Boston

*New England Medical Center, Boston

St. Elizabeth's Hospital, Boston

*University Hospital, Boston

University of Massachusetts Medical Center, Worcester

MICHIGAN

*Harper Hospital, Detroit

Henry Ford Hospital, Detroit

St. Joseph Mercy Hospital, Ann Arbor

University of Michigan Hospitals, Ann Arbor

William Beaumont Hospital,
Royal Oak

MINNESOTA
Mayo Clinic, Rochester

Rochester Methodist Hospital,
Rochester

*St. Mary's Hospital, Rochester

Regions Hospital, St. Paul

**University of Minnesota Hospital
and Clinic, Minneapolis**

MISSISSIPPI
Mississippi Baptist Medical Center,
Jackson

**University of Mississippi Medical
Center University Hospitals and
Clinics, Jackson**

MISSOURI
*Barnes-Jewish Hospital, St. Louis

St. John's Mercy Medical Center,
St. Louis

***St. Louis University Medical
Center, St. Louis**

St. Mary's Health Center, St. Louis

**University Hospital and Clinics,
Columbia**

NEBRASKA
AMI St. Joseph Hospital, Omaha

Methodist Hospital, Omaha

**University of Nebraska Medical
Center, Omaha**

NEW HAMPSHIRE
Dartmouth-Hitchcock Medical
Center, Hanover

NEW JERSEY
Hackensack Medical Center,
Hackensack

Medical Center at Princeton,
Princeton

***Robert Wood Johnson University
Hospital, New Brunswick**

**University of Medicine and
Dentistry of New Jersey University
Hospital, Newark**

NEW MEXICO
Lovelace Medical Center,
Albuquerque

University Hospital, Albuquerque

NEW YORK
***Albany Medical Center Hospital,
Albany**

**Bellevue Hospital Center,
New York**

Beth Israel Medical Center,
New York

Bronx Municipal Hospital Center,
Bronx

Brookdale Hospital Medical
Center, Brooklyn

*Buffalo General Hospital, Buffalo

Cabrini Medical Center, New York

Coney Island Hospital, Brooklyn

Crouse-Irving Memorial Hospital,
Syracuse

Elmhurst Hospital Center, Flushing

**Erie County Medical Center,
Buffalo**

Genesee Hospital, Rochester

**Kings County Hospital Center,
Brooklyn**

La Guardia Hospital, Forest Hills

Lenox Hill Hospital, New York

Lincoln Medical and Mental
Health Center, Bronx

Long Island College Hospital,
Brooklyn

Long Island Jewish Medical Center,
New Hyde Park

Maimonides Medical Center,
Brooklyn

Memorial Sloan-Kettering Cancer
Center, New York

Metropolitan Hospital Center,
New York

***Montefiore Medical Center Henry
and Lucy Moses Division, Bronx**

Montefiore Medical Center Jack D.
Weiler Hospital of the Albert
Einstein College of Medicine,
Bronx

***Mt. Sinai Medical Center,
New York**

***New York Hospital-Cornell
Medical Center, New York**

***New York University Medical
Center, New York**

North Central Bronx Hospital,
Bronx

Our Lady of Mercy Medical Center,
Bronx

***Presbyterian Hospital in the City
of New York Columbia-
Presbyterian Medical Center,
New York**

Queens Hospital Center, Jamaica

Rochester General Hospital,
Rochester

Roswell Park Cancer Institute,
Buffalo

St. Joseph's Hospital Health Center,
Syracuse

St. Luke's-Roosevelt Hospital
Center Roosevelt Division,
New York

St. Luke's-Roosevelt Hospital
Center St. Luke's Division,
New York

**State University of New York
Health Science Center University
Hospital, Syracuse**

**State University of New York
Health Science Center at Brooklyn
University Hospital of Brooklyn,
Brooklyn**

***Strong Memorial Hospital of the
University of Rochester, Rochester**

**Westchester County Medical
Center, Valhalla**

NORTH CAROLINA
***Duke University Medical Center,
Durham**

Forsyth Memorial Hospital,
Winston-Salem

***North Carolina Baptist Hospital,
Winston-Salem**

**University of North Carolina
Hospitals, Chapel Hill**

Wake Medical Center, Raleigh

OHIO
Akron City Hospital, Akron

Akron General Medical Center,
Akron

Cleveland Clinic, Cleveland

Medical College of Ohio Hospital, Toledo

MetroHealth Medical Center, Cleveland

Ohio State University Hospitals, Columbus

Riverside Methodist Hospitals, Columbus

St. Vincent Medical Center, Toledo

Toledo Hospital, Toledo

*University Hospitals of Cleveland, Cleveland

University of Cincinnati Hospital, Cincinnati

OKLAHOMA

Oklahoma Medical Center, Oklahoma City

OREGON

Oregon Health Sciences University University Hospital, Portland

PENNSYLVANIA

Abington Memorial Hospital, Abington

*Allegheny General Hospital, Pittsburgh

Bryn Mawr Hospital, Bryn Mawr

Geisinger Medical Center, Danville

*Hospital of the Medical College of Pennsylvania, Philadelphia

*Hospital of the University of Pennsylvania, Philadelphia

Lancaster General Hospital, Lancaster

Montefiore University Hospital, Pittsburgh

Penn State University Hospital The Milton S. Hershey Medical Center, Hershey

Pennsylvania Hospital, Philadelphia

*Presbyterian University Hospital, Pittsburgh

*Temple University Hospital, Philadelphia

*Thomas Jefferson University Hospital, Philadelphia

PUERTO RICO

University Hospital, San Juan

RHODE ISLAND

*Rhode Island Hospital, Providence

Roger Williams Hospital, Providence

SOUTH CAROLINA

Charleston Memorial Hospital, Charleston

Medical Center of Medical University of South Carolina, Charleston

TENNESSEE

Baptist Hospital, Nashville

Baptist Memorial Hospital, Memphis

Methodist Hospitals of Memphis Central Unit, Memphis

Metropolitan Nashville General Hospital, Nashville

Regional Medical Center at Memphis, Memphis

*Vanderbilt University Hospital and Clinic, Nashville

TEXAS

Baylor University Medical Center, Dallas

Bexar County Hospital District Medical Center Hospital, San Antonio

Dallas County Hospital District Parkland Memorial Hospital, Dallas

Harris County Hospital District Ben Taub General Hospital, Houston

*Hermann Hospital, Houston

Humana Hospital-San Antonio, San Antonio

*Methodist Hospital, Houston

*Scott and White Memorial Hospital, Temple

St. Joseph Hospital, Houston

St. Luke's Episcopal Hospital, Houston

University of Texas M. D. Anderson Cancer Center, Houston

University of Texas Medical Branch Hospitals, Galveston

UTAH

LDS Hospital, Salt Lake City

University of Utah Hospital and Clinics, Salt Lake City

VERMONT

Fanny Allen Hospital, Colchester

*Fletcher Allen Healthcare MCHV Campus, Burlington

VIRGINIA

Fairfax Hospital, Falls Church

Memorial Hospital of Danville, Danville

Sentara Leigh Hospital, Norfolk

Sentara Norfolk General Hospital, Norfolk

University of Virginia Medical Center, Charlottesville

Virginia Commonwealth University Medical College of Virginia Hospitals, Richmond

WASHINGTON

Harborview Medical Center, Seattle

University of Washington Medical Center, Seattle

Virginia Mason Medical Center, Seattle

WEST VIRGINIA

Ohio Valley Medical Center, Wheeling

*West Virginia University Hospitals, Morgantown

WISCONSIN

*Froedtert Memorial Lutheran Hospital, Milwaukee

Lutheran Hospital-La Crosse, La Crosse

John L. Doyne Hospital, Milwaukee

University of Wisconsin Hospital and Clinics, Madison

Health Problems of Women

ALABAMA

Carraway Methodist Medical Center, Birmingham

Cooper Green Hospital, Birmingham

University of Alabama Hospitals, Birmingham

University of South Alabama Medical Center, Mobile

ARIZONA

Good Samaritan Regional Medical Center, Phoenix

Kino Community Hospital, Tucson

Maricopa Medical Center, Phoenix

St. Joseph's Hospital and Medical Center, Phoenix

*University Medical Center, Tucson

ARKANSAS

University Hospital of Arkansas, Little Rock

CALIFORNIA

California Medical Center-Los Angeles, Los Angeles

Cedars-Sinai Medical Center, Los Angeles

Glendale Adventist Medical Center, Glendale

Kaiser Foundation Hospital, Fontana

Kaiser Foundation Hospital, Los Angeles

Kaiser Foundation Hospital, Oakland

Kaiser Foundation Hospital, Sacramento

Kaiser Foundation Hospital, San Diego

Kaiser Foundation Hospital, San Francisco

Kaiser Foundation Hospital, Santa Clara

Kern Medical Center, Bakersfield

*Loma Linda University Medical Center, Loma Linda

Long Beach Memorial Medical Center, Long Beach

Los Angeles County Harbor-University of California, Los Angeles Medical Center, Torrance

Los Angeles County-King-Drew Medical Center, Los Angeles

Los Angeles County-University of Southern California Medical Center, Los Angeles

Mt. Zion Medical Center of University of California, San Francisco, San Francisco

Olive View Medical Center, Sylmar

Riverside General Hospital University Medical Center, Riverside

San Bernardino County Medical Center, San Bernardino

San Francisco General Hospital and Medical Center, San Francisco

Santa Clara Valley Medical Center, San Jose

*Stanford University Hospital, Stanford

Sutter General Hospital, Sacramento

Sutter Memorial Hospital, Sacramento

University of California, Los Angeles Medical Center, Los Angeles

University of California, Davis Medical Center, Sacramento

University of California, Irvine Medical Center, Orange

University of California, San Diego Medical Center, San Diego

University of California, San Francisco Medical Center, San Francisco

Valley Medical Center of Fresno, Fresno

White Memorial Medical Center, Los Angeles

COLORADO

Denver Health and Hospitals, Denver

Presbyterian-St. Luke's Medical Center, Denver

Rose Medical Center, Denver

St. Joseph Hospital, Denver

University of Colorado Health Sciences Center University Hospital, Denver

CONNECTICUT

Bridgeport Hospital, Bridgeport

Danbury Hospital, Danbury

Hartford Hospital, Hartford

Mt. Sinai Hospital, Hartford

New Britain General Hospital, New Britain

St. Francis Hospital and Medical Center, Hartford

Stamford Hospital, Stamford

University of Connecticut Health Center John Dempsey Hospital, Farmington

*Yale-New Haven Hospital, New Haven

DELAWARE

Medical Center of Delaware, Wilmington

DISTRICT OF COLUMBIA

District of Columbia General Hospital, Washington

*George Washington University Hospital, Washington

*Georgetown University Hospital, Washington

Greater Southeast Community Hospital, Washington

*Howard University Hospital, Washington

Providence Hospital, Washington

Washington Hospital Center, Washington

FLORIDA

Baptist Hospital, Pensacola

Baptist Medical Center, Jacksonville

Bayfront Medical Center, St. Petersburg

Jackson Memorial Hospital, Miami

Orlando Regional Medical Center, Orlando

Sacred Heart Hospital of Pensacola, Pensacola

*Shands Hospital at the University of Florida, Gainesville

Tampa General Hospital, Tampa

University Medical Center, Jacksonville

GEORGIA

*Crawford Long Hospital of Emory University, Atlanta

*Emory University Hospital, Atlanta

Georgia Baptist Medical Center, Atlanta

Grady Memorial Hospital, Atlanta

Medical Center of Central Georgia, Macon

Medical College of Georgia Hospital and Clinics, Augusta

Memorial Medical Center, Savannah

University Hospital, Augusta

HAWAII

Kapiolani Medical Center for Women and Children, Honolulu

Queen's Medical Center, Honolulu

ILLINOIS

Christ Hospital and Medical Center, Oak Lawn

Columbus Hospital, Chicago

Cook County Hospital, Chicago

Evanston Hospital, Evanston

Humana Hospital-Michael Reese, Chicago

Illinois Masonic Medical Center, Chicago

*Loyola University of Chicago Foster G. McGaw Hospital, Maywood

Lutheran General Hospital, Chicago

MacNeal Hospital, Berwyn

Memorial Medical Center, Springfield

Mercy Hospital and Medical Center, Chicago

Mt. Sinai Hospital Medical Center of Chicago, Chicago

Northwestern Memorial Hospital Prentice Women's Hospital, Chicago

Resurrection Medical Center, Chicago

*Rush-Presbyterian-St. Luke's Medical Center, Chicago

St. Cabrini Hospital, Chicago

St. Francis Hospital of Evanston, Evanston

St. Francis Medical Center, Peoria

St. John's Hospital, Springfield

St. Joseph Hospital and Health Care Center, Chicago

*University of Chicago Hospitals, Chicago

University of Illinois Hospital and Clinics, Chicago

INDIANA

Indiana University Medical Center, Indianapolis

Methodist Hospital of Indiana, Indianapolis

St. Vincent Hospital and Health Care Center, Indianapolis

William N. Wishard Memorial Hospital, Indianapolis

IOWA

University of Iowa Hospitals and Clinics, Iowa City

KANSAS

HCA Wesley Medical Center, Wichita

University of Kansas Hospital, Kansas City

KENTUCKY

Central Baptist Hospital, Lexington

Humana Hospital-University of Louisville, Louisville

Norton Hospital, Louisville

University of Kentucky Hospital Albert B. Chandler Medical Center, Lexington

LOUISIANA

Dr. Walter Olin Moss Regional Hospital, Lake Charles

E. A. Conway Memorial Hospital, Monroe

Earl K. Long Memorial Hospital, Baton Rouge

Huey P. Long Regional Medical Center, Pineville

Lallie Kemp Hospital, Independence

Louisiana State University Hospital, Shreveport

Medical Center of Louisiana at New Orleans, New Orleans

Ochsner Foundation Hospital, New Orleans

South Louisiana Medical Center, Houma

*Tulane University Hospital and Clinics, New Orleans

University Medical Center, Lafayette

MAINE

Maine Medical Center, Portland

MARYLAND

Francis Scott Key Medical Center, Baltimore

Franklin Square Hospital Center, Baltimore

Greater Baltimore Medical Center, Baltimore

Harbor Hospital Center, Baltimore

Holy Cross Hospital of Silver Spring, Silver Spring

*Johns Hopkins Hospital, Baltimore

Maryland General Hospital, Baltimore

Mercy Medical Center, Baltimore

Sinai Hospital of Baltimore, Baltimore

Union Memorial Hospital, Baltimore

*University of Maryland Medical System, Baltimore

MASSACHUSETTS

Baystate Medical Center, Springfield

Berkshire Medical Center, Pittsfield

*Beth Israel Hospital, Boston

Boston Medical Center, Boston

*Brigham and Women's Hospital, Boston

Metrowest Medical Center, Framingham

Malden Hospital, Malden

*Massachusetts General Hospital, Boston

Medical Center of Central Massachusetts, Worcester

*New England Medical Center, Boston

St. Mary's Women & Infant Center, Boston

St. Vincent Hospital, Worcester

University of Massachusetts Medical Center, Worcester

MICHIGAN

Blodgett Memorial Medical Center, Grand Rapids

Butterworth Hospital, Grand Rapids

Detroit Receiving Hospital and University Health Center, Detroit

*Grace Hospital, Detroit

*Harper Hospital, Detroit

Henry Ford Hospital, Detroit

Hurley Medical Center, Flint

Hutzel Hospital, Detroit

Oakwood Hospital, Dearborn

North Oakland Medical Centers, Pontiac

Providence Hospital, Southfield

Saginaw General Hospital, Saginaw

Sinai Hospital, Detroit

Sparrow Hospital, Lansing

St. John Hospital and Medical Center, Detroit

St. Joseph Mercy Hospital, Ann Arbor

St. Mary's Health Services, Grand Rapids

University of Michigan Hospitals, Ann Arbor

William Beaumont Hospital, Royal Oak

MINNESOTA

Hennepin County Medical Center, Minneapolis

Mayo Clinic, Rochester

Rochester Methodist Hospital, Rochester

*St. Mary's Hospital, Rochester

Regions Hospital, St. Paul

University of Minnesota Hospital and Clinic, Minneapolis

MISSISSIPPI

University of Mississippi Medical Center University Hospitals and Clinics, Jackson

MISSOURI

*Barnes-Jewish Hospital, St. Louis

Deaconess Hospital, St. Louis

Menorah Medical Center, Kansas City

St. John's Mercy Medical Center, St. Louis

St. Louis Regional Medical Center, St. Louis

*St. Louis University Medical Center, St. Louis

St. Luke's Hospital, Kansas City

St. Mary's Health Center, St. Louis

Truman Medical Center-West, Kansas City

University Hospital and Clinics, Columbia

NEBRASKA

AMI St. Joseph Hospital, Omaha

Bergan Mercy Medical Center, Omaha

University of Nebraska Medical Center, Omaha

NEVADA

University Medical Center of Southern Nevada, Las Vegas

Women's Hospital, Las Vegas

NEW JERSEY

Cooper Hospital-University Medical Center, Camden

Englewood Hospital, Englewood

Hackensack Medical Center, Hackensack

Jersey City Medical Center, Jersey City

Jersey Shore Medical Center, Neptune

Monmouth Medical Center, Long Branch

Morristown Memorial Hospital, Morristown

Muhlenberg Regional Medical Center, Plainfield

Newark Beth Israel Medical Center, Newark

*Robert Wood Johnson University Hospital, New Brunswick

St. Barnabas Medical Center, Livingston

St. James Hospital of Newark, Newark

St. Joseph's Hospital and Medical Center, Paterson

St. Michael's Medical Center, Newark

St. Peter's Medical Center, New Brunswick

University of Medicine and Dentistry of New Jersey University Hospital, Newark

NEW MEXICO

University Hospital, Albuquerque

NEW YORK

*Albany Medical Center Hospital, Albany

Bellevue Hospital Center, New York

Beth Israel Medical Center, New York

New York Hospital Medical Center of Queens, Flushing

Bronx-Lebanon Hospital Center, Bronx

Bronx Municipal Hospital Center, Bronx

Brookdale Hospital Medical Center, Brooklyn

Brooklyn Hospital Center, Brooklyn

*Buffalo General Hospital, Buffalo

Coney Island Hospital, Brooklyn

Crouse-Irving Memorial Hospital, Syracuse

Elmhurst Hospital Center, Flushing

Erie County Medical Center, Buffalo

Flushing Hospital Medical Center, Flushing

Genesee Hospital, Rochester

Harlem Hospital Center, New York

Highland Hospital of Rochester, Rochester

Interfaith Medical Center, Brooklyn

Jamaica Hospital, Jamaica

Kings County Hospital Center, Brooklyn

Lenox Hill Hospital, New York

Lincoln Medical and Mental Health Center, Bronx

Long Island College Hospital, Brooklyn

Long Island Jewish Medical Center, New Hyde Park

Lutheran Medical Center, Brooklyn

Maimonides Medical Center, Brooklyn

Mary Immaculate Hospital, Jamaica

Mercy Hospital, Rockville Centre

Metropolitan Hospital Center, New York

Millard Fillmore Hospitals, Buffalo

*Montefiore Medical Center Henry and Lucy Moses Division, Bronx

Montefiore Medical Center Jack D. Weiler Hospital of the Albert Einstein College of Medicine, Bronx

*Mt. Sinai Medical Center, New York

Nassau County Medical Center, East Meadow

*New York Hospital-Cornell Medical Center, New York

New York Infirmary-Beekman Downtown Hospital, New York

*New York University Medical Center, New York

North Central Bronx Hospital, Bronx

North Shore University Hospital, Manhasset

Our Lady of Lourdes Medical Center, Camden

Our Lady of Mercy Medical Center, Bronx

*Presbyterian Hospital in the City of New York Columbia-Presbyterian Medical Center, New York

Queens Hospital Center, Jamaica

Rochester General Hospital, Rochester

Sisters of Charity Hospital of Buffalo, Buffalo

St. John's Episcopal Hospital-South Shore, Far Rockaway

St. John's Queens Hospital, Elmhurst

St. Joseph's Hospital Health Center, Syracuse

St. Luke's-Roosevelt Hospital Center Roosevelt Division, New York

St. Luke's-Roosevelt Hospital Center St. Luke's Division, New York

St. Mary's Hospital, Brooklyn

St. Peter's Hospital, Albany

St. Vincent's Hospital and Medical Center of New York, New York

St. Vincent's Medical Center of Richmond, Staten Island

State University of New York at Stony Brook University Hospital, Stony Brook

State University of New York Health Science Center University Hospital, Syracuse

State University of New York Health Science Center at Brooklyn University Hospital of Brooklyn, Brooklyn

Staten Island University Hospital, Staten Island

*Strong Memorial Hospital of the University of Rochester, Rochester

Westchester County Medical Center, Valhalla

Winthrop-University Hospital, Mineola

NORTH CAROLINA

Carolinas Medical Center, Charlotte

*Duke University Medical Center, Durham

Forsyth Memorial Hospital, Winston-Salem

New Hanover Regional Medical Center, Wilmington

*North Carolina Baptist Hospital, Winston-Salem

Pitt County Memorial Hospital, Greenville

University of North Carolina Hospitals, Chapel Hill

Wake Medical Center, Raleigh

OHIO

Akron City Hospital, Akron

Akron General Medical Center, Akron

Aultman Hospital, Canton

Bethesda Oak Hospital, Cincinnati

Christ Hospital, Cincinnati

Good Samaritan Hospital, Cincinnati

Grant Medical Center, Columbus

Medical College of Ohio Hospital, Toledo

MetroHealth Medical Center, Cleveland

Miami Valley Hospital, Dayton

Mt. Carmel Medical Center, Columbus

Mt. Sinai Medical Center, Cleveland

Ohio State University Hospitals, Columbus

Riverside Methodist Hospitals, Columbus

St. Ann's Hospital of Columbus, Westerville

St. Elizabeth Hospital Medical Center, Youngstown

St. Luke's Hospital, Cleveland

St. Vincent Medical Center, Toledo

Toledo Hospital, Toledo

*University Hospitals of Cleveland, Cleveland

University of Cincinnati Hospital, Cincinnati

OKLAHOMA

Hillcrest Medical Center, Tulsa

Oklahoma Medical Center, Oklahoma City

St. Francis Hospital, Tulsa

St. John Medical Center, Tulsa

OREGON

Emanuel Hospital and Health Center, Portland

Good Samaritan Hospital and Medical Center, Portland

Oregon Health Sciences University University Hospital, Portland

PENNSYLVANIA

Abington Memorial Hospital, Abington

Albert Einstein Medical Center, Philadelphia

*Allegheny General Hospital, Pittsburgh

The Allentown Hospital-Lehigh Valley Hospital Center, Allentown

Chestnut Hill Hospital, Philadelphia

Crozer-Chester Medical Center, Upland

Frankford Hospital of the City of Philadelphia, Philadelphia

Geisinger Medical Center, Danville

Germantown Hospital and Medical Center, Philadelphia

*Hahnemann University Hospital, Philadelphia

Harrisburg Hospital, Harrisburg

*Hospital of the Medical College of Pennsylvania, Philadelphia

*Hospital of the University of Pennsylvania, Philadelphia

Lankenau Hospital, Wynnewood

Lower Bucks Hospital, Bristol

Magee-Womens Hospital, Pittsburgh

Methodist Hospital, Philadelphia

Penn State University Hospital The Milton S. Hershey Medical Center, Hershey

Pennsylvania Hospital, Philadelphia

Reading Hospital and Medical Center, Reading

St. Luke's Hospital, Bethlehem

*Temple University Hospital, Philadelphia

*Thomas Jefferson University Hospital, Philadelphia

Western Pennsylvania Hospital, Pittsburgh

York Hospital, York

PUERTO RICO

Caguas Regional Hospital, Caguas

Dr. Ramon E. Betances Hospital-Mayaguez Medical Center Branch, Mayaguez

Ponce Regional Hospital, Ponce

San Juan Municipal Hospital, Rio Piedras

University Hospital, San Juan

RHODE ISLAND

*Rhode Island Hospital, Providence

Women and Infants Hospital of Rhode Island, Providence

SOUTH CAROLINA

Charleston Memorial Hospital, Charleston

Greenville Memorial Hospital, Greenville

Medical Center of Medical University of South Carolina, Charleston

Richland Memorial Hospital, Columbia

TENNESSEE

Baptist Hospital, Nashville

Erlanger Medical Center, Chattanooga

Metropolitan Nashville General Hospital, Nashville

Regional Medical Center at Memphis, Memphis

University of Tennessee Medical Center, Memphis

University of Tennessee Memorial Hospital, Knoxville

*Vanderbilt University Hospital and Clinic, Nashville

TEXAS

Baylor University Medical Center, Dallas

Bexar County Hospital District Medical Center Hospital, San Antonio

Brackenridge Hospital, Austin

Dallas County Hospital District Parkland Memorial Hospital, Dallas

Harris County Hospital District Ben Taub General Hospital, Houston

Harris County Hospital District Lyndon B. Johnson General Hospital, Houston

Harris Methodist Fort Worth, Fort Worth

*Hermann Hospital, Houston

High Plains Baptist Hospital, Amarillo

Medical Center Hospital, Odessa

Methodist Medical Center, Dallas

Northwest Texas Hospital, Amarillo

R. E. Thomason General Hospital, El Paso

*Scott and White Memorial Hospital, Temple

St. Joseph Hospital, Houston

St. Paul Medical Center, Dallas

Tarrant County Hospital District John Peter Smith Hospital, Fort Worth

University Medical Center, Lubbock

University of Texas Medical Branch Hospitals, Galveston

UTAH

LDS Hospital, Salt Lake City

University of Utah Hospital and Clinics, Salt Lake City

VERMONT

***Fletcher Allen Healthcare
MCHV Campus, Burlington**

VIRGINIA

Depaul Medical Center, Norfolk

Fairfax Hospital, Falls Church

Portsmouth General Hospital,
Portsmouth

Riverside Regional Medical Center,
Newport News

Roanoke Memorial Hospitals,
Roanoke

Sentara Norfolk General Hospital,
Norfolk

**University of Virginia Medical
Center, Charlottesville**

**Virginia Commonwealth University
Medical College of Virginia
Hospitals, Richmond**

WASHINGTON

Swedish Hospital Medical Center,
Seattle

**University of Washington Medical
Center, Seattle**

WEST VIRGINIA

Charleston Area Medical Center
Women and Children's Hospital
of West Virginia, Charleston

Ohio Valley Medical Center,
Wheeling

***West Virginia University
Hospitals, Morgantown**

Wheeling Hospital, Wheeling

WISCONSIN

Meriter Hospital, Madison

John L. Doyne Hospital, Milwaukee

Sinai Samaritan Medical Center-
Mt. Sinai Campus, Milwaukee

St. Marys Hospital Medical Center,
Madison

**University of Wisconsin Hospital
and Clinics, Madison**

Mental Health

ALABAMA

Searcy Hospital, Mt. Vernon

**University of Alabama Hospitals,
Birmingham**

**University of South Alabama
Medical Center, Mobile**

ARIZONA

Good Samaritan Regional Medical
Center, Phoenix

Kino Community Hospital, Tucson

Maricopa Medical Center, Phoenix

*University Medical Center, Tucson

ARKANSAS

Arkansas State Hospital, Little Rock

**University Hospital of Arkansas,
Little Rock**

CALIFORNIA

California-Pacific Medical Center,
San Francisco

Camarillo State Hospital and
Development Center, Camarillo

Cedars-Sinai Medical Center,
Los Angeles

Community Mental Health
Services, Greenbrae

Kaiser Foundation Hospital,
Santa Clara

Kings View Hospital, Reedley

Langley Porter Psychiatric Hospital
and Clinics, San Francisco

***Loma Linda University Medical
Center, Loma Linda**

**Los Angeles County Harbor-
University of California, Los
Angeles Medical Center, Torrance**

Los Angeles County-King-Drew
Medical Center, Los Angeles

**Los Angeles County-University
of Southern California Medical
Center, Los Angeles**

Napa State Hospital, Napa

Olive View Medical Center, Sylmar

**San Francisco General Hospital
and Medical Center, San Francisco**

San Mateo County General
Hospital, San Mateo

Solano County Mental Health
Clinic, Fairfield

***Stanford University Hospital,
Stanford**

University of California, Los
Angeles Neuropsychiatric Hospital,
Los Angeles

**University of California, Davis
Medical Center, Sacramento**

**University of California, Irvine
Medical Center, Orange**

**University of California, San Diego
Medical Center, San Diego**

**University of California, San
Francisco Medical Center,
San Francisco**

Valley Medical Center of Fresno,
Fresno

Ventura County Mental Health
Center, Ventura

COLORADO

Denver Health and Hospitals,
Denver

**University of Colorado Health
Sciences Center University
Hospital, Denver**

CONNECTICUT

Connecticut Mental Health Center,
New Haven

Connecticut Valley Hospital,
Middletown

Danbury Hospital, Danbury

Greenwich Hospital, Greenwich

Hartford Hospital, Hartford

Hospital of St. Raphael, New Haven

Institute of Living, Hartford

Mt. Sinai Hospital, Hartford

Norwalk Hospital, Norwalk

Norwich Hospital, Norwich

St. Francis Hospital and Medical
Center, Hartford

Stamford Hospital, Stamford

**University of Connecticut Health
Center John Dempsey Hospital,
Farmington**

William W. Buckus Hospital,
Norwich

*Yale-New Haven Hospital,
New Haven

Yale Psychiatric Institute,
New Haven

DELAWARE

Delaware State Hospital,
New Castle

Medical Center of Delaware,
Wilmington

DISTRICT OF COLUMBIA

*George Washington University
Hospital, Washington

*Georgetown University Hospital,
Washington

*Howard University Hospital,
Washington

St. Elizabeth's Hospital
DC Commission on Mental Health
Services, Washington

FLORIDA

Jackson Memorial Hospital, Miami

The Manors, Tarpon Springs

*Shands Hospital at the University
of Florida, Gainesville

Tampa General Hospital, Tampa

University of South Florida
Psychiatry Center, Tampa

GEORGIA

Brawner Psychiatric Institute,
Smyrna

*Emory University Hospital,
Atlanta

Georgia Regional Hospital
at Atlanta, Decatur

Grady Memorial Hospital, Atlanta

HCA West Paces Ferry Hospital,
Atlanta

Medical College of Georgia
Hospital and Clinics, Augusta

Ridgeview Institute, Smyrna

HAWAII

Queen's Medical Center, Honolulu

St. Francis Medical Center,
Honolulu

ILLINOIS

Andrew McFarland Mental Health
Center, Springfield

Choate Mental Health and
Developmental Center, Anna

Cook County Hospital, Chicago

Decatur Memorial Hospital,
Decatur

Evanston Hospital, Evanston

Humana Hospital-Michael Reese,
Chicago

*Loyola University of Chicago
Foster G. McGaw Hospital,
Maywood

Lutheran General Hospital,
Chicago

Memorial Medical Center,
Springfield

Mt. Sinai Hospital Medical Center
of Chicago, Chicago

*Northwestern Memorial Hospital,
Chicago

*Rush-Presbyterian-St. Luke's
Medical Center, Chicago

St. John's Hospital, Springfield

*University of Chicago Hospitals,
Chicago

University of Illinois Hospital
and Clinics, Chicago

INDIANA

Indiana University Medical Center,
Indianapolis

Larue D. Carter Memorial
Hospital, Indianapolis

Lifespring Mental Health Services,
Jeffersonville

William N. Wishard Memorial
Hospital, Indianapolis

IOWA

University of Iowa Hospitals
and Clinics, Iowa City

KANSAS

C. F. Menninger Memorial
Hospital, Topeka

St. Joseph Medical Center, Wichita

Topeka State Hospital, Topeka

University of Kansas Hospital,
Kansas City

KENTUCKY

Humana Hospital-University
of Louisville, Louisville

Norton Hospital, Louisville

University of Kentucky Hospital
Albert B. Chandler Medical Center,
Lexington

LOUISIANA

Medical Center of Louisiana
at New Orleans, New Orleans

Ochsner Foundation Hospital,
New Orleans

River Oaks Psychiatric Hospital,
New Orleans

Touro Infirmary, New Orleans

*Tulane University Hospital
and Clinics, New Orleans

MAINE

Maine Medical Center, Portland

MARYLAND

Crownsville Hospital Center,
Crownsville

Francis Scott Key Medical Center,
Baltimore

Franklin Square Hospital Center,
Baltimore

*Johns Hopkins Hospital,
Baltimore

Sheppard and Enoch Pratt
Hospital, Baltimore

Spring Grove Hospital Center,
Catonsville

Springfield Hospital Center,
Sykesville

*University of Maryland Medical
System, Baltimore

Walter P. Carter Center, Baltimore

MASSACHUSETTS

Austen Riggs Center, Stockbridge

*Beth Israel Hospital, Boston

Boston Medical Center, Boston

Cambridge Hospital, Cambridge

Charles River Hospital, Wellesley

Dr. Solomon Carter Fuller Mental
Health Center, Boston

Erich Lindemann Mental Health Center, Boston

Faulkner Hospital, Boston

Lemuel Shattuck Hospital, Boston

Lemuel Shattuck Hospital Bay Cove Mental Health Center, Boston

*Massachusetts General Hospital, Boston

Massachusetts Mental Health Center, Boston

May Behavioral Health, Roslindale

McLean Hospital, Belmont

*New England Medical Center, Boston

St. Elizabeth's Hospital, Boston

Tewksbury State Hospital, Tewksbury

*University Hospital, Boston

University of Massachusetts Medical Center, Worcester

Worcester State Hospital, Worcester

MICHIGAN

Detroit Psychiatric Institute, Detroit

*Harper Hospital, Detroit

Hawthorn Center, Northville

Henry Ford Hospital, Detroit

Kent Community Hospital Complex, Grand Rapids

Northville Regional Psychiatric Hospital, Northville

Pine Rest Christian Hospital, Grand Rapids

Providence Hospital, Southfield

Sinai Hospital, Detroit

St. Lawrence Hospital and Healthcare Services, Lansing

St. Mary's Health Services, Grand Rapids

University of Michigan Hospitals, Ann Arbor

MINNESOTA

Hennepin County Medical Center, Minneapolis

Lakeland Mental Health Center, Inc., Moorhead

Mayo Clinic, Rochester

*St. Mary's Hospital, Rochester

Regions Hospital, St. Paul

University of Minnesota Hospital and Clinic, Minneapolis

MISSISSIPPI

Mississippi State Hospital, Whitfield

University of Mississippi Medical Center University Hospitals and Clinics, Jackson

MISSOURI

*Barnes-Jewish Hospital, St. Louis

St. Louis Psyche Rehab Center, St. Louis

Mid-Missouri Mental Health Center, Columbia

*St. Louis University Medical Center, St. Louis

University Hospital and Clinics, Columbia

Western Missouri Mental Health Center, Kansas City

NEBRASKA

AMI St. Joseph Center for Mental Health, Omaha

University of Nebraska Medical Center, Omaha

NEW HAMPSHIRE

Dartmouth-Hitchcock Medical Center, Hanover

New Hampshire Hospital, Concord

NEW JERSEY

Bergen Pines County Hospital, Paramus

Camden County Health Services Center, Blackwood

Cooper Hospital-University Medical Center, Camden

Greater Trenton Community Mental Health Center, Trenton

Hackensack Medical Center, Hackensack

Overlook Hospital, Summit

St. Barnabas Medical Center, Livingston

Trenton Psychiatric Hospital, Trenton

University of Medicine and Dentistry of New Jersey University Hospital, Newark

University of Medicine and Dentistry of New Jersey Community Mental Health Center at Piscataway, Piscataway

NEW MEXICO

University Hospital, Albuquerque

University of New Mexico Mental Health Center, Albuquerque

NEW YORK

*Albany Medical Center Hospital, Albany

Bellevue Hospital Center, New York

Beth Israel Medical Center, New York

Bronx-Lebanon Hospital Center, Bronx

Bronx Municipal Hospital Center, Bronx

Bronx Psychiatric Center, Bronx

Brookdale Hospital Medical Center, Brooklyn

Cabrini Medical Center, New York

Capital District Psychiatric Center, Albany

Creedmoor Psychiatric Center, Queens Village

Elmhurst Hospital Center, Flushing

Erie County Medical Center, Buffalo

Harlem Hospital Center, New York

Kings County Hospital Center, Brooklyn

Kingsboro Psychiatric Center, Brooklyn

Lincoln Medical and Mental Health Center, Bronx

Long Island Jewish Medical Center, New Hyde Park

Long Island Jewish Medical Center Hillside Hospital, Glen Oaks

Maimonides Medical Center, Brooklyn

Manhattan Psychiatric Center-Ward's Island, New York

Metropolitan Hospital Center, New York

Middletown Psychiatric Center, Middletown

*Montefiore Medical Center Henry and Lucy Moses Division, Bronx

*Mt. Sinai Medical Center, New York

Nassau County Medical Center, East Meadow

*New York Hospital-Cornell Medical Center, New York

New York Hospital Payne Whitney Psychiatric Clinic, New York

New York Hospital Westchester Div., White Plains

New York State Psychiatric Institute, New York

*New York University Medical Center, New York

North Shore University Hospital, Manhasset

*Presbyterian Hospital in the City of New York Columbia-Presbyterian Medical Center, New York

Queens Hospital Center, Jamaica

Richard H. Hutchings Psychiatric Center, Syracuse

St. Luke's-Roosevelt Hospital Center St. Luke's Division, New York

St. Vincent's Hospital and Medical Center of New York, New York

St. Vincent's Hospital and Medical Center of New York Westchester Branch, Harrison

St. Vincent's Medical Center of Richmond, Staten Island

State University of New York at Stony Brook University Hospital, Stony Brook

State University of New York Health Science Center University Hospital, Syracuse

State University of New York Health Science Center at Brooklyn University Hospital of Brooklyn, Brooklyn

*Strong Memorial Hospital of the University of Rochester, Rochester

Westchester County Medical Center, Valhalla

NORTH CAROLINA

Cherry Hospital, Goldsboro

Dorothea Dix Hospital, Raleigh

*Duke University Medical Center, Durham

*North Carolina Baptist Hospital, Winston-Salem

Pitt County Memorial Hospital, Greenville

Pitt County Mental Health Center, Greenville

University of North Carolina Hospitals, Chapel Hill

NORTH DAKOTA

Southeast Human Services Center, Fargo

St. Luke's Hospitals-Meritcare, Fargo

OHIO

Akron General Medical Center, Akron

Cleveland Clinic, Cleveland

Cleveland Psychiatric Institute, Cleveland

Cleveland Psychoanalytic Institute, Cleveland

Good Samaritan Hospital and Health Center, Dayton

Grant Medical Center, Columbus

Harding Hospital, Worthington

Kettering Medical Center, Kettering

Medical College of Ohio Hospital, Toledo

MetroHealth Medical Center, Cleveland

Mt. Carmel Medical Center, Columbus

Mt. Sinai Medical Center, Cleveland

Ohio State University Hospitals, Columbus

Riverside Methodist Hospitals, Columbus

St. Thomas Medical Center, Akron

St. Vincent Medical Center, Toledo

Toledo Mental Health Center, Toledo

*University Hospitals of Cleveland, Cleveland

University of Cincinnati Hospital, Cincinnati

OKLAHOMA

Griffin Memorial Hospital, Norman

Hillcrest Medical Center, Tulsa

Oklahoma Medical Center, Oklahoma City

Tulsa Psychiatric Center, Tulsa

OREGON

Oregon Health Sciences University University Hospital, Portland

PENNSYLVANIA

Abington Memorial Hospital, Abington

Albert Einstein Medical Center, Philadelphia

Crozer-Chester Medical Center, Upland

Friends Hospital, Philadelphia

*Hahnemann University Hospital, Philadelphia

*Hospital of the Medical College of Pennsylvania, Philadelphia

*Hospital of the University of Pennsylvania, Philadelphia

Mercy Catholic Medical Center Fitzgerald Mercy Division, Philadelphia

Montefiore University Hospital, Pittsburgh

Norristown State Hospital, Norristown

Northwestern Institute, Fort Washington

Penn State University Hospital The Milton S. Hershey Medical Center, Hershey

Pennsylvania Hospital, Philadelphia

*Presbyterian University Hospital, Pittsburgh

St. Francis Medical Center, Pittsburgh

*Temple University Hospital, Philadelphia

*Thomas Jefferson University Hospital, Philadelphia

Western Psychiatric Institute and Clinic, Pittsburgh

PUERTO RICO

University Hospital, San Juan

RHODE ISLAND

Butler Hospital, Providence

Emma Pendleton Bradley Hospital, East Providence

Miriam Hospital, Providence

Providence Center for Counseling and Psychiatric Services, Providence

*Rhode Island Hospital, Providence

SOUTH CAROLINA

Charleston Memorial Hospital, Charleston

Medical Center of Medical University of South Carolina, Charleston

William S. Hall Psychiatric Institute, Columbia

SOUTH DAKOTA

McKennan Hospital, Sioux Falls

Southeastern Mental Health Center, Sioux Falls

TENNESSEE

*George W. Hubbard Hospital of Meharry Medical College, Nashville

Johnson City Medical Center Hospital, Johnson City

Memphis Mental Health Institute, Memphis

Middle Tennessee Mental Health Institute, Nashville

Regional Medical Center at Memphis, Memphis

University of Tennessee Medical Center, Memphis

*Vanderbilt University Hospital and Clinic, Nashville

Watauga Area Mental Health Center, Johnson City

Woodridge Hospital, Johnson City

TEXAS

Austin State Hospital, Austin

Austin-Travis County Mental Health Center, Austin

Baylor University Medical Center, Dallas

Bexar County Hospital District Medical Center Hospital, San Antonio

Brackenridge Hospital, Austin

Dallas County Hospital District Parkland Memorial Hospital, Dallas

Harris County Hospital District Ben Taub General Hospital, Houston

Harris County Psychiatric Center, Houston

*Hermann Hospital, Houston

*Methodist Hospital, Houston

Presbyterian Hospital of Dallas, Dallas

R. E. Thomason General Hospital, El Paso

St. Mary of the Plains Hospital, Lubbock

Terrell State Hospital, Terrell

Timberlawn Psychiatric Hospital, Dallas

University Medical Center, Lubbock

University of Texas M. D. Anderson Cancer Center, Houston

University of Texas Medical Branch Hospitals, Galveston

UTAH

Salt Lake Valley Mental Health, Salt Lake City

University of Utah Hospital and Clinics, Salt Lake City

Western Institute of Neuropsychiatry, Salt Lake City

VERMONT

Brattleboro Retreat, Brattleboro

*Fletcher Allen Healthcare MCHV Campus, Burlington

VIRGINIA

Fairfax Hospital, Falls Church

Department of Psychiatry and Behavioral Sciences, Norfolk

Sentara Norfolk General Hospital, Norfolk

University of Virginia Medical Center, Charlottesville

Virginia Commonwealth University Medical College of Virginia Hospitals, Richmond

WASHINGTON

Harborview Medical Center, Seattle

University of Washington Medical Center, Seattle

WEST VIRGINIA

Charleston Area Medical Center, Charleston

*West Virginia University Hospitals, Morgantown

WISCONSIN

Columbia Hospital, Milwaukee

*Froedtert Memorial Lutheran Hospital, Milwaukee

Mercy Medical Center, Oshkosh

Meriter Hospital, Madison

John L. Doyne Hospital, Milwaukee

Milwaukee Psychiatric Hospital, Milwaukee

Sinai Samaritan Medical Center-Mt. Sinai Campus, Milwaukee

University of Wisconsin Hospital and Clinics, Madison

Winnebago Mental Health Institute, Winnebago

In talking with your friends and family about choosing the right hospital for the treatment of your disorder, you will no doubt hear of lists compiled by the popular press. To expand on the comprehensive lists of hospitals already presented in the Directory, we would like to share with you some of the results of two surveys: One compiled by *U.S. News & World Report* in 1998 and another from the book *The Best in Medicine*.

When reviewing these lists, remember that they are not definitive. The right hospital for you is not necessarily among these names. As we said in the introduction to the Directory, choosing a hospital should be a decision made by you and your physician. There are very specific criteria that you should use to make your final selection, criteria that probably were not considered in compiling these lists. The methods used to conduct the surveys are not foolproof, and because physicians were polled for their opinions, the results are, of course, subjective.

What makes these surveys interesting is that they are able to do what no individual can—consult hundreds of physicians across the country about the hospitals that they believe are among the best in their specialty.

Because these hospitals enjoy good reputations among doctors, you may want to include them on your list of potential hospitals, but do not exclude others just because they are not listed here. By including these surveys in the Directory, we by no means endorse their methods or conclusions.

U.S. NEWS & WORLD REPORT SURVEY

The ninth annual *U.S. News & World Report* ranking of America's best hospitals draws on a groundbreaking mathematical model that combines the last three years' worth of reputational surveys by the magazine, federal death rate statistics, and nine categories of hard data, such as the ratio of registered nurses to number of beds. The model was developed in 1993 and updated last year by analysts at the National Opinion Research Center (NORC), a social science research group at the University of Chicago.

A total of 1,985 hospitals met the initial criteria for inclusion in the ranking. Qualifying hospitals had to be affiliated with a medical school, be a member of the Council of Teaching Hospitals, or have readily available a minimum of nine of 17 key technologies. Simply performing transplants or being classified as a trauma center by the American Hospital Association did not qualify a hospital for inclusion. One hundred thirty-two hospitals made the final ranking.

Reputational results were based on a mail survey of a geographic cross section of 2,400 doctors—150 board certified specialists in each of 16 specialties (13 of which are covered here, corresponding to those disorders covered in the Handbook). The physicians were asked to name the top five hospitals in their specialty without considering location or expense. Each hospital was then matched against a master list, assembled by NORC, of the nation's major academic hospitals and specialized medical centers.

In most of the specialties, reputation counted for one third of a hospital's total score. The death rate, based on pooled 1996-98 data from the federal Health Care Financing Administration, counted for another third. The final third comprised a specialty-specific combination of nine quality indicators, which ranged from the ratio of nurses to beds to the amount of discharge planning offered. The top hospitals in these specialties were assigned a score of 100.

In ophthalmology and psychiatry, rankings were based solely on reputation (death rates and other indicators of quality were inapplicable, unavailable, or unreliable). The scores for these hospitals simply reflect the percentage of doctors who rated them among the best.

The only significant change in the 1998 model was the elimination of AIDS care ratings. According to the magazine, people with HIV or AIDS now tend to receive care as outpatients, making the rankings in this specialty increasingly less relevant.

The Top Hospitals

The following hospitals were on at least four of the specialty lists from U.S. News & World Report.

Johns Hopkins Hospital
Baltimore, MD
16 specialties

Mayo Clinic
Rochester, MN
16 specialties

Duke University Medical Center
Durham, NC
15 specialties

UCLA Medical Center
Los Angeles, CA
14 specialties

Barnes-Jewish Hospital
St. Louis, MO
14 specialties

Stanford University Hospital
Stanford, CA
14 specialties

Massachusetts General Hospital
Boston, MA
13 specialties

Cleveland Clinic
Cleveland, OH
13 specialties

University of California, San Francisco Medical Center
San Francisco, CA
13 specialties

Brigham and Women's Hospital
Boston, MA
11 specialties

University of Washington Medical Center
Seattle, WA
7 specialties

Memorial Sloan-Kettering Cancer Center
New York, NY
5 specialties

University of Texas M. D. Anderson Cancer Center
Houston, TX
5 specialties

The Best Hospitals by Specialty

Cancer

Memorial Sloan-Kettering Cancer Center
New York, NY — 100.0

University of Texas M. D. Anderson Cancer Center
Houston, TX — 94.7

Johns Hopkins Hospital
Baltimore, MD — 58.7

Mayo Clinic
Rochester, MN — 48.3

Dana-Farber Cancer Institute
Boston, MA — 48.1

Duke University Medical Center
Durham, NC — 33.9

Stanford University Medical Center
Stanford, CA — 31.1

University of Washington Medical Center
Seattle, WA — 29.6

University of Chicago Hospitals
Chicago, IL — 28.6

UCLA Medical Center
Los Angeles, CA — 25.9

Cardiology

Cleveland Clinic
Cleveland, OH — 100.0

Mayo Clinic
Rochester, MN — 94.3

Massachusetts General Hospital
Boston, MA — 60.9

Duke University Medical Center
Durham, NC — 53.9

St. Luke's Episcopal Hospital (Texas Heart Institute)
Houston, TX — 52.2

Brigham and Women's Hospital
Boston, MA — 50.1

Emory University Hospital
Atlanta, GA — 47.0

Johns Hopkins Hospital
Baltimore, MD — 43.7

Stanford University Hospital
Stanford, CA — 43.2

Barnes-Jewish Hospital
St. Louis, MO — 34.6

Endocrinology

Mayo Clinic
Rochester, MN   100.0

Massachusetts General Hospital
Boston, MA   91.6

Johns Hopkins Hospital
Baltimore, MD   48.1

Barnes-Jewish Hospital
St. Louis, MO   39.7

Brigham and Women's Hospital
Boston, MA   35.5

University of Chicago Hospitals
Chicago, IL   35.4

**University of Virginia,
Health Sciences Center**
Charlottesville, VA   33.3

UCLA Medical Center
Los Angeles, CA   28.8

**Duke University
Medical Center**
Durham, NC   27.9

Beth Israel Deaconess Hospital
Boston, MA   25.9

Gastroenterology

Mayo Clinic
Rochester, MN   100.0

Cleveland Clinic
Cleveland, OH   52.2

Johns Hopkins Hospital
Baltimore, MD   52.2

Massachusetts General Hospital
Boston, MA   51.5

Mt. Sinai Medical Center
New York, NY   44.0

University of Chicago Hospitals
Chicago, IL   36.7

UCLA Medical Center
Los Angeles, CA   35.0

**University of California,
San Francisco Medical Center**
San Francisco, CA   34.8

Duke University Medical Center
Durham, NC   30.5

Brigham and Women's Hospital
Boston, MA   28.7

Gynecology

Johns Hopkins Hospital
Baltimore, MD   100.0

Mayo Clinic
Rochester, MN   79.8

Massachusetts General Hospital
Boston, MA   72.1

**University of Texas
M. D. Anderson Cancer Center**
Houston, TX   70.9

Brigham and Women's Hospital
Boston, MA   61.1

**Memorial Sloan-Kettering
Cancer Center**
New York, NY   56.7

Duke University Medical Center
Durham, NC   52.5

UCLA Medical Center
Los Angeles, CA   43.0

**Columbia-Presbyterian
Medical Center**
New York, NY   39.4

Northwestern Memorial Hospital
Chicago, IL   38.9

Neurology

Mayo Clinic
Rochester, MN   100.0

Massachusetts General Hospital
Boston, MA   93.3

Johns Hopkins Hospital
Baltimore, MD   82.7

**Columbia-Presbyterian
Medical Center**
New York, NY   63.1

**University of California,
San Francisco Medical Center**
San Francisco, CA   55.8

Cleveland Clinic
Cleveland, OH   42.3

UCLA Medical Center
Los Angeles, CA   40.5

**Duke University
Medical Center**
Durham, NC   34.2

**Hospital of the University
of Pennsylvania**
Philadelphia, PA   32.9

**New York Hospital-
Cornell Medical Center**
New York, NY   31.5

Ophthalmology

*(Rankings based solely on reputational scores
from physician surveys.)*

**University of Miami
Bascom Palmer Eye Institute**
Miami, FL   74.4%

**Johns Hopkins Hospital
Wilmer Eye Institute**
Baltimore, MD   72.5%

Wills Eye Hospital
Philadelphia, PA   61.5%

**Massachusetts Eye and
Ear Infirmary**
Boston, MA   48.8%

**UCLA Medical Center,
Jules Stein Eye Institute**
Los Angeles, CA   28.1%

**University of Iowa
Hospitals and Clinics**
Iowa City, IA   21.2%

**University of California
San Francisco Medical Center**
San Francisco, CA   10.8%

Doheny Eye Institute
Los Angeles, CA   10.3%

Duke University Medical Center
Durham, NC   8.7%

Mayo Clinic
Rochester, MN   7.6%

Orthopedics

Mayo Clinic
Rochester, MN   100.0

Hospital for Special Surgery
New York, NY   93.8

Massachusetts General Hospital
Boston, MA   67.5

Johns Hopkins Hospital
Baltimore, MD   45.0

Cleveland Clinic
Cleveland, OH   35.2

Duke University Medical Center
Durham, NC   32.8

University of Washington
Medical Center
Seattle, WA — 29.3

University of Iowa
Hospitals and Clinics
Iowa City, IA — 27.1

UCLA Medical Center
Los Angeles, CA — 26.9

Brigham and Women's
Hospital
Boston, MA — 24.7

Otolaryngology

Johns Hopkins Hospital
Baltimore, MD — 100.0

University of Iowa Hospitals
and Clinics
Iowa City, IA — 84.2

University of Michigan Hospitals
Ann Arbor, MI — 60.4

Barnes-Jewish Hospital
St. Louis, MO — 56.4

University of Pittsburgh
Medical Center
Pittsburgh, PA — 55.5

UCLA Medical Center
Los Angeles, CA — 53.7

Mayo Clinic
Rochester, MN — 51.0

University of Washington
Medical Center
Seattle, WA — 42.6

University of Texas
M. D. Anderson Cancer Center
Houston, TX — 42.3

University of California,
San Francisco Medical Center
San Francisco, CA — 42.1

Psychiatry

*(Rankings based solely on reputational scores
from physician surveys.)*

Massachusetts General Hospital
Boston, MA — 24.3%

C. F. Menninger Memorial Hospital
Topeka, KS — 23.4%

McLean Hospital
Belmont, MA — 19.4%

Johns Hopkins Hospital
Baltimore, MD — 13.5%

New York Hospital-
Cornell Medical Center
New York, NY — 11.8%

Mayo Clinic
Rochester, MN — 9.4%

UCLA Neuropsychiatric Hospital
Los Angeles, CA — 9.3%

Columbia-Presbyterian
Medical Center
New York, NY — 8.9%

Sheppard and Enoch Pratt Hospital
Baltimore, MD — 8.3%

Yale-New Haven Hospital
New Haven, CT — 8.0%

Pulmonary Disease

National Jewish Center
Denver, CO — 100.0

Mayo Clinic
Rochester, MN — 75.9

Barnes-Jewish Hospital
St. Louis, MO — 51.4

Johns Hopkins Hospital
Baltimore, MD — 47.0

Massachusetts General Hospital
Boston, MA — 40.5

University of California,
San Francisco Medical Center
San Francisco, CA — 40.4

University Hospital
Denver, CO — 37.3

Duke University
Medical Center
Durham, NC — 34.2

Cleveland Clinic
Cleveland, OH — 28.2

UCLA Medical Center
Los Angeles, CA — 24.5

Rheumatology

Mayo Clinic
Rochester, MN — 100.0

Johns Hopkins Hospital
Baltimore, MA — 76.7

Hospital for Special Surgery
New York, NY — 72.0

Brigham and Women's Hospital
Boston, MA — 60.9

University of Alabama
Hospital at Birmingham
Birmingham, AL — 60.0

UCLA Medical Center
Los Angeles, CA — 58.3

Massachusetts General Hospital
Boston, MA — 54.9

Cleveland Clinic
Cleveland, OH — 53.6

University of Michigan
Medical Center
Ann Arbor, MI — 40.9

Duke University Medical Center
Durham, NC — 39.3

Urology

Johns Hopkins Hospital
Baltimore, MD — 100.0

Mayo Clinic
Rochester, MN — 65.8

UCLA Medical Center
Los Angeles, CA — 51.7

Cleveland Clinic
Cleveland, OH — 46.9

Duke University Medical Center
Durham, NC — 39.0

Massachusetts General Hospital
Boston, MA — 37.4

Stanford University Hospital
Stanford, CA — 33.0

Barnes-Jewish Hospital
St. Louis, MO — 32.8

Memorial Sloan-Kettering
Cancer Center
New York, NY — 30.2

University of Texas
M. D. Anderson Cancer Center
Houston, TX — 29.0

© July 27, 1998 U.S. News & World Report.

THE BEST IN MEDICINE SURVEY

Herbert J. Dietrich, M.D., and Virginia H. Biddle, the authors of the book *The Best in Medicine,* sent questionnaires to 10 representative physicians in each of 25 medical specialty categories. Each doctor was asked to list 10 hospitals of outstanding excellence for his or her own specialty, excluding his or her own base of operation and regardless of location. The physicians were then asked to specifiy three areas of expertise for each hospital they selected.

In addition, the authors personally interviewed a number of doctors who specialize in those fields not covered in sufficient detail in the questionnaires. They then consulted statistics pertaining to the postgraduate training programs of those medical institutions that are accredited by the Accreditation Council for Graduate Medical Education. Using the data from all these sources, they compiled a list of 25 medical centers that are outstanding in each category.

The 25 Best Medical Centers in the United States

The following hospitals scored high marks for at least eight departments in general medicine and surgery. The reader should remember that a center's exact position on the list is less important than the fact that these are peer institutions. Differences are often reflected in the particular emphasis given to certain aspects of a specialty.

Mayo Clinic
Rochester, MN

Massachusetts General Hospital
Boston, MA

University of Alabama Hospitals
Birmingham, AL

Johns Hopkins Hospital
Baltimore, MD

Baylor College of Medicine and Hospitals
Houston, TX
(Principal affiliated Teaching Hospitals are Methodist Hospital and Harris County Hospital District-Ben Taub General Hospital.)

University of Washington Medical Center
Seattle, WA

Cleveland Clinic
Cleveland, OH

Hospital of the University of Pennsylvania
Philadelphia, PA

Duke University Medical Center
Durham, NC

University of California, San Francisco Medical Center
San Francisco, CA

New York Hospital-Cornell Medical Center
New York, NY

University of Michigan Hospitals
Ann Arbor, MI

Brigham and Women's Hospital
Boston, MA

Yale-New Haven Hospital
New Haven, CT

Vanderbilt University Hospital and Clinic
Nashville, TN

University of Miami Affiliated Hospitals
Miami, FL
(Principal affiliated Teaching Hospital is Jackson Memorial Hospital.)

University of Minnesota Hospital and Clinic
Minneapolis, MN

University of Texas-Southwestern Medical Center
Dallas, TX
(Principal affiliated Teaching Hospital is Parkland Memorial Hospital.)

Northwestern Memorial Hospital
Chicago, IL

Barnes-Jewish Hospital
St. Louis, MO

University of Pittsburgh Medical and Health Care Division
Pittsburgh, PA
(Principal affiliated Teaching Hospitals are Western Psychiatric Institute and Clinic, Montefiore University Hospital, and Presbyterian University Hospital.)

University of Colorado Health Sciences Center
Denver, CO

Stanford University Hospital
Stanford, CA

Presbyterian Hospital in the City of New York, Columbia-Presbyterian Medical Center
New York, NY

University of California at Los Angeles Medical Center
Los Angeles, CA

The Best Hospitals by Specialty

These are the specialties not covered by the U.S. News & World Report Survey.

Dermatology

ALABAMA
University of Alabama Hospitals
Birmingham

CALIFORNIA
Stanford University Hospital
Stanford

COLORADO
University of Colorado Health Sciences Center
Denver

CONNECTICUT
Yale-New Haven Hospital
New Haven

FLORIDA
Jackson Memorial Hospital
Miami

GEORGIA
Emory University Hospital
Atlanta

ILLINOIS
University of Illinois Hospital and Clinics
Chicago

MASSACHUSETTS
Massachusetts General Hospital
Boston

MICHIGAN
University of Michigan Hospitals
Ann Arbor

MINNESOTA
Mayo Clinic
Rochester

NEW HAMPSHIRE
Dartmouth-Hitchcock Medical Center
Hanover

NEW YORK
New York Hospital-Cornell Medical Center
New York

Presbyterian Hospital in the City of New York, Columbia-Presbyterian Medical Center
New York

NORTH CAROLINA
Duke University Medical Center
Durham

OHIO
Cleveland Clinic
Cleveland

OKLAHOMA
University of Oklahoma Health Sciences Center
Oklahoma City
(Principal affiliated Teaching Hospitals are Oklahoma Medical Center and Presbyterian Hospital.)

PENNSYLVANIA
Hospital of the University of Pennsylvania
Philadelphia

TEXAS
University of Texas-Southwestern Medical Center
Dallas
(Principal affiliated Teaching Hospital is Parkland Memorial Hospital.)

Baylor College of Medicine and Hospitals
Houston
(Principal affiliated Teaching Hospitals are Methodist Hospital and Harris County Hospital District-Ben Taub General Hospital.)

VIRGINIA
Virginia Commonwealth University, Medical College of Virginia Hospitals
Richmond

Hematology

ALABAMA
University of Alabama Hospitals
Birmingham

CALIFORNIA
Green Hospital of Scripps Clinic
La Jolla

University of California, San Francisco Medical Center
San Francisco

CONNECTICUT
Yale-New Haven Hospital
New Haven

DISTRICT OF COLUMBIA
George Washington University Hospital
Washington

FLORIDA
University of South Florida Medical Center
Tampa
(Principal affiliated Teaching Hospital is Tampa General Hospital.)

University of Miami Affiliated Hospitals
Miami
(Principal affiliated Teaching Hospital is Jackson Memorial Hospital.)

ILLINOIS
University of Illinois Hospital and Clinics
Chicago

MARYLAND
Johns Hopkins Hospital
Baltimore

MASSACHUSETTS
Brigham and Women's Hospital
Boston

New England Medical Center
Boston

Dana-Farber Cancer Institute
Boston

MINNESOTA
University of Minnesota Hospital and Clinic
Minneapolis

MISSOURI
University Hospital and Clinics
Columbia

NEW YORK
**St. Luke's-Roosevelt Hospital
Center, St. Luke's Division**
New York

**State University of New York
Health Science Center,
University Hospital**
Syracuse

NORTH CAROLINA
**University of North Carolina
Hospitals**
Chapel Hill

Duke University Medical Center
Durham

PENNSYLVANIA
**Hospital of the University
of Pennsylvania**
Philadelphia

TEXAS
**University of Texas-
Southwestern Medical Center**
Dallas
*(Principal affiliated Teaching Hospital is
Parkland Memorial Hospital.)*

UTAH
**University of Utah Hospital
and Clinics**
Salt Lake City

Pulmonary Medicine

ALABAMA
University of Alabama Hospitals
Birmingham

ARKANSAS
University Hospital of Arkansas
Little Rock

CALIFORNIA
**University of California,
Davis Medical Center**
Sacramento

COLORADO
**University of Colorado Health
Sciences Center**
Denver

CONNECTICUT
**Yale-New Haven Hospital,
Winchester Chest Clinic**
New Haven

ILLINOIS
University of Chicago Hospitals
Chicago

INDIANA
Indiana University Medical Center
Indianapolis

MARYLAND
Johns Hopkins Hospital
Baltimore

MASSACHUSETTS
University Hospital
Boston

Brigham and Women's Hospital
Boston

MICHIGAN
University of Michigan Hospitals
Ann Arbor

MINNESOTA
Mayo Clinic and Foundation
Rochester

NEW YORK
Bellevue Hospital Center
New York

NORTH CAROLINA
Duke University Medical Center
Durham

PENNSYLVANIA
**Hospital of the University
of Pennsylvania**
Philadelphia

Presbyterian University Hospital
Pittsburgh

TENNESSEE
**Vanderbilt University Hospital
and Clinic**
Nashville

TEXAS
**Baylor College of Medicine
and Hospitals**
Houston
*(Principal affiliated Teaching Hospitals are
Methodist Hospital and Harris County
Hospital District-Ben Taub General
Hospital.)*

**University of Texas-Southwestern
Medical Center**
Dallas
*(Principal affiliated Teaching Hospital is
Parkland Memorial Hospital.)*

UTAH
**University of Utah Hospital
and Clinics**
Salt Lake City

WASHINGTON
**University of Washington
Medical Center**
Seattle

© 1986, Herbert J. Dietrich, M.D., and Virginia H.
Biddle. Reprinted by permission of Harmony Books,
a division of Crown Publishers, Inc.

Health Information and Support Organizations

The organizations in this section are listed first by disorder, then alphabetically, according to whether they are a Health Information Organization or a Support Group. Each listing gives you the organization's name, address, and phone number.

If you cannot find an organization that covers your needs, turn to page 617 and look under the section called General Organizations.

Cancer

HEALTH INFORMATION ORGANIZATIONS

AMC Cancer Research Center
1600 Pierce St.
Denver, CO 80214
800-525-3777
303-233-6501 in CO

American Cancer Society, Inc.
2200 Lake Blvd.
Atlanta, GA 30319
800-ACS-2345
404-816-7800

American College of Radiology
1891 Preston White Dr.
Reston, VA 20191
703-648-8900

Bloch Cancer Hotline
4410 Main St.
Kansas City, MO 64111
816-932-8453

Cancer Research Institute, Inc.
681 Fifth Ave.
New York, NY 10022
212-688-7515

Centers for Disease Control Office on Smoking and Health
Public Information Branch
4770 Buford Highway, NE
Mailstop K-50
Atlanta, GA 30341-3724
770-488-5705

Leukemia Society of America
600 Third Ave.
New York, NY 10016
212-573-8484

National Alliance of Breast Cancer Organizations
9 E. 37th St., 10th Fl.
New York, NY 10016
212-889-0606

National Cancer Care Foundation, Inc./Cancer Care, Inc.
1180 Avenue of the Americas
New York, NY 10036
212-221-3300

National Cancer Institute
Public Inquiries Office
Office of Cancer Communications
Bldg. 31, Rm. 10A24
Bethesda, MD 20892
800-422-6237
301-496-5583

National Coalition for Cancer Survivorship
1010 Wayne Ave., 5th Fl.
Silver Spring, MD 20910
301-650-8868

Patient Advocates for Advanced Cancer Treatment
1143 Parmelee, NW
Grand Rapids, MI 49504
616-453-1477

Rose Kushner Breast Cancer Advisory Center
PO Box 224
Kensington, MD 20895
Please contact by mail.

Skin Cancer Foundation
245 Fifth Ave., Suite 1403
New York, NY 10016
212-725-5176

United Ostomy Association
36 Executive Park, Suite 120
Irvine, CA 92714-6744
800-826-0826

Y-ME
National Organization for Breast Cancer Information and Support
212 W. Van Buren
Chicago, IL 60607
800-221-2141

YWCA
ENCORE
610 Lexington Ave.
New York, NY 10022
212-755-4500
Fax: 212-759-3158

SUPPORT GROUPS

AMC Cancer Research Center
1600 Pierce St.
Denver, CO 80214
800-525-3777
303-233-6501 in CO

American Cancer Society, Inc.
2200 Lake Blvd.
Atlanta, GA 30319
800-ACS-2345
404-816-7800

Cancer Caring Center
4117 Liberty Ave.

Pittsburgh, PA 15224
412-622-1212

Cancer Lifeline
Second & Seneca Bldg.
1191 Second Ave., Suite 680
Seattle, WA 98101
206-461-4542

Cancer Wellness Center
215 Revere Dr.
Northbrooke, IL 60062
847-509-9595 (hotline)

**Intestinal Multiple Polyposis &
Colorectal Cancer (IMPACC)**
c/o Mrs. Dolores Boone
1008-101 Brinker Dr.
Hagerstown, MD 21740
301-791-7526

Let's Face It
PO Box 711
Concord, MA 01742
978-371-3186

Leukemia Society of America
600 Third Ave.
New York, NY 10016
212-573-8484

**National Alliance of Breast Cancer
Organizations**
9 E. 37th St., 10th Fl.
New York, NY 10016
212-889-0606

**National Coalition for Cancer
Survivorship**
1010 Wayne Ave., 5th Fl.
Silver Spring, MD 20910
301-650-8868

**Patient Advocates for Advanced
Cancer Treatment**
1143 Parmelee, NW
Grand Rapids, MI 49504
616-453-1477

United Ostomy Association
36 Executive Park, Suite 120
Irvine, CA 92714-6744
800-826-0826

Y-ME
National Organization for Breast
Cancer Information and Support
212 W. Van Buren
Chicago, IL 60607
800-221-2141

YWCA
ENCORE
610 Lexington Ave.
New York, NY 10022
212-755-4500
Fax: 212-759-3158

The Blood

HEALTH INFORMATION ORGANIZATIONS

**Sickle Cell Disease Association
of America**
200 Corporate Pointe, Suite 495
Culver City, CA 90230-7633
800-421-8453
203-736-5455 in CA

**National Heart, Lung, and Blood
Institute**
Information Center
PO Box 30105
Bethesda, MD 20824-0105
301-251-1222

SUPPORT GROUPS

**Sickle Cell Disease Association
of America**
200 Corporate Pointe, Suite 495
Culver City, CA 90230-7633
800-421-8453
203-736-5455 in CA

The Brain and Nervous System

HEALTH INFORMATION ORGANIZATIONS

Acoustic Neuroma Association
PO Box 12402
Atlanta, GA 30355
404-237-8023

**Alzheimer's Disease Education
and Referral Center**
PO Box 8250-JML
Silver Spring, MD 20907-8250
301-495-3311

Alzheimer's Association, Inc.
919 N. Michigan Ave.
Suite 1000
Chicago, IL 60611-1676
800-272-3900
312-335-8700 (office)

Alzheimer's Association
6465 S. Yale Ave., Suite 206
Tulsa, OK 74136-7810
918-481-7741

**American Association of
Neurological Surgeons**
22 S. Washington St.
Park Ridge, IL 60068

847-692-9501
Fax: 847-692-2589

American Brain Tumor Association
2720 River Rd.
Des Plaines, IL 60018
800-886-2282 (patient services)
708-827-9910

**American Chronic Pain
Association, Inc.**
PO Box 850
Rocklin, CA 95677
916-632-0922

**American Council for Headache
Education**
875 Kings Hwy., Suite 200
Woodbury, NJ 08096
800-255-ACHE
609-845-0322

**American Parkinson's Disease
Association**
1250 Hylan Blvd., Suite 4B
Staten Island, NY 10305
800-223-2732

**American Society of
Anesthesiologists**
520 N. Northwest Hwy.
Park Ridge, IL 60068
847-825-5586

The Brain Injury Association
105 N. Alfred St.
Alexandria, VA 22314
800-444-6443
703-236-6000

Brain Tumor Information Service
University of Chicago
5841 S. Maryland Ave.
Rm. J341
Chicago, IL 60637
312-944-6800

Brain Tumor Society
84 Seattle St.
Boston, MA 02134
617-783-0340

**Commission on Accreditation
of Rehabilitation Facilities**
4891 E. Grant Rd.
Tuscon, AZ 85712
520-325-1044
Fax: 602-571-1601

Epilepsy Foundation of America
4351 Garden City Dr., Suite 500
Landover, MD 20785
800-EFA-1000
301-459-3700

**Huntington's Disease Society
of America**
140 W. 22nd St., 6th Fl.
New York, NY 10012-2420
800-345-4372
212-242-1968

National Ataxia Foundation
15500 Wayzata Blvd., Suite 750
Wayzata, MN 55391
612-473-7666

National Brain Tumor Foundation
785 Market St., Suite 1600
San Francisco, CA 94103
800-934-CURE
415-284-0208

**National Foundation for Brain
Research**
1250 24th St., NW, Suite 300
Washington, DC 20037
202-293-5453

National Headache Foundation
428 W. St. James Pl., 2nd Fl.
Chicago, IL 60614
800-843-2256
312-878-7715

**National Institute of Neurological
Disorders and Stroke**
Office of Scientific and Health
Reports
9000 Rockville Pike, Bldg. 31 8A-06
Bethesda, MD 20892
800-352-9424
301-496-5751

National Parkinson Foundation
1501 N.W. Ninth Ave./
Bob Hope Rd.
Miami, FL 33136-1494
800-327-4545
800-433-7022 in FL

**National Spinal Cord Injury
Association**
545 Concord Ave., Suite 29
Cambridge, MA 02135
800-962-9629

**Parkinson Support Groups
of America**
11376 Cherry Hill Rd., Apt. 204
Beltsville, MD 20705
301-937-1545

Parkinson's Disease Foundation
710 W. 168th St.
New York, NY 10032
800-457-6676
212-923-4700

United Parkinson Foundation
833 W. Washington Blvd.
Chicago, IL 60607
312-733-1893

Vestibular Disorders Association
PO Box 4467
Portland, OR 97208-4467
503-229-7705 (answering machine)
Fax: 503-229-8064

SUPPORT GROUPS

Acoustic Neuroma Association
PO Box 12402
Atlanta, GA 30355
404-237-8023

Alzheimer's Association, Inc.
919 N. Michigan Ave.
Suite 1000
Chicago, IL 60611-1676
800-272-3900
312-335-8700 (office)

Alzheimer's Association
6465 S. Yale., Suite 206
Tulsa, OK 74136-7810
918-481-7741

**American Chronic Pain
Association, Inc.**
PO Box 850
Rocklin, CA 95677
916-632-0922

**American Council for Headache
Education**
875 Kings Hwy., Suite 200
Woodbury, NJ 08096
800-255-ACHE
609-845-0322

American Paralysis Association
Spinal Cord Injury Hotline
2200 Kernan Dr.
Baltimore, MD 21207
800-526-3456

**American Parkinson's Disease
Association**
1250 Hylan Blvd., Suite 4B
Staten Island, NY 10305
800-223-2732

The Brain Injury Association
105 N. Alfred St.
Alexandria, VA 22314
800-444-6443
703-236-6000

Brain Tumor Information Service
University of Chicago
5841 S. Maryland Ave.
Rm. J341
Chicago, IL 60637
312-944-6800

Brain Tumor Society
84 Seattle St.
Boston, MA 02134
617-783-0340

Epilepsy Foundation of America
4351 Garden City Dr., Suite 500
Landover, MD 20785
800-EFA-1000
301-459-3700

**Huntington's Disease Society
of America**
140 W. 22nd St., 6th Fl.
New York, NY 10012-2420
800-345-4372
212-242-1968

National Ataxia Foundation
15500 Wayzata Blvd., Suite 750
Wayzata, MN 55391
612-473-7666

National Brain Tumor Foundation
785 Market St., Suite 1600
San Francisco, CA 94103
800-934-CURE
415-284-0208

National Parkinson Foundation
1501 N.W. Ninth Ave./
Bob Hope Rd.
Miami, FL 33136-1494
800-327-4545
800-433-7022 in FL

**National Spinal Cord Injury
Association**
545 Concord Ave., Suite 29
Cambridge, MA 02135
800-962-9629

**Parkinson Support Groups
of America**
11376 Cherry Hill Rd., Apt. 204
Beltsville, MD 20705
301-937-1545

Parkinson's Disease Foundation
710 W. 168th St.
New York, NY 10032
800-457-6676
212-923-4700

United Parkinson Foundation
833 W. Washington Blvd.
Chicago, IL 60607
312-733-1893

Vestibular Disorders Association
PO Box 4467
Portland, OR 97208-4467
503-229-7705 (answering machine)
Fax: 503-229-8064

Dental and Oral Disorders

HEALTH INFORMATION ORGANIZATIONS

American Association of Endodontists
211 E. Chicago Ave., Suite 1100
Chicago, IL 60611-2691
800-USA-ENDO

American Association of Oral and Maxillofacial Surgeons
9700 W. Bryn Mawr Ave.
Rosemont, IL 60018
800-467-5268

American Board of Oral Pathology
PO Box 25915
Tampa, FL 33622-5915
813-286-2444

American Board of Orthodontics
401 N. Lindbergh Blvd.
Suite 308
St. Louis, MO 63141
314-432-6130

American Board of Periodontology
666 W. Baltimore St.
Pasadena, MD 21201
410-437-3749

American Board of Prosthodontics
PO Box 8437
Atlanta, GA 30306
Please contact by mail.

American Dental Association
Department of Public Information and Education
211 E. Chicago Ave.
Chicago, IL 60611
Please contact by mail.

American Society for Geriatric Dentistry
211 E. Chicago Ave., Suite 1616
Chicago, IL 60611
Please contact by mail.

Centers for Disease Control
Division of Oral Health
1600 Clifton Rd.
Atlanta, GA 30333
404-639-3311

National Institute of Dental Research
Bldg. 31, Rm. 2C-35
31 Center Dr. MSC 2290
Bethesda, MD 20892-2290
301-496-4261

The Digestive System

HEALTH INFORMATION ORGANIZATIONS

American Liver Foundation
1425 Pompton Ave.
Cedar Grove, NJ 07009
800-223-0179
201-256-2550
Fax: 201-256-3214

Center for Ulcer Research and Education Foundation
UCLA-CURE/VA Wadsworth
Bldg. 115, Rm. 115
Los Angeles, CA 90073
213-825-3187

Crohn's & Colitis Foundation of America, Inc.
386 Park Ave. South
New York, NY 10016
800-343-3637
212-685-3440

Digestive Disease National Coalition
507 Capitol Ct., NE, Suite 200
Washington, DC 20002
202-544-7497

Gastro-Intestinal Research Foundation
70 E. Lake St., Suite 1015
Chicago, IL 60601-5907
312-332-1350

Intestinal Disease Foundation, Inc.
1323 Forbes Ave., Suite 200
Pittsburgh, PA 15219
412-261-5888

National Digestive Diseases Information Clearinghouse
2 Information Way
Bethesda, MD 20892
Please contact by mail.

SUPPORT GROUPS

American Liver Foundation
1425 Pompton Ave.
Cedar Grove, NJ 07009
800-223-0179
201-256-2550
Fax: 201-256-3214

Crohn's & Colitis Foundation of America, Inc.
386 Park Ave. South
New York, NY 10016
800-343-3637
212-685-3440

The Ears, Nose, and Throat

HEALTH INFORMATION ORGANIZATIONS

American Academy of Otolaryngology-Head and Neck Surgery
1 Prince St.
Alexandria, VA 22314
703-836-4444
Fax: 703-683-5100

American Hearing Research Foundation
55 E. Washington St., Suite 2022
Chicago, IL 60602
312-726-9670

American Speech-Language-Hearing Association
10801 Rockville Pike
Rockville, MD 20852
800-638-8255
301-897 5700
Fax: 301-571-0457

American Tinnitus Association
1618 S.W. First Ave., Suite 417
Portland, OR 97201
503-248-9985

Alexander Graham Bell Association for the Deaf, Inc.
3417 Volta Place, NW
Washington, DC 20007-2778
202-337-5220

Better Hearing Institute
PO Box 1840
Washington, DC 20013
800-327-9355

Deafness Research Foundation
575 Fifth Ave., 11th Fl.
New York, NY 10017
800-535-3323

Dial a Hearing Test
PO Box 1880
Media, PA 19063
800-222-EARS

Hearing Aid Helpline
16880 Middlebelt Rd., Suite 4
Livonia, MI 48154
800-521-5247

National Association of the Deaf
814 Thayer Ave.
Silver Spring, MD 20910
301-587-1788
301-587-1789 (TDD)

**National Information Center
on Deafness**
Gallaudet University
800 Florida Ave., NE
Washington, DC 20002
202-651-5051 (voice)
202-651-5052 (TDD)

**National Institute on Deafness and
Other Communication Disorders**
31 Center Dr., Bldg. 31, MSC 2320
Bethesda, MD 20892
301-496-7243
301-402-0252 (TDD)
Fax: 301-402-0018

**Self-Help for Hard of Hearing
People, Inc.**
7910 Woodmont Ave., Suite 1200
Bethesda, MD 20814
301-657-2248 (voice)
301-657-2249 (TDD)

Vestibular Disorders Association
PO Box 4467
Portland, OR 97208-4467
503-229-7705 (answering machine)
Fax: 503-229-8064

SUPPORT GROUPS

**American Academy of
Otolaryngology-Head and Neck
Surgery**
1 Prince St.
Alexandria, VA 22314
703-836-4444
Fax: 703-683-5100

**American Hearing Research
Foundation**
55 E. Washington St., Suite 2022
Chicago, IL 60602
312-726-9670

American Tinnitus Association
1618 S.W. First Ave., Suite 417
Portland, OR 97201
503-248-9985

Better Hearing Institute
PO Box 1840
Washington, DC 20013
800-327-9355

Deafness Research Foundation
575 Fifth Ave., 11th Fl.
New York, NY 10017
800-535-3323

**International Association of
Laryngectomies**
7440 N. Shadeland Ave.
Suite 100
Indianapolis, IN 46250
317-570-4568

**National Information Center
on Deafness**
Gallaudet University
800 Florida Ave., NE
Washington, DC 20002
202 651 5051 (voice)
202-651-5052 (TDD)

**Self-Help for Hard of Hearing
People, Inc.**
7910 Woodmont, Suite 1200
Bethesda, MD 20814
301-657-2248 (voice)
301-657-2249 (TDD)

Vestibular Disorders Association
PO Box 4467
Portland, OR 97208-4467
503-229-7705 (answering machine)
Fax: 503-229-8064

The Endocrine System

HEALTH INFORMATION
ORGANIZATIONS

American Diabetes Association
1660 Duke St.
Alexandria, VA 22314
800-ADA-DISC
703-549-1500
Fax: 703-683-2890

American Dietetic Association
216 W. Jackson Blvd., Suite 800
Chicago, IL 60606-6995
800-745-0775
312-899-0040

Joslin Diabetes Center, Inc.
1 Joslin Place
Boston, MA 02115
617-732-2440
Fax: 617-732-2664

The National Agricultural Library
Food and Nutrition Information
Center
10301 Baltimore Blvd.
Beltsville, MD 20705-2351
301-504-5719
Fax: 301-504-5472

National Dairy Council
10255 W. Higgins Rd., Suite 900
Rosemont, IL 60018-5616
708-803-2000 ext. 220
Fax: 708-803-2077

**National Diabetes Information
Clearinghouse**
Box NDIC
9000 Rockville Pike

Bethesda, MD 20892
Please contact by mail.

National Federation of the Blind
Diabetics Division
811 Cherry St., Suite 309-1
Columbia, MO 65201
573-875-8911

**The Thyroid Foundation
of America, Inc.**
Ruth Sleeper Hall, RSL 350
40 Parkman St.
Boston, MA 02114-2698
617-726-8500
Fax: 617-726-4136

SUPPORT GROUPS

American Diabetes Association
1660 Duke St.
Alexandria, VA 22314
800-ADA-DISC
703-549-1500
Fax: 703-683-2890

**The Thyroid Foundation
of America, Inc.**
Ruth Sleeper Hall, RSL 350
40 Parkman St.
Boston, MA 02114-2698
617-726-8500
Fax: 617-726-4136

The Eyes

HEALTH INFORMATION
ORGANIZATIONS

**American Academy
of Ophthalmology**
Inquiry Clerk
655 Beach St.
San Francisco, CA 94109
415-561-8500
Fax: 415-561-8567

American Council of the Blind
1155 15th St., NW, Suite 720
Washington, DC 20005
800-424-8666
202-467-5081
Fax: 202-467-5085

American Foundation for the Blind
11 Penn Plaza, Suite 300
New York, NY 10001
800-232-5463
212-502-7600
Fax: 212-620-2105

American Optometric Association
Communications Center
243 N. Lindbergh Blvd.
St. Louis, MO 63141
314-991-4100
Fax: 314-991-4101

Associated Services for the Blind
919 Walnut St.
Philadelphia, PA 19107
215-627-0600
Fax: 215-922-0692

**Association for Macular
Diseases, Inc.**
210 E. 64th St.
New York, NY 10021
212-605-3719

**Benign Essential Blepharospasm
Research Foundation, Inc.**
PO Box 12468
Beaumont, TX 77726-2468
409-832-0788

Eye Bank Association of America
1001 Connecticut Ave., NW
Suite 601
Washington, DC 20036
202-775-4999

Glaucoma Research Foundation
200 Pine Street, Suite 200
San Francisco, CA 94104
415-986-3162

Guiding Eyes for the Blind, Inc.
611 Granite Springs Rd.
Yorktown Heights, NY 10598
914-245-4024

Library of Congress
National Library Service for the
Blind and Physically Handicapped
1291 Taylor St., NW
Washington, DC 20542
800-424-8567
202-707-9275 (reference)

**Lighthouse National Center
for Vision and Aging**
111 E. 59th St.
New York, NY 10022
800-334-5497 (TDD)
212-821-9200 (TDD)

**National Association for the
Visually Handicapped**
22 W. 21st St., 6th Fl.
New York, NY 10010
212-889-3141

**National Eye Care Project
Help Line**
PO Box 429098
San Francisco, CA 94142-9098
800-222-EYES

National Eye Institute
Information Office
Bldg. 31, Rm. 6A-32
Bethesda, MD 20892
301-496-5248

**National Retinitis Pigmentosa
Foundation, Inc.**
1401 Mt. Royal Ave., 4th Fl.
Baltimore, MD 21217
800-683-5555

Prevent Blindness America
500 E. Remington Rd.
Schaumburg, IL 60173
800-331-2020

Vision Foundation
818 Mt. Auburn St.
Watertown, MA 02472
617-926-4232

SUPPORT GROUPS

**American Academy of
Ophthalmology**
Inquiry Clerk
655 Beach St.
San Francisco, CA 94109
415-561-8500
Fax: 415-561-8567

American Council of the Blind
1155 15th St., NW, Suite 720
Washington, DC 20005
800-424-8666
202-467-5081
Fax: 202-467-5085

American Foundation for the Blind
11 Penn Plaza, Suite 300
New York, NY 10001
800-232-5463
212-502-7600
Fax: 212-620-2105

**Association for Macular
Diseases, Inc.**
210 E. 64th St.
New York, NY 10021
212-605-3719

**Benign Essential Blepharospasm
Research Foundation, Inc.**
PO Box 12468
Beaumont, TX 77726-2468
409-832-0788

**Council of Citizens With Low
Vision**
International Organization
1859 N. Washington Ave.
Clearwater, FL 33755
800-733-2258
727-443-0350
Fax: 800-733-2258

Glaucoma Research Foundation
200 Pine St., Suite 200
San Francisco, CA 94104
415-986-3162

**Lighthouse National Center
for Vision and Aging**
111 E. 59th St.
New York, NY 10022
800-334-5497 (TDD)
212-821-9200 (TDD)

**National Association for the
Visually Handicapped**
22 W. 21st St., 6th Fl.
New York, NY 10010
212-889-3141

National Federation of the Blind
1800 Johnson St.
Baltimore, MD 21230
410-659-9314

**National Retinitis Pigmentosa
Foundation, Inc.**
1401 Mt. Royal Ave., 4th Fl.
Baltimore, MD 21217
800-683-5555

Vision Foundation
818 Mt. Auburn St.
Watertown, MA 02472
617-926-4232

The Heart and Blood Vessels

HEALTH INFORMATION
ORGANIZATIONS

**American Association of
Neurological Surgeons**
22 S. Washington St.
Park Ridge, IL 60068
847-692-9501
Fax: 847-692-2589

American College of Cardiology
9111 Old Georgetown Rd.
Bethesda, MD 20814-1699
800-253-4636
301-897-5400
Fax: 301-897-9745

American Heart Association
7272 Greenville Ave.
Dallas, TX 75231-4596
214-373-6300
Fax: 214-706-1341

**American Occupational Therapy
Association, Inc.**
PO Box 31220
4720 Montgomery Lane

Bethesda, MD 20824-1220
301-652-2682
Fax: 301-948-5529

American Physical Therapy Association
1111 N. Fairfax St.
Alexandria, VA 22314
703-684-2782
Fax: 703-684-7343

Citizens for Public Action on Blood Pressure and Cholesterol
PO Box 30374
Bethesda, MD 20824
301-770-1711
Fax: 301-770-1713

Commission on Accreditation of Rehabilitation Facilities
4891 E. Grant Rd.
Tuscon, AZ 85712
520-325-1044
Fax: 520-571-1601

National Aphasia Association
PO Box 1887, Murray Hill Station
New York, NY 10156-0611
800-922-4NAA

National Heart, Lung, and Blood Institute
Information Center
PO Box 30105
Bethesda, MD 20824-0105
301-251-1222

National Institute of Neurological Disorders and Stroke
Office of Scientific and Health Reports
9000 Rockville Pike
Bldg. 31 8A-06
Bethesda, MD 20892
800-352-9424
301-496-5751

National Rehabilitation Information Center
8455 Colesville Rd., Suite 935
Silver Spring, MD 20910-3319
800-346-2742
301-588-9284

National Stroke Association
8480 E. Orchard Rd., Suite 1000
Englewood, CO 80111-5015
800-787-6537
303-771-1700
Fax: 303-762-1190

United States Department of Education
National Institute on Disability and Rehabilitation Research
330 C St., SW, Rm. 3060
Washington, DC 20202-2572
202-205-8134

SUPPORT GROUPS

Citizens for Public Action on Blood Pressure and Cholesterol
PO Box 30374
Bethesda, MD 20824
301-770-1711
Fax: 301-770-1713

Coronary Club, Inc.
9500 Euclid Ave., Rm. E4-15
Cleveland, OH 44195
216-444-3690

Mended Hearts
7272 Greenville Ave.
Dallas, TX 75231
214-706-1442

National Aphasia Association
PO Box 1887, Murray Hill Station
New York, NY 10156-0611
800-922-4NAA

National Heart, Lung, and Blood Institute
Information Center
PO Box 30105
Bethesda, MD 20824-0105
301-251-1222

National Rehabilitation Information Center
8455 Colesville Rd., Suite 935
Silver Spring, MD 20910-3319
800-346-2742
301-588-9284

National Stroke Association
8480 E. Orchard Rd., Suite 1000
Englewood, CO 80111-5015
800-787-6537
303-771-1700
Fax: 303-762-1190

The Kidneys and Urinary Tract

HEALTH INFORMATION ORGANIZATIONS

American Association of Kidney Patients
100 S. Ashley Dr., Suite 280
Tampa, FL 33602

800-749-2257
813-223-7099
Fax: 813-223-0001

American Foundation for Urologic Disease
300 W. Pratt St., Suite 401
Baltimore, MD 21201
800-242-2383
410-727-2908
Fax: 410-528-0550

American Kidney Fund
6110 Executive Blvd., Suite 1010
Rockville, MD 20852
800-638-8299
301-881-3052
Fax: 301-881-0898

American Urological Association
1120 N. Charles St.
Baltimore, MD 21201
410-727-1100

The National Kidney and Urologic Diseases Information Clearinghouse
PO Box NKUDIC
9000 Rockville Pike
Bethesda, MD 20892
Please contact by mail.

National Kidney Foundation
30 E. 33rd St.
New York, NY 10016
800-622-9010
212-889-2210
Fax: 212-689-9261

SUPPORT GROUPS

American Association of Kidney Patients
100 S. Ashley Dr., Suite 280
Tampa, FL 33602
800-749-2257
813-223-7099
Fax: 813-223-0001

American Foundation for Urologic Disease
300 W. Pratt St., Suite 401
Baltimore, MD 21201
800-242-2383
410-727-2908
Fax: 410-528-0550

American Kidney Fund
6110 Executive Blvd., Suite 1010
Rockville, MD 20852
800-638-8299
301-881-3052
Fax: 301-881-0898

Transplant Recipients International Organization
1000 16th St., NW, Suite 602
Washington, DC 20036
202-293-0980
Fax: 202-293-0973

The Lungs and Respiratory System

HEALTH INFORMATION ORGANIZATIONS

American Academy of Allergy and Immunology
611 E. Wells St.
Milwaukee, WI 53202
800-822-2762
414-272-6071

American Allergy Association
PO Box 7273
Menlo Park, CA 94026
415-322-1663
Fax: 415-328-2295

American Lung Association
1740 Broadway
New York, NY 10019
212-315-8700
Fax: 212-265-5642

Asthma and Allergy Foundation of America
1125 15th St., NW, Suite 502
Washington, DC 20005
800-7ASTHMA
202-466-7643
Fax: 202-466-8940

Emphysema Anonymous, Inc.
PO Box 3224
Seminole, FL 34642
813-391-9977

National Heart, Lung, and Blood Institute
Information Center
PO Box 30105
Bethesda, MD 20824-0105
301-251-1222

National Institute of Allergy and Infectious Diseases
Bldg. 31, Rm. 7A-50
31 Center Dr., MSC 2520
Bethesda, MD 20892-2520
301-656-0003

National Jewish Center for Immunology and Respiratory Medicine
Lung Line
1400 Jackson St.
Denver, CO 80206
800-222-LUNG

SUPPORT GROUPS

American Academy of Allergy and Immunology
611 E. Wells St.
Milwaukee, WI 53202
800-822-2762
414-272-6071

American Allergy Association
PO Box 7273
Menlo Park, CA 94026
415-322-1663
Fax: 415-328-2295

American Lung Association
1740 Broadway
New York, NY 10019
212-315-8700
Fax: 212-265-5642

Asthma and Allergy Foundation of America
1125 15th St., NW, Suite 502
Washington, DC 20005
800-7ASTHMA
202-466-7643
Fax: 202-466-8940

Emphysema Anonymous, Inc.
PO Box 3224
Seminole, FL 34642
813-391-9977

The Muscles and Bones

HEALTH INFORMATION ORGANIZATIONS

American Academy of Orthopaedic Surgeons
6300 N. River Rd.
Rosemont, IL 60018-4262
800-346-AAOS
847-823-7186
Fax: 847-823-8125

American Podiatric Medical Association
9312 Old Georgetown Rd.
Bethesda, MD 20814-1621
800-FOOT-CARE
301-571-9200
Fax: 301-530-2752

Ankylosing Spondylitis Association
PO Box 5872
Sherman Oaks, CA 91413
800-777-8189
310-652-0609 in CA

Arthritis Foundation
1330 W. Peachtree St.
Atlanta, GA 30309
800-283-7800
404-872-7100
Fax: 404-872-0457

Lupus Foundation of America
1300 Piccard Dr., Suite 200
Rockville, MD 20850
800-558-0121
301-670-9292

National Arthritis and Musculoskeletal and Skin Diseases Information Clearinghouse
1 AMS Circle
Bethesda, MD 20892-3675
301-495-4484

National Osteoporosis Foundation
1150 17th St., NW, Suite 500
Washington, DC 20036
202-223-2226

Sjögren's Syndrome Foundation
333 N. Broadway, Suite 2000
Jericho, NY 11753
516-933-6365

SUPPORT GROUPS

Arthritis Foundation
1330 W. Peachtree St.
Atlanta, GA 30309
800-283-7800
404-872-7100
Fax: 404-872-0457

Lupus Foundation of America
1300 Piccard Dr., Suite 200
Rockville, MD 20850
800-558-0121
301-670-9292

National Osteoporosis Foundation
1150 17th St., NW, Suite 500
Washington, DC 20036
202-223-2226

The Skin

HEALTH INFORMATION ORGANIZATIONS

American Academy of Dermatology
930 N. Meacham Rd.
Schaumburg, IL 60173-4695

708-330-0230
Fax: 708-330-0050

National Alopecia Areata Foundation
710 C St., Suite 11
San Rafael, CA 94901
415-456-4644

National Arthritis and Musculo-skeletal and Skin Diseases Information Clearinghouse
1 AMS Circle
Bethesda, MD 20892-36754
301-495-4484

National Institute of Allergy and Infectious Diseases
Bldg. 31, Rm. 7A-50
31 Center Dr., MSC 2520
Bethesda, MD 20892-2520
301-496-5717

National Psoriasis Foundation
6600 S.W. 92nd Ave., Suite 300
Portland, OR 97223-7195
503-297-1545
Fax: 503-245-0626

The Skin Cancer Foundation
245 Fifth Ave., Suite 1403
New York, NY 10016
212-725-5176

SUPPORT GROUPS

American Academy of Dermatology
930 N. Meacham Rd.
Schaumburg, IL 60173-4695
708-330-0230
Fax: 708-330-0050

National Alopecia Areata Foundation
710 C St., Suite 11
San Rafael, CA 94901
415-456-4644

National Psoriasis Foundation
6600 S.W. 92nd Ave., Suite 300
Portland, OR 97223-7195
503-297-1545
Fax: 503-245-0626

Health Problems of Men

HEALTH INFORMATION ORGANIZATIONS

American College of Surgeons
Office of Public Information
633 N. St. Clair St.
Chicago, IL 60611
312-202-5000

American Foundation for Urologic Disease
300 W. Pratt St., Suite 401
Baltimore, MD 21201
800-242-2383
410-727-2908
Fax: 410-528-0550

American Urological Association
1120 N. Charles St.
Baltimore, MD 21201
410-727-1100

Brady Urological Institute
John Hopkins Hospital
600 N. Wolfe St.
Baltimore, MD 21287-2101
410-955-6100

Continence Restored, Inc.
24 E. 12th St., Suite 2-1
New York, NY 10003
212-879-3131

Help for Incontinent People
PO Box 8310
Spartanburg, SC 29305-8310
800-BLADDER
843-579-7900
Fax: 843-579-7902

Impotence Institute of America
PO Box 401
Bowie, MD 20718-0410
800-669-1603
301-577-0660

The National Kidney and Urologic Diseases Information Clearinghouse
PO Box NKUDIC
9000 Rockville Pike
Bethesda, MD 20892
Please contact by mail.

Recovery of Male Potency
27211 Lahser Rd., Suite 208
Southfield, MI 48034
800-835-7667
313-357-1216

SUPPORT GROUPS

American Foundation for Urologic Disease
300 W. Pratt St., Suite 401
Baltimore, MD 21201
800-242-2383
410-727-2908
Fax: 410-528-0550

Continence Restored, Inc.
24 E. 12th St., Suite 2-1
New York, NY 10003
212-879-3131

Help for Incontinent People
PO Box 8310
Spartanburg, SC 29305-8310
800-BLADDER
843-579-7900
Fax: 843-579-7902

Impotents Anonymous
PO Box 410
Bowie, MD 20718-0410
800-669-1603

Health Problems of Women

HEALTH INFORMATION ORGANIZATIONS

American College of Obstetricians and Gynecologists
Resource Center
409 12th St., SW
Washington, DC 20024
202-638-5577
Fax: 202-484-5107

American College of Surgeons
Office of Public Information
633 N. St. Clair St.
Chicago, IL 60611
312-202-5000

American Urological Association
1120 N. Charles St.
Baltimore, MD 21201
410-727-1100

Continence Restored, Inc.
24 E. 12th St., Suite 2-1
New York, NY 10003
212-879-3131

Help for Incontinent People
PO Box 8310
Spartanburg, SC 29305-8310
800-BLADDER
843-579-7900
Fax: 843-579-7902

Hysterectomy Educational Resources and Services Foundation
422 Bryn Mawr Ave.
Bala Cynwyd, PA 19004
610-667-7757

National Cancer Institute
Public Inquiries Office
Office of Cancer Communications
Bldg. 31, Rm. 10A24
Bethesda, MD 20892
800-422-6237
301-496-5583

National Women's Health Network
514 10th St., NW, Suite 400
Washington, DC 20004
202-347-1140
Fax: 202-347-1168

Women's Sports Foundation
Eisenhower Park
East Meadow, NY 11554
800-227-3988
516-542-4700

SUPPORT GROUPS

Continence Restored, Inc.
24 E. 12th St., Suite 2-1
New York, NY 10003
212-879-3131

Help for Incontinent People
PO Box 8310
Spartanburg, SC 29305-8310
800-BLADDER
843-579-7900
Fax: 843-579-7902

Hysterectomy Educational Resources and Services Foundation
422 Bryn Mawr Ave.
Bala Cynwyd, PA 19004
610-667-7757

National Women's Health Network
514 10th St., NW, Suite 400
Washington, DC 20004
202-347-1140
Fax: 202-347-1168

Older Women's League
666 11th St., NW, Suite 700
Washington, DC 20001
202-783-6686
Fax: 202-638-2356

Mental Health

HEALTH INFORMATION ORGANIZATIONS

Al-Anon Family Group Headquarters
1600 Corporate Landing Pkwy.
Virginia Beach, VA 23454
800-356-9996
757-563-1600

American Mental Health Counselors Association
801 N. Fairfax Ave.
Suite 304
Alexandria, VA 22314
800-326-2642
703-548-6003

American Psychiatric Association
1400 K St., NW
Washington, DC 20005
202-682-6000
Fax: 202-682-6114

American Psychological Association
750 First St., NE
Washington, DC 20002
202-336-5500

American Sleep Apnea Association
1424 K St., Suite 302
Washington, DC 20005
202-293-3650
Please contact by mail.

American Sleep Disorders Association
6301 Bandel Rd., Suite 101
Rochester, MN 55901
507-287-6006
Fax: 507-287-6008

Depression and Related Affective Disorders Association
Johns Hopkins Hospital
600 N. Wolfe St., Meyer 3-181
Baltimore, MD 21287-7381
410-955-4647

Depression Awareness Recognition & Treatment Program
5600 Fishers Lane
Parklawn Bldg., Rm. 1085
Rockville, MD 20857
800-421-4211
301-443-3720

Emotions Anonymous
PO Box 4245
St. Paul, MN 55104-0245
651-647-9712

National Alliance for the Mentally Ill
200 N. Glebe Rd., Suite 1015
Arlington, VA 22203-3754
800-950-6264
703-524-7600

National Association of Private Psychiatric Hospitals
1317 F St., NW, Suite 301
Washington, DC 20004
202-393-6700

National Council on Alcoholism and Drug Dependence
12 W. 21st St.
New York, NY 10010
212-206-6770

National Depressive and Manic-Depressive Association
730 N. Franklin, Suite 501

Chicago, IL 60610
312-642-0049
Fax: 312-642-7243

National Institute of Mental Health
Mental Health Public Inquiries
5600 Fishers Lane, Rm. 7C-02
Rockville, MD 20857
301-443-4513 (publications)

National Mental Health Association
1021 Prince St.
Alexandria, VA 22314-2971
800-969-6977
703-684-7722
Fax: 703-684-5968

National Sleep Foundation
122 S. Robertson Blvd.
Suite 201
Los Angeles, CA 90048
Please contact by mail.

Well Spouse Foundation
610 Lexington Ave., Suite 208
New York, NY 10022
800-838-0879
212-644-1241

SUPPORT GROUPS

Al-Anon Family Group Headquarters
1600 Corporate Landing Pkwy.
Virginia Beach, VA 23454
800-356-9996
757-563-1600

Alcoholics Anonymous
475 Riverside Dr.
New York, NY 10115
212-870-3400

American Sleep Apnea Association
1424 K St., Suite 302
Washington, DC 20005
202-293-3650
Please contact by mail.

Council on Anxiety Disorders
PO Box 17011
Winston-Salem, NC 27116
336-722-7760

Emotional Health Anonymous
PO Box 429
Glendale, CA 91209
818-377-4341

Emotions Anonymous
PO Box 4245
St. Paul, MN 55104-0245
651-647-9712

National Alliance for the Mentally Ill
200 N. Glebe Rd., Suite 1015

Arlington, VA 22203-3754
800-950-6264
703-524-7600

National Depressive and Manic-Depressive Association
730 N. Franklin, Suite 501
Chicago, IL 60610
312-642-0049
Fax: 312-642-7243

National Mental Health Association
1021 Prince St.
Alexandria, VA 22314-2971
800-969-6977
703-684-7722
Fax: 703-684-5968

National Mental Health Consumer Self-Help Clearinghouse
1211 Chestnut St.
Philadelphia, PA 19107
800-688-4226
215-751-1810

Recoveries Anonymous
PO Box 1212
Hewitt Square Station
East Northport, NY 11731
516-261-1212

Recovery, Inc.
802 N. Dearborn St.
Chicago, IL 60610
312-337-5661

General Health Information and Support Organizations

GENERAL HEALTH INFORMATION ORGANIZATIONS

Aerobics and Fitness Foundation
15250 Ventura Blvd., Suite 200
Sherman Oaks, CA 91403
800-BE-FIT-86

Alcohol, Drug Abuse, and Mental Health Administration
Office of the Administrator
5600 Fishers Lane
Parklawn Bldg., Rm. 12-105
Rockville, MD 20857
301-443-4795

American Association of Retired Persons
601 E St., NW
Washington, DC 20049
202-434-2277

American Association of Retired Persons
Pharmacy Service
500 Montgomery St.
Alexandria, VA 22314
800-456-4636
703-684-0244

American College of Surgeons
Office of Public Information
633 N. St. Clair St.
Chicago, IL 60611
312-202-5000

American Dietetic Association
216 W. Jackson Blvd., Suite 800
Chicago, IL 60606-6995
800-745-0775
312-899-0040

American Geriatrics Society
770 Lexington Ave., Suite 300
New York, NY 10021
212-308-1414

American Health Foundation
1 Dana Rd.
Valhalla, NY 10595
212-953-1900
Fax: 914-592-6317

American Hospital Association
1 N. Franklin St., Suite 2700
Chicago, IL 60606
800-242-2626
312-422-3000

American Medical Association
515 N. State St.
Chicago, IL 60610
800-262-3211
312-464-5000

American Music Therapy Association
8455 Colesville Rd., Suite 1000
Silver Spring, MD 20910
301-589-3300

American Nurses Association
600 Maryland Ave., SW, Suite 100
Washington, DC 20024-2571
800-444-5720
202-651-7000

American Red Cross
430 17th St., NW
Washington, DC 20006
202-737-8300

American Society of Internal Medicine
2011 I St., Suite 800
Washington, DC 20006
800-338-ASIM
202-835-2746
Fax: 202-682-8659

American Society of Plastic and Reconstructive Surgeons
444 E. Algonquin Rd.
Arlington Heights, IL 60005
847-228-9900

American Society on Aging
833 Market St., Suite 511
San Francisco, CA 94103
415-974-9600

American Trauma Society
8903 Presidential Pkwy.
Suite 512
Upper Marlboro, MD 20772-2656
800-556-7890
301-420-4189

Association of American Medical Colleges
2450 N St., NW
Washington, DC 20037
202-828-0400
Fax: 202-828-1125

Center for Medical Consumers
237 Thompson St.
New York, NY 10012
212-674-7105

Centers for Disease Control
Center for Chronic Disease Prevention and Health Promotion
1600 Clifton Rd., NE
Bldg. 1, SSB249, MS A 34
Atlanta, GA 30333
404-639-3311

Centers for Disease Control
Office of Public Affairs
1600 Clifton Rd., NE
Atlanta, GA 30333
404-639-3311
404-639-3534 (publications)

Choice in Dying
475 Riverside Dr.
New York, NY 10115
212-870-2003
800-989-9455

Community Health Accreditation Program, Inc.
61 Broadway, 33rd Fl.
New York, NY 10006
800-669-1656
212-363-5555 ext. 242

Congress of the United States
Office of Technology Assessment
Washington, DC 20510-8025
202-653-7188

Consumer Health Information Research Institute/National Council for Reliable Health Information
300 E. Pink Hill Rd.
Independence, MO 64057
816-228-4595

Consumer Information Center
Pueblo, CO 81009
719-948-3334

Council of Better Business Bureaus
4200 Wilson Blvd., Suite 800
Arlington, VA 22203
703-276-0100

Department of Health and Human Services
Administration on Aging
200 Independence Ave., SW
Hubert Humphrey Bldg., Rm. 309-F
Washington, DC 20201
202-401-4541

Department of Health and Human Services
Public Health Service
200 Independence Ave., SW
Hubert Humphrey Bldg., Rm. 716-G
Washington, DC 20201
202-690-7694

Food and Drug Administration
Center for Biologics Evaluation and Research
1401 Rockville Pike
Bethesda, MD 20852-1448
301-827-0548

Food and Drug Administration
Center for Devices and Radiological Health
9200 Corporate Blvd.
Rockville, MD 20857
301-443-4690

Food and Drug Administration
Center for Drug Evaluation and Research
5600 Fishers Lane
Rockville, MD 20857
301-594-6740

Food and Drug Administration
Office of Consumer Affairs
5600 Fishers Lane, HFE 88
Rockville, MD 20857
301-463-6332

Foundation for Hospice and Home Care
519 C St., NE
Washington, DC 20002
202-547-5263

Gerontological Society of America
Information Service
1030 15th St., NW, Suite 250
Washington, DC 20005-4006
202-842-1275
Fax: 202-842-1150

Gray Panthers Project Fund
733 15th St., NW, Suite 437
Washington, DC 20005
202-737-6637

Health Care Financing Administration
7500 Security Blvd.
Baltimore, MD 21244
410-786-3000

Health Care Financing Administration
Office of Prepaid Health Care
330 Independence Ave., SW
Wilbur J. Cohen Bldg., Rm. 4360
Washington, DC 20201
202-619-0815
Fax: 202-619-2011

Health Resources and Services Administration
Office of the Administrator
5600 Fishers Lane
Parklawn Bldg., Rm. 14-05
Rockville, MD 20857
301-443-2216

Hospice Education Institute
Hospicelink
190 Westbrook Rd.
Essex, CT 06426-1511
800-331-1620
860-767-1620 in CT

IBM National Support Center for Persons with Disabilities
PO Box 2150-HO6R1
Atlanta, GA 30301
800-426-4832

Joint Commission on Accreditation of Health Care Organizations
Department of Corporate Relations
1 Renaissance Blvd.
Oakbrook Terrace, IL 60181
630-792-5000
Fax: 630-916-5644

Library of Congress
Science and Technology Division
101 Independence Ave., SE
Adams Bldg., 5th Fl.
Washington, DC 20540
202-707-5664

The Living Bank
PO Box 6725
Houston, TX 77265
800-528-2971
713-528-2971 in TX

Lupus Foundation of America
1300 Piccard Dr., Suite 200
Rockville, MD 20850
800-558-0121
301-670-9292

National Agricultural Library
Food and Nutrition Information Center
10301 Baltimore Blvd.
Beltsville, MD 20705-2351
301-504-5719
Fax: 301-504-5472

National Association for Home Care
228 Seventh St., SE
Washington, DC 20003
202-547-7424

National Association of Area Agencies on Aging
927 15th St., NW, 6th Fl.
Washington, DC 20005
202-296-8130

National Association of State Units on Aging
1225 I St., NW, Suite 725
Washington, DC 20006
202-898-2578

National Consumers League
1701 K St., NW, Suite 1200
Washington, DC 20006
202-835-3323

National Council Against Health Fraud Resource Center
300 E. Pink Hill Rd.
Independence, MO 64057
816-228-4595

National Council of Senior Citizens
1331 F St., NW
Washington, DC 20004-1171
202-289-6976

National Council on Disability
1331 F St., NW, Suite 1050
Washington, DC 20004-1107
202-272-2004

National Council on the Aging, Inc.
409 Third St., SW
Washington, DC 20024
800-424-9046

National Council on the Aging, Inc.
National Institute of Adult
Day Care
409 Third St., SW
Washington, DC 20024
202 479 6654

National Hospice Organization
1901 N. Moore St., Suite 901
Arlington, VA 22209
800-658-8898
703-243-5900

National Institute of General Medical Sciences
45 Center Dr.
Bethesda, MD 20892-6200
301-496-7301

National Institute on Aging
Public Information Office
9000 Rockville Pike
Bldg. 31, Rm. 5C27
Bethesda, MD 20892
301-496-1752

National Institutes of Health
9000 Rockville Pike
Bethesda, MD 20892
301-496-4461
Fax: 301-496-0017

National Interfaith Coalition on Aging
c/o NCOA
409 Third St., SW
Washington, DC 20024
202-479-6689

National League for Nursing
350 Hudson St.
New York, NY 10014
800-669-1656
212-363-5555

National Organization for Rare Disorders
PO Box 8923
New Fairfield, CT 06812
800-447-6673
203-746-6518

Office of Disease Prevention and Health Promotion
National Health Information
Center
PO Box 1133
Washington, DC 20013-1133
800-336-4797
301-565-4167 in MD

Office of Health Facilities
5600 Fishers Lane
Parklawn Bldg., Rm. 11-25
Rockville, MD 20857
800-638-0742 (Hill-Burton Program)

The President's Committee on Employment of People with Disabilities
1331 F St., NW, Suite 300
Washington, DC 20004-1107
202-376-6200
202-376-6205 (TDD)
Fax: 202-376-6219

President's Council on Physical Fitness and Sports
200 Independence Ave., SW
Hubert Humphrey Bldg., Rm. 738-H
Washington, DC 20201-0004
202-690-9000

Scleroderma Foundation
89 Newbury St.
Danvers, MA 01923
800-722-HOPE
978-750-4499

Sjögren's Syndrome Foundation
333 N. Broadway, Suite 2000
Jericho, NY 11753
516-933-6365

United Network for Organ Sharing
PO Box 13770
1100 Boulders Pkwy., Suite 500
Richmond, VA 23225-8770
800-24-DONOR

United States Department of Education
Clearinghouse on Disability
Information
330 C St., SW, Rm. 3132
Washington, DC 20202-2524
202-205-5465

United States Department of Education
National Institute on Disability and
Rehabilitation Research
330 C St., SW, Rm. 3060
Washington, DC 20202-2572
202-205-8134

United States Government Printing Office
710 N. Capital St., NW
Washington, DC 20401
202-512-1800 (orders/information)

United Way of America
701 N. Fairfax St.
Alexandria, VA 22314-2045
703-836-7100

Very Special Arts USA
The John F. Kennedy Center for
Performing Arts, Education Office
Washington, DC 20004
800-933-8721
202-628-2800 (TDD)

Visiting Nurse Associations of America
11 Beacon St., Suite 910
Boston, MA 02108
800-426-2547

Warren Grant Magnuson Clinical Center
Office of Clinical Center
Communications
9000 Rockville Pike
Bldg. 10, Rm. 1C-255
Bethesda, MD 20892
301-496-4891 (referrals)

NATIONAL SELF-HELP
CLEARINGHOUSES

American Self-Help Clearinghouse
Northwest Covenant Medical Center
25 Pocono Rd.
Denville, NJ 07834
973-586-0276

National Self-Help Clearinghouse
Graduate School and University
Center of the City University of
New York
25 W. 43rd St., Rm. 620
New York, NY 10036
212-642-2944

GENERAL ORGANIZATIONS

This section contains the General Health Information Organizations that do not easily fit under the disorders covered by the Handbook. They are ordered alphabetically, and each listing gives you the organization's name, address, and phone number. Also in this section are National and Regional Self-Help Clearinghouses, beginning on page 619.

To find a Health Information Organization by Disorder, turn to page 604.

GENERAL HEALTH INFORMATION ORGANIZATIONS

Aerobics and Fitness Foundation
15250 Ventura Blvd., Suite 200
Sherman Oaks, CA 91403
800-BE-FIT-86

Alcohol, Drug Abuse, and Mental Health Administration
Office of the Administrator
5600 Fishers Lane
Parklawn Bldg., Rm. 12-105
Rockville, MD 20857
301-443-4795

American Association of Retired Persons
601 E St., NW
Washington, DC 20049
202-434-2277

American Association of Retired Persons
Pharmacy Service
500 Montgomery St.
Alexandria, VA 22314
800-456-4636
703-684-0244

American College of Surgeons
Office of Public Information
633 N. St. Clair St.
Chicago, IL 60611
312-202-5000

American Dietetic Association
216 W. Jackson Blvd., Suite 800
Chicago, IL 60606-6995
800-745-0775
312-899-0040

American Geriatrics Society
770 Lexington Ave., Suite 300
New York, NY 10021
212-308-1414

American Health Foundation
1 Dana Rd.
Valhalla, NY 10595
212-953-1900
Fax: 914-592-6317

American Hospital Association
1 N. Franklin St., Suite 2700
Chicago, IL 60606
800-242-2626
312-422-3000

American Medical Association
515 N. State St.
Chicago, IL 60610
800-262-3211
312-464-5000

American Music Therapy Association
8455 Colesville Rd., Suite 1000
Silver Spring, MD 20910
301-589-3300

American Nurses Association
600 Maryland Ave., SW, Suite 100
Washington, DC 20024-2571
800-444-5720
202-651-7000

American Red Cross
430 17th St., NW
Washington, DC 20006
202-737-8300

American Society of Internal Medicine
2011 I St., Suite 800
Washington, DC 20006
800-338-ASIM
202-835-2746
Fax: 202-682-8659

American Society of Plastic and Reconstructive Surgeons
444 E. Algonquin Rd.
Arlington Heights, IL 60005
847-228-9900

American Society on Aging
833 Market St., Suite 511
San Francisco, CA 94103
415-974-9600

American Trauma Society
8903 Presidential Pkwy.
Suite 512
Upper Marlboro, MD 20772-2656
800-556-7890
301-420-4189

Association of American Medical Colleges
2450 N St., NW
Washington, DC 20037
202-828-0400
Fax: 202-828-1125

Center for Medical Consumers
237 Thompson St.
New York, NY 10012
212-674-7105

Centers for Disease Control
Center for Chronic Disease Prevention and Health Promotion
1600 Clifton Rd., NE
Bldg. 1, SSB249, MS A 34
Atlanta, GA 30333
404-639-3311

Centers for Disease Control
Office of Public Affairs
1600 Clifton Rd., NE
Atlanta, GA 30333
404-639-3311
404-639-3534 (publications)

Choice in Dying
475 Riverside Dr.
New York, NY 10115
212-870-2003
800-989-9455

Community Health Accreditation Program, Inc.
61 Broadway, 33rd Fl.
New York, NY 10006
800-669-1656
212-363-5555 ext. 242

Congress of the United States
Office of Technology Assessment
Washington, DC 20510-8025
202-653-7188

**Consumer Health Information
Research Institute/National
Council for Reliable Health
Information**
300 E. Pink Hill Rd.
Independence, MO 64057
816-228-4595

Consumer Information Center
Pueblo, CO 81009
719-948-3334

Council of Better Business Bureaus
4200 Wilson Blvd., Suite 800
Arlington, VA 22203
703-276-0100

**Department of Health and Human
Services**
Administration on Aging
200 Independence Ave., SW
Hubert Humphrey Bldg., Rm. 309-F
Washington, DC 20201
202-401-4541

**Department of Health and Human
Services**
Public Health Service
200 Independence Ave., SW
Hubert Humphrey Bldg., Rm. 716-G
Washington, DC 20201
202-690-7694

Food and Drug Administration
Center for Biologics Evaluation
and Research
1401 Rockville Pike
Bethesda, MD 20852-1448
301-827-0548

Food and Drug Administration
Center for Devices and
Radiological Health
9200 Corporate Blvd.
Rockville, MD 20857
301-443-4690

Food and Drug Administration
Center for Drug Evaluation and
Research
5600 Fishers Lane
Rockville, MD 20857
301-594-6740

Food and Drug Administration
Office of Consumer Affairs
5600 Fishers Lane, HFE 88
Rockville, MD 20857
301-463-6332

**Foundation for Hospice
and Home Care**
519 C St., NE
Washington, DC 20002
202-547-5263

Gerontological Society of America
Information Service
1030 15th St., NW, Suite 250
Washington, DC 20005-4006
202-842-1275
Fax: 202-842-1150

Gray Panthers Project Fund
733 15th St., NW, Suite 437
Washington, DC 20005
202-737-6637

**Health Care Financing
Administration**
7500 Security Blvd.
Baltimore, MD 21244
410-786-3000

**Health Care Financing
Administration**
Office of Prepaid Health Care
330 Independence Ave., SW
Wilbur J. Cohen Bldg., Rm. 4360
Washington, DC 20201
202-619-0815
Fax: 202-619-2011

**Health Resources and Services
Administration**
Office of the Administrator
5600 Fishers Lane
Parklawn Bldg., Rm. 14-05
Rockville, MD 20857
301-443-2216

Hospice Education Institute
Hospicelink
190 Westbrook Rd.
Essex, CT 06426-1511
800-331-1620
860-767-1620 in CT

**IBM National Support Center
for Persons with Disabilities**
PO Box 2150-HO6R1
Atlanta, GA 30301
800-426-4832

**Joint Commission on Accreditation
of Health Care Organizations**
Department of Corporate Relations
1 Renaissance Blvd.
Oakbrook Terrace, IL 60181
630-792-5000
Fax: 630-916-5644

Library of Congress
Science and Technology Division
101 Independence Ave., SE
Adams Bldg., 5th Fl.
Washington, DC 20540

202-707-5664

The Living Bank
PO Box 6725
Houston, TX 77265
800-528-2971
713-528-2971 in TX

Lupus Foundation of America
1300 Piccard Dr., Suite 200
Rockville, MD 20850
800-558-0121
301-670-9292

National Agricultural Library
Food and Nutrition Information
Center
10301 Baltimore Blvd.
Beltsville, MD 20705-2351
301-504-5719
Fax: 301-504-5472

**National Association
for Home Care**
228 Seventh St., SE
Washington, DC 20003
202-547-7424

**National Association of Area
Agencies on Aging**
927 15th St., NW, 6th Fl.
Washington, DC 20005
202-296-8130

**National Association of State
Units on Aging**
1225 I St., NW, Suite 725
Washington, DC 20006
202-898-2578

National Consumers League
1701 K St., NW, Suite 1200
Washington, DC 20006
202-835-3323

**National Council Against Health
Fraud Resource Center**
300 E. Pink Hill Rd.
Independence, MO 64057
816-228-4595

National Council of Senior Citizens
1331 F St., NW
Washington, DC 20004-1171
202-289-6976

National Council on Disability
1331 F St., NW, Suite 1050
Washington, DC 20004-1107
202-272-2004

National Council on the Aging, Inc.
409 Third St., SW
Washington, DC 20024
800-424-9046

National Council on the Aging, Inc.
National Institute of Adult
Day Care
409 Third St., SW
Washington, DC 20024
202-479-6654

National Hospice Organization
1901 N. Moore St., Suite 901
Arlington, VA 22209
800-658-8898
703-243-5900

**National Institute of General
Medical Sciences**
45 Center Dr.
Bethesda, MD 20892-6200
301-496-7301

National Institute on Aging
Public Information Office
9000 Rockville Pike
Bldg. 31, Rm. 5C27
Bethesda, MD 20892
301-496-1752

National Institutes of Health
9000 Rockville Pike
Bethesda, MD 20892
301-496-4461
Fax: 301-496-0017

**National Interfaith Coalition
of Aging**
c/o NCOA
409 Third St., SW
Washington, DC 20024
202-479-6689

National League for Nursing
350 Hudson St.
New York, NY 10014
800-669-1656
212-363-5555

**National Organization for Rare
Disorders**
PO Box 8923
New Fairfield, CT 06812
800-447-6673
203-746-6518

**Office of Disease Prevention
and Health Promotion**
National Health Information
Center
PO Box 1133
Washington, DC 20013-1133
800-336-4797
301-565-4167 in MD

Office of Health Facilities
5600 Fishers Lane
Parklawn Bldg., Rm. 11-25
Rockville, MD 20857
800-638-0742 (Hill-Burton Program)

**The President's Committee
on Employment of People
with Disabilities**
1331 F St., NW, Suite 300
Washington, DC 20004-1107
202-376-6200
202-376-6205 (TDD)
Fax: 202-376-6219

**President's Council on Physical
Fitness and Sports**
200 Independence Ave., SW
Hubert Humphrey Bldg., Rm. 738-H
Washington, DC 20201-0004
202-690-9000

Scleroderma Foundation
89 Newbury St.
Danvers, MA 01923
800-722-HOPE
978-750-4499

Sjögren's Syndrome Foundation
333 N. Broadway, Suite 2000
Jericho, NY 11753
516-933-6365

United Network for Organ Sharing
PO Box 13770
1100 Boulders Pkwy., Suite 500
Richmond, VA 23225-8770
800-24-DONOR

**United States Department
of Education**
Clearinghouse on Disability
Information
330 C St., SW, Rm. 3132
Washington, DC 20202-2524
202-205-5465

**United States Department
of Education**
National Institute on Disability and
Rehabilitation Research
330 C St., SW, Rm. 3060
Washington, DC 20202-2572
202-205-8134

**United States Government
Printing Office**
710 N. Capital St., NW
Washington, DC 20401
202-512-1800 (orders/information)

United Way of America
701 N. Fairfax St.
Alexandria, VA 22314-2045
703-836-7100

Very Special Arts USA
The John F. Kennedy Center for
Performing Arts, Education Office
Washington, DC 20004
800-933-8721
202-628-2800 (TDD)

**Visiting Nurse Associations
of America**
11 Beacon St., Suite 910
Boston, MA 02108
800-426-2547

**Warren Grant Magnuson
Clinical Center**
Office of Clinical Center
Communications
9000 Rockville Pike
Bldg. 10, Rm. 1C-255
Bethesda, MD 20892
301-496-4891 (referrals)

NATIONAL SELF-HELP
CLEARINGHOUSES

American Self-Help Clearinghouse
Northwest Covenant Medical Center
25 Pocono Rd.
Denville, NJ 07834
973-586-0276

National Self-Help Clearinghouse
Graduate School and University
Center of the City University of
New York
25 W. 43rd St., Rm. 620
New York, NY 10036
212-642-2944

REGIONAL SELF-HELP
CLEARINGHOUSES

CALIFORNIA

Concord

**Mental Health Association
of Contra Costa County**
1070 Concord Ave., Suite 170
Concord, CA 94520
510-603-1212

Davis

**Mental Health Association
of Yolo County**
219 East St., Suite B
Davis, CA 95617
530-756-8181

Fresno

**Fresno County Information
Referral Network**
2420 Mariposa St.
Fresno, CA 93721
209-488-3857

Los Angeles

University of California Los Angeles
California Self-Help Center
405 Hilgard Ave.
Los Angeles, CA 90024
800-222-LINK in CA
310-305-8878

Merced

Mental Health Association of Merced County
480 E. 13th St.
Merced, CA 95340
209-381-6800

CONNECTICUT

New Haven

Self-Help Mutual Support Network Consultation Center
389 Whitney Ave.
New Haven, CT 06511
203-789-7645
Fax: 203-562-6355

ILLINOIS

Champaign

Family Services of Champaign County
405 S. State St.
Champaign, IL 61820
217-352-0099
Fax: 217-352-9512

INDIANA

Indianapolis

Information and Referral Network
3901 N. Meridian St., Suite 300
Indianapolis, IN 46208
317-921-1305

KANSAS

Wichita

Kansas Self-Help Network
Wichita State University
Campus Box 34
1845 Fairmount St.
Wichita, KS 67260-0034
316-978-3843

MASSACHUSETTS

Amherst

Massachusetts Clearinghouse of Mutual Help Groups
113 Skinner Hall
University of Massachusetts
Amherst, MA 01003
413-545-2313
Fax: 413-545-4410

MICHIGAN

Benton Harbor

Center for Self-Help
Riverwood Center
PO Box 547
1485 S. M-139
Benton Harbor, MI 49022
800-336-0341
616-925-0585

Lansing

Michigan Protection and Advocacy Service
Michigan Self-Help Clearinghouse
106 W. Allegan, Suite 300
Lansing, MI 48933
800-752-5858 in MI
517-484-7373

MINNESOTA

St. Paul

United Way
First Call for Help
166 E. Fourth St., Suite 310
St. Paul, MN 55101-1448
651-224-1133

MISSOURI

St. Louis

Mental Health Association of St. Louis
1905 S. Grand Blvd.
St. Louis, MO 63104
314-773-1399
Fax: 314-773-5930

NEW HAMPSHIRE

Concord

New Hampshire Division of Mental Health and Developmental Services
105 Pleasant St.
State Office Park South
Concord, NH 03301

603-271-5060

NEW JERSEY

Denville

Self-Help Clearinghouse
St. Clare's Health Services
25 Pocono Rd.
Denville, NJ 07834
973-625-7101
800-367-6274 in NJ

NEW YORK

Albany

New York State Council on Children and Families
5 Empire State Plaza, Suite 2810
Corning Tower
Albany, NY 12223
518-473-3652
Fax: 518-473-2570

Bath

Institute for Human Services
6666 County Road 11
Bath, NY 14810
800-346-2211 (24-hour help line)
607-776-9467

Buffalo

Mental Health Association of Erie County Inc.
999 Delaware Ave.
Buffalo, NY 14209
716-886-1242

Central Islip

New York Institute of Technology
Long Island Self-Help Clearinghouse
Central Islip Campus
Central Islip, NY 11722
516-348-3000

Elmira

Economic Opportunity Program, Inc.
318 Madison Ave.
Elmira, NY 14901
607-734-6174

Schuyline/Info Line
462 W. Church St.
Elmira, NY 14901
800-348-0448
607-737-2077

Fulton

Catholic Charities in Oswego County
365 W. First St.
Fulton, NY 13069
315-598-3980

Gloversville

Family Counseling Center
11-21 Broadway
Gloversville, NY 12078
518-725-4310

Goshen

Mental Health Association in Orange County, Inc.
Tri-County Self-Help Clearinghouse
20 John St.
Goshen, NY 10924
914-294-9355

Ithaca

Mental Health Association in Tompkins County
225 S. Fulton St., Suite B
Ithaca, NY 14850
607-273-9250

Kingston

Mental Health Association in Ulster County
MHA Self-Help Clearinghouse
PO Box 2304
221 Tuyten Bridge Rd.
Kingston, NY 12402
914-336-4747

Lockport

Mental Health Association in Niagara County, Inc.
Niagara County Self-Help Clearinghouse
151 East Ave.
Lockport, NY 14094
716-433-3780

New City

Mental Health Association of Rockland
Rockland County Self-Help Clearinghouse and Information Center
20 Squadron Blvd.
New City, NY 10956
914-639-7400

Olean

Cattaraugus County Self-Help Clearinghouse
Crosstics
American Red Cross-Olean Branch
528 N. Barry St.
Olean, NY 14760
716-372-5800

Plattsburgh

Fulton County Self-Help Clearinghouse
CEF Crisis/Helpline
36 Brinkerhoff St.
Plattsburgh, NY 12901
518-561-2330

Potsdam

Reachout of St. Lawrence County, Inc.
PO Box 5051
Potsdam, NY 13676-5051
315-265-2422

Poughkeepsie

United Way of Dutchess County, Inc.
Dutchess County Self-Help Clearinghouse
PO Box 832
75 Market St.
Poughkeepsie, NY 12601
914-473-1500

Rochester

Mental Health Association of Rochester/Monroe
Monroe County Self-Help Clearinghouse
339 East Ave., Suite 201
Rochester, NY 14604
716-325-3145
Fax: 716-256-2732

Schenectady

Human Services Planning Council of Schenectady County, Inc.
Schenectady County Self-Help Clearinghouse
152 Barrett St., 2nd Fl.
Schenectady, NY 12305
518-374-2244

Syracuse

The Volunteer Center, Inc.
Onondaga County Self-Help Clearinghouse
518 James St., 2nd Fl.
Syracuse, NY 13203
315-474-7011
Fax: 315-479-6772

Utica

Voluntary Action Center of Greater Utica
401 Columbia St.
Utica, NY 13502
315-735-4463

White Plains

Westchester Self-Help Clearinghouse
456 North St.
White Plains, NY 10605
914-949-6301

NORTH CAROLINA

Charlotte

Supportworks
1012 Kings Dr., Suite 923
Charlotte, NC 28283
704-331-9500

OHIO

Dayton

Ohio Self-Help Clearinghouse
Family Service Association
184 Salem Ave.
Dayton, OH 45406
937-225-3004
Fax: 937-222-3710

OREGON

Portland

Northwest Regional Self-Help Clearinghouse
PO Box 637
Portland, OR 97207
503-222-5555

PENNSYLVANIA

Scranton

Voluntary Action Center of Northeast Pennsylvania
Self-Help Information and Networking Exchange
538 Spruce St.
Scranton Life Bldg., Suite 420
Scranton, PA 18503
717-961-1234
Fax: 717-341-5816

SOUTH CAROLINA

West Columbia

The Support Group Network
Lexington Medical Center
2720 Sunset Blvd.
West Columbia, SC 29169
803-791-9227
803-791-2800

TENNESSEE

Knoxville

**Mental Health Association
of Knox County**
Support Group Clearinghouse
PO Box 52405
Knoxville, TN 37950-2405
423-584-9125

TEXAS

Dallas

**Mental Health Association
of Dallas County**
Dallas Self-Help Clearinghouse
2929 Carlisle St., Suite 350
Dallas, TX 75204-1058
214-871-2420

Fort Worth

**Tarrant County Mental Health
Association**
Tarrant County Self-Help
Clearinghouse
3136 W. Fourth St.
Fort Worth, TX 76107
817-335-5405

Houston

**Mental Health Association in
Houston and Harris County**
Houston Self-Help Clearinghouse
2211 Norfolk St., Suite 810
Houston, TX 77098
713-523-8963

San Antonio

**Mental Health Association
in Greater San Antonio**
Greater San Antonio Self-Help
Clearinghouse
901 N.E. Loop 410, Suite 504
San Antonio, TX 78209
210-826-2288

VIRGINIA

Annandale

**Mental Health Association
of Northern Virginia**
3340 Woodburn Rd.
Annandale, VA 22003
703-573-5679

**Self-Help Clearinghouse
of Greater Washington**
7630 Little River Tpk.
Suite 206
Annandale, VA 22003
703-941-5465

WASHINGTON

Olympia

**Crisis Clinic/Thurston
and Mason Counties**
PO Box 2463
Olympia, WA 98507
800-627-2211
360-586-2800

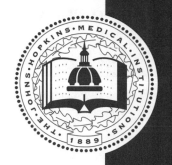

ACKNOWLEDGMENTS
AND INDEX

ACKNOWLEDGMENTS

We wish to thank the following organizations which so generously gave us permission to reprint material from their publications. Grouped by Handbook chapter title, those publications are acknowledged below, preceded by the respective subject entry name as it appears in the Handbook:

CANCER

OVERVIEW—*What You Need To Know About Cancer,* revised April 1993, The National Cancer Institute.

BLADDER CANCER—*What You Need To Know About Bladder Cancer,* revised February 1997, The National Cancer Institute.

BREAST CANCER—*What You Need To Know About Breast Cancer,* revised August 1995, The National Cancer Institute.

CERVICAL CANCER—*What You Need To Know About Cancer of the Cervix,* revised July 1994, The National Cancer Institute.

COLORECTAL CANCER—*What You Need To Know About Cancer of the Colon and Rectum,* revised August 1993, reprinted April 1994, The National Cancer Institute.

HODGKIN'S DISEASE—*What You Need To Know About Hodgkin's Disease,* revised August 1991, reprinted December 1992, The National Cancer Institute.

KIDNEY CANCER—*What You Need To Know About Kidney Cancer,* revised June 1996, The National Cancer Institute.

LEUKEMIA—*What You Need To Know About Leukemia,* revised December 1994, The National Cancer Institute.

LUNG CANCER—*What You Need To Know About Lung Cancer,* revised June 1993, reprinted September 1997, The National Cancer Institute.

MULTIPLE MYELOMA—*What You Need To Know About Multiple Myeloma,* revised December 1991, reprinted April 1995, The National Cancer Institute.

NON-HODGKIN'S LYMPHOMAS—*What You Need To Know About Non-Hodgkin's Lymphomas,* revised August 1991, reprinted October 1992, The National Cancer Institute.

ORAL CANCER—*What You Need To Know About Oral Cancer,* revised November 1996, The National Cancer Institute.

OVARIAN CANCER—*What You Need To Know About Ovarian Cancer,* revised October 1993, The National Cancer Institute.

PANCREATIC CANCER—*What You Need To Know About Cancer of the Pancreas,* revised October 1989, printed August 1992, The National Cancer Institute.

PROSTATE CANCER—*What You Need To Know About Prostate Cancer,* revised June 1996, The National Cancer Institute.

SKIN CANCER—*What You Need To Know About Skin Cancer,* revised January 1995, The National Cancer Institute.

STOMACH CANCER—*What You Need To Know About Cancer of the Stomach,* revised November 1993, The National Cancer Institute.

UTERINE CANCER—*What You Need To Know About Cancer of the Uterus,* revised September 1997, The National Cancer Institute.

CHAPTER 2

THE BLOOD

VITAMIN AND MINERAL DEFICIENCY ANEMIAS—*The Johns Hopkins Medical Letter HEALTH AFTER 50,* Volume 2 Issue 12, © 1991 Medletter Associates, Inc.

SICKLE CELL ANEMIA—*Sickle Cell Anemia,* June 1990, The Warren Grant Magnuson Clinical Center.

THE BRAIN AND NERVOUS SYSTEM

DEMENTIA—*The Dementias: Hope Through Research,* printed 1983, The National Institute of Neurological Disorders and Stroke.

ALZHEIMER'S DISEASE—*Alzheimer's Disease,* printed 1990, revised 1994, The National Institute of Mental Health.

NORMAL CHANGES IN THE AGING BRAIN—*The Johns Hopkins Medical Letter HEALTH AFTER 50,* Volume 3 Issue 8, © 1991 Medletter Associates, Inc.

CHRONIC PAIN—*Chronic Pain: Hope Through Research,* November 1989, reprinted September 1998, The National Institute of Neurological Disorders and Stroke.

HEADACHE—*Headache: Hope Through Research,* October 1996, The National Institute of Neurological Disorders and Stroke.

BRAIN TUMORS—*Brain Tumors: Hope Through Research,* March 1993, The National Institute of Neurological Disorders and Stroke.

DIZZINESS—*Dizziness: Hope Through Research,* September 1986, The National Institute of Neurological Disorders and Stroke.

EPILEPSY—*Epilepsy: Hope Through Research,* July 1981, The National Institute of Neurological Disorders and Stroke.

PARKINSON'S DISEASE—*Parkinson's Disease: Hope Through Research,* September 1994, The National Institute of Neurological Disorders and Stroke.

SHINGLES—*Shingles: Hope Through Research,* November 1981, The National Institute of Neurological Disorders and Stroke.

DENTAL AND ORAL DISORDERS

TOOTH DECAY—*Age Page: Taking Care of Your Teeth and Mouth,* revised October 1989, The National Institute on Aging.

PERIODONTAL DISEASE—*Periodontal (Gum) Disease,* The National Institute of Dental Research.

COSMETIC DENTAL OPTIONS—*The Johns Hopkins Medical Letter HEALTH AFTER 50,* Volume 2 Issue 3, © 1990 Medletter Associates, Inc.

DRY MOUTH (XEROSTOMIA)—*Dry Mouth (Xerostomia),* revised1991, The National Institute of Dental Research.

DENTURES/DENTAL IMPLANTS—*The Johns Hopkins Medical Letter HEALTH AFTER 50,* Volume 1 Issues 1/7, © 1989 Medletter Associates, Inc.

THE DIGESTIVE SYSTEM

OVERVIEW—*Your Digestive System and How It Works,* August 1992, The National Institute of Diabetes and Digestive and Kidney Diseases.

GASTROESOPHAGEAL REFLUX DISEASE—*Gastroesophageal Reflux Disease (Heartburn and Hiatal Hernia),* September 1994, The National Institute of Diabetes and Digestive and Kidney Diseases.

H. PYLORI AND PEPTIC ULCER—*H. Pylori and Peptic Ulcer,* October 1997, The National Institute of Diabetes and Digestive and Kidney Diseases.

PANCREATITIS—*Pancreatitis,* July 1992, The National Institute of Diabetes and Digestive and Kidney Diseases.

CIRRHOSIS OF THE LIVER—*Cirrhosis of the Liver,* reprinted November 1991, The National Institute of Diabetes and Digestive and Kidney Diseases.

VIRAL HEPATITIS—*Viral Hepatitis: Everybody's Problem?* © 1997 The American Liver Foundation.

GALLSTONES—*Gallstones: A National Health Problem,* © 1997 The American Liver Foundation.

CROHN'S DISEASE—*Crohn's Disease,* February 1998, The National Institute of Diabetes and Digestive and Kidney Diseases.

ULCERATIVE COLITIS—*Ulcerative Colitis,* April 1998, The National Institute of Diabetes and Digestive and Kidney Diseases.

IRRITABLE BOWEL SYNDROME—*Irritable Bowel Syndrome,* October 1992, The National Institute of Diabetes and Digestive and Kidney Diseases.

DIVERTICULOSIS AND DIVERTICULITIS—*Diverticulosis and Diverticulitis,* October 1996, The National Institute of Diabetes and Digestive and Kidney Diseases.

CONSTIPATION—*Constipation,* July 1995, The National Institute of Diabetes and Digestive and Kidney Diseases.

DIARRHEA—*The Johns Hopkins Medical Letter HEALTH AFTER 50,* Volume 1 Issue 5, © 1989 Medletter Associates, Inc.

HEMORRHOIDS—*Hemorrhoids,* May 1994, The National Institute of Diabetes and Digestive and Kidney Diseases.

THE EARS, NOSE, AND THROAT

HEARING LOSS AND AGING—*Hearing and Older People,* reprinted 1995, The National Institute on Deafness and Other Communication Disorders.

SINUSITIS—*Is It More Than Just a Cold?* © 1997 The American Academy of Otolaryngology–Head and Neck Surgery.

SMELL AND TASTE DISORDERS—*Smell and Taste Disorders,* © 1996 The American Academy of Otolaryngology–Head and Neck Surgery.

SORE THROAT—*Sore Throats: Causes and Cures,* © 1996 The American Academy of Otolaryngology–Head and Neck Surgery.

THE ENDOCRINE SYSTEM

DIABETES MELLITUS—*What You Need To Know About Diabetes,* reprinted December 1990, © 1984 The American Diabetes Association; *Basic Information Series,* Numbers 1-22, © 1993, 1994 The American Diabetes Association.

OBESITY—*Obesity and Energy Metabolism,* printed February 1984, The Warren Grant Magnuson Clinical Center.

LOSING WEIGHT AND KEEPING IT OFF—*The Johns Hopkins Medical Letter HEALTH AFTER 50,* Volume 3 Issue 3, © 1991 Medletter Associates, Inc.

THYROID DISEASE—*Thyroid Disease in the Elderly,* revised 1994, © The Thyroid Foundation of America.

THE EYES

CATARACT—*Cataract,* © 1996 The American Academy of Ophthalmology.

GLAUCOMA—*Glaucoma,* © 1997 The American Academy of Ophthalmology.

MACULAR DEGENERATION—*Macular Degeneration,* © 1997 The American Academy of Ophthalmology.

THE BEST SUNGLASSES—*The Johns Hopkins Medical Letter HEALTH AFTER 50,* Volume 3 Issue 5, © 1991 Medletter Associates, Inc.

REFRACTIVE ERRORS—*Refractive Errors,* © 1998 The American Academy of Ophthalmology.

THE CAROTID ARTERY AND THE EYE—*The Carotid Artery and the Eye,* © 1998 The American Academy of Ophthalmology.

FLOATERS AND FLASHES—*Floaters and Flashes,* © 1993 The American Academy of Ophthalmology.

ACKNOWLEDGMENTS

THE HEART AND BLOOD VESSELS

ATHEROSCLEROSIS—*1996 Heart and Stroke Facts,* © 1995 The American Heart Association.

HIGH BLOOD PRESSURE—*1996 Heart and Stroke Facts,* © 1995 The American Heart Association.

HEART ATTACK AND ANGINA—*1996 Heart and Stroke Facts,* © 1995 The American Heart Association.

ARRHYTHMIAS AND SUDDEN CARDIAC DEATH—*1996 Heart and Stroke Facts,* © 1995 The American Heart Association.

STROKE—*1996 Heart and Stroke Facts,* © 1995 The American Heart Association.

CONGENITAL HEART DEFECTS—*1996 Heart and Stroke Facts,* © 1995 The American Heart Association.

RHEUMATIC HEART DISEASE—*1996 Heart and Stroke Facts,* © 1995 The American Heart Association.

CONGESTIVE HEART FAILURE—*1996 Heart and Stroke Facts,* © 1995 The American Heart Association.

BACTERIAL ENDOCARDITIS—*1996 Heart and Stroke Facts,* © 1995 The American Heart Association.

PERIPHERAL VASCULAR DISEASE—*The Johns Hopkins Medical Letter HEALTH AFTER 50,* Volume 3 Issue 7, © 1991 Medletter Associates, Inc.

VARICOSE VEINS—*The Johns Hopkins Medical Letter HEALTH AFTER 50,* Volume 1 Issue 11, © 1990 Medletter Associates, Inc.

THE KIDNEYS AND URINARY TRACT

OVERVIEW—*Your Kidneys: Master Chemists of the Body,* revised 1996 © 1989 The National Kidney Foundation.

DIALYSIS TREATMENTS—*Dialysis,* © 1991, 1992 The National Kidney Foundation.

URINARY TRACT INFECTIONS—*Urinary Tract Infections,* © 1995 Medletter Associates, Inc.

KIDNEY STONES—*Kidney Stones,* © 1995 Medletter Associates, Inc.

GLOMERULONEPHRITIS—*Glomerulonephritis,* revised 1998 © 1992 The National Kidney Foundation.

THE LUNGS AND RESPIRATORY SYSTEM

OVERVIEW—*How To Keep Your Lungs Healthy,* February 1990, © 1990 The American Lung Association.

ASTHMA—*Asthma,* © 1995 Medletter Associates, Inc.

CHRONIC BRONCHITIS—*Facts About Chronic Bronchitis,* December 1989, © 1989 The American Lung Association.

EMPHYSEMA—*Facts About Emphysema,* January 1990, © 1990 The American Lung Association.

PNEUMONIA—*Facts About Pneumonia,* June 1992, © 1992 The American Lung Association.

INFLUENZA—*Facts About Influenza (Flu),* July 1991, © 1991 The American Lung Association.

THE MUSCLES AND BONES

OSTEOPOROSIS—*Osteoporosis,* © 1995 Medletter Associates, Inc.

OSTEOARTHRITIS—*Osteoarthritis,* © 1995 Medletter Associates, Inc.

RHEUMATOID ARTHRITIS—*Rheumatoid Arthritis,* © 1995 Medletter Associates, Inc.

FIBROMYALGIA—*The Johns Hopkins Medical Letter HEALTH AFTER 50,* Volume 6 Issue 9, © 1994 Medletter Associates, Inc.

CARPAL TUNNEL SYNDROME—*The Johns Hopkins Medical Letter HEALTH AFTER 50,* Volume 5 Issue 4, © 1993 Medletter Associates, Inc.

BURSITIS—*Bursitis,* © 1995 Medletter Associates, Inc.

TENDINITIS—*Tendinitis,* © 1995 Medletter Associates, Inc.

FOOT PROBLEMS—*The Johns Hopkins Medical Letter HEALTH AFTER 50,* Volume 2 Issue 3, © 1990 Medletter Associates, Inc.

THE SKIN

SKIN AND AGING—*Aging Skin,* © 1997 The American Academy of Dermatology.

SKIN LESIONS—*Aging Skin,* © 1997 The American Academy of Dermatology.

SKIN DISEASES—*Aging Skin,* © 1997 The American Academy of Dermatology.

MOLE INSPECTION—LEARNING YOUR ABCD'S—*The Johns Hopkins Medical Letter HEALTH AFTER 50,* Volume 2 Issue 4, © 1990 Medletter Associates, Inc.

HEALTH PROBLEMS OF MEN

ERECTILE DYSFUNCTION—*The Johns Hopkins Medical Letter HEALTH AFTER 50,* Volume 2 Issue 1, © 1990 Medletter Associates, Inc.

PROSTATE ENLARGEMENT—*Treating Your Enlarged Prostate,* February 1994, The U.S. Department of Health and Human Services.

CHAPTER 15

HEALTH PROBLEMS OF WOMEN

BENIGN BREAST CONDITIONS—*Understanding Breast Changes: A Health Guide For All Women,* printed September 1997, The National Cancer Institute.

MENOPAUSE—*Menopause,* printed 1995, The National Institute on Aging.

URINARY INCONTINENCE—*The Johns Hopkins Medical Letter HEALTH AFTER 50,* Volume 3 Issue 3, © 1991 Medletter Associates.

VAGINITIS—*Vaginitis: Causes and Treatments,* April 1997, © The American College of Obstetricians and Gynecologists.

MENTAL HEALTH

DEPRESSION—*Let's Talk Facts About Depression,* © 1998 The American Psychiatric Association.

ANXIETY DISORDERS—*Let's Talk Facts About Anxiety Disorders,* © 1993 The American Psychiatric Association.

MANIC-DEPRESSIVE DISORDER—*Let's Talk Facts About Manic-Depressive Disorders,* © 1993 The American Psychiatric Association.

SLEEP DISORDERS—*Sleep as We Grow Older,* © 1997 The American Sleep Disorders Association.

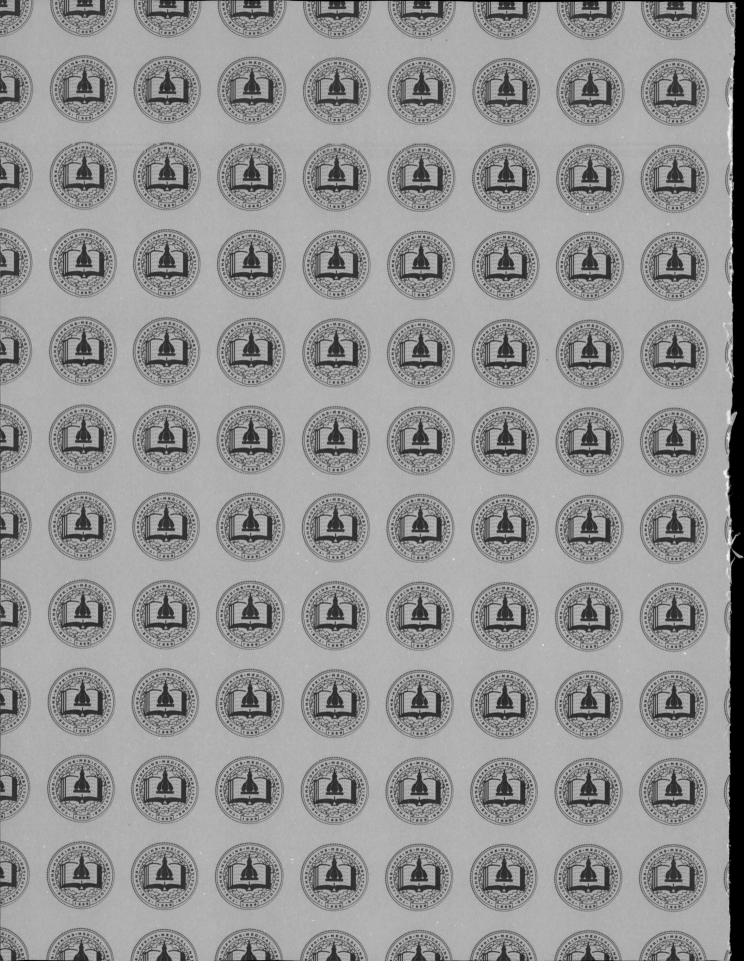